Clinical Manual of Addiction Psychopharmacology

THIRD EDITION

Clinical Manual of Addiction Psychopharmacology

THIRD EDITION

EDITED BY

Jeffrey DeVido, M.D., M.T.S.
Carla Marienfeld, M.D.
Henry R. Kranzler, M.D.
Petros Levounis, M.D., M.A.

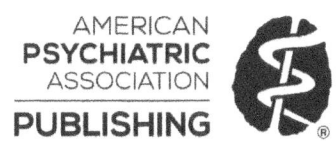

Note: The authors have worked to ensure that all information in this book is accurate at the time of publication and consistent with general psychiatric and medical standards, and that information concerning drug dosages, schedules, and routes of administration is accurate at the time of publication and consistent with standards set by the U.S. Food and Drug Administration and the general medical community. As medical research and practice continue to advance, however, therapeutic standards may change. Moreover, specific situations may require a specific therapeutic response not included in this book. For these reasons and because human and mechanical errors sometimes occur, we recommend that readers follow the advice of physicians directly involved in their care or the care of a member of their family.

Books published by American Psychiatric Association Publishing represent the findings, conclusions, and views of the individual authors and do not necessarily represent the policies and opinions of American Psychiatric Association Publishing or the American Psychiatric Association.

Copyright © 2025 American Psychiatric Association.
ALL RIGHTS RESERVED. Unless authorized in writing by the APA, no part of this book may be reproduced or used in a manner inconsistent with APA's copyright. This prohibition applies to unauthorized uses or reproductions in any form, including electronic applications. For inquiries about permissions or licensing please contact the Permissions and Licensing department at the address below or submit inquiries online at www.appi.org/Support/Customer-Information/Permissions.

If you wish to buy 50 or more copies of the same title, please visit www.appi.org/specialdiscounts for more information.

Third Edition
Manufactured in the United States of America on acid-free paper
29 28 27 26 25   5 4 3 2 1
American Psychiatric Association Publishing
800 Maine Avenue SW, Suite 900
Washington, DC 20024-2812
www.appi.org

Library of Congress Cataloging-in-Publication Data
Names: DeVido, Jeffrey editor | Marienfeld, Carla editor | Kranzler, Henry R., 1950- editor | Levounis, Petros editor
Title: Clinical manual of addiction psychopharmacology / [edited by] Jeffrey DeVido, M.D., M.T.S., Carla Marienfeld, M.D., Henry R. Kranzler, M.D., Petros Levounis, M.D., M.A.
Description: Third edition. | Washington, D.C. : American Psychiatric Association Publishing, [2025] | Revised edition of: Clinical manual of addiction psychopharmacology / edited by Henry R. Kranzler, M.D., Domenic A. Ciraulo, M.D., Leah R. Zindel, R.Ph., M.A.L.S. Washington, DC : American Psychiatric Publishing, a division of American Psychiatric Association, [2014] | Includes bibliographical references and index.
Identifiers: LCCN 2025013568 (print) | LCCN 2025013569 (ebook) | ISBN 9781615374465 paperback | ISBN 9781615374472 ebook
Subjects: LCSH: Substance abuse--Chemotherapy--Handbooks, manuals, etc. | Psychopharmacology--Handbooks, manuals, etc.
Classification: LCC RC564.15 .C56 2025 (print) | LCC RC564.15 (ebook) | DDC 362.29--dc23/eng/20250621
LC record available at https://lccn.loc.gov/2025013568
LC ebook record available at https://lccn.loc.gov/2025013569

British Library Cataloguing in Publication Data
A CIP record is available from the British Library.

EU GPSR Authorized Representative: LOGOS EUROPE, 9 rue Nicolas Poussin, 17000, LA ROCHELLE, France; E-mail: Contact@logoseurope.eu

This book is dedicated to all individuals with an addictive disorder: those who are no longer with us, those whose recovery continues to inspire us, and those who continue to suffer. This book is also dedicated to researchers, clinicians, families, friends, educators, and all those who have supported them, whose tireless efforts to advance our understanding and treatment of addictive disorders deserve our thanks.

Finally, the editors thank all the chapter authors for contributing their time, expertise, energy, and passion, without which this book would not have been possible.

Contents

Contributors ix
Preface xv

1 Treatment of Substance Use Disorders 1

2 Nicotine and Tobacco 33

3 Alcohol Use Disorder 71

4 Cannabis and Cannabinoids 151

5 Opioids 191

6 Stimulants 275

7 Sedatives, Hypnotics, or Anxiolytics 327

8 Hallucinogens and Phencyclidine 369

9 Club Drugs and Inhalants 431

10 Behavioral Addictions 477

11 Integrative Medicine Approaches to
Addiction Treatment 501

12 Circuit-Based Interventions for Substance
Use Disorders 527

Index 557

Contributors

Aurelia I. Andreiev, M.D.
Psychiatrist, Halton Healthcare, Oakville, Ontario, Canada

Hewa Artin, M.D.
Assistant Clinical Professor, Department of Psychiatry and Biobehavioral Sciences, University of California, Los Angeles, California

Christopher Blazes, M.D.
Associate Professor, Department of Psychiatry, Oregon Health and Science University, Portland, Oregon

Zafiris Daskalakis, M.D., Ph.D.
Dr. Igor and JoAnn Grant Endowed Chair and Professor, Department of Psychiatry, University of California San Diego School of Medicine, La Jolla, California

Jeffrey DeVido, M.D., M.T.S.
Assistant Clinical Professor—Volunteer, Department of Psychiatry and Behavioral Sciences, Weill Institute for Neurosciences and University of California, San Francisco; Chief of Addiction Services, Marin County, California, Department of Health and Human Services, Behavioral Health and Recovery Services Division; Behavioral Health Clinical Director, Partnership HealthPlan of California, Fairfield, California; Staff Psychiatrist, Mind Therapy Clinic, Corte Madera, California

Martin Epson, M.D., J.D., M.T.S.
Staff Psychiatrist, Marin County (California) Department of Health and Human Services, Behavioral Health and Recovery Services, San Rafael, California; Psychiatrist, Mind Therapy Clinic; Volunteer Assistant Clinical Professor, Department of Psychiatry and Behavioral Sciences, Weill Institute for Neurosciences, University of California San Francisco, California

Luis C. Farhat, M.D.
Postdoctoral Fellow, Faculdade de Medicina da Universidade de São Paulo, São Paulo, Brazil

Tony P. George, M.D.
Professor of Psychiatry, Temerty Faculty of Medicine, University of Toronto; Clinician-Scientist, Centre for Addiction and Mental Health, Toronto, Ontario, Canada

Emily Hartwell, Ph.D.
Staff Psychologist, Crescenz Veterans Affairs Medical Center; Assistant Professor of Psychiatry, University of Pennsylvania, Philadelphia, Pennsylvania

Kyle Kampman, M.D.
Professor, Department of Psychiatry, Perelman School of Medicine, Philadelphia, Pennsylvania

Kristopher A. Kast, M.D.
Assistant Professor, Department of Psychiatry and Behavioral Sciences, Vanderbilt University Medical Center, Nashville, Tennessee

Gali Katznelson, M.D.
Psychiatry Resident, University of Toronto, Toronto, Ontario, Canada

Clifford Knapp, Ph.D.
Adjunct Associate Professor of Pharmacology, Touro College of Osteopathic Medicine, New York, New York

Contributors xi

Kendra Kobrin, M.D., Ph.D.
Staff Psychiatrist Outpatient, Cape Cod Healthcare, Boston, Massachusetts

Henry R. Kranzler, M.D.
Professor of Psychiatry and Director of the Center for Studies of Addiction, Perelman School of Medicine, University of Pennsylvania; Co-Associate Director for Research, VISN4 MIRECC, Philadelphia Veterans Affairs Medical Center, Philadelphia, Pennsylvania

Stephen Leung, M.D.
Health Sciences Assistant Clinical Professor, Department of Psychiatry and Behavioral Sciences, University of California San Francisco, California

Petros Levounis, M.D., M.A.
Professor and Chair, Department of Psychiatry; Associate Dean, Professional Development, Rutgers New Jersey Medical School; Chief of Service, University Hospital, Newark, New Jersey

David Marcovitz, M.D.
Associate Professor of Psychiatry and Behavioral Sciences and Director, Middle TN SOR Hub, Department of Psychiatry and Behavioral Sciences, Vanderbilt University Medical Center, Nashville, Tennessee

Carla Marienfeld, M.D.
Clinical Professor and Addiction Psychiatry Fellowship Director, Department of Psychiatry, University of California San Diego, San Diego, California

R. Kathryn McHugh, Ph.D.
Chief of Psychology, McLean Hospital, Belmont, Massachusetts; Associate Professor, Department of Psychiatry, Harvard Medical School, Boston, Massachusetts

Marc N. Potenza, M.D., Ph.D.
Professor, Department of Psychiatry, Yale School of Medicine, New Haven, Connecticut

John A. Renner, Jr., M.D.
Professor of Psychiatry, Chobanian & Avedisian School of Medicine, Boston University, Boston, Massachusetts

Richard N. Rosenthal, M.D.
Arthur J. Antenucci Professor of Psychiatry, Columbia University College of Physicians & Surgeons; Chairman, Department of Psychiatry, St. Luke's Roosevelt Hospital Center, New York, New York

Thanos Rossopoulos, M.D.
Resident Physician, Department of Psychiatry, Department of Family Medicine, University of California San Diego School of Medicine, La Jolla, California

Marina Tsoy-Podosenin, M.D., Ph.D.
Medical Director, Mercy Hospital Behavioral Health Outpatient Clinic, Catholic Health of Long Island, New York, New York

Maya Vijayaraghavan, M.D.
Professor of Medicine; Steven A. Schroeder Distinguished Professor of Health and Health Care; Director, Smoking Cessation Leadership Center, UCSF Division of General Internal Medicine, San Francisco General Hospital, San Francisco, California

Sita Yerramsetti, M.D., M.P.H.
Private Practice, La Jolla, California

Disclosures

The following contributors have indicated a financial interest in or other affiliation with a commercial supporter, manufacturer of a commercial product, and/or provider of a commercial service as listed below:

Jeffrey DeVido, M.D., M.T.S.
Equity shareholder: Philip Morris/Altria Group, Merck, Cigna

Luis C. Farhat, M.D.
Scholarly stipend: #2021/08540-0 São Paulo Research Foundation (FAPESP)

Henry R. Kranzler, M.D.
Scientific advisory board member: Altimmune, Clearmind Medicine
Consultant: Altimmune, Clearmind Medicine, Sobrera Pharma, Lilly Pharmaceuticals
Grant/research support: Alkermes, Altimmune
Inventor: U.S. provisional patent, "Multi-ancestry Genome-wide Association Meta-analysis of Buprenorphine Treatment Response"

Marc N. Potenza, M.D., Ph.D.
Support: Mohegan Sun, Connecticut Council on Problem Gambling
Consultant/advisor: Opiant Pharmaceuticals (Indivior), Idorsia, BariaTek, AXA, Game Day Data, Addiction Policy Forum
Patent application: Yale University, Novartis

John A. Renner, Jr., M.D.
Employment: VA Boston Health Care
Royalties: American Psychiatric Association Publishing
Honoraria: American Psychiatric Association
Officer/director/trustee/executive: Spectrum Health Systems

The following contributors stated that they had no competing interests during the year preceding manuscript submission:
Hewa Artin, M.D.; Christopher Blazes, M.D.; Martin Epson, M.D., J.D., M.T.S.; Tony P. George, M.D.; Emily Hartwell, Ph.D.; Kyle Kampman, M.D.; Kristopher A. Kast, M.D.; Gali Katznelson, M.D.; Clifford Knapp, Ph.D.; Stephen Leung, M.D.; Petros Levounis, M.D., M.A.; David Marcovitz, M.D.; Carla Marienfeld, M.D.; R. Kathryn McHugh, Ph.D.; Richard N. Rosenthal, M.D.; Thanos Rossopoulos, M.D.; Maya Vijayaraghavan, M.D.; Sita Yerramsetti, M.D., M.P.H.

The following contributors did not supply information regarding disclosures:
Aurelia I. Andreiev, M.D.; Zafiris Daskalakis, M.D.; Kendra Kobrin, M.D., Ph.D.; Marina Tsoy-Podosenin, M.D., Ph.D.

Preface

Since the publication of the previous edition of this book in 2015, our understanding of addictive disorders and their treatment has advanced significantly. During the same span, the need for behavioral health expertise has exploded: the intervening years have been marked by crises in public health, inequitable access to care, climate change, mental health, and technology-enabled isolation, to name a few. At first glance, these crises may seem unrelated, but as health care providers we have witnessed a complex relationship among these events that has affected our individual and collective social well-being, a manifestation of which is the current devastating epidemic of substance use and overdose/poisoning.

Therefore, one thing is certain: The urgency of the moment requires that health care providers and systems of care better understand, communicate about, and (most importantly) treat substance misuse and addictive disorders. With this imperative, this book takes as its starting point the supposition that although substance misuse and addictive disorders develop from (and are sustained by) a complex set of social, environmental, economic, and biological factors, they are nonetheless inherently treatable conditions.

Fortunately, there is growing interest in the fields of clinical addiction medicine and addiction psychiatry, fields that as subspecialties were relegated to the margins of health care. There are now more than 5,000[1]

---

[1] This number represents approximately 3,800 Addiction Medicine Diplomates, 500 American Osteopathic Addiction Medicine Diplomates, and 1,400 Addiction Psychiatry Diplomates. Some of these diplomates are concurrently certified by multiple boards, making the estimated total number less than the sum total of the individual board-certified numbers.

specialty-certified addiction specialists and countless others who, although not certified, have undertaken additional training to support the clinical needs of their patients and communities. This is encouraging and reflects a growing sense of mainstream health care ownership of (and responsibility over) the assessment and management of substance misuse and addictive disorders. The overarching goal of this book, therefore, is to provide updated support for this emerging workforce to keep pace with the rapid advancements in our understanding and treatment of these conditions. The expert authors assembled herein aim to summarize and translate the scientific advancements in our understanding of how misused substances impact the individuals who use them, and they describe the psychopharmacological and neurobiological bases for the treatments available to manage these conditions.

Unfortunately, advances in pharmacotherapies for addictive disorders have not occurred at a comparable pace across substances, as evidenced by the lack of FDA-approved pharmacotherapies for most substance use disorders (SUDs). Some substances, such as stimulants, represent an explosive area of public health concern, and the lack of FDA-approved pharmacotherapies constrains community treatment efforts. However, the substantial insights into the pharmacology of the various addictive substances that are discussed in detail in this book provide a solid basis for medication development across the spectrum of addictive disorders. In parallel, advances in pharmacogenetics have provided additional potential targets for medication development that may one day provide a basis for more personalized treatment of addictive disorders. Interventional approaches other than pharmacotherapies, such as transcranial magnetic stimulation and deep brain stimulation, also offer emerging research that is advancing in parallel with pharmacotherapy and pharmacogenetics. Altogether, the future landscape of addictive disorder treatment is bright.

The structure of this book remains, as in the previous edition, largely organized by substance type, because this approach is essential to an understanding of the neurobiological and pharmacodynamic characteristics of these substances and their treatments. In this edition, chapters have been added to reflect additional emerging treatment approaches that transcend specific substances, such as integrative medicine and interventional approaches that include transcranial magnetic stimulation and deep brain stimulation. Each chapter is organized to provide a foundational neuropharmacological

Table P.2 DSM-5-TR criteria for substance use disorders

Group	Criterion
Impaired control	1: The individual may take the substance in larger amounts or over a longer period than was originally intended.
	2: The individual may express a persistent desire to cut down or regulate substance use and may report multiple unsuccessful efforts to decrease or discontinue use.
	3: The individual may spend a great deal of time obtaining the substance, using the substance, or recovering from its effects.
	4: *Craving* is manifested by an intense desire or urge for the drug that may occur at any time but is more likely when in an environment where the drug previously was obtained or used.
Social impairment	5: Recurrent substance use may result in a failure to fulfill major role obligations at work, school, or home.
	6: The individual may continue substance use despite having persistent or recurrent social or interpersonal problems caused or exacerbated by the effects of the substance.
	7: Important social, occupational, or recreational activities may be given up or reduced because of substance use.
Risky use	8: Risky use may take the form of recurrent substance use in situations in which it is physically hazardous.
	9: The individual may continue substance use despite knowledge of having a persistent or recurrent physical or psychological problem that is likely to have been caused or exacerbated by the substance.

case of gambling disorder, no substance is consumed, so naturally there is no substance-induced syndrome described.)

SUDs are characterized by "a cluster of cognitive, behavioral, and physiological symptoms indicating that the individual continues using the substance despite significant substance-related problems" (American Psychiatric Association 2022, p. 544). The diagnosis of an SUD can be applied to all 10 classes of substances, with the exception of caffeine. Neurobiologically, SUDs are marked by fundamental changes in brain circuitry (especially those involved in reward processing, memory formation, emotion processing, and executive top-down control of thinking and behavior), which may persist long after the substances are discontinued. These neurobiological changes manifest in the form of pathological patterns of behavior related to the use of a substance. The 11 criteria for the diagnosis of SUD are broadly organized into four groups: *impaired control, social impairment, risky use,* and *pharmacological criteria* (see Table P.2). Of note, the term *addiction* was removed in the update from DSM-IV-TR to DSM-5 (American Psychiatric Association 2000, 2013) in favor of the more neutral term *substance use disorder*, which also is defined with more certainty and has a less negative connotation. However, the term *addiction* is still used widely in countries outside of the United States, and even in the United States it is used by some researchers and clinicians to denote severe addictive illness. As a result, the terms *SUD* and *addiction* may be used interchangeably at times in this book, and this is an attempt to preserve the original language preferences of the researchers, clinicians, and authors who contributed to this work or to whom the authors make reference.

An SUD diagnosis is made when an individual has symptoms that meet at least 2 of the 11 criteria presented in Table P.2. The severity of each disorder is further characterized by the number of symptoms that meet the diagnostic criteria: the presence of two to three symptoms meeting DSM-5-TR criteria is defined as *mild*, four to five is *moderate*, and six or more is *severe*. It is noteworthy that the pharmacological criteria are neither necessary nor sufficient to make a diagnosis of SUD. Therefore, the behavioral criteria carry greater emphasis, which fits with clinical experience.

SUDs can be further characterized by the use of modifiers that denote where an individual may be in the course of their chronic SUD condition. *Early remission* refers to when an individual's symptoms no longer meet full criteria for the SUD for longer than 3 months but less than 12 months, factors (and behavior-specific factors, as in gambling disorder or other behavioral addictions) that may uniquely characterize the different substances. This Preface highlights the broader conceptual framework of principles that guide the diagnostic undertaking that is universal to all substance-related and addictive disorders.

DSM-5-TR identifies 10 classes of substances, all of which, when taken in excess, directly activate the brain reward system (see Table P.1) and as a result can lead to substance-related and addictive disorders. In addition, DSM-5-TR also describes one *behavioral addiction* (gambling disorder) in which engaging in certain activities, rather than consumption of a particular substance, results in similar reward system activation. Other behavioral addictions have been described (e.g., sex addiction, exercise addiction, shopping addiction), but the evidence base does not yet support their inclusion as distinct diagnoses.

DSM-5-TR separates substance-related and addictive disorders into two broad categories: substance-induced disorders (intoxication, withdrawal, other substance/medication-induced mental disorders) and SUDs. (In the

Table P.1 Classes of substances included in DSM-5-TR

Alcohol

Caffeine

Cannabis

Hallucinogens (with separate categories for phencyclidine [or similarly acting arylcyclohexylamines] and other hallucinogens)

Inhalants

Opioids

Sedatives, hypnotics, or anxiolytics

Stimulants (amphetamine-type substances, cocaine, and other or unspecified stimulants)

Tobacco

Other (or unknown) substances

Source. American Psychiatric Association 2022.

explanation of how various substances affect the individuals who use them, including the clinical manifestations of intoxication and withdrawal syndromes (as are relevant). This foundation is followed by an updated review of the evidence for various psychopharmacological therapies and approaches for treating special populations (as are available), such as those with noteworthy co-occurring psychiatric or medical disorders and pregnant individuals. Epidemiological review has been intentionally minimized in favor of providing a practical neuropharmacological background, description of clinical phenomenology, and treatment guidance.

With this organizational structure, it is important to underscore that substance misuse and addictive disorders themselves transcend specific substances. Rather, these conditions represent the culmination of the maladaptive behavioral relationship that individuals have developed with various substances. Therefore, we begin the book with a newly reworked chapter ("Treatment of Substance Use Disorders") that views the pharmacotherapy of addictive disorders through a broader social and system-based lens.

Confronting substance misuse and addictive disorders, and the complex set of environmental, economic, social, and biological factors from which they emerge and that sustain them, is the purview of all health care providers. Unfortunately, stigma against both individuals with addictive disorders and the treatments of these disorders themselves remains widespread in health care. Familiarity counteracts stigma, however, as is commonly argued. This book, therefore, has as a secondary aim: reducing stigma through education and thereby empowering providers to tackle the current epidemic of substance use and overdose/poisoning.

DSM-5-TR Preface

In compiling chapters of this book, it became apparent that the inclusion of DSM-5-TR diagnostic criteria (American Psychiatric Association 2022) for each addictive disorder covered here would result in considerable content overlap. Therefore, rather than repeat the discussion of diagnostic criteria in each chapter, we provide here a brief, overarching review of the DSM-5-TR diagnostic criteria for substance-related and addictive disorders to which readers can refer as needed.

DSM-5-TR offers both a broad framework of principles to guide the diagnosis of substance-related and addictive disorders and substance-specific

Table P.2 DSM-5-TR criteria for substance use disorders *(continued)*

Group	Criterion
Pharmacological criteria	10: *Tolerance* is signaled by requiring a markedly increased dose of the substance to achieve the desired effect or a markedly reduced effect when the usual dose is consumed.
	11: *Withdrawal* is a syndrome that occurs when blood or tissue concentrations of a substance decline in an individual who had maintained prolonged heavy use of the substance.

Source. American Psychiatric Association 2022, pp. 544, 546.

sustained remission is when an individual's symptoms no longer meet full criteria for longer than 12 months, and *in a controlled environment* refers to when a person is in an environment wherein access to the substance is restricted. Of note, *craving* is excepted from these symptom determinations, because it may persist indefinitely.

Specific manifestations of substance-induced disorders (intoxication, withdrawal, other substance/medication-induced mental disorders) vary by substance. Each chapter in this book that discusses a specific substance reviews the pharmacological properties of that substance, along with its intoxication and withdrawal syndromes (if any).

Substance intoxication is marked by the "development of a reversible substance-specific syndrome due to the recent ingestion of a substance" (American Psychiatric Association 2022, p. 548) and can result from ingestion of a substance in any of the 10 classes listed in Table P.1, with the exception of tobacco. This syndrome manifests as clinically significant problematic behavioral or psychological changes that are attributable to the physiological effects of that substance on the CNS and are not the result of another medical condition or mental disorder.

Similarly, substance withdrawal is specific to a particular substance, with some substances (e.g., alcohol, opioids, tobacco) having more pronounced withdrawal syndromes than others (e.g., hallucinogens, inhalants).

Substance withdrawal is marked by a "problematic behavioral change, with physiological and cognitive concomitants, that is due to the cessation of, or reduction in, heavy and prolonged substance use" (American Psychiatric Association 2022, p. 548). Withdrawal manifests as clinically significant distress or impairments in function (e.g., social, occupational) that are not due to another medical condition or mental disorder.

Finally, substance/medication-induced mental disorders are those potentially severe, usually temporary, but sometimes persisting syndromes that develop during the use of substances, medications, or toxins and that mirror those of other mental disorders (e.g., psychosis resembling schizophrenia resulting from methamphetamine use). A careful history, including collateral information and longitudinal observation, may be required to differentiate a substance/medication-induced mental disorder from a substance-independent mental disorder.

A Note About Different Editions of DSM

DSM has undergone multiple revisions since its introduction in 1952 (sequentially: DSM, DSM-II, DSM-III, DSM-III-R, DSM-IV, DSM-IV-TR, DSM-5, DSM-5-TR [American Psychiatric Association 1952, 1968, 1980, 1987, 1994, 2000, 2013, 2022]). These revisions reflect our evolving understanding of mental disorders, including substance-related and addictive disorders, culminating in the publication of DSM-5-TR in 2022. Some revisions have made major changes in the diagnostic criteria for substance-related and addictive disorders, whereas others have not. For example, in the transition from DSM-IV-TR to DSM-5, the concepts of *substance abuse* and *substance dependence* were eliminated in favor of *substance use disorder*, which represented a major evolution in how we diagnose substance-related and addictive disorders. Conversely, the transition from DSM-5 to DSM-5-TR yielded no changes to the diagnostic criteria for substance-related and addictive disorders.

Because much of the research related to substance-related and addictive disorders has been tied to the prevailing DSM version in use at the time the research was undertaken, it is therefore understandable that it can be difficult (if not impossible) to directly compare research results tied to different editions of DSM. This does not, however, mean that earlier research is invalid. Rather, this means that readers must take this into consideration when evaluating research findings that might span several decades.

In this book, we have sought to use DSM-5 and DSM-5-TR terms and diagnostic classifications as much as possible. In some instances, however, the reader will find that different terminologies, diagnostic clarifications, and DSM editions will be used or referenced. In doing this, we aim to remain adherent to the original clinical and research language used by the authors of those works, while simultaneously alerting the reader to the unavoidable (and often confusing) dilemma that arises from having quality research and clinical experience spanning a great breadth of evolution in our overall conceptualization and understanding of substance-related and addictive disorders.

References

American Psychiatric Association: Diagnostic and Statistical Manual: Mental Disorders. Washington, DC, American Psychiatric Association, 1952

American Psychiatric Association: Diagnostic and Statistical Manual of Mental Disorders, 2nd Edition. Washington, DC, American Psychiatric Association, 1968

American Psychiatric Association: Diagnostic and Statistical Manual of Mental Disorders, 3rd Edition. Washington, DC, American Psychiatric Association, 1980

American Psychiatric Association: Diagnostic and Statistical Manual of Mental Disorders, 3rd Edition, Revised. Washington, DC, American Psychiatric Association, 1987

American Psychiatric Association: Diagnostic and Statistical Manual of Mental Disorders, 4th Edition. Washington, DC, American Psychiatric Association, 1994

American Psychiatric Association: Diagnostic and Statistical Manual of Mental Disorders, 4th Edition, Text Revision. Washington, DC, American Psychiatric Association, 2000

American Psychiatric Association: Diagnostic and Statistical Manual of Mental Disorders, 5th Edition. Arlington, VA, American Psychiatric Association, 2013

American Psychiatric Association: Diagnostic and Statistical Manual of Mental Disorders, 5th Edition, Text Revision. Washington, DC, American Psychiatric Association, 2022

Treatment of Substance Use Disorders

Kristopher A. Kast, M.D.
R. Kathryn McHugh, Ph.D.
David E. Marcovitz, M.D.

The treatment of individuals with substance use and addictive disorders involves layers of complexity beyond prescribing effective pharmacotherapy. Multiple behavioral and other psychosocial interventions have demonstrated effectiveness for substance use disorder (SUD)–related outcomes, both in combination with pharmacotherapy and as monotherapy. These nonpharmacological approaches will be briefly reviewed here.

Furthermore, these treatments exist within a context that itself has meaningful effects on individual and population outcomes. Such factors include significant stigma against individuals with SUDs, a discontinuous system of addiction care that varies by geography and sociodemography, an accumulating burden of social drivers of health (SDOH), and historical tension between heterogeneous therapeutic philosophies. These factors may significantly affect an individual's ability to access and benefit from evidence-based therapies. Contextualizing SUD treatment within these frames allows effective individual treatment planning as well as meaningful advocacy for population-level interventions to improve outcomes and heal communities.

Above all, we seek here to represent a "multiple pathways" approach—the complexity of an individual patient's experience necessitates a striving yet flexible approach to care. Diverse patients need diverse and comprehensive treatment offerings.

Epidemiology and the Treatment Gap

The 12-month prevalence of SUDs in the U.S. general population is 17.1%, with alcohol, tobacco, and cannabis use disorders being most prevalent (Substance Abuse and Mental Health Services Administration 2024). Notable epidemiological trends include the following: a closing gender gap, with the historically greater prevalence of substance use and SUDs in men relative to women narrowing or even possibly reversing (as in the case of young adult women with binge alcohol use); increasing prevalence of cannabis use as tobacco use and underage alcohol use decline; and rising use of electronic nicotine (or cannabinoid) delivery systems (ENDS; more commonly known as electronic cigarettes, e-cigarettes, or vapes) (Substance Abuse and Mental Health Services Administration 2024).

The U.S. health care system has been experiencing an escalating overdose crisis since 2000. Rising rates of overdose deaths have been driven by three waves of opioid use: 1) diverted and illicitly manufactured prescription opioids, followed by 2) nonprescribed diacetylmorphine (heroin) and 3) high-potency synthetic opioids, including fentanyl. More than 100,000 drug overdose deaths were reported annually between 2021 and 2023, the highest annual tolls at the time of this writing, with a hopeful 26.9% decline in 2024 to ~80,000 deaths; the majority of those deaths involved an opioid (Ahmad et al. 2025; National Center for Health Statistics 2021; Substance Abuse and Mental Health Services Administration 2024). Stimulants including methamphetamines are also increasingly implicated in overdose deaths, with stimulant-associated rates rising 180% from 2015 to 2019 (Kariisa et al. 2019; National Institute for Health Care Management Foundation 2021). Overdose deaths have been approaching the annual rate of alcohol-related deaths (~ 178,000/year), although both remain behind the rate of annual tobacco-related deaths (~480,000/year) (Esser 2024; National Center for Chronic Disease Prevention and Health Promotion Office on Smoking and Health 2014).

Most individuals with SUDs in the general population are not engaged in treatment. This treatment gap is illustrated across epidemiological surveys, with the most recent survey reporting that only 23.6% of individuals with SUDs access care (Substance Abuse and Mental Health Services Administration 2024). Among the >75% of individuals not receiving treatment, more than 95% did not believe they needed it (Substance Abuse and Mental Health Services Administration 2024). Individuals' experience of systemic stigma or judgment by individual health care providers may further contribute to the low perceived need for treatment. For those seeking treatment, significant barriers to engagement were identified, including elevated rates of uninsured or underinsured status (Substance Abuse and Mental Health Services Administration 2024).

Despite low engagement in addiction care, individuals with SUDs present to nonaddiction settings across medical specialties, in part because of the deleterious effects of SUDs on nearly every organ system, with resulting elevated rates of health care utilization, psychiatric disorders, acute and chronic infectious diseases, obstetrical and neonatal complications, and mortality (Peacock et al. 2018; Walley et al. 2012). This care-seeking mismatch leads to a need for alternative approaches to reach individuals in the treatment gap, including population-level harm-reduction interventions, lower barriers to accessing care, and addiction-specialist consultative services in general medical settings where individuals with SUDs present for non-SUD complaints (McNeely et al. 2019).

Furthermore, among individuals entering SUD treatment, multiple concurrent substance exposures are common. The mean number of substance types used is 3.5, with a limited evidence base guiding treatment for individuals experiencing polysubstance use (Compton et al. 2021; Onyeka et al. 2012). Polysubstance use is an urgent research need, given the consistent evidence for worsened outcomes among this population (Crummy et al. 2020).

In addition to multiple substances used, individuals entering SUD treatment experience elevated rates of co-occurring psychiatric and medical diagnoses (Substance Abuse and Mental Health Services Administration 2024). Such comorbidities have also consistently been associated with worsened outcomes (National Institute on Drug Abuse 2020). The need for integrated care to address this burden of comorbidity—ranging from remote collaboration to colocation to health home models—has been voiced since the 1990s (American Psychiatric Association and Academy of Psychosomatic Medicine 2016). Nonetheless, fully integrated models and a full level-of-care (LOC) spectrum are rare in the U.S. health care system (Sterling et al. 2011).

Stigma and the U.S. Historical, Cultural, and Legal Context

Contemporary clinicians consistently demonstrate significant stigma and unconscious bias against individuals with SUDs presenting for care (Avery and Avery 2019). Individuals with SUDs are viewed as poorly motivated, manipulative, aggressive, and less important than other patients, resulting in avoidance, low-empathy care, and therapeutic pessimism that affect patient outcomes (Avery et al. 2019; van Boekel et al. 2013). This perception of individuals with SUDs reflects a recurring theme across the U.S. historical context.

Stigmatizing and racialized views of individuals with SUDs were present in the post–Civil War period. Depictions of Black men as violent "cocaine fiends" in medical journals were followed by state-level legislation criminalizing cocaine use (Jackson et al. 2022). Although prescribed morphine was the most commonly used opioid at the turn of the twentieth century, inaccurate depictions of Chinese "opium dens" as major sources of opioid-related social problems preceded the 1906 Pure Food and Drug Act, leading to exclusion of opium and cocaine import (Hansen et al. 2020; Jackson et al. 2022). The 1914 Harrison Narcotics Act was interpreted in case law as excluding opioid use from illnesses warranting medical treatment, thereby prohibiting prescription of opioid agonists for the treatment of opioid addiction—a practice previously common in morphine maintenance clinics in the post–Civil War era (Musto and Ramos 1981; Terry 1915). Subsequent prosecution of thousands of physicians was followed by a decades-long period of separation between the health care system and treatments for addiction. Subsequently, cannabis use and "reefer madness" were linked to the Mexican immigrant population in the Southwest, leading to criminalization of cannabis possession and perpetuation of the racialized bogey-person stereotype of individuals with SUDs (Jackson et al. 2022). The 1935 opening of the United States Narcotic Farm in Lexington, Kentucky, symbolized the shift to a carceral system–based approach to SUD treatment (Kosten and Gorelick 2002).

Peer-based recovery communities—including 12-step–based programs and therapeutic communities emerging in the 1930s—grew outside traditional health care settings and often espoused antagonistic views toward increasingly carceral system–based medical interventions, encouraging individuals to avoid psychotropic medications in an era where few effective medications were available (Avery and Kast 2019). This peer-based recovery system persists today, with slow-developing changes in acceptance of medical treatment and pharmacotherapy (Avery and Kast 2019).

The Nixon administration's 1971 declaration of illicit drug use as "public enemy number one" was followed by a wave of legislation that increased incarceration for drug-related offenses, with new mandatory minimum sentencing and disparate penalties for specific substance formulations (Jackson et al. 2022). For example, the 100:1 mandatory minimum setencing disparity between crack cocaine and powder cocaine resulted in dramatic increases in the carceral system population, with gross overrepresentation of Black and Latinx individuals (Jackson et al. 2022).

Contemporaneous legislation in 1970 also reopened agonist-based and non-carceral system–based treatment for opioid addiction, with the creation of opioid treatment programs, colloquially known as methadone clinics. Significant federal regulation restricted access to methadone-based treatment, leading to underutilization despite significant evidence for efficacy (Madras et al. 2020). With further neurobiological understanding of SUDs and shifting perceptions of the population of individuals struggling with SUDs (from the criminalized bogey-person to suburban youth) (Hansen et al. 2020; Jackson et al. 2022), legislation in 2000 created a less restrictive option for office-based buprenorphine treatment of opioid use disorder. These separate legislative acts and their historical contexts continue to shape access to methadone- and buprenorphine-based treatments, which varies by geography and sociodemography, with significant racial disparities—furthering the historical interaction between systemic racism and SUD treatment in the U.S. context (Hansen et al. 2020; Jackson et al. 2022).

Structural Competency and the System of Care for Individuals With Substance Use Disorders

Harm-Reduction Interventions in the Treatment Gap

For the >75% of individuals with SUDs in the treatment gap (i.e., those not voluntarily seeking engagement in SUD treatment), multiple effective interventions to mitigate harms associated with substance use have been assessed and deployed to improve public health (Riley and Pates 2012). These harm-reduction approaches include efforts to reduce overdose deaths, prevent and treat infectious complications of injection drug use, and address SDOH that limit care access.

Evidence shows that overdose education and naloxone distribution reduce overdose deaths by increasing bystander opioid overdose reversal with this μ opioid receptor antagonist, notably without a compensatory increase in opioid use (Jones et al. 2017; Walley et al. 2013). Public health approaches to increasing access to naloxone have included low-cost or no-cost standing prescriptions at local pharmacies and pharmacist-driven programs (Smart et al. 2021). Supervised consumption sites and prescribed diacetylmorphine/hydromorphone treatment are novel (and controversial) harm-reduction approaches to reach individuals in the treatment gap and thus reduce harms associated with unsupervised use, including overdose deaths, infectious complications from unsafe injection practices, criminal activity, and complications from adulterated illicit substance supplies (DeBeck et al. 2011; Oviedo-Joekes et al. 2009). These programs have been piloted outside the U.S. health care system, although efforts to create supervised consumption sites are ongoing in some jurisdictions.

Syringe-needle access programs also have evidence for reducing infectious complications in people who inject drugs (Aspinall et al. 2014; Peters et al. 2016). HIV preexposure prophylaxis and hepatitis C direct-acting antiviral therapy also demonstrate efficacy in people who inject drugs, reducing risk of transmission and individuals' disease burden (Choopanya et al. 2013; Norton et al. 2017).

Housing First initiatives prioritize rehousing for individuals with SUDs before other treatment goals are met, which is a reversal of prior requirements for abstinence/recovery ahead of rehousing (Appel et al. 2012; Srebnik et al. 2013). These programs are building evidence for reduced acute-care utilization, increased employment rates, and reduced overall burden of SDOH (Ly and Latimer 2015).

Substance Use Disorder Treatment in the Legal and Carceral Systems

Individuals with SUDs are disproportionately involved in legal and carceral systems. Some jurisdictions have created specialized drug courts, with highly supervised periods of SUD treatment as a diversion from incarceration that demonstrate reduced recidivism and societal cost (Bright and Martire 2013; Finigan et al. 2007; Klag et al. 2005; Miller and Flaherty 2000). For individuals entering the carceral system, there are significant differences in SUD treatment access and variability in available treatment modalities (Substance Abuse and Mental Health Services Administration 2019). Notably, access to first-line agonist-based medication for opioid use disorder (MOUD) is significantly limited in some carceral settings. Abstinence-based psychosocial approaches (e.g., prison-based therapeutic communities) or second-line antagonist-based treatment (with extended-release naltrexone) are overrepresented in carceral system–based SUD treatment, often owing to concerns about diversion of agonist treatments. This disparity in MOUD access for a vulnerable population represents a missed opportunity to reduce the elevated overdose death rates following carceral system release (Binswanger et al. 2020; Joudrey et al. 2019).

Engagement During Non–Substance Use Disorder General Medical Care

Individuals with SUDs experience significant medical comorbidity that leads to care-seeking in outpatient and inpatient settings (Walley et al. 2012). Access to consultation with addiction specialists during these encounters offers an opportunity for engagement and intervention that may improve outcomes, including increased MOUD initiation rates, improved linkage to outpatient care, and reductions in inpatient and emergency department admissions (Kast et al. 2024; Ober et al. 2025; Wakeman et al. 2017; Weinstein et al. 2018). Notably, less-intensive interventions, such as SBIRT (Screening, Brief Intervention, and Referral to Treatment), appear effective only for subsyndromal at-risk alcohol use, suggesting that individuals with SUDs may require more intensive assessment and treatment during acute care (Barata et al. 2017). Transitions from acute-care settings are problematic, with significant dropout between referral and engagement in SUD specialty care (Marcovitz et al. 2021; Schwarz et al. 2019; Sullivan et al. 2021). SUD pharmacotherapy initiated during acute care may improve subsequent engagement, as demonstrated with buprenorphine in emergency department settings (D'Onofrio et al. 2015).

Variable Access to Involuntary Treatment

Additional variability in SUD treatment access is present for individuals meeting legally defined criteria for involuntary hospitalization. Statutory law for involuntary treatment varies by state jurisdiction, with many states explicitly excluding SUDs from qualifying psychiatric disorders (National Judicial Opioid Task Force 2018). Ethical concerns regarding involuntary treatment for SUDs, alongside potential harmful effects, have also been raised (Evans et al. 2020; Messinger and Beletsky 2021; Nicolini et al. 2018). However, there is evidence for individuals with grave disability attributable to SUDs experiencing symptom response to this escalated LOC despite initial involuntary status (Boit et al. 2019; Vuong et al. 2021).

American Society of Addiction Medicine Patient Placement Criteria, Levels of Care, and Treatment Duration for Substance Use Disorders

Individuals with SUDs voluntarily seeking addiction treatment present with wide-ranging degrees of acuity and comorbidity. Escalating LOCs for SUD treatment—ranging from outpatient to residential to inpatient medical care—match acute medical and psychiatric needs. Each LOC differs in the scope of services offered, including housing, psychosocial treatments, nursing and medical supervision, intensity of medical monitoring, and availability of consultation with other medical specialties. The American Society of Addiction Medicine (ASAM) patient placement criteria assist in matching a patient to the appropriate LOC, which has demonstrated benefit for patient outcomes and appropriate resource utilization (Gastfriend and Mee-Lee 2003; Sharon et al. 2003; Stallvik et al. 2015). The ASAM criteria provide a framework for assessing acute intoxication/withdrawal risk, medical and psychiatric comorbidity, relapse risk, patient-level motivation, and recovery environment (Mee-Lee et al. 2013).

Available length of stay (LOS) has decreased markedly for more intensive treatment levels. Early abstinence-based therapeutic community models recommended treatment periods of 2 years or longer to allow for full rehabilitation, development of new social and work skills, and complex changes in social networks and community (Avery and Kast 2019; Vanderplasschen et al. 2013). Inpatient admissions for medically supervised withdrawal typically last fewer than 7 days and infrequently transition to further residential treatment, which has shortened to a duration of approximately 4 weeks. These changes attempt to reduce care costs, although they may conflict with evidence that the highest-risk period for relapse is within the first 90 days of recovery and that engagement in SUD treatment for more than 6 months correlates with improved outcomes (Simpson 1979, 1981; Simpson et al. 1997; Vanderplasschen et al. 2013). Notably, there is limited evidence for residential care improving SUD outcomes with these reductions in LOS. Older observational data from long-term therapeutic communities suggested improved outcomes with an LOS longer than 6 or 12 months compared with shorter stays (Simpson 1979, 1981; Simpson et al. 1997).

Access to the full spectrum of LOCs varies widely by geographic and sociodemographic variables, leading to many higher-acuity patients receiving care in lower-acuity settings or in nonspecialty settings (Medicaid and CHIP Payment and Access Commission 2018). Disparities in insurance coverage for SUD treatment, as well as a large proportion of individuals with SUDs living without insurance (≤60% of individuals presenting for SUD treatment), further affect access (Medicaid and CHIP Payment and Access Commission 2018; Olfson et al. 2021; Orgera and Tolbert 2016; Substance Abuse and Mental Health Services Administration 2014a). Additionally, the full continuum of care rarely exists within a single system, and transitions often involve risk of treatment dropout between facilities (Medicaid and CHIP Payment and Access Commission 2018).

Unfortunately, there are also concerning and unethical practices in the landscape of SUD care. The worst of these include predatory treatment facilities, characterized by aggressive patient recruitment practices, grossly inadequate or substandard care, and excessive billing or even insurance fraud (Rao-Patel et al. 2018).

Treatment Goals for Individuals With Substance Use Disorders

Tension between harm-reduction and abstinence-based treatment goals persists in the current system (Collins et al. 2016; Henwood et al. 2014; Taylor et al. 2021). Misalignment between patient and treatment provider goals may lead to therapeutic alliance rupture and care disengagement, risking relapse and associated adverse outcomes (Collins et al. 2016). Additionally, individuals with SUDs entering treatment facilities may encounter opposing treatment philosophies that limit access to evidence-based interventions. This barrier is most evident for agonist-based MOUD (Madras et al. 2020).

Abstinence-based housing or treatment facilities often do not accept or do not provide agonist-based MOUD. This decision may be driven by administrative concerns over the cost of offering MOUD (requiring medical staff with prescribing privileges), stigma and bias against agonist-based MOUD (viewed as trading one drug for another), or divergent treatment philosophies favoring nonmedication approaches. However, consistent and replicated evidence for risks associated with abstinence-based approaches to opioid use disorder—including the risk of relapse and overdose death in the context of the overdose crisis—raises ethical concerns for programs prohibiting agonist-based MOUD (Brezel et al. 2020; Madras et al. 2020). This concern has extended to programs for medical professionals with SUDs, with state physician health programs facing scrutiny for historical avoidance of agonist-based MOUD (Beletsky et al. 2019). More recent guidance from the U.S. Department of Justice has clarified that the Americans with Disabilities Act protects from discrimination individuals with opioid use disorder receiving MOUD, including protection from being denied access to housing or treatment facilities because of their MOUD treatment (Civil Rights Division 2022).

Widening the scope of meaningful outcomes beyond abstinence opens clinical attention to other meaningful effects for patients, including lower quantities of use, less injection use, reduced overdose risk, lessened comorbidity burden, fewer acute care visits, increased return to education or work, increased social network support, and more frequent rehousing (Riley and Pates 2012; Taylor et al. 2021). These outcomes are also achievable even without prioritizing abstinence (although not ruling out abstinence). As an example within alcohol use disorder, decreases in alcohol intake that move patients to lower World Health Organization risk categories have demonstrated meaningful reductions in mental health problems and drinking consequences (Witkiewitz et al. 2020).

Further treatment complications arise when individuals present with co-occurring SUDs and achieve abstinence for one substance but not others—as in the case of persistent cannabis, benzodiazepine, or cocaine use despite remission of opioid use while receiving MOUD treatment. This situation is common given the prevalence of co-use and leads to divergent responses from treatment programs, with some discontinuing MOUD treatment. Given strong evidence for reduced harms (including reduced overdoses, injection use, and criminal activity) despite persistent use of other substances, the 2015 ASAM national practice guideline explicitly stated that this co-use should not be a reason to suspend opioid use disorder treatment (Kampman and Jarvis 2015).

Clinical Approach to the Patient

Motivational interviewing is a foundational clinical approach to treating individuals with SUDs (Levounis et al. 2017). This collaborative interpersonal style attends to the patient's language of behavior change and is designed to strengthen internal motivation for shared treatment goals (Miller and Rollnick 2012). Clinicians apply motivational interviewing by first communicating acceptance of and partnership with individuals entering treatment, embodying the global approach or spirit of motivational interviewing that is more closely correlated with improved outcomes than specific motivational interviewing techniques (Apodaca and Longabaugh 2009; Levounis et al. 2017; Miller and Rollnick 2012). Internal reasons for change are evoked and selectively reflected by the clinician, whereas normative clinical responses to reasons for sustaining SUD behaviors are avoided (Levounis et al. 2017; Miller and Rollnick 2012). Clinician behavior consistent with motivational interviewing increases patient change talk, resulting in improved SUD treatment engagement and likelihood of positive change (Levounis et al. 2017; Miller and Rollnick 2012).

A patient's culturally acquired explanations and understanding of illness and healing—especially for addictive behavior—may differ markedly from the medical or neurobiological model assumed by clinical teams. Clinician cultural competency and humility is another core skill for SUD treatment that reflects the ability to maintain an interpersonal stance that is open to aspects of cultural identity and influence most important to the patient and their recovery (Hook et al. 2013). Healthy tension between knowing and not knowing allows clinicians to avoid pitfalls associated with making simplified assumptions about the effect of cultural identity, either by denying impact or by total attribution (Hook et al. 2013). Gaps in specific cultures between ideal norms (e.g., near abstinence) and behavioral norms of substance use (e.g., actual binge-pattern use) sometimes lead to dissonance, shame, and secrecy that may exacerbate SUD prevalence (El-Guebaly and Kim 2021; Westermeyer and Dickmann 2019). Family-specific behavioral patterns are also often idiosyncratic and differ from culturally transmitted rules, further complicating assumptions regarding population-level norms and generalizations about culture (Gross et al. 2019). Subculture membership according to sexuality, substance use, or other shared experiences also affects cultural identity (El-Guebaly and Kim 2021; Westermeyer and Dickmann 2019). The intersection of a patient's culture, family system, and subcultures introduces significant complexity to the impact of culture on clinical care. Inclusion of cultural formulation in diagnostic and therapeutic thinking may assist in identification of barriers and facilitate cultural recovery, with regained viable identity, affiliation, vocation, and recreation within the patient's culture (Westermeyer et al. 2006).

Trauma exposure is prevalent among many individuals seeking SUD treatment, ranging from adverse childhood experiences to PTSD (Brown et al. 1999; Cabanis et al. 2021; Felitti et al. 1998). Accordingly, essential components of SUD care include knowledge about and assessment of the effects of trauma exposure, as well as integrated trauma-focused treatment where possible and applicable. A trauma-informed approach calls for revising the organizational climate to promote awareness of the psychological effects of trauma exposure and to structure environments and services to mitigate exacerbation of traumatic stress exposure sequelae in the treatment environment (Raja et al. 2015; Substance Abuse and Mental Health Services Administration 2014a). Specific organizational changes should aim to emphasize physical and psychological safety and may include gender-responsive services (particularly important given historically male-predominant populations in SUD treatment settings), transparency around organizational policy with active peer or patient representation in policy-making, shared decision-making, a strengths-based approach in treatment planning, and peer supports involved in care (Substance Abuse and Mental Health Services Administration 2014a).

Assessing an Individual Presenting for Substance Use Disorder Treatment

Assessment of the patient presenting for SUD care aims to 1) ensure immediate medical and physical safety, 2) form initial hypotheses regarding symptoms and underlying diagnoses, and 3) cocreate an initial treatment plan (Barnhill 2018). Each component is discussed here.

Immediate safety concerns include risk of emergent withdrawal states, with withdrawal from alcohol, sedative-hypnotics, and opioids being most salient. This risk assessment allows for referral to the appropriate LOC if medically supervised withdrawal is indicated. Standardized instruments—such as the Prediction of Alcohol Withdrawal Severity Scale, the Clinical Institute Withdrawal Assessment for Alcohol Scale, and the Clinical Opiate Withdrawal Scale—assist clinicians in quantifying the risk of emergent withdrawal and the severity of withdrawal symptoms (Kast et al. 2025). Identifying and stabilizing opioid withdrawal with agonist-based MOUD is an emerging priority, given the high risk of treatment dropout, relapse, and unintentional overdose with other opioid withdrawal management approaches, such as clonidine (Weiss et al. 2011; Ziaaddini et al. 2012).

The clinical interview provides necessary data to support any diagnosis of SUD. Information is obtained on the range of substance categories used, age at onset of use, pattern and quantity of use across time, routes of administration (with particular attention to high-risk methods, including injection and intranasal use), experience of withdrawal phenomena (including complicated alcohol-withdrawal states, such as seizures or delirium), overdose events, and other functional sequelae of use. Prior treatment experiences and periods of recovery/abstinence inform treatment planning, as do co-occurring psychiatric and medical diagnoses. Patient-completed screening instruments (e.g., Patient Health Questionnaire-9 and Generalized Anxiety Disorder-7) are useful in identifying symptoms but require follow-up clinical assessment to clarify underlying diagnoses.

Often, this breadth of information is not obtained in a single visit. The clinical setting and immediate treatment needs prioritize variable information-gathering in the initial encounter. As the treatment relationship develops, new information may become available that reframes diagnostic thinking, as with the emergence of co-occurring psychiatric symptoms previously not disclosed because of anticipated stigma.

Objective data to balance the clinical interview include physical and mental status examinations, toxicology/drug testing, review of the prescription drug monitoring program and prior health records, and collateral information-gathering with patient consent. Although these data points are considered objective, each has limitations, including imperfect sensitivity and specificity for clinically relevant problems. Discordant findings against the patient's subjective report should be evaluated with equipoise, considering possible inaccuracies on both sides. Conducting a nonjudgmental review of discordant findings directly with patients ensures process transparency and allows for collaborative decision-making in considering changes to a treatment plan (Kampman and Jarvis 2015).

As indicated by the breadth of factors informing the ASAM patient placement criteria, biopsychosocial formulation remains the gold standard for organizing a comprehensive treatment plan that incorporates neurobiological, psychological, and social understanding of complex patients (Engel 1977). For example, an individual presenting with opioid use disorder and generalized anxiety disorder leading to recent job loss may benefit from pharmacotherapy targeting stabilization of the mesolimbic reward circuits, stress-response system, and extended amygdala, while also experiencing a response to evidence-based behavioral treatment to address persistent anxiety symptoms and their effects on substance use. Behavioral treatment may be particularly indicated for people with significant functional impairment, for those with conditions that often do not respond adequately to medication, or in circumstances in which a behavioral treatment has superior evidence compared with pharmacotherapy (e.g., insomnia, OCD). Furthermore, in our example, this individual's recent unemployment may affect access to these treatments, and facilitated engagement with available social resources may improve outcomes. The degree of comorbidity and SDOH burden in this population underscores the importance of including psychiatrists, clinical psychologists, and interdisciplinary team members from social work, nursing, case management, and peer recovery specialist backgrounds in the assessment and management of SUDs.

Pharmacotherapy Treatment Frame and Nonpharmacological Treatments

In addition to evidence-based pharmacotherapy, SUD treatment occurs within a specialized treatment frame. At treatment entry, frequency of visits and toxicology/drug testing is usually weekly (or more frequent for an intensive outpatient/partial hospital LOC), with stepwise de-escalation as recovery goals are met and rapid reescalation in response to peri-lapse or relapse (Kampman and Jarvis 2015).

Prescribing controlled substances—such as methadone, buprenorphine, benzodiazepines, or psychostimulant therapy—often requires a more formalized treatment agreement that outlines expectations and requirements for continued safe prescribing in the current LOC as well as standardized responses to nonadherence. The quantity of controlled medication prescribed and dispensed often mirrors the visit frequency, deescalating and escalating in response to stability.

The chronic, relapsing course of SUD creates a need for transitions between different LOCs, including referrals to higher LOCs for individuals experiencing relapse with severe sequelae that are unresponsive to treatment plan adjustments at the current LOC. For example, a patient receiving buprenorphine MOUD who experiences relapsed injection opioid use and does not adhere to the treatment agreement despite escalation to weekly visits may require either of the following: 1) referral to an intensive outpatient/partial hospital program or residential treatment facility to attempt stabilization with additional psychosocial interventions or 2) transition to daily-observed methadone dosing through a federally regulated opioid treatment program.

Medical management approaches to SUD have been studied, with evidence for alcohol and opioid use disorders (Bhatraju et al. 2017; Frances 2007; Weiss et al. 2011). These approaches attempt to reduce several identified barriers to SUD treatment, including the cost and complexity of providing multiple treatment modalities beyond pharmacotherapy. Typical medical management involves prescribing evidence-based medication, health education, motivational interviewing–based goal-setting facilitation, referral to peer-based recovery supports (e.g., Alcoholics Anonymous [AA], Narcotics Anonymous), and frequent visits (Frances 2007; Weiss et al. 2011). A significant proportion of individuals with SUDs may experience symptom response to medical management alone. The ability to provide low-barrier medical management within a primary care practice may increase access to effective treatments, particularly where specialty care or psychosocial treatment modalities are limited (Bhatraju et al. 2017). Additional expansion of telehealth-based delivery of medical management, specifically focused on MOUD treatment, has further reduced some barriers to accessing SUD care, although unequal access to technology and internet service remains a challenge (Mahmoud et al. 2022).

Multiple psychological treatment modalities have demonstrated efficacy for SUD, with cognitive-behavioral therapy (CBT) approaches most studied across diagnoses. CBT approaches demonstrate robust efficacy, with some evidence of greater treatment response in certain SUDs (e.g., cannabis use disorder) (Magill and Ray 2009). Increasingly, psychological treatment development has taken a transdiagnostic approach, seeking to integrate treatment principles for co-occurring disorders (e.g., alcohol use disorder and PTSD) within a single intervention, with initial evidence for efficacy of these approaches for both targeted conditions (Mehta et al. 2021). Large randomized controlled trials comparing specific psychotherapies—including CBT, motivational interviewing, 12-step facilitation, supportive-expressive (psychodynamic) therapy, and drug counseling—have shown robust effects for substance use and associated sequelae (Crits-Christoph et al. 1999; Mattson et al. 1998). Both individual and group settings have supporting evidence, with significant benefits for cost and access in group treatment and no substantive decrease in efficacy (Epstein et al. 2018; Sobell et al. 2009). Furthermore, behavioral therapies that involve supportive others (e.g., couples or family-based therapies) demonstrate particularly robust effects (Powers et al. 2008; Roozen et al. 2004). Contingency management—a behavioral intervention in which desired behaviors (e.g., negative urine drug screen results, treatment attendance) are rewarded—has demonstrated strong efficacy, including for disorders for which no gold-standard medication is currently available (e.g., stimulant use disorder) (Petry 2011; Petry et al. 2005). Barriers to viable reimbursement models have long limited use of contingency management outside funded studies, although several states now use Medicaid 1115 demonstration waivers, federal grants, and opioid settlement funds to implement programs (Amaya et al. 2025).

The transdiagnostic efficacy of these interventions has led to their inclusion across pharmacological studies. In the treatment of some SUDs (alcohol use disorder, tobacco use disorder), improved efficacy is observed with the combination of CBT and pharmacotherapy (Ray et al. 2020; U.S. Preventive Services Task Force et al. 2021). In contrast, results of the addition of behavioral therapy to MOUD have been mixed, with evidence for improvements in outcomes when added to methadone but less clear findings when added to buprenorphine (Weiss et al. 2014). This difference may be attributable in part to a possible ceiling effect from medication management (Carroll and Weiss 2017). In the case of MOUD, in which the effect size from medication is significant, several trials failing to demonstrate an additional benefit from behavioral therapy have led many in the field to recommend a medication-first approach in which behavioral therapy is not required or in many cases not even offered. Others caution that these failed trials included an intensity of medical management unmatched in the real-world setting (Carroll and Weiss 2017). Initial evidence suggests that there may be individual differences in treatment response, with some people experiencing an adequate symptom response to buprenorphine alone and other subgroups (e.g., people with PTSD) benefiting from the combination with behavioral therapy (McHugh et al. 2021; Weiss et al. 2014). Regardless, more research is needed to match patients receiving MOUD to behavioral therapy and to evaluate stepped care in which behavioral therapies are more strongly encouraged when MOUD alone is insufficient (Carroll and Weiss 2017).

Peer-based recovery programs—ranging from the meetings-based AA and SMART Recovery to residential settings including therapeutic communities—are also associated with improved outcomes, best studied in abstinence-related outcomes for 12-step programs targeting alcohol use disorder (Kelly et al. 2020). Individuals presenting for SUD treatment are more likely to engage in peer recovery programs if specifically prescribed by their medical providers, and psychotherapeutic interventions facilitating 12-step involvement (along with other behavioral intervention components) improve outcomes similarly to other psychotherapies (Crits-Christoph et al. 1999; Kelly et al. 2020). Regarding mediators of 12-step program effects, a literature review suggests that common mechanisms, such as enhancing self-efficacy and coping skills and facilitating adaptive social network changes, may have greater relation to enhanced abstinence than AA-specific processes or spiritual mechanisms (Kelly et al. 2009). Indeed, others have compared mechanisms of recovery in AA with those found in professional psychotherapies and found significant theoretical overlap (Marcovitz et al. 2020).

Peer recovery support and recovery coaching are additional emerging interventions involving mentoring, education, and support from a trained peer with lived experience in SUDs (Eddie et al. 2019). Recovery coaches may be integrated into multiple LOCs, including spaces where access to traditional peer recovery meetings is limited. In addition to improved substance use outcomes, this unique peer role may facilitate improved relationships with providers and social networks, increase retention, and lead to greater treatment satisfaction (Eddie et al. 2019).

Additional SUD treatment approaches with emerging evidence include digital therapeutics and neuromodulation. Novel digital therapeutics have begun to incorporate contingency management within other treatment modalities; for example, the combination of digital application–delivered CBT and contingency management has emerging evidence for improving retention in buprenorphine-treated individuals with opioid use disorder (Maricich et al. 2021). Neuromodulation, including transcranial magnetic stimulation (TMS), also has new evidence demonstrating possible efficacy in treating SUD-specific symptoms, including craving, with FDA clearance for one TMS system for tobacco smoking cessation in 2020 (Tang et al. 2023; Terraneo et al. 2016).

Assessing Treatment Response and Outcomes

The primary outcome domains of relevance to SUD care include substance use and other symptoms of SUD, treatment retention and adherence, functional outcomes, and mechanistic outcomes. The assessment of substance use is challenging for many reasons, including the absence of means to define quantity for most substances (except for alcohol and pharmaceutically manufactured substances), variability in the detection window for toxicology and drug testing across substances (as well as the cost of these tests), and disincentives for accurate self-report (e.g., fear of treatment discontinuation or hospitalization). Several steps can help optimize accurate assessment, including the use of multiple methods of measurement (e.g., toxicology and self-report), the use of memory aids to support accurate recall of substance use (e.g., a calendar-based method with anchoring to salient events), and clear communication about nonpunitive clinic or provider policies regarding self-reports of use.

Toxicology and drug testing results demonstrate changes in patterns of use in response to treatment, allowing for early detection of relapse, external accountability and monitoring, and treatment plan modification (Baxter et al. 2017). Screening immunoassays are lower in cost and available at the point of care to allow immediate interpretation and treatment planning in real time. Limitations in sensitivity and specificity and in the breadth of substance categories assessed by screening immunoassays sometimes require use of costlier confirmatory testing, where expected or unexpected presumptive results are reassessed using gas or liquid chromatography and mass spectrometry. Notably, in the third wave of the opioid epidemic, fentanyl and other high-potency synthetic opioids are often not assessed by screening immunoassays designed to detect chemical structures similar to naturally derived opiates such as heroin and morphine (Tabarra et al. 2019). Rapid shifts in population substance use patterns and emergence of novel synthetic substances continually challenge the utility and interpretability of drug testing results, requiring iterative updates to testing panels to provide clinically useful data.

Treatment retention is a central outcome for SUD care. Although overall retention rates are similar to general psychiatric and medical treatment, consequences of early treatment discontinuation are grave for the population with SUDs, risking relapse, medical and socioeconomic sequelae, overdose, and death (Onken et al. 1997; Stark 1992). Some interventions for SUDs have shown promise in improving retention, including contingency management, community reinforcement, and motivational interviewing approaches (Carroll et al. 2006; Higgins et al. 1994; Meyers et al. 2011; Petry et al. 2005). Among SUD pharmacotherapies, agonist-based MOUD consistently and dramatically increases retention (Kelly et al. 2011; Lee et al. 2018). Psychiatric comorbidity further complicates treatment retention, and strategies targeting concurrent treatment of psychiatric disorders have been effective for some retention outcomes, including treatment of co-occurring ADHD with stimulant therapy (Brown et al. 1999; Cacciola et al. 2001; Kast et al. 2021; Kelly et al. 2012; Mangrum et al. 2006).

Patient-reported outcome measures can allow for more detailed clinical assessment of meaningful outcomes beyond retention and abstinence, including substance-related behaviors, medical and mental health, legal system involvement, social network regrowth, return to education or work, and financial and housing security. Standardized instruments, including the Addiction Severity Index and the Brief Addiction Monitor, provide a framework for iterative reassessment across treatment to direct clinical attention to problem areas that may predispose to relapse or limit recovery goals (Cacciola et al. 2013; McLellan et al. 1992). Patient access to electronic health records allows for asynchronous completion of these metrics ahead of appointments, increasing the breadth of assessment despite limited time in a single office visit.

Patient-reported outcome measures may also include assessment of purported mechanisms of treatment outcome. For example, treatments may target reduction of substance craving or enhancement of coping skills. Measures of these mechanistic outcomes can provide valuable information about treatment progress and whether the chosen treatment approach is successfully modifying its target. Consideration of such outcomes can also identify opportunities to modify interventions or leverage augmentation strategies (e.g., adding CBT to medication treatment, encouraging mutual help engagement).

Key Points

- Pharmacotherapy represents one of several layers of complexity that define treatment of substance use disorders (SUDs) and addictive disorders. In addition, nonpharmacological approaches, as well as broader contextual factors such as stigma, sociodemography, and social drivers of health, are important to appreciate when considering treatment of SUDs.
- Less than 25% of individuals with an SUD receive specialty addiction treatment. Of the >75% of individuals with an SUD who do not access treatment, more than 95% report not wanting treatment, which constitutes a significant treatment gap.
- Stigma against individuals with SUDs exists today, has historical foundations (which have been highly racialized), and contributes to the variable treatment access seen in primary medical and carceral settings.
- Harm-reduction approaches, such as syringe exchange programs, Housing First programs, overdose education, and naloxone distribution, represent strategies for decreasing morbidity and mortality among those who are not actively interested in formal SUD treatment.
- The American Society of Addiction Medicine has codified the array of different SUD treatment settings into a framework of levels of care meant to facilitate appropriate matching of patient needs with treatment venue. However, access to these levels of care can be influenced by nonclinical factors, such as insurance coverage and patient predation by unscrupulous providers. Moreover, myriad treatment philosophies can pervade even providers supplying similar levels of care, making the process of patient matching even more confusing.
- Patient-centered approaches to working with patients with SUDs that are sensitive to cultural and trauma factors can be more efficacious than confrontational and punitive approaches. Motivational

interviewing represents one manner of engagement that is patient centered and avoids unhelpful outright confrontation.
- The assessment of individuals with SUDs should begin by determining medical or psychiatric acute risk, forming initial hypotheses about symptoms and the underlying diagnoses, and cocreating a treatment plan.
- Treatment of SUDs occurs in a specialized treatment frame that may include structural components (e.g., toxicology screening, medication agreements and contracts, frequent check-ins, and fluid transitions between different levels of care) and behavioral or psychological interventions (e.g., cognitive-behavioral therapy, contingency management, 12-step facilitation, and peer-based programs such as Alcoholics Anonymous), in addition to addiction psychopharmacological interventions.
- The primary outcome domains of relevance to SUD care include use of substances and other symptoms of SUD, treatment retention and adherence, functional outcomes, and mechanistic outcomes.

References

Ahmad FB, Cisewski JA, Rossen LM, et al: Provisional drug overdose death counts. National Center for Health Statistics, 2025. Available at: https://dx.doi.org/10.15620/cdc/20250305008. Accessed May 22, 2025.

Amaya D, Saunders H, Hinton E: Section 1115 Waiver Watch: A Look at the Use of Contingency Management to Address Stimulant Use Disorder. Policy Watch, Kaiser Family Foundation, 2025. Available at: https://www.kff.org/policy-watch/section-1115-waiver-watch-a-look-at-the-use-of-contingency-management-to-address-stimulant-use-disorder/. Accessed May 22, 2025.

American Psychiatric Association, Academy of Psychosomatic Medicine: Dissemination of Integrated Care Within Adult Primary Care Settings: The Collaborative Care Model. 2016. Available at: https://www.psychiatry.org/File%20Library/Psychiatrists/Practice/Professional-Topics/Integrated-Care/APA-APM-Dissemination-Integrated-Care-Report.pdf. Accessed January 28, 2025.

Apodaca TR, Longabaugh R: Mechanisms of change in motivational interviewing: a review and preliminary evaluation of the evidence. Addiction 104(5):705–715, 2009 19413785

Appel PW, Tsemberis S, Joseph H, et al: Housing First for severely mentally ill homeless methadone patients. J Addict Dis 31(3):270–277, 2012 22873188

Aspinall EJ, Nambiar D, Goldberg DJ, et al: Are needle and syringe programmes associated with a reduction in HIV transmission among people who inject drugs: a systematic review and meta-analysis. Int J Epidemiol 43(1):235–248, 2014 24374889

Avery JD, Avery JJ (eds): The Stigma of Addiction: An Essential Guide. Cham, Switzerland, Springer Nature, 2019

Avery JD, Kast KA (eds): The Opioid Epidemic and the Therapeutic Community Model: An Essential Guide. Cham, Switzerland, Springer Nature, 2019

Avery J, Knoepflmacher D, Mauer E, et al: Improvement in residents' attitudes toward individuals with substance use disorders following an online training module on stigma. HSS J 15(1):31–36, 2019 30863230

Barata IA, Shandro J, Montgomery M, et al: Effectiveness of SBIRT for alcohol use disorders in the emergency department: a systematic review. West J Emerg Med 18(6):1143–1152, 2017 29085549

Barnhill JW: The initial interview, in Co-Occurring Mental Illness and Substance Use Disorders: A Guide to Diagnosis and Treatment. Arlington, VA, American Psychiatric Association Publishing, 2018, pp 3–12

Baxter L, Brown L, Pating D, et al: Appropriate use of drug testing in clinical addiction medicine. J Addict Med 11(Suppl):1–56, 2017

Beletsky L, Wakeman SE, Fiscella K: Practicing what we preach: ending physician health program bans on opioid-agonist therapy. N Engl J Med 381(9):796–798, 2019 31461593

Bhatraju EP, Grossman E, Tofighi B, et al: Public sector low threshold office-based buprenorphine treatment: outcomes at year 7. Addict Sci Clin Pract 12(1):7, 2017 28245872

Binswanger IA, Nguyen AP, Morenoff JD, et al: The association of criminal justice supervision setting with overdose mortality: a longitudinal cohort study. Addiction 115(12):2329–2338, 2020 32267585

Boit H, Palmer GA, Olson SA: A comparison between the involuntary and voluntary treatment of patients with alcohol use disorder in a residential rehabilitation treatment program. J Addict Nurs 30(1):57–60, 2019 30830001

Brezel ER, Powell T, Fox AD: An ethical analysis of medication treatment for opioid use disorder (MOUD) for persons who are incarcerated. Subst Abus 41(2):150–154, 2020 31800376

Bright DA, Martire KA: Does coerced treatment of substance-using offenders lead to improvements in substance use and recidivism? A review of the treatment efficacy literature. Aust Psychol 48(1):69–81, 2013

Brown PJ, Stout RL, Mueller T: Substance use disorder and posttraumatic stress disorder comorbidity: addiction and psychiatric treatment rates. Psychol Addict Behav 13(2):115–122, 1999

Cabanis M, Outadi A, Choi F: Early childhood trauma, substance use and complex concurrent disorders among adolescents. Curr Opin Psychiatry 34(4):393–399, 2021 33993169

Cacciola JS, Alterman AI, Rutherford MJ, et al: The relationship of psychiatric comorbidity to treatment outcomes in methadone maintained patients. Drug Alcohol Depend 61(3):271–280, 2001 11164691

Cacciola JS, Alterman AI, Dephilippis D, et al: Development and initial evaluation of the Brief Addiction Monitor (BAM). J Subst Abuse Treat 44(3):256–263, 2013 22898042

Carroll KM, Weiss RD: The role of behavioral interventions in buprenorphine maintenance treatment: a review. Am J Psychiatry 174(8):738–747, 2017 27978771

Carroll KM, Ball SA, Nich C, et al: Motivational interviewing to improve treatment engagement and outcome in individuals seeking treatment for substance abuse: a multisite effectiveness study. Drug Alcohol Depend 81(3):301–312, 2006 16169159

Choopanya K, Martin M, Suntharasamai P, et al: Antiretroviral prophylaxis for HIV infection in injecting drug users in Bangkok, Thailand (the Bangkok Tenofovir Study): a randomised, double-blind, placebo-controlled phase 3 trial. Lancet 381(9883):2083–2090, 2013 23769234

Civil Rights Division, U.S. Department of Justice: The Americans with Disabilities Act and the opioid crisis: combating discrimination against people in treatment or recovery. White paper, U.S. DOJ, 2022. Available at: https://archive.ada.gov/opioid_guidance.pdf. Accessed May 22, 2025.

Collins SE, Jones CB, Hoffmann G, et al: In their own words: content analysis of pathways to recovery among individuals with the lived experience of homelessness and alcohol use disorders. Int J Drug Policy 27:89–96, 2016 26364078

Compton WM, Valentino RJ, DuPont RL: Polysubstance use in the U.S. opioid crisis. Mol Psychiatry 26(1):41–50, 2021 33188253

Crits-Christoph P, Siqueland L, Blaine J, et al: Psychosocial treatments for cocaine dependence: National Institute on Drug Abuse Collaborative Cocaine Treatment Study. Arch Gen Psychiatry 56(6):493–502, 1999 10359461

Crummy EA, O'Neal TJ, Baskin BM, et al: One is not enough: understanding and modeling polysubstance use. Front Neurosci 14:569, 2020 32612502

DeBeck K, Kerr T, Bird L, et al: Injection drug use cessation and use of North America's first medically supervised safer injecting facility. Drug Alcohol Depend 113(2–3):172–176, 2011 20800976

D'Onofrio G, O'Connor PG, Pantalon MV, et al: Emergency department–initiated buprenorphine/naloxone treatment for opioid dependence: a randomized clinical trial. JAMA 313(16):1636–1644, 2015 25919527

Eddie D, Hoffman L, Vilsaint C, et al: Lived experience in new models of care for substance use disorder: a systematic review of peer recovery support services and recovery coaching. Front Psychol 10:1052, 2019 31263434

El-Guebaly N, Kim H: Cross-cultural aspects of substance-related and addictive disorders, in Textbook of Substance Use Disorder Treatment. Edited by Brady KT, Levin FR, Galanter M, et al. Washington, DC, American Psychiatric Association Publishing, 2021, pp 609–628

Engel GL: The need for a new medical model: a challenge for biomedicine. Science 196(4286):129–136, 1977 847460

Epstein EE, McCrady BS, Hallgren KA, et al: Individual versus group female-specific cognitive behavior therapy for alcohol use disorder. J Subst Abuse Treat 88:27–43, 2018 29606224

Esser MB, Sherk A, Liu Y, et al: Deaths from Excessive Alcohol Use—United States, 2016–2021. MMWR Morb Mortal Wkly Rep 73:154–161, 2024

Evans EA, Harrington C, Roose R, et al: Perceived benefits and harms of involuntary civil commitment for opioid use disorder. J Law Med Ethics 48(4):718–734, 2020 33404337

Felitti VJ, Anda RF, Nordenberg D, et al: Relationship of childhood abuse and household dysfunction to many of the leading causes of death in adults: the Adverse Childhood Experiences (ACE) study. Am J Prev Med 14(4):245–258, 1998 9635069

Finigan MW, Carey SM, Cox A: Impact of a Mature Drug Court Over 10 Years of Operation: Recidivism and Costs. Washington, DC, National Institute of Justice, July 2007. Available at: https://www.ojp.gov/pdffiles1/nij/grants/219225.pdf. Accessed January 28, 2025.

Frances RJ: Combined pharmacotherapies and behavioral interventions for alcohol dependence: the COMBINE study: a randomized controlled trial. Yearbook of Psychiatry and Applied Mental Health 2007:95–96, 2007

Gastfriend DR, Mee-Lee D: The ASAM patient placement criteria: context, concepts and continuing development. J Addict Dis 22(Suppl 1):1–8, 2003 15991586

Gross KA, Lagos ME, Yessengaliyeva E, et al: Family involvement in addiction, treatment, and recovery, in The ASAM Principles of Addiction Medicine, 6th Edition. New York, Wolters Kluwer, 2019, pp 2378–2416

Hansen H, Parker C, Netherland J: Race as a ghost variable in (white) opioid research. Sci Technol Human Values 45(5):848–876, 2020

Henwood BF, Padgett DK, Tiderington E: Provider views of harm reduction versus abstinence policies within homeless services for dually diagnosed adults. J Behav Health Serv Res 41(1):80–89, 2014 23404076

Higgins ST, Budney AJ, Bickel WK, et al: Incentives improve outcome in outpatient behavioral treatment of cocaine dependence. Arch Gen Psychiatry 51(7):568–576, 1994 80311230

Hook JN, Davis DE, Owen J, et al: Cultural humility: measuring openness to culturally diverse clients. J Couns Psychol 60(3):353–366, 2013 23647387

Jackson DS, Nguemeni Tiako MJ, et al: Disparities in addiction treatment: learning from the past to forge an equitable future. Med Clin North Am 106(1):29–41, 2022 34823733

Jones JD, Campbell A, Metz VE, et al: No evidence of compensatory drug use risk behavior among heroin users after receiving take-home naloxone. Addict Behav 71:104–106, 2017 28325710

Joudrey PJ, Khan MR, Wang EA, et al: A conceptual model for understanding post-release opioid-related overdose risk. Addict Sci Clin Pract 14(1):17, 2019 30982468

Kampman K, Jarvis M: American Society of Addiction Medicine (ASAM) National Practice Guideline for the Use of Medications in the Treatment of Addiction Involving Opioid Use. J Addict Med 9(5):358–367, 2015 26406300

Kariisa M, Scholl L, Wilson N, et al: Drug overdose deaths involving cocaine and psychostimulants with abuse potential—United States, 2003–2017. MMWR Morb Mortal Wkly Rep 68(17):388–395, 2019 31048676

Kast KA, Rao V, Wilens TE: Pharmacotherapy for attention-deficit/hyperactivity disorder and retention in outpatient substance use disorder treatment: a retrospective cohort study. J Clin Psychiatry 82(2):20m13598, 2021

Kast KA, Le TDV, Stewart LS, et al: Impact of inpatient addiction psychiatry consultation on opioid use disorder outcomes. Am J Addict 33(5):543–550, 2024

Kast KA, Sidelnik SA, Nejad SH, et al: Management of alcohol withdrawal syndromes in general hospital settings. BMJ 388:e080461, 2025

Kelly JF, Magill M, Stout RL: How do people recover from alcohol dependence? A systematic review of the research on mechanisms of behavior change in Alcoholics Anonymous. Addict Res Theory 17(3):236–259, 2009

Kelly JF, Humphreys K, Ferri M: Alcoholics Anonymous and other 12-step programs for alcohol use disorder. Cochrane Database Syst Rev 3(3):CD012880, 2020 32159228

Kelly SM, O'Grady KE, Mitchell SG, et al: Predictors of methadone treatment retention from a multi-site study: a survival analysis. Drug Alcohol Depend 117(2–3):170–175, 2011 21310552

Kelly TM, Daley DC, Douaihy AB: Treatment of substance abusing patients with comorbid psychiatric disorders. Addict Behav 37(1):11–24, 2012 21981788

Klag S, O'Callaghan F, Creed P: The use of legal coercion in the treatment of substance abusers: an overview and critical analysis of thirty years of research. Subst Use Misuse 40(12):1777–1795, 2005 16419556

Kosten TR, Gorelick DA: The Lexington narcotic farm. Am J Psychiatry 159(1):22, 2002 11772684

Lee JD, Nunes EV Jr, Novo P, et al: Comparative effectiveness of extended-release naltrexone versus buprenorphine-naloxone for opioid relapse prevention (X:BOT): a multicentre, open-label, randomised controlled trial. Lancet 391(10118):309–318, 2018 29150198

Levounis P, Arnaout B, Marienfeld C (eds): Motivational Interviewing for Clinical Practice. Arlington, VA, American Psychiatric Association Publishing, 2017

Ly A, Latimer E: Housing First impact on costs and associated cost offsets: a review of the literature. Can J Psychiatry 60(11):475–487, 2015 26720505

Madras BK, Ahmad NJ, Wen J, et al: Improving access to evidence-based medical treatment for opioid use disorder: strategies to address key barriers within the treatment system. NAM Perspect April 27, 2020 35291732

Magill M, Ray LA: Cognitive-behavioral treatment with adult alcohol and illicit drug users: a meta-analysis of randomized controlled trials. J Stud Alcohol Drugs 70(4):516–527, 2009 19515291

Mahmoud H, Naal H, Whaibeh E, et al: Telehealth-based delivery of medication-assisted treatment for opioid use disorder: a critical review of recent developments. Curr Psychiatry Rep 24(9):375–386, 2022 35895282

Mangrum LF, Spence RT, Lopez M: Integrated versus parallel treatment of co-occurring psychiatric and substance use disorders. J Subst Abuse Treat 30(1):79–84, 2006 16377455

Marcovitz DE, McHugh KR, Roos C, et al: Overlapping mechanisms of recovery between professional psychotherapies and Alcoholics Anonymous. J Addict Med 14(5):367–375, 2020 32058337

Marcovitz DE, White KD, Sullivan W, et al: Bridging Recovery Initiative Despite Gaps in Entry (BRIDGE): study protocol for a randomized controlled trial of a bridge clinic compared with usual care for patients with opioid use disorder. Trials 22(1):757, 2021 34717736

Maricich YA, Bickel WK, Marsch LA, et al: Safety and efficacy of a prescription digital therapeutic as an adjunct to buprenorphine for treatment of opioid use disorder. Curr Med Res Opin 37(2):167–173, 2021 33140994

Mattson ME, Del Boca FK, Carroll KM, et al: Compliance with treatment and follow-up protocols in project MATCH: predictors and relationship to outcome. Alcohol Clin Exp Res 22(6):1328–1339, 1998 9756050

McHugh RK, Hilton BT, Chase AM, et al: Do people with opioid use disorder and posttraumatic stress disorder benefit from adding individual opioid drug counseling to buprenorphine? Drug Alcohol Depend 228:109084, 2021 34607194

McLellan AT, Kushner H, Metzger D, et al: The Fifth Edition of the Addiction Severity Index. J Subst Abuse Treat 9(3):199–213, 1992 1334156

McNeely J, Troxel AB, Kunins HV, et al: Study protocol for a pragmatic trial of the Consult for Addiction Treatment and Care in Hospitals (CATCH) model for engaging patients in opioid use disorder treatment. Addict Sci Clin Pract 14(1):5, 2019 30777122

Medicaid and CHIP Payment and Access Commission: Access to Substance Use Disorder Treatment in Medicaid. Washington, DC, MACPAC, June 2018. Available at: https://www.macpac.gov/publication/access-to-substance-use-disorder-treatment-in-medicaid/. Accessed January 28, 2025.

Mee-Lee D, Shulman G, Fishman M, et al: The ASAM Criteria: Treatment Criteria for Addictive, Substance-Related, and Co-Occurring Conditions, 3rd Edition. Carson City, NV, The Change Companies, 2013

Mehta K, Hoadley A, Ray LA, et al: Cognitive-behavioral interventions targeting alcohol or other drug use and co-occurring mental health disorders: a meta-analysis. Alcohol Alcohol 56(5):535–544, 2021 33778869

Messinger J, Beletsky L: Involuntary commitment for substance use: addiction care professionals must reject enabling coercion and patient harm. J Addict Med 15(4):280–282, 2021 33989262

Meyers RJ, Roozen HG, Smith JE: The community reinforcement approach: an update of the evidence. Alcohol Res Health 33(4):380–388, 2011 23580022

Miller NS, Flaherty JA: Effectiveness of coerced addiction treatment (alternative consequences): a review of the clinical research. J Subst Abuse Treat 18(1):9–16, 2000 10636601

Miller WR, Rollnick S: Motivational Interviewing: Helping People Change, 3rd Edition. New York, Guilford, 2012

Musto DF, Ramos MR: Notes on American medical history: a follow-up study of the New Haven morphine maintenance clinic of 1920. N Engl J Med 304(18):1071–1077, 1981 7010175

National Center for Chronic Disease Prevention and Health Promotion Office on Smoking and Health: The Health Consequences of Smoking: 50 Years of Progress: A Report of the Surgeon General. Atlanta, GA, Centers for Disease Control and Prevention, 2014. Available at: https://www.ncbi.nlm.nih.gov/books/n/surgsmoke50/pdf/. Accessed January 28, 2025.

National Center for Health Statistics: Drug Overdose Deaths in the U.S. Top 100,000 Annually. Atlanta, GA, Centers for Disease Control and Prevention, 2021. Available at: https://www.cdc.gov/nchs/pressroom/nchs_press_releases/2021/20211117.htm. Accessed January 28, 2025.

National Institute for Health Care Management Foundation: Stimulant Deaths on the Rise, Compounded by Rise in Synthetic Opioids. Washington, DC, NIHCM Foundation, June 17, 2021. Available at: https://nihcm.org/publications/stimulant-deaths-on-the-rise-compounded-by-rise-in-synthetic-opioids. Accessed March 21, 2022.

National Institute on Drug Abuse: Common Comorbidities With Substance Use Disorders Research Report. Bethesda, MD, National Institute on Drug Abuse, 2020

National Judicial Opioid Task Force: Involuntary Commitment and Guardianship Laws for Persons With a Substance Use Disorder. Conference of Chief Justices, Conference of State Court Administrators, State Justice Institute, National Center for State Courts, 2018. Available at: https://www.ncsc.org/__data/assets/pdf_file/0028/18478/inv-comm-and-guard-laws-for-sud-final.pdf. Accessed January 28, 2025.

Nicolini M, Vandenberghe J, Gastmans C: Substance use disorder and compulsory commitment to care: a care-ethical decision-making framework. Scand J Caring Sci 32(3):1237–1246, 2018 29193265

Norton BL, Fleming J, Bachhuber MA, et al: High HCV cure rates for people who use drugs treated with direct acting antiviral therapy at an urban primary care clinic. Int J Drug Policy 47:196–201, 2017 28811158

Ober AJ, Murray-Krezan C, Page K, et al: Hospital addiction consultation service and opioid use disorder treatment: the START randomized clinical trial. JAMA Intern Med 185(6):624–633, 2025

Olfson M, Wall MM, Barry CL, et al: Effects of the ACA on health care coverage for adults with substance use disorders. Psychiatr Serv 72(8):905–911, 2021 33957766

Onken LS, Blaine JD, Boren JJ: Beyond the Therapeutic Alliance: Keeping the Drug-Dependent Individual in Treatment. Rockville, MD, National Institutes of Health, 1997

Onyeka IN, Uosukainen H, Korhonen MJ, et al: Sociodemographic characteristics and drug abuse patterns of treatment-seeking illicit drug abusers in Finland, 1997–2008: the Huuti study. J Addict Dis 31(4):350–362, 2012 23244554

Orgera K, Tolbert J: Key Facts About Uninsured Adults With Opioid Use Disorder. San Francisco, CA, Kaiser Family Foundation, 2016

Oviedo-Joekes E, Brissette S, Marsh DC, et al: Diacetylmorphine versus methadone for the treatment of opioid addiction. N Engl J Med 361(8):777–786, 2009 19692689

Peacock A, Leung J, Larney S, et al: Global statistics on alcohol, tobacco and illicit drug use: 2017 status report. Addiction 113(10):1905–1926, 2018 29749059

Peters PJ, Pontones P, Hoover KW, et al: HIV infection linked to injection use of oxymorphone in Indiana, 2014–2015. N Engl J Med 375(3):229–239, 2016 27468059

Petry NM: Contingency management: what it is and why psychiatrists should want to use it. Psychiatrist 35(5):161–163, 2011 22558006

Petry NM, Peirce JM, Stitzer ML, et al: Effect of prize-based incentives on outcomes in stimulant abusers in outpatient psychosocial treatment programs: a National Drug Abuse Treatment Clinical Trials Network study. Arch Gen Psychiatry 62(10):1148–1156, 2005 16203960

Powers MB, Vedel E, Emmelkamp PMG: Behavioral couples therapy (BCT) for alcohol and drug use disorders: a meta-analysis. Clin Psychol Rev 28(6):952–962, 2008 18374464

Raja S, Hasnain M, Hoersch M, et al: Trauma informed care in medicine: current knowledge and future research directions. Fam Community Health 38(3):216–226, 2015 26017000

Rao-Patel A, Adelberg M, Arsenault S, et al: Fraud's Newest Hot Spot: The Opioid Epidemic and the Corresponding Rise of Unethical Addiction Treatment Providers. Health Affairs Forefront, April 26, 2018. Available at: https://www.healthaffairs.org/do/10.1377/forefront.20180423.449595/full/. Accessed January 28, 2025.

Ray LA, Meredith LR, Kiluk BD, et al: Combined pharmacotherapy and cognitive behavioral therapy for adults with alcohol or substance use disorders: a systematic review and meta-analysis. JAMA Netw Open 3(6):e208279, 2020 32558914

Riley D, Pates R: Harm Reduction in Substance Use and High-Risk Behaviour. New York, Wiley, 2012

Roozen HG, Boulogne JJ, van Tulder MW, et al: A systematic review of the effectiveness of the community reinforcement approach in alcohol, cocaine and opioid addiction. Drug Alcohol Depend 74(1):1–13, 2004 15072802

Schwarz A-S, Nielsen B, Søgaard J, et al: Making a bridge between general hospital and specialised community-based treatment for alcohol use disorder: a pragmatic randomised controlled trial. Drug Alcohol Depend 196:51–56, 2019 30665152

Sharon E, Krebs C, Turner W, et al: Predictive validity of the ASAM patient placement criteria for hospital utilization. J Addict Dis 22(Suppl 1):79–93, 2003 15991591

Simpson DD: The relation of time spent in drug abuse treatment to posttreatment outcome. Am J Psychiatry 136(11):1449–1453, 1979 495799

Simpson DD: Treatment for drug abuse: follow-up outcomes and length of time spent. Arch Gen Psychiatry 38(8):875–880, 1981 7259424

Simpson DD, Joe GW, Broome KM, et al: Program diversity and treatment retention rates in the Drug Abuse Treatment Outcome Study (DATOS). Psychol Addict Behav 11(4):279–293, 1997

Smart R, Pardo B, Davis CS: Systematic review of the emerging literature on the effectiveness of naloxone access laws in the United States. Addiction 116(1):6–17, 2021 32533570

Sobell LC, Sobell MB, Agrawal S: Randomized controlled trial of a cognitive-behavioral motivational intervention in a group versus individual format for substance use disorders. Psychol Addict Behav 23(4):672–683, 2009 20025373

Srebnik D, Connor T, Sylla L: A pilot study of the impact of housing first-supported housing for intensive users of medical hospitalization and sobering services. Am J Public Health 103(2):316–321, 2013 23237150

Stallvik M, Gastfriend DR, Nordahl HM: Matching patients with substance use disorder to optimal level of care with the ASAM criteria software. J Subst Use 20(6):389–398, 2015

Stark MJ: Dropping out of substance abuse treatment: a clinically oriented review. Clin Psychol Rev 12(1):93–116, 1992

Sterling S, Chi F, Hinman A: Integrating care for people with co-occurring alcohol and other drug, medical, and mental health conditions. Alcohol Res Health 33(4):338–349, 2011 23580018

Substance Abuse and Mental Health Services Administration: SAMHSA's Concept of Trauma and Guidance for a Trauma-Informed Approach (HHS Publ No 14-4884). Rockville, MD, Office of Policy, Planning, and Innovation, 2014a. Available at: https://ncsacw.acf.hhs.gov/userfiles/files/SAMHSA_Trauma.pdf. Accessed January 28, 2025.

Substance Abuse and Mental Health Services Administration: The TEDS Report: Health Insurance Status of Adult Substance Abuse Treatment Admissions Aged 26 or Older: 2011. Rockville, MD, Substance Abuse and Mental Health Services Administration, February 6, 2014b. Available at: https://www.samhsa.gov/data/sites/default/files/sr134-health-insurance-2014/sr134-health-insurance-2014/sr134-health-insurance-2014.htm. Accessed January 28, 2025.

Substance Abuse and Mental Health Services Administration: Use of Medication-Assisted Treatment for Opioid Use Disorder in Criminal Justice Settings (HHS Publ No PEP19-MATUSECJS). Rockville, MD, Center for Behavioral Health Statistics and Quality, Substance Abuse and Mental Health Services Administration, 2019. Available at: https://store.samhsa.gov/sites/default/files/d7/priv/pep19-matusecjs.pdf. Accessed January 28, 2025.

Substance Abuse and Mental Health Services Administration: Key Substance Use and Mental Health Indicators in the United States: Results From the 2023 National Survey on Drug Use and Health (HHS Publication No. PEP24-07-021, NSDUH Series H-59). Rockville, MD, Center for Behavioral Health Statistics and Quality, Substance Abuse and Mental Health Services Administration, 2024. Available at: https://www.samhsa.gov/data/sites/default/files/reports/rpt47095/National%20Report/National%20Report/2023-nsduh-annual-national.pdf. Accessed May 22, 2025.

Sullivan RW, Szczesniak LM, Wojcik SM: Bridge clinic buprenorphine program decreases emergency department visits. J Subst Abuse Treat 130:108410, 2021 34118702

Tabarra I, Soares S, Rosado T, et al: Novel synthetic opioids: toxicological aspects and analysis. Forensic Sci Res 4(2):111–140, 2019 31304442

Tang VM, Goud R, Zawertailo L, et al: Repetitive transcranial magnetic stimulation for smoking cessation: next steps for translation and implementation into clinical practice. Psychiatry Res 326:115340, 2023

Taylor JL, Johnson S, Cruz R, et al: Integrating harm reduction into outpatient opioid use disorder treatment settings: harm reduction in outpatient addiction treatment. J Gen Intern Med 36(12):3810–3819, 2021 34159545

Terraneo A, Leggio L, Saladini M, et al: Transcranial magnetic stimulation of dorsolateral prefrontal cortex reduces cocaine use: a pilot study. Eur Neuropsychopharmacol 26(1):37–44, 2016 26655188

Terry CE: The Harrison Anti-Narcotic Act. Am J Public Health 5(6):518, 1915

U.S. Preventive Services Task Force; Krist AH, Davidson KW, Mangione CM, et al: Interventions for tobacco smoking cessation in adults, including pregnant persons: US Preventive Services Task Force Recommendation Statement. JAMA 325(3):265–279, 2021 33464343

van Boekel LC, Brouwers EPM, van Weeghel J, et al: Stigma among health professionals towards patients with substance use disorders and its consequences for healthcare delivery: systematic review. Drug Alcohol Depend 131(1–2):23–35, 2013 23490450

Vanderplasschen W, Colpaert K, Autrique M, et al: Therapeutic communities for addictions: a review of their effectiveness from a recovery-oriented perspective. ScientificWorldJournal 2013:427817, 2013 23401669

Vuong T, Gillies M, Larney S, et al: The association between involuntary alcohol treatment and subsequent emergency department visits and hospitalizations: a Bayesian analysis of treated patients and matched controls. Addiction 117(6):1589–1597, 2021 34817096

Wakeman SE, Metlay JP, Chang Y, et al: Inpatient addiction consultation for hospitalized patients increases post-discharge abstinence and reduces addiction severity. J Gen Intern Med 32(8):909–916, 2017 28526932

Walley AY, Paasche-Orlow M, Lee EC, et al: Acute care hospital utilization among medical inpatients discharged with a substance use disorder diagnosis. J Addict Med 6(1):50–56, 2012 21979821

Walley AY, Xuan Z, Hackman HH, et al: Opioid overdose rates and implementation of overdose education and nasal naloxone distribution in Massachusetts: interrupted time series analysis. BMJ 346:f174, 2013 23372174

Weinstein ZM, Wakeman SE, Nolan S: Inpatient addiction consult service: expertise for hospitalized patients with complex addiction problems. Med Clin North Am 102(4):587–601, 2018 29933817

Weiss RD, Potter JS, Fiellin DA, et al: Adjunctive counseling during brief and extended buprenorphine–naloxone treatment for prescription opioid dependence: a 2-phase randomized controlled trial. Arch Gen Psychiatry 68(12):1238–1246, 2011 22065255

Weiss RD, Griffin ML, Potter JS, et al: Who benefits from additional drug counseling among prescription opioid-dependent patients receiving buprenorphine-naloxone and standard medical management? Drug Alcohol Depend 140:118–122, 2014 24831754

Westermeyer J, Dickmann P: Cultural issues in addiction medicine, in The ASAM Principles of Addiction Medicine, 6th Edition. New York, Wolters Kluwer, 2019, pp 1388–1405

Westermeyer J, Mellman L, Alarcon R: Cultural competence in addiction psychiatry. Addict Disord Their Treat 5(3):107–119, 2006

Witkiewitz K, Heather N, Falk DE, et al: World Health Organization risk drinking level reductions are associated with improved functioning and are sustained among patients with mild, moderate and severe alcohol dependence in clinical trials in the United States and United Kingdom. Addiction 115(9):1668–1680, 2020 32056311

Ziaaddini H, Nasirian M, Nakhaee N: Comparison of the efficacy of buprenorphine and clonidine in detoxification of opioid-dependents. Addict Health 4(3–4):79–86, 2012 24494140

Nicotine and Tobacco[1]

Aurelia I. Andreiev, M.D.
Gali Katznelson, M.D.
Maya Vijayaraghavan, M.D.
Tony P. George, M.D.

Tobacco use disorder (TUD) continues to be a major health issue worldwide. The prevalence of nicotine and tobacco use is approximately 15% in the United States (Cornelius et al. 2023); many of these smokers have tried to quit numerous times. Moreover, in the past 15 years, there has been a tremendous increase in the use of electronic cigarettes (e-cigarettes), which now represent about 35% of the nicotine product market (George 2024). In this chapter, we review the clinical features of nicotine and tobacco use

---

[1] This chapter was supported in part by National Institutes of Health grants R21-DA-043949 (to Dr. George) and R37-CA-248448-01A1 (to Dr. Vijayaraghavan).

and addiction and discuss the three approved pharmacotherapies (nicotine replacement therapies [NRTs], sustained-release [SR] bupropion, and varenicline). We then discuss non-FDA-approved tobacco pharmacotherapies, which are often used for treatment-resistant TUD, and deep transcranial magnetic stimulation (TMS), which was approved by the FDA in 2020 for tobacco cessation. (See Table 2.1 for a list of FDA-approved, FDA-cleared, and non-FDA-approved pharmacotherapies, along with nonpharmacotherapeutic interventions.) Finally, we discuss the subspecialty approach to vulnerable populations of smokers, such as individuals with co-occurring mental health disorders and addictions, smokers with medical illness, and smokers who are pregnant or experiencing homelessness. Our goal is to give the reader an up-to-date, comprehensive, and integrated approach to using pharmacotherapies and related biological therapies to treat TUD, wherein medications are often needed in combination with behavioral supports to reduce or quit nicotine and tobacco use.

Phenomenology of Tobacco Use Disorder and Clinical Aspects of Withdrawal

The primary addictive substance in cigarette smoke is nicotine. Cigarette smoking is a very efficient nicotine delivery system because nicotine is aerosolized and subsequently absorbed through the pulmonary vasculature. Consequently, smoking produces high arterial nicotine concentrations compared with venous concentrations (Benowitz 2010). These high arterial concentrations deliver a bolus of nicotine 1–3 mg rapidly to the brain (i.e., within seconds) per smoked cigarette (Benowitz 2010). A number of neurotransmitters are released with nicotinic receptor activation, including dopamine, norepinephrine, serotonin, and endogenous opioids. The immediate positive reinforcing effects of smoking include reduced anxiety and increased alertness and concentration. Nicotine's half-life is 60–90 minutes, so repeated administration is needed throughout the day for continued effects. Consequently, daily smokers usually smoke at frequent intervals to maintain a narrow range of nicotine levels. Chronic administration of nicotine increases the number of nicotinic receptors, presumably resulting from chronic nicotinic receptor desensitization and inactivation. An increased number of receptors may play a role in the withdrawal symptoms many

Table 2.1 Pharmacological and neuromodulation treatments for tobacco use disorder

Treatment	Description	Evidence rating[a]	Dosage
NRT[b]			
Gum (OTC)	Slow nicotine absorption gradually reduces nicotine craving and withdrawal	1	2 mg ($\leq$20 cigarettes/d) to 4 mg every 1–2 h (fixed dosing better than ad libitum)
Transdermal nicotine patch (OTC)	Slow nicotine absorption gradually reduces nicotine craving and withdrawal	1	15 mg/16 h, 7–22 mg/24 h; steady state after 2–3 d; highest dosing for $\geq$10 cigarettes/d
Lozenge (OTC)	Slow nicotine absorption gradually reduces nicotine craving and withdrawal	1	2–4 mg every 1–2 h × 2–4 wk, then every 2–4 h thereafter; 25% higher serum level vs. gum
Vapor inhaler (prescription)	Fast nicotine absorption leads to stimulation of the nAChR, which rapidly reduces nicotine craving and withdrawal	1	6–16 cartridges/d (4 mg/cartridge); not for people with asthma
Nasal spray (prescription)	Fast nicotine absorption leads to stimulation of the nAChR, which reduces craving and withdrawal	1	10 mg/mL (0.5 mg/spray); 1 spray per nostril 1–2 times/h; quickest onset of all NRTs

Table 2.1 Pharmacological and neuromodulation treatments for tobacco use disorder *(continued)*

Treatment	Description	Evidence rating[a]	Dosage
Non-nicotine pharmacotherapy			
Bupropion SR[b]	Blocks reuptake of dopamine and norepinephrine; high-affinity, noncompetitive nAChR antagonism reduces nicotine reinforcement, withdrawal, and craving	1	Set quit date within 2 wk of starting; 150 mg qam × 3 d, then 150 mg bid × 7–12 wk; often combined with NRT
Varenicline[b]	Acts as a partial agonist of $\alpha_4\beta_2$ nAChRs	1	Set quit date 8–35 d after starting; 0.5 mg qd × 3 d, then 0.5 mg bid × 4–7 d, then 1 mg bid × 12 wk; studies show safety in range of psychopathologies
Nortriptyline	Blocks reuptake of norepinephrine and 5-HT; probably reduces withdrawal symptoms and comorbid depressive symptoms; side effects limit utility	1–2	Not FDA-approved indication; set quit date 1 wk after starting; 75–100 mg (divided or once daily) × 6–14 wk

Table 2.1 Pharmacological and neuromodulation treatments for tobacco use disorder *(continued)*

Treatment	Description	Evidence rating[a]	Dosage
Clonidine	α_2-Adrenoreceptor agonist reduces nicotine withdrawal symptoms	2	Not FDA-approved indication; 0.1–0.4 mg/d × 2–6 wk; watch for rebound hypertension on discontinuation
Naltrexone	Minimal evidence that this μ opioid peptide receptor antagonist improves smoking cessation outcomes alone or in combination with transdermal nicotine. It may reduce alcohol use and obviate cessation-induced weight gain.	3	Not FDA-approved indication; 25 mg/d PO × 1 wk, then increase to 50 mg/d (to decrease gastrointestinal distress)
Cytisine	Nicotinic partial agonist appears to be safe and efficacious for smoking cessation	2	Not FDA-approved indication; six 1.5-mg tablets/d (every 2 h) on days 1–3; five 1.5-mg tablets/d (every 2.5 h) on days 4–12; four 1.5-mg tablets/d (every 3 h) on days 13–16; three 1.5-mg tablets/d (every 4 h) on days 17–20; and, finally, two 1.5-mg tablets/d (every 6 h) on days 21–25. This assumes a daily 12-h awake period.

Table 2.1 Pharmacological and neuromodulation treatments for tobacco use disorder *(continued)*

Treatment	Description	Evidence rating[a]	Dosage
Nicotine vaccine	Limited evidence of efficacy for smoking cessation in early human trials, and Phase III trials have been negative	3	
Neuromodulation techniques[c]			
Deep rTMS	Modest evidence that deep rTMS using the H-coil directed to the bilateral insula may improve smoking cessation success rates	2	

Note. 5-HT = 5-hydroxytryptamine (serotonin); nAChR = nicotinic acetylcholine receptor; NRT = nicotine replacement therapy; OTC = over the counter; rTMS = repetitive transcranial magnetic stimulation; SR = sustained release.
[a]Effectiveness rating: 1 = strong evidence to support efficacy; 2 = moderate evidence to support efficacy; 3 = little evidence to support efficacy.
[b]Approved by the FDA.
[c]Cleared by the FDA.

smokers experience with prolonged cigarette abstinence (Dani and Balfour 2011). Withdrawal symptoms include dysphoria or depressed mood, insomnia, irritability, anxiety, frustration, difficulty concentrating, and increased appetite with weight gain. Withdrawal symptoms typically peak within 24–36 hours after cessation and usually diminish after 1 week of abstinence, but prolonged withdrawal may occur in some individuals (George 2024). Thus, individuals may continue to smoke cigarettes to avoid the negative symptoms of withdrawal (dysphoria, insomnia, anxiety) (Polosa and Benowitz 2011). It is likely that both the primary, positively reinforcing effects of smoking and the avoidance of withdrawal symptoms sustain tobacco use in most smokers. It is important to note that higher plasma levels of nicotine generally correlate with higher reinforcement and withdrawal symptom attenuation, which may explain why faster-onset nicotine replacement formulations (e.g., nicotine nasal spray and inhaler) lead to improved smoking cessation outcomes (George 2024).

Psychopharmacological Approaches to Management of Tobacco Use Disorder

Nicotine Replacement Therapies

NRTs were designed to enhance efficacy rates during smoking cessation by providing partial replacement of the nicotine usually delivered by smoking (George 2024). FDA-approved NRTs for smoking cessation include nicotine polacrilex gum (2 and 4 mg), nicotine lozenge (2 and 4 mg), transdermal nicotine (7–22 mg), nicotine nasal spray, and nicotine inhaler formulations. The choice of NRT for an individual patient depends on the patient's preference, the adverse-effect profile of the NRT, the presence of other medical conditions, and previous treatment success or failure with a certain type of NRT. The odds ratios for individual NRTs are increased approximately twofold compared with placebo (George 2024; Nagano et al. 2019).

Nicotine Gum

Nicotine gum was the first NRT marketed for smoking cessation. Two dose forms (2 and 4 mg) are available for over-the-counter purchase. Nicotine gum contains nicotine bound to an ion-exchange resin, polacrilex. The nicotine is released slowly into the mouth and absorbed through the buccal mucosa. Nicotine gum is most beneficial with concurrent behavioral therapy and when used on a fixed schedule (i.e., chewing one piece every 1–2 hours) rather than ad libitum dosing (unless combined with other forms of NRT such as transdermal applications, as described later in the subsection "Combined Nicotine Replacement Therapy Formulations"). The usual treatment duration for nicotine gum is 6–14 weeks; however, benefits may occur with a longer duration (Fiore et al. 2008).

Nicotine gum should be chewed slowly, with intermittent parking of the gum at the side of the mouth to allow for buccal absorption and to avoid adverse effects (e.g., hiccups, heartburn, stomach upset) and poor bioavailability if swallowed. Only 50% of the nicotine in a piece of gum is systemically absorbed. Nicotine concentrations peak approximately 30 minutes after the onset of chewing (Benowitz 2010). The starting dose for individuals who smoke fewer than 20 cigarettes per day is 2 mg, whereas the 4-mg dose is recommended for heavier smokers (George 2024).

Nicotine Lozenge

The nicotine lozenge contains nicotine bound to a polacrilex ion-exchange resin (similar to that in nicotine gum). It is available for over-the-counter purchase in 2- and 4-mg dose forms. Because the nicotine lozenge does not require chewing, it may be preferable to nicotine gum for patients with dental problems or who dislike chewing gum. The lozenge formulations release 25% more nicotine than an equal dose of the gum (George 2024). In a large randomized controlled trial (RCT), low-dependence smokers (i.e., who waited >30 minutes on awakening to have their first cigarette) were randomly assigned to receive the 2-mg lozenge or a matching placebo, and highly dependent smokers (i.e., who had their first cigarette ≤30 minutes on awakening) were randomly assigned to receive the 4-mg lozenge or placebo for at least 24 weeks (Shiffman et al. 2002). Participants in the active lozenge group had a significantly higher 28-day abstinence rate at 6 weeks, compared with the placebo group, for both the 2-mg (46% vs. 29.7%; $P < 0.001$) and 4-mg (48.7% vs. 20.8%; $P < 0.001$) doses. Efficacy of the medication was sustained through 1-year follow-up.

Patients who use the lozenge for smoking cessation should use one nicotine lozenge every 1–2 hours for the first 2–4 weeks, decreasing the interval to every 2–4 hours thereafter. Common adverse effects with the nicotine lozenge are related to inadvertent swallowing and include heartburn, hiccups, and nausea (Shiffman et al. 2002). Because the product contains phenylalanine, the lozenge should not be used for smoking cessation by individuals with phenylketonuria.

Transdermal Nicotine Patch

Transdermal nicotine is also available over the counter for smoking cessation. This form of nicotine delivery may be especially useful for smoking cessation because a constant delivery of nicotine may aid in adherence to NRT. Eight weeks of treatment is generally sufficient for smoking cessation (Fiore et al. 2008). Compared with other NRTs, transdermal nicotine probably has the lowest misuse potential because of its low plasma levels and slow absorption, few to no withdrawal symptoms after treatment has ended, and lack of patient control over nicotine delivery.

Transdermal nicotine has been available in various formulations and dosing schedules (e.g., 15 mg/16 hours, 7 mg/24 hours, 14 mg/24 hours, and 21 mg/24 hours). Currently, in the United States, only the 24-hour transdermal patches (7 mg, 14 mg, and 21 mg) are available; in several other countries, 16-hour formulations and 22-mg/24-hour formulations are available. Historically, research has used a range of transdermal products, which is why the dosage ranges listed in this chapter may not correspond directly with those dosages and products that are currently commercially available. Peak nicotine concentrations for the various systems are reached 2–6 hours after application, and steady-state conditions occur 2–3 days after continued patch use (Benowitz 2010). The highest-dose nicotine patch (i.e., 21 mg/24 hours, 22 mg/24 hours, or 15 mg/16 hours) delivers approximately 0.9 mg/hour transdermally (Benowitz 2010).

The transdermal system is applied in the morning and removed either at bedtime or the next morning. Among individuals smoking 10 or more cigarettes per day, the highest-dose patch should be used to start; a lower dose can be used if the patient smokes fewer than 10 cigarettes per day (Benowitz 2010). Although dosage reduction with most formulations is usually recommended after 2–4 weeks to taper the NRT because of clinical concerns about nicotine withdrawal from transdermal nicotine, one meta-analysis showed no benefit of dosage reduction on patch efficacy (Fiore et al. 2008). In fact, there is little evidence for clinically significant nicotine withdrawal syndrome after transdermal nicotine discontinuation. Transdermal nicotine should not be used for patients with skin conditions that could be exacerbated by the patch.

Nicotine Nasal Spray

Nicotine nasal spray delivers nicotine through the nasal mucosa. One advantage of this formulation is that it relieves nicotine cravings more quickly than more slowly absorbed buccal or transdermally administered formulations. In one study, the nicotine nasal spray was 2.6 times more likely to produce smoking cessation than placebo at 1 year (George 2024). The nicotine spray was most beneficial among highly dependent smokers.

The nasal spray is available only by prescription. One spray to each nostril constitutes a dose. Although one dose delivers approximately 1 mg of nicotine, only 0.5 mg of nicotine is systemically absorbed. The nasal spray delivers nicotine rapidly, with venous nicotine concentrations peaking 5–10 minutes after administration. Nicotine nasal spray most closely approximates the pharmacokinetic profile of nicotine following smoked cigarettes. Because this form of NRT is administered nasally, patients with rhinitis, nasal polyps, or sinusitis should avoid its use for smoking cessation. The nasal spray produces some initial irritation of the nasal mucosa at the dosage formulation that is available commercially (10 mg/mL), but this effect subsides with repeated dosing.

Nicotine Inhaler

Nicotine (vapor) inhalers, which are used by puffing through a cartridge inhaler, may be useful for smoking cessation for some patients because their use is similar to the smoking ritual (i.e., holding the device, with repeated hand-to-mouth activity, and puffing on the device replicate many of the sensory and motoric aspects of smoking), and they deliver nicotine rapidly (although not as rapidly as the nasal spray). In one placebo-controlled study, in which subjects were allowed to use an inhaler for up to 6 months, quit rates at 1 year remained higher in the nicotine inhaler group than in the placebo inhaler group (George 2024).

The inhaler is only available by prescription (George 2024). The usual treatment period is up to 24 weeks. When the product is used as directed, the patient will likely use 6–16 inhaler cartridges per day. This form of NRT is contraindicated in patients with known hypersensitivity to nicotine or menthol. The inhaler should be used with caution in people with asthma because although most of the nicotine is absorbed through the buccal mucosa and is not delivered to the lungs, nicotine by inhalation may produce bronchial constriction.

Combined Nicotine Replacement Therapy Formulations

One way to improve efficacy further is to combine a passive and continuous nicotine delivery system (patch) with an active and intermittent delivery system (e.g., gum, inhaler, or spray) (George 2024). The rationale for combined treatment is that smokers may need a constant delivery of nicotine to alleviate withdrawal symptoms, and they may also need an ad libitum nicotine medication that can be used to control smoking urges and further relieve withdrawal symptoms (Sweeney et al. 2001). Moreover, two nicotine replacement products may provide a more closely matched degree of nicotine substitution than monotherapy.

Combination regimens may increase effectiveness of the nicotine patch. In particular, the patch (>14 weeks) plus either ad libitum nicotine gum or nasal spray had an estimated odds ratio of 1.9 (95% CI, 1.3–2.7) for success of the combined therapy compared with the patch alone. Of note, ad libitum use of the gum or spray in these studies ranged from 26 to 52 weeks. For comparison, bupropion SR combined with transdermal nicotine had an estimated odds ratio of 1.3 (95% CI, 1.0–1.8) compared with transdermal nicotine alone (George 2024).

Non-nicotine Pharmacotherapies

Not all smokers respond well to NRTs. Furthermore, many smokers have co-occurring symptoms, suggesting that mechanisms independent of the nicotinic receptor may increase vulnerability to TUD. Thus, there has been considerable interest in non-nicotine medications to treat nicotine dependence, either alone or in combination with NRTs. Observations that the antidepressant bupropion has potential as a treatment for smoking cessation and that other antidepressants (e.g., tricyclic antidepressants and selective serotonin reuptake inhibitors [SSRIs]) may modify smoking behaviors have catalyzed intensive research on medications that act on dopamine, norepinephrine, serotonin, glutamate, GABA, nicotinic, cannabinoid, or opioid receptors. We review here the safety and efficacy of bupropion, varenicline, and other non-nicotine therapies. Of the non-nicotine medications for smoking cessation, only bupropion SR and varenicline are considered first-line treatment for cigarette smokers.

Sustained-Release Bupropion

The phenyl aminoketone atypical antidepressant agent bupropion in the SR formulation is a first-line pharmacological treatment for tobacco smokers.

The mechanism of action of this antidepressant in the treatment of TUD likely involves blockade of dopamine and norepinephrine reuptake as well as antagonism of high-affinity nicotinic acetylcholine receptors (nAChRs) (George 2024). The goals of bupropion therapy for TUD are 1) cessation of smoking behavior and 2) reduction of nicotine withdrawal symptoms.

A pivotal study by Hurt et al. (1997) established the efficacy and safety of bupropion SR for treatment of TUD, which led to its approval by the FDA for this indication in 1997. This study was a 7-week, double-blind, placebo-controlled multicenter trial of three dosages of bupropion SR (100, 150, or 300 mg/day in divided doses) and enrolled 615 cigarette smokers who smoked at least 15 cigarettes per day. The medication was administered in combination with weekly individual cessation counseling. End-of-trial 7-day point prevalence cessation rates were 19.0% for placebo, 28.8% for bupropion 100 mg/day, 38.6% for 150 mg/day, and 44.2% for 300 mg/day. At 1-year follow-up, cessation rates were 12.4% for placebo, 19.6% for bupropion 100 mg/day, 22.9% for 150 mg/day, and 23.1% for 300 mg/day. Bupropion treatment dose-dependently reduced weight gain associated with smoking cessation and significantly reduced nicotine withdrawal symptoms at the 150- and 300-mg/day dosages. In this study, the major adverse effects associated with bupropion, compared with placebo, were insomnia and dry mouth. Accordingly, the target dosage for bupropion treatment of TUD is 300 mg/day (150 mg bid). The target quit date is typically set on the eighth day of bupropion treatment, when bupropion levels are at steady-state concentrations.

The combination of bupropion SR with the transdermal patch was evaluated in a double-blind, double placebo–controlled, randomized multicenter trial (Jorenby et al. 1999). A total of 893 cigarette smokers who smoked at least 15 cigarettes per day were randomly assigned to one of four groups: 1) placebo bupropion (0 mg/day) plus placebo patch, 2) bupropion (300 mg/day) plus placebo patch, 3) placebo bupropion plus nicotine patch (21 mg/day for 4 weeks, followed by 14 mg/day for 2 weeks and 7 mg/day for 2 weeks), and 4) bupropion (300 mg/day) plus the nicotine patch (21 mg/day for 4 weeks, followed by 14 mg/day for 2 weeks and 7 mg/day for 2 weeks). Treatment with bupropion was initiated 1 week before the target quit date (day 8), at which time patch treatment was added for a total of 8 weeks. All subjects received weekly individual smoking cessation counseling. Cessation rates at the 1-year follow-up assessment were 15.6%

for placebo, 16.4% for the active nicotine transdermal patch alone, 30.3% for bupropion alone, and 35.5% for the patch and bupropion combination. The rates for the group receiving bupropion plus the patch and the group receiving bupropion only were significantly better than those for the placebo group and the patch-only group; however, the rate for the combination was not significantly better than that for bupropion only. Weight suppression after cessation was most robust in the combination therapy group. The combination was well tolerated, with adverse effects being those expected from the patch and bupropion. It is noteworthy that the patch-only treatment was significantly different from placebo at the end of the trial but not at the follow-up assessments. Approximately 6% of participants in the trial developed hypertension, but most had preexisting blood pressure problems. The combination of transdermal nicotine and bupropion has been approved by the FDA for smoking cessation. In a previous study, bupropion SR and transdermal nicotine had an estimated odds ratio of 1.3 (95% CI, 1.0–1.8) compared with the nicotine patch alone (George 2024). Thus, the clinical utility of combining bupropion SR and the nicotine patch is unclear.

The primary adverse effects reported with bupropion SR administration in cigarette smokers are headache, dry mouth, nausea and vomiting, insomnia, and activation. Seizures occur very rarely (incidence <0.2%) at dosages of 300 mg/day or less, which is comparable to rates seen with most SSRI antidepressants (Finkelstein et al. 2018).

Varenicline

Varenicline tartrate, an $\alpha_4\beta_2$ nAChR partial agonist, was approved as a first-line smoking cessation agent by the FDA in 2006 and was approved in Canada and Europe in 2007. The initial Phase II trials of varenicline established its safety and efficacy compared with placebo, and they suggested an optimal dosage of 2 mg/day (Oncken et al. 2006), with dosage titration during the first week before the quit date. Two identical but independent 12-week Phase III trials comparing varenicline (2 mg/day) to bupropion SR (300 mg/day) were then conducted (Gonzales et al. 2006; Jorenby et al. 2006). Quit rates for the two studies were similar for continuous abstinence over the last 4 weeks (weeks 9–12), with rates of 43.9% versus 44.0% for varenicline, 29.8% versus 29.5% for bupropion SR, and 17.6% vs 17.7% for placebo. Quit rates were significantly higher for participants taking varenicline than those taking bupropion SR alone, and both medications individually resulted in significantly higher quit rates than placebo. Participants taking varenicline continued to show a higher rate of abstinence than participants taking bupropion or placebo. In addition, varenicline has been found to be more effective in smoking relapse prevention compared with placebo (Tonstad et al. 2006).

Varenicline reduces nicotine cravings and smoking satisfaction, and it is generally well tolerated. The most common adverse events reported in the initial studies were nausea and insomnia. Since approval of varenicline, however, concerns have arisen over treatment-emergent neuropsychiatric events, including agitation, suicidal and homicidal ideation, mania, and psychosis (McClure et al. 2010). In fact, in 2008, a black box warning about the safety of varenicline in psychiatric populations was issued, then later revoked. In support of its safety, Williams and colleagues (2012) documented the safety and efficacy of varenicline in schizophrenia, and Chengappa and colleagues (2014) showed similar outcomes in bipolar disorder. Moreover, the EAGLES trial, which was conducted with approximately 8,000 smokers with and without severe or any mental illness, demonstrated the safety and efficacy of varenicline in people with a wide range of mental illnesses, including mood and anxiety disorders, psychosis, and personality disorders (Anthenelli et al. 2016). Nonetheless, close monitoring of smokers, especially those with a history of psychiatric illness, has been strongly advised when prescribing this agent.

Relapse Prevention Studies

Although many studies have examined the use of pharmacotherapy for smoking cessation, far fewer have studied its use in preventing smoking relapse over the longer term. The paucity of reports on the extended use of NRTs for the prevention of smoking relapse may be related to the low number of studies examining the safety of long-term use. However, for a patient who reports prolonged urges to smoke or nicotine withdrawal symptoms, the clinician should consider extending the current approved pharmacotherapy or adding an additional pharmacotherapy (Fiore et al. 2008). If there is concern that weight gain may threaten a patient's risk of relapse, continued use of bupropion SR, varenicline, or nicotine gum is warranted, because these treatments have been shown to delay weight gain (George 2024).

Bupropion SR was evaluated by Hays et al. (2001) in a previous study. The authors compared the effects of bupropion with placebo for the prevention of smoking relapse in 784 cigarette smokers who achieved smoking abstinence after a 7-week open-label trial of bupropion (300 mg/day). Abstinent smokers were randomly assigned to receive bupropion (300 mg/day) or placebo for a total of 52 weeks. The majority of the smokers (58.8%) enrolled in the open-label phase of the trial quit smoking. Significantly more smokers were abstinent at the end of the 52-week treatment period in the bupropion group than in the placebo group (55.1% vs. 42.3%; $P < 0.01$), but no difference was evident at the 1-year posttreatment follow-up assessment. In addition, the number of days to smoking relapse was greater in the bupropion group compared with the placebo group (156 vs. 65 days; $P < 0.05$). Weight gain was significantly less in the bupropion group, both at the end of treatment and at the 1-year follow-up. The results of this study support the efficacy of bupropion SR in preventing smoking relapse, but the question of how long bupropion therapy can be continued as a maintenance treatment requires further study.

Similarly, a large placebo-controlled trial of varenicline (2 mg/day) for 12 weeks after initial abstinence also showed that this agent delays relapse to smoking compared with placebo (Tonstad et al. 2006). On the basis of that study, an additional 12 weeks of varenicline was approved by the FDA for tobacco relapse prevention.

Other Non-nicotine Pharmacotherapies

Findings from studies of several non-FDA-approved non-nicotine pharmacotherapies for nicotine dependence are summarized in the following sections.

Nortriptyline

Nortriptyline, a tricyclic antidepressant, has been shown in randomized, double-blind, placebo-controlled trials to be superior to placebo for smoking cessation (Prochazka et al. 1998). Nortriptyline appears to have efficacy comparable to that of bupropion for smoking cessation (Hall et al. 2002). The efficacy of this agent may be improved with more intensive behavioral therapies (Hall et al. 1998). Nortriptyline's mechanism of action may relate to its noradrenergic and serotonergic reuptake blockade, two neurotransmitters that have been implicated in the neurobiology of physiological nicotine dependence. Adverse effects of nortriptyline are typical of tricyclic antidepressants and include dry mouth, blurred vision, constipation, and orthostatic hypotension. Although it appears to have some utility for smokers with a history of major depression and can be recommended as a second-line agent after NRTs and bupropion, more study of nortriptyline is needed.

Clonidine
Clonidine dampens sympathetic activity originating at the locus coeruleus by stimulation of presynaptic α_2-adrenergic receptors in the sympathetic chain (Covey and Glassman 1991; Hughes et al. 1994). Clonidine appears to have some efficacy for alcohol and opioid withdrawal and thus was evaluated for the treatment of nicotine withdrawal as well (Covey and Glassman 1991; Hughes et al. 1994). Clinical trials have used oral or transdermal clonidine in dosages of 0.1–0.4 mg/day for 2–6 weeks. Behavioral counseling was offered to participants in five of the six trials. The pooled odds ratio for smoking cessation with clonidine versus placebo was 1.89 (95% CI, 1.30–2.74). There was a high incidence of dose-dependent side effects, particularly dry mouth and sedation (Gourlay et al. 2004). One study showed that clonidine was more effective in women than in men (58% vs. 20% 7-day point prevalence quit rates at 12 weeks) (Hilleman et al. 1993); however, other studies have failed to find this association. In general, the effects of clonidine are not as robust as those of NRTs (George 2024), and this agent should be considered a second-line therapy for smokers for whom treatment with first-line pharmacotherapies fails.

Naltrexone
Naltrexone is an orally bioactive form of the opioid antagonist naloxone. The rationale for using naltrexone for smoking cessation is that the performance-enhancing and other positive effects of nicotine may be mediated by action on opioid receptors (Pomerleau and Pomerleau 1984). Most (but not all) studies have shown that naltrexone increases smoking (interpreted as an attempt to overcome blockade) (Hughes et al. 1994; Sutherland et al. 1995); a trial in patients recovering from alcohol use disorder showed that naltrexone may reduce smoking by about 5 cigarettes per day, even though it appeared to have little utility in smoking cessation (Rohsenow et al. 2003).

The adverse effects of oral naltrexone include nausea and blockade of analgesia from narcotic pain relievers (Hughes et al. 1994). There is little evidence to support the efficacy of naltrexone alone for smoking cessation (Sutherland et al. 1995), and results are conflicting as to whether adding it to the nicotine patch enhances efficacy (Covey et al. 1999; Krishnan-Sarin et al. 2003; O'Malley et al. 2006). To date, there have been no published trials on the use of depot naltrexone for smoking cessation.

Selective Serotonin Reuptake Inhibitors

There is little available evidence supporting the use of SSRIs for smoking cessation, either alone (Niaura et al. 2002) or in combination with NRTs. Placebo-controlled trials of fluoxetine combined with the nicotine inhaler (Blondal et al. 1999) and of paroxetine combined with the nicotine patch (Killen et al. 2000) failed to show that either of these combinations is superior to NRTs plus placebo for smoking cessation. Thus, the use of SSRIs for smoking cessation alone is not recommended.

Monoamine Oxidase Inhibitors

Inhibition of monoamine oxidases A and B (MAO-A and -B) theoretically could be helpful for smoking cessation. These inhibitors block the metabolism of neurotransmitters involved in the biology of TUD, including dopamine (MAO-B inhibitors) and serotonin and norepinephrine (MAO-A inhibitors), leading to increases in their synaptic levels, which are reduced during acute nicotine withdrawal. The net effect of treatment with these agents could be to reverse the effects of withdrawal, thereby ameliorating withdrawal symptoms and the risk of a relapse to smoking.

In a preliminary trial of the MAO-A inhibitor moclobemide, the active medication resulted in a higher short-term rate of self-reported smoking cessation than placebo in a sample of 88 smokers (Berlin et al. 1995). Moreover, a preliminary trial by George et al. (2003) in 40 smokers provided support for the short-term efficacy of the MAO-B inhibitor selegiline hydrochloride for smoking cessation. However, larger trials of selegiline in both oral (Weinberger et al. 2010) and transdermal (Kahn et al. 2012) formulations failed to support the efficacy of this MAO-B inhibitor for smoking cessation.

Cytisine

Cytisine, an alkaloid extracted from the seeds of *Cytisus laburnum*, is a partial agonist of the $\alpha_4\beta_2$ receptor (similar to varenicline). Cytisine has been sold under the trade name Tabex for many years in many European countries and over the internet, and it is much less expensive than other pharmacotherapies for smoking cessation (at the time of this writing, cytisine is not approved by the FDA for this indication). In a placebo-controlled study (West et al. 2011), a 25-day standard treatment course resulted in a sustained 12-month abstinence rate of 8.4% in the cytisine group and 2.4% in the placebo group ($P = 0.001$). Seven-day point prevalence rates at 12 months were 13.2% in the cytisine group and 7.3% in the placebo group. Gastrointestinal adverse events were observed more frequently in the cytisine group than in the placebo group, and serious adverse events were few and similar between groups. In the study by West et al. (2011), cytisine was effective for smoking cessation, with an odds ratio similar to that of NRT.

Cytisine may be particularly useful in low- to middle-income countries, where tobacco use rates are rising and the cost of standard pharmacotherapies is high (West et al. 2011). It was shown in a large multisite trial (Courtney et al. 2021) to be nearly as effective for smoking cessation as varenicline, with fewer side effects. Cytisine is available as tablets, capsules, and oral strips.

Nicotine Vaccine

Nicotine vaccines have been developed for smoking cessation (Fagerström and Balfour 2006). They are designed to stimulate an antibody response to nicotine, binding nicotine in the plasma and reducing brain exposure to nicotine. Although nicotine is not immunogenic, it stimulates an immune response when linked to an appropriate carrier protein (e.g., cholera B toxin, *Pseudomonas* exotoxin A) (Fagerström and Balfour 2006). A gradual reduction in the brain's exposure to nicotine could facilitate smoking cessation. Although early studies provided proof of concept for the vaccine (i.e., a greater antibody response was associated with higher cessation rates), large-scale Phase III trials have not shown its efficacy (Hatsukami et al. 2011). Further research is needed to establish the safety and efficacy of the different vaccine formulations.

Neuromodulation

Modest evidence suggests that deep repetitive transcranial magnetic stimulation (rTMS) directed to the insula bilaterally may promote smoking cessation and reduction (Dinur-Klein et al. 2014), although other studies have not demonstrated positive effects (Kozak et al. 2018). In addition, studies suggest that rTMS targeting the dorsolateral prefrontal cortex may be beneficial in increasing abstinence rates and latency to relapse (Pripfl et al. 2014; Sheffer et al. 2018). This novel neuroscience-based method was cleared by the FDA for the indication of smoking cessation in 2020. However, further research, including refinement of treatment protocols (e.g., duration, targets, strength) and use of other noninvasive neuromodulation methods (e.g., transcranial direct-current stimulation and theta-burst rTMS) to facilitate smoking cessation, is warranted (Addicott et al. 2024; Coles et al. 2018; Wing et al. 2013). The authors of a 2024 systematic review of RCTs concluded that noninvasive brain stimulation techniques including TMS seem to be safe and well tolerated relative to other possible treatments, are more effective than sham treatments in research studies, compare favorably with other established smoking reduction or cessation pharmacotherapies, and have results that persist when cessation/reduction is achieved (although longer-term follow-up studies are needed) (Iannuzzo et al. 2024). Additional information is available in Chapter 12 ("Circuit-Based Interventions for Substance Use Disorders").

Pharmacogenetic and Pharmacogenomic Approaches
The promise of pharmacogenetic and pharmacogenomic approaches may lead to personalized medicine approaches to tobacco cessation, as has been demonstrated in early randomized trials (Lerman et al. 2015), but further study is required.

Electronic Nicotine Delivery Systems

Electronic nicotine delivery systems (ENDS), also more commonly known as electronic cigarettes, e-cigarettes, or vapes, were invented in 2003 and quickly increased in popularity. By 2015, ENDS constituted an approximately $10 billion global market, with around 56% of this market based in the United States. Additional literature reports a significant increase in the prevalence of e-cigarette use among adults in the United States regardless of smoking level, age, race, sex, or education level (Rigotti et al. 2015). For instance, between 2020 and 2021 alone, adult use of e-cigarettes increased from 3.7% to 4.5% (Cornelius et al. 2023). The CDC reported that as of 2024, e-cigarettes have become the most commonly used tobacco product among middle and high school students in the United States, with 1.63 million students (5.9%) reporting being current users of these products (Jamal et al. 2024; Park-Lee et al. 2024).

E-cigarettes are handheld devices consisting of a cartridge in which the nicotine-containing liquid (e-liquid) is stored, a heating element, and a battery. The liquid usually contains propylene glycol or glycerol, distilled water, nicotine, flavoring, and other optional additives. The process starts with the user pressing a button or inhaling through the mouthpiece, mimicking a cigarette. The mechanism of action of these devices includes rapid heating and cooling of the nicotine solution, such that aerosolized particles are generated and inhaled through the mouthpiece, much like the therapeutic nicotine inhaler. The level of nicotine and pH, as well as additive content, can vary among e-liquids (Lowe et al. 2019).

An important reported trend is the use of vaping for cannabis (tetrahydrocannabinol [THC]) consumption, with reusable third-generation e-cigarettes. A significant risk that exists with cannabis vaping is that THC levels can exceed combustion-produced methods 4- to 30-fold, increasing the incidence of neuropsychiatric side effects (e.g., anxiety, paranoia, thought disorder) (Motooka et al. 2018).

Compared with a tobacco cigarette, the plasma concentration delivered with an e-cigarette is lower overall (~18 vs. ~25 ng/mL) (Etter and Bullen 2011). Risk for nicotine physiological dependence via e-cigarettes varies with the model of the device, nicotine concentration used, and inhalation technique but is lower overall than the risk posed by tobacco cigarettes (Etter and Bullen 2011; Rigotti et al. 2015).

Although toxin levels are generally lower in e-cigarettes compared with tobacco cigarettes (Lowe et al. 2019), there are several other concerns with ENDS, including mouth and throat irritation, nausea, headache, dizziness, and dry cough (Etter and Bullen 2011). Topical injury from e-liquids, fires, and explosions are other means of harm to users. One concerning aspect of ENDS that has been reported in the literature has been addition of other agents to the e-liquid, including erectile dysfunction or weight loss medications, which come with their own potential for adverse reactions. Long-term health consequences of e-cigarette use or vaping are still unknown. In a systematic review, Wasfi et al. (2022) determined that there were nonsignificant to mixed impacts on various organ systems, and they cautioned that the certainty of the evidence remains very low.

E-cigarette or vaping use–associated lung injury (E-VALI) occurs in the hospital setting. The usual presentation of this condition is with cough and fever; chest radiographs show bilateral infiltrates. E-VALI is characterized by acute lung injury, which is sometimes severe and typically associated with constitutional and gastrointestinal symptoms in the most severe cases. The mortality rate was reported in the literature at 2.3% (Heinzerling et al.

2020). Interestingly, vitamin E acetate, a common additive to vaping products containing THC, was found in the bronchial lavage of more than 90% of patients with E-VALI. Since the removal of vitamin E acetate from vaping products, the incidence of E-VALI has significantly decreased (Ranpara et al. 2021).

Although ENDS appear to aid in smoking cessation (Eisenberg et al. 2020; Hajek et al. 2019) among prior tobacco smokers, physiological nicotine dependence and even use disorder attributable to initial vaping of e-cigarettes in nonsmokers may result in a sizable number of new tobacco smokers (Motooka et al. 2018; Rigotti et al. 2015; Zhong et al 2016). In a more recent systematic review and meta-analysis, the authors concluded that among those attempting to quit smoking, nicotine e-cigarettes may be more efficacious than traditional nicotine replacement and behavioral therapies and may help reduce smoking-related health risks (Levett et al. 2023).

Special Populations

Co-occurring Cardiovascular Problems

In general, for smokers with cardiovascular disease, the benefits of NRTs outweigh the potential risks.

Bupropion SR is generally well tolerated in smokers with cardiovascular disease (Rigotti et al. 2006). Because rare cases of elevated blood pressure can occur with bupropion use (Fiore et al. 2008), it is prudent to monitor blood pressure during bupropion treatment in individuals with cardiovascular disease.

A multicenter randomized, placebo-controlled study of the safety and efficacy of varenicline was conducted in 714 individuals with cardiovascular disease (Rigotti et al. 2015). Although the sample size was too small to make definitive conclusions about safety, there was an approximately 1% greater risk of nonfatal myocardial infarction and need for coronary cardiovascularization with varenicline treatment versus placebo. In addition, there was a 0.5% greater risk of new diagnosis or need for a procedure for peripheral arterial disease. Consequently, the FDA required the addition of a new safety warning to the package insert for varenicline, highlighting its potential to increase the risk of certain cardiovascular events in people with cardiovascular disease.

Co-occurring Psychiatric Disorders

Several studies have suggested that bupropion SR may be useful for smoking cessation or smoking reduction in psychiatric patients who smoke or in substance-misusing smokers. In a secondary analysis of data from the study by Hurt et al. (1997), Hayford et al. (1999) found that bupropion SR was efficacious for smoking cessation in smokers irrespective of a history of major depression or alcoholism. Kalman and colleagues (2011) showed that bupropion SR is safe in cigarette smokers who are in recovery from alcohol use disorder. In another study, the EAGLES investigators did not show a significant increase in neuropsychiatric adverse events as a result of treatment with bupropion SR relative to placebo or the nicotine patch in individuals with or without psychiatric comorbidities (Anthenelli et al. 2016).

Studies have examined the safety and effectiveness of bupropion SR for smoking cessation in patients with major depression (Chengappa et al. 2001), bipolar disorder (Chengappa et al. 2014), and PTSD (McFall et al. 2005, 2010). Interestingly, Correa et al. (2021) reanalyzed data from the EAGLES trial and found that having multiple psychiatric diagnoses may be linked to more severe neuropsychiatric adverse events when attempting to quit smoking.

Bupropion SR has been evaluated in several trials involving patients with schizophrenia, including an open-label trial of 300 mg/day (Weiner et al. 2001) and placebo-controlled trials of 150 mg/day (Evins et al. 2001) and 300 mg/day (George et al. 2002). In a 12-week double-blind trial, Evins et al. (2001) found that among 18 patients with schizophrenia who were smokers, bupropion (150 mg/day) led to a 40%–50% reduction in expired-breath carbon monoxide levels compared with placebo. One of nine subjects in the bupropion group versus zero of nine in the placebo group had achieved smoking cessation by the end of the trial. During the trial, bupropion reduced both positive and negative symptoms of schizophrenia. George et al. (2002) conducted a 10-week double-blind, placebo-controlled trial of bupropion SR (300 mg/day) in a sample of 32 nicotine-dependent smokers with schizophrenia or schizoaffective disorder. Trial end-point cessation rates (confirmed by expired-breath carbon monoxide level <10 ppm) were 8 of 16 (50%) in the bupropion group and 2 of 16 (12.5%) in the placebo group ($P < 0.05$). Positive symptoms of schizophrenia were not affected, but negative symptom scores were reduced by approximately 15% in the bupropion group. Moreover, treatment with second-generation versus first-generation antipsychotics was associated with better cessation outcome, as observed in a previous study (George et al. 2000).

Accordingly, results from the preliminary studies described in this section suggest the following: 1) smoking reduction or cessation with bupropion SR is possible in patients with schizophrenia (with end-point cessation rates ranging from 11% to 50%); 2) exacerbation of psychotic symptoms is unlikely, and negative symptoms of schizophrenia may be reduced; and 3) the medication's efficacy for smoking cessation may be greater at higher doses in this population. Similarly, subsequent studies from Evins et al. (2007) and George et al. (2008) demonstrated the safety and efficacy of NRTs in combination with bupropion SR in smokers with schizophrenia.

Controlled trials have evaluated the use of varenicline in smokers with serious mental illness. Evins and colleagues (2014) showed that after 52 weeks of pharmacotherapy with varenicline and cognitive-behavioral therapy (CBT) in a relapse prevention paradigm, tobacco abstinence was significantly improved compared with placebo plus CBT. They also noted no psychiatric adverse events and no significant treatment effects on ratings of psychiatric symptoms. Another study (Williams et al. 2012) also showed that smokers with a diagnosis of schizophrenia or schizoaffective disorder who received varenicline as part of a 12-week double-blind, randomized multicenter trial reported significantly higher smoking cessation rates. Varenicline was well tolerated, with no exacerbation of positive or negative symptoms of schizophrenia.

Pregnant Smokers

Tobacco smoking in pregnancy is associated with a range of adverse pregnancy outcomes that include perinatal mortality, premature rupture of membranes, fetal growth restriction, birth defects, sudden infant death syndrome, and respiratory, endocrine, neurological, and behavioral effects in the child. Pregnancy is thought to be the life event that motivates most women to attempt smoking cessation (Cooper et al. 2017) and thus presents a key time for intervention. It is generally accepted that NRTs expose the fetus and the mother to less harm than smoking (Bar-Zeev et al. 2018). Guidelines from Australia, Canada, and the United Kingdom support the use of NRTs for pregnant people who have been unable to quit otherwise. However, the U.S. Preventive Services Task Force stated that current evidence is insufficient to make this recommendation (Krist et al. 2021) and instead recommended a shared decision-making approach for clinicians that takes into account patient tobacco dependence level.

Efficacy studies of NRT use in pregnancy reveal mixed results but overall favor NRTs. In a 2020 Cochrane meta-analysis of nine trials, Claire et al. (2020) found low-certainty evidence that NRTs as an adjunct to behavioral intervention can increase smoking cessation in late pregnancy. NRTs increased smoking cessation (RR 1.37; 95% CI, 1.08–1.74; I^2 = 34%; N = 2,336 women), but the effect was less evident when evaluating only placebo-controlled randomized trials (RR 1.21; 95% CI, 0.95–1.55; I^2 = 0%; N = 2,063 women). There was no evidence that patch or fast-acting NRTs were more effective, and there was no evidence for altered birth outcomes. Notably, adherence to NRTs was low.

Unlike many other teratogens, nicotine seems to be most dangerous in the third trimester (Holbrook 2016). In addition, quitting in the first trimester may have great benefits, such as reducing rates of preterm birth and small-for-gestational-age infants (McCowan et al. 2009). Thus, introducing an NRT as early in pregnancy as possible is recommended. It is generally accepted that using the lowest possible dose of nicotine is prudent, including using a short-acting NRT whenever possible and removing the patch at night. However, evidence showing poor adherence to NRTs in pregnancy suggests that higher doses should be studied (Claire et al. 2020).

Because nicotine metabolism is increased in pregnancy, the lower concentrations of nicotine from NRTs may not adequately substitute for smoking (Claire et al. 2020). This finding may explain why NRTs seem less effective in pregnancy than in nonpregnancy (Hartmann-Boyce et al. 2018). Correlational data suggest that using a short-acting oral product in combination with a patch increases the odds of quitting (Brose et al. 2013).

There is a perception that ENDS are safer in pregnancy than cigarettes (DeVito et al. 2021), and this is endorsed by the U.K. National Health Service. However, there have been no ENDS safety or efficacy trials in pregnant people to date, whereas animal studies have suggested teratogenicity (Cardenas et al. 2019).

Bupropion and varenicline also hold promise for benefit in pregnancy, but the evidence is scant. A systematic review of 18 studies of bupropion and varenicline in pregnancy did not suggest harms in terms of congenital anomalies, birthweight, or premature birth but found no strong evidence to suggest safety (Turner et al. 2019). No professional society recommends the use of bupropion or varenicline in pregnancy.

The safety and efficacy of pharmacotherapies for smoking cessation during pregnancy are not well established. In the absence of such data, no definitive recommendations can be made for the use of NRTs, ENDS, bupropion SR, or varenicline in pregnant people who wish to reduce or quit smoking. Individual decisions to promote smoking cessation during pregnancy should be made by the clinician in collaboration with the patient during a thorough discussion of the risks and benefits.

People Experiencing Homelessness

The prevalence of tobacco use among people experiencing homelessness is estimated to be between 57% and 82% (Baggett et al. 2013b; Soar et al. 2020). TUD is the leading preventable cause of mortality (Schroeder and Morris 2010). People experiencing homelessness are three to five times more likely to die prematurely than those not facing homelessness (Baggett et al. 2013a), and tobacco-related cancer and heart disease are the leading causes of death among people older than 50 years experiencing homelessness. Moreover, the incidence of these conditions among those younger than 50 is higher than in the age-matched general population (Baggett et al. 2013a).

Epidemiological studies show that most people experiencing homelessness initiate smoking at a young age (Arnsten et al. 2004) and smoke 10–13 cigarettes per day on average. Moreover, one-third report smoking within 30 minutes of waking (Vijayaraghavan and Pierce 2015; Vijayaraghavan et al. 2016, 2018). More than two-thirds of people experiencing homelessness report concurrent use of alternative tobacco products, with e-cigarettes, smokeless tobacco, and cigars being the most common forms (Alizaga et al. 2020; Baggett et al. 2016b; Durazo et al. 2021; Neisler et al. 2018).

Many people experiencing homelessness use tobacco as a coping mechanism for stressors of homelessness (Chen et al. 2016), increasing the challenge of smoking cessation. Limited access to tobacco cessation treatment in homeless service sites and lack of permanent smoke-free housing are other barriers to smoking cessation (Vijayaraghavan et al. 2015). High levels of TUD and co-occurring substance use disorders are associated with a low likelihood of quit attempts and sustained abstinence (Vijayaraghavan et al. 2014), and PTSD is positively associated with smoking among people experiencing homelessness (Baggett et al. 2016a).

Despite these barriers, people experiencing homelessness make quit attempts at the same rate as people with stable housing (Baggett and Rigotti 2010; Connor et al. 2002), although they are less successful at quitting smoking (quit ratio of 9% compared with 61% in the general population) (Baggett and Rigotti 2010; Creamer et al. 2019).

Ten RCTs of smoking cessation interventions for people experiencing homelessness have included some combination of behavioral counseling and pharmacotherapy, with adjunctive treatments such as contingent reinforcements or e-cigarettes. Three small single-arm trials examined behavioral counseling and pharmacotherapy, and two trials offered adjunctive financial incentives for tobacco cessation (abstinence rates at 6 months were 12%–45%). Most of the RCTs offered counseling (group and one-on-one) (Burling et al. 2001; Ojo-Fati et al. 2015) in the form of motivational interviewing, CBT, or both. All but two studies offered some form of pharmacotherapy. One trial offered e-cigarette liquid for 4 weeks (Dawkins et al. 2020) with brief advice to quit. All other trials offered an NRT in the form of gum or the patch (Baggett et al. 2019; Burling et al. 2001; Ojo-Fati et al. 2015; Okuyemi et al. 2006, 2013; Rash et al. 2018), with modest cessation outcomes.

Estimates of smoking abstinence varied significantly between those studies. However, none of the trials showed differences in abstinence between intervention and control groups. Measures of biochemically verified abstinence differed between trials, with one reporting estimates of abstinence at 4 weeks (Spector et al. 2007), one at 8 weeks (Baggett et al. 2018, 2019), and others at 6 months of follow-up. Studies that used behavioral counseling and pharmacotherapy reported rates of abstinence of 9%–17% at 6 months of follow-up (Okuyemi et al. 2006, 2013).

Studies that used contingent reinforcements for smoking cessation reported generally higher abstinence rates compared with studies that did not use contingent reinforcements: 22% at 4 weeks of follow-up (Rash et al. 2018) and 48% at 8 weeks of follow-up (Baggett et al. 2018). However, these trials were limited by small sample sizes and need to be replicated in larger RCTs. The study that used e-cigarettes reported a sustained abstinence rate of 6% at 24 weeks of follow-up (Dawkins et al. 2020), substantially lower than those observed in the general population (30%–40%) (Fiore et al. 2008).

In a Cochrane Review that included the 10 aforementioned trials, Vijayaraghavan et al. (2020) concluded that there was insufficient evidence to assess the effects of any tobacco cessation intervention for people experiencing homelessness. Interestingly, based on this Cochrane Review, trials that used contingent reinforcements were no more effective than those that did not use reinforcements. There was low certainty of evidence to suggest that more intensive interventions (i.e., greater number of sessions) were more effective than brief support. None of the trials or the effects on quit attempts had a measurable impact on psychiatric or substance use outcomes. Although standard smoking cessation supports, such as behavioral counseling and pharmacotherapy, are likely to be effective for people experiencing homelessness, Vijayaraghavan et al. (2020) concluded that larger, higher-quality studies that better address the challenges that people experiencing homelessness face daily are needed to engage this population in smoking cessation treatments, retain individuals for longer follow-ups, address social and environmental triggers of smoking, and assess the impact of smoking cessation treatment on psychiatric and substance use outcomes.

Key Points

- The prevalence of nicotine and tobacco use has been decreasing to approximately 15% in the U.S. population. Electronic cigarettes comprise an increasing portion of the market and have even been considered as a method to quit tobacco smoking.
- There are three FDA-approved tobacco cessation treatments: nicotine replacement therapies, sustained-release bupropion, and varenicline. All of these pharmacotherapies significantly increase smoking cessation rates; however, the majority of smokers are unable to achieve long-term abstinence, and absolute 1-year quit rates remain low. Further study is needed to determine whether combination pharmacotherapies or longer-term pharmacotherapies may increase these abstinence rates.
- Seven first-line agents are recommended for smoking cessation: transdermal nicotine patch, nicotine gum, nicotine lozenge, nicotine inhaler, and nicotine nasal spray formulations and sustained-release bupropion and varenicline (see Table 2.1).
- Second-line nonapproved pharmacotherapies such as nortriptyline and cytisine show promise, but their efficacy for smoking cessation has not been fully established.

- Pharmacotherapies should be used for the treatment of tobacco use disorder, with optimal results produced by the combination of medications with behavioral support. More study is needed to determine how the intensity of behavioral treatments interacts with different pharmacotherapeutic agents.
- Deep repetitive transcranial magnetic stimulation (neuroscience-based targeting of deep brain reward structures) has been cleared by the FDA for smoking cessation, but its feasibility and external validity require further study.
- We describe an approach to address treatment resistance in special populations of smokers, including smokers with medical illness and psychiatric comorbidities, pregnant smokers, and people experiencing homelessness. Well-controlled, large-scale studies are also needed to identify specific therapies that are safe and effective for smoking cessation in these populations.

References

Addicott MA, Kinney KR, Saldana S, et al: A randomized controlled trial of intermittent theta burst stimulation to the medial prefrontal cortex for tobacco use disorder: clinical efficacy and safety. Drug Alcohol Depend 258:111278, 2024 38579605

Alizaga NM, Hartman-Filson M, Elser H, et al: Alternative flavored and unflavored tobacco product use and cigarette quit attempts among current smokers experiencing homelessness. Addict Behav Rep 12:100280, 2020 32637560

Anthenelli RM, Benowitz NL, West R, et al: Neuropsychiatric safety and efficacy of varenicline, bupropion, and nicotine patch in smokers with and without psychiatric disorders (EAGLES): a double-blind, randomised, placebo-controlled clinical trial. Lancet 387(10037):2507–2520, 2016 27116918

Arnsten JH, Reid K, Bierer M, et al: Smoking behavior and interest in quitting among homeless smokers. Addict Behav 29(6):1155–1161, 2004 15236817

Baggett TP, Rigotti NA: Cigarette smoking and advice to quit in a national sample of homeless adults. Am J Prev Med 39(2):164–172, 2010 20621264

Baggett TP, Hwang SW, O'Connell JJ, et al: Mortality among homeless adults in Boston: shifts in causes of death over a 15-year period. JAMA Intern Med 173(3):189–195, 2013a 23318302

Baggett TP, Tobey ML, Rigotti NA: Tobacco use among homeless people: addressing the neglected addiction. N Engl J Med 369(3):201–204, 2013b 23863048

Baggett TP, Campbell EG, Chang Y, et al: Other tobacco product and electronic cigarette use among homeless cigarette smokers. Addict Behav 60:124–130, 2016a 27128808

Baggett TP, Campbell EG, Chang Y, et al: Posttraumatic stress symptoms and their association with smoking outcome expectancies among homeless smokers in Boston. Nicotine Tob Res 18(6):1526–1532, 2016b 26508393

Baggett TP, Chang Y, Yaqubi A, et al: Financial incentives for smoking abstinence in homeless smokers: a pilot randomized controlled trial. Nicotine Tob Res 20(12):1442–1450, 2018 29059442

Baggett TP, McGlave C, Kruse GR, et al: SmokefreeTXT for homeless smokers: pilot randomized controlled trial. JMIR Mhealth Uhealth 7(6):e13162, 2019 31165717

Bar-Zeev Y, Lim LL, Bonevski B, et al: Nicotine replacement therapy for smoking cessation during pregnancy. Med J Aust 208(1):46–51, 2018 29320660

Benowitz NL: Nicotine addiction. N Engl J Med 362(24):2295–2303, 2010 20554984

Berlin I, Saïd S, Spreux-Varoquaux O, et al: A reversible monoamine oxidase A inhibitor (moclobemide) facilitates smoking cessation and abstinence in heavy, dependent smokers. Clin Pharmacol Ther 58(4):444–452, 1995 7586937

Blondal T, Gudmundsson LJ, Tomasson K, et al: The effects of fluoxetine combined with nicotine inhalers in smoking cessation: a randomized trial. Addiction 94(7):1007–1015, 1999 10707439

Brose LS, McEwen A, West R: Association between nicotine replacement therapy use in pregnancy and smoking cessation. Drug Alcohol Depend 132(3):660–664, 2013 23680076

Burling TA, Burling AS, Latini D: A controlled smoking cessation trial for substance-dependent inpatients. J Consult Clin Psychol 69(2):295–304, 2001 11393606

Cardenas VM, Fischbach LA, Chowdhury P: The use of electronic nicotine delivery systems during pregnancy and the reproductive outcomes: a systematic review of the literature. Tob Induc Dis 17:52, 2019 31582941

Chen JS, Nguyen AH, Malesker MA, et al: High-risk smoking behaviors and barriers to smoking cessation among homeless individuals. Respir Care 61(5):640–645, 2016 26860400

Chengappa KN, Kambhampati RK, Perkins K, et al: Bupropion sustained release as a smoking cessation treatment in remitted depressed patients maintained on treatment with selective serotonin reuptake inhibitor antidepressants. J Clin Psychiatry 62(7):503–508, 2001 11488359

Chengappa KNR, Perkins KA, Brar JS, et al: Varenicline for smoking cessation in bipolar disorder: a randomized, double-blind, placebo-controlled study. J Clin Psychiatry 75(7):765–772, 2014 25006684

Claire R, Chamberlain C, Davey MA, et al: Pharmacological interventions for promoting smoking cessation during pregnancy. Cochrane Database Syst Rev 3(3):CD010078, 2020 32129504

Coles AS, Kozak K, George TP: A review of brain stimulation methods to treat substance use disorders. Am J Addict 27(2):71–91, 2018 29457674

Connor SE, Cook RL, Herbert MI, et al: Smoking cessation in a homeless population: there is a will, but is there a way? J Gen Intern Med 17(5):369–372, 2002 12047734

Cooper S, Orton S, Leonardi-Bee J, et al: Smoking and quit attempts during pregnancy and postpartum: a longitudinal UK cohort. BMJ Open 7(11):e018746, 2017 29146659

Cornelius ME, Loretan CG, Jamal A, et al: Tobacco product use among adults—United States, 2021. MMWR Morb Mortal Wkly Rep 72(18):475–483, 2023 37141154

Correa JB, Lawrence D, McKenna BS, et al: Psychiatric comorbidity and multimorbidity in the EAGLES trial: descriptive correlates and associations with neuropsychiatric adverse events, treatment adherence, and smoking cessation. Nicotine Tob Res 23(10):1646–1655, 2021 33788933

Courtney RJ, McRobbie H, Tutka P, et al: Effect of cytisine vs varenicline on smoking cessation: a randomized clinical trial. JAMA 326(1):56–64, 2021 34228066

Covey LS, Glassman AH: A meta-analysis of double-blind placebo-controlled trials of clonidine for smoking cessation. Br J Addict 86(8):991–998, 1991 1833003

Covey LS, Glassman AH, Stetner F: Naltrexone effects on short-term and long-term smoking cessation. J Addict Dis 18(1):31–40, 1999 10234561

Creamer MR, Wang TW, Babb S, et al: Tobacco product use and cessation indicators among adults—United States, 2018. MMWR Morb Mortal Wkly Rep 68(45):1013–1019, 2019 31725711

Dani JA, Balfour DJ: Historical and current perspective on tobacco use and nicotine addiction. Trends Neurosci 34(7):383–392, 2011 21696833

Dawkins L, Bauld L, Ford A, et al: A cluster feasibility trial to explore the uptake and use of e-cigarettes versus usual care offered to smokers attending homeless centres in Great Britain. PLoS One 15(10):e0240968, 2020 33095798

DeVito EE, Fagle T, Allen AM, et al: Electronic nicotine delivery systems (ENDS) use and pregnancy I: ENDS use behavior during pregnancy. Curr Addict Rep 8(3):347–365, 2021 34513567

Dinur-Klein L, Dannon P, Hadar A, et al: Smoking cessation induced by deep repetitive transcranial magnetic stimulation of the prefrontal and insular cortices: a prospective, randomized controlled trial. Biol Psychiatry 76(9):742–749, 2014 25038985

Durazo A, Hartman-Filson M, Elser H, et al: E-cigarette use among current smokers experiencing homelessness. Int J Environ Res Public Health 18(7):3691, 2021 33916203

Eisenberg MJ, Hébert-Losier A, Windle SB, et al: Effect of e-cigarettes plus counseling vs counseling alone on smoking cessation: a randomized clinical trial. JAMA 324(18):1844–1854, 2020 33170240

Etter JF, Bullen C: Electronic cigarette: users profile, utilization, satisfaction and perceived efficacy. Addiction 106(11):2017–2028, 2011 21592253

Evins AE, Mays VK, Rigotti NA, et al: A pilot trial of bupropion added to cognitive behavioral therapy for smoking cessation in schizophrenia. Nicotine Tob Res 3(4):397–403, 2001 11694208

Evins AE, Cather C, Culhane MA, et al: A 12-week double-blind, placebo-controlled study of bupropion SR added to high-dose dual nicotine replacement therapy for smoking cessation or reduction in schizophrenia. J Clin Psychopharmacol 27(4):380–386, 2007 7632223

Evins AE, Cather C, Pratt SA, et al: Maintenance treatment with varenicline for smoking cessation in patients with schizophrenia and bipolar disorder: a randomized clinical trial. JAMA 311(2):145–154, 2014 24399553

Fagerström K, Balfour DJ: Neuropharmacology and potential efficacy of new treatments for tobacco dependence. Expert Opin Investig Drugs 15(2):107–116, 2006 16433591

Finkelstein Y, Macdonald EM, Li P, et al: Second-generation anti-depressants and risk of new-onset seizures in the elderly. Clin Toxicol (Phila) 56(12):1179–1184, 2018 29989445

Fiore MC, Jaen CR, Baker TB, et al: Treating Tobacco Use and Dependence: 2008 Update. Clinical Practice Guideline. Rockville, MD, U.S. Dept of Health and Human Services, Public Health Service, 2008

George TP: Nicotine and tobacco, in Goldman-Cecil Medicine, 27th Edition. Edited by Goldman L, Cooney KA. New York, Elsevier, 2024, pp 2349–2352

George TP, Ziedonis DM, Feingold A, et al: Nicotine transdermal patch and atypical antipsychotic medications for smoking cessation in schizophrenia. Am J Psychiatry 157(11):1835–1842, 2000 11058482

George TP, Vessicchio JC, Termine A, et al: A placebo controlled trial of bupropion for smoking cessation in schizophrenia. Biol Psychiatry 52(1):53–61, 2002 12079730

George TP, Vessicchio JC, Termine A, et al: A preliminary placebo-controlled trial of selegiline hydrochloride for smoking cessation. Biol Psychiatry 53(2):136–143, 2003 12547469

George TP, Vessicchio JC, Sacco KA, et al: A placebo-controlled trial of bupropion combined with nicotine patch for smoking cessation in schizophrenia. Biol Psychiatry 63(11):1092–1096, 2008 18096137

Gonzales D, Rennard SI, Nides M, et al: Varenicline, an alpha4beta2 nicotinic acetylcholine receptor partial agonist, vs sustained-release bupropion and placebo for smoking cessation: a randomized controlled trial. JAMA 296(1):47–55, 2006 16820546

Gourlay SG, Stead LF, Benowitz NL: Clonidine for smoking cessation. Cochrane Database Syst Rev (3):CD000058, 2004 15266422

Hajek P, Phillips-Waller A, Przulj D, et al: A randomized trial of e-cigarettes versus nicotine-replacement therapy. N Engl J Med 380(7):629–637, 2019 30699054

Hall SM, Reus VI, Muñoz RF, et al: Nortriptyline and cognitive-behavioral therapy in the treatment of cigarette smoking. Arch Gen Psychiatry 55(8):683–690, 1998 9707377

Hall SM, Humfleet GL, Reus VI, et al: Psychological intervention and antidepressant treatment in smoking cessation. Arch Gen Psychiatry 59(10):930–936, 2002 12365880

Hartmann-Boyce J, Chepkin SC, Ye W, et al: Nicotine replacement therapy versus control for smoking cessation. Cochrane Database Syst Rev 5(5):CD000146, 2018 29852054

Hatsukami DK, Jorenby DE, Gonzales D, et al: Immunogenicity and smoking-cessation outcomes for a novel nicotine immunotherapeutic. Clin Pharmacol Ther 89(3):392–399, 2011 21270788

Hayford KE, Patten CA, Rummans TA, et al: Efficacy of bupropion for smoking cessation in smokers with a former history of major depression or alcoholism. Br J Psychiatry 174:173–178, 1999 10211174

Hays JT, Hurt RD, Rigotti NA, et al: Sustained-release bupropion for pharmacologic relapse prevention after smoking cessation: a randomized, controlled trial. Ann Intern Med 135(6):423–433, 2001 11560455

Heinzerling A, Armatas C, Karmarkar E, et al: Severe lung injury associated with use of e-cigarette, or vaping, products: California, 2019. JAMA Intern Med 180(6):861–869, 2020 32142111

Hilleman DE, Mohiuddin SM, Delcore MG, et al: Randomized, controlled trial of transdermal clonidine for smoking cessation. Ann Pharmacother 27(9):1025–1028, 1993 8219431

Holbrook BD: The effects of nicotine on human fetal development. Birth Defects Res C Embryo Today 108(2):181–192, 2016 27297020

Hughes JR, Higgins ST, Bickel WK: Nicotine withdrawal versus other drug withdrawal syndromes: similarities and dissimilarities. Addiction 89(11):1461–1470, 1994 7841857

Hurt RD, Sachs DP, Glover ED, et al: A comparison of sustained-release bupropion and placebo for smoking cessation. N Engl J Med 337(17):1195–1202, 1997 9337378

Iannuzzo F, Crudo S, Basile GA, et al: Efficacy and safety of non-invasive brain stimulation techniques for the treatment of nicotine addiction: a systematic review of randomized controlled trials. AIMS Neurosci 11(3):212–225, 2024 39431276

Jamal A, Park-Lee E, Birdsey J, et al: Tobacco product use among middle and high school students—National Youth Tobacco Survey, United States. MMWR Morb Mortal Wkly Rep 73(41):917–924, 2024 39418216

Jorenby DE, Leischow SJ, Nides MA, et al: A controlled trial of sustained-release bupropion, a nicotine patch, or both for smoking cessation. N Engl J Med 340(9):685–691, 1999 10053177

Jorenby DE, Hays JT, Rigotti NA, et al: Efficacy of varenicline, an alpha4beta2 nicotinic acetylcholine receptor partial agonist, vs placebo or sustained-release bupropion for smoking cessation: a randomized controlled trial. JAMA 296(1):56–63, 2006 16820547

Kahn R, Gorgon L, Jones K, et al: Selegiline transdermal system (STS) as an aid for smoking cessation. Nicotine Tob Res 14(3):377–382, 2012 21846661

Kalman D, Herz L, Monti P, et al: Incremental efficacy of adding bupropion to the nicotine patch for smoking cessation in smokers with a recent history of alcohol dependence: results from a randomized, double-blind, placebo-controlled study. Drug Alcohol Depend 118(2–3):111–118, 2011 21507585

Killen JD, Fortmann SP, Schatzberg AF, et al: Nicotine patch and paroxetine for smoking cessation. J Consult Clin Psychol 68(5):883–889, 2000 11068974

Kozak K, Sharif-Razi M, Morozova M, et al: Effects of short-term, high-frequency repetitive transcranial magnetic stimulation to bilateral dorsolateral prefrontal cortex on smoking behavior and cognition in patients with schizophrenia and non-psychiatric controls. Schizophr Res 197:441–443, 2018 29486960

Krishnan-Sarin S, Meandzija B, O'Malley S: Naltrexone and nicotine patch smoking cessation: a preliminary study. Nicotine Tob Res 5(6):851–857, 2003 14750508

Krist AH, Davidson KW, Mangione CM, et al: Interventions for tobacco smoking cessation in adults, including pregnant persons: US Preventive Services Task Force recommendation statement. JAMA 325(3):265–279, 2021 33464343

Lerman C, Schnoll RA, Hawk LW Jr, et al: Use of the nicotine metabolite ratio as a genetically informed biomarker of response to nicotine patch or varenicline for smoking cessation: a randomised, double-blind placebo-controlled trial. Lancet Respir Med 3(2):131–138, 2015 25588294

Levett JY, Filion KB, Reynier P, et al: Efficacy and safety of e-cigarette use for smoking cessation: a systematic review and meta-analysis of randomized controlled trials. Am J Med 136(8):804.e4–813.e4, 2023 37148992

Lowe DJE, Coles AS, George TP, et al: E-cigarettes, in The Assessment and Treatment of Addiction: Best Practices and New Frontiers. Edited by Danovitch I, Mooney LJ. New York, Elsevier, 2019, pp 43–56

McClure JB, Swan GE, Catz SL, et al: Smoking outcome by psychiatric history after behavioral and varenicline treatment. J Subst Abuse Treat 38(4):394–402, 2010 20363092

McCowan LM, Dekker GA, Chan E, et al: Spontaneous preterm birth and small for gestational age infants in women who stop smoking early in pregnancy: prospective cohort study. BMJ 338:b1081, 2009 19325177

McFall M, Saxon AJ, Thompson CE, et al: Improving the rates of quitting smoking for veterans with posttraumatic stress disorder. Am J Psychiatry 162(7):1311–1319, 2005 15994714

McFall M, Saxon AJ, Malte CA, et al: Integrating tobacco cessation into mental health care for posttraumatic stress disorder: a randomized controlled trial. JAMA 304(22):2485–2493, 2010 21139110

Motooka Y, Matsui T, Slaton RM, et al: Adverse events of smoking cessation treatments (nicotine replacement therapy and non-nicotine prescription medication) and electronic cigarettes in the Food and Drug Administration Adverse Event Reporting System, 2004–2016. SAGE Open Med 6:2050312118777953, 2018 29844912

Nagano T, Katsurada M, Yasuda Y, et al: Current pharmacologic treatments for smoking cessation and new agents undergoing clinical trials. Ther Adv Respir Dis 13:1753466619875925, 2019 31533544

Neisler J, Reitzel LR, Garey L, et al: Concurrent nicotine and tobacco product use among homeless smokers and associations with cigarette dependence and other factors related to quitting. Drug Alcohol Depend 185:133–140, 2018 29448145

Niaura R, Spring B, Borrelli B, et al: Multicenter trial of fluoxetine as an adjunct to behavioral smoking cessation treatment. J Consult Clin Psychol 70(4):887–896, 2002 12182272

Ojo-Fati O, John F, Thomas J, et al: Integrating smoking cessation and alcohol use treatment in homeless populations: study protocol for a randomized controlled trial. Trials 16:385, 2015 26320081

Okuyemi KS, Thomas JL, Hall S, et al: Smoking cessation in homeless populations: a pilot clinical trial. Nicotine Tob Res 8(5):689–699, 2006 17008196

Okuyemi KS, Goldade K, Whembolua GL, et al: Motivational interviewing to enhance nicotine patch treatment for smoking cessation among homeless smokers: a randomized controlled trial. Addiction 108(6):1136–1144, 2013 23510102

O'Malley SS, Cooney JL, Krishnan-Sarin S, et al: A controlled trial of naltrexone augmentation of nicotine replacement therapy for smoking cessation. Arch Intern Med 166(6):667–674, 2006 16567607

Oncken C, Gonzales D, Nides M, et al: Efficacy and safety of the novel selective nicotinic acetylcholine receptor partial agonist, varenicline, for smoking cessation. Arch Intern Med 166(15):1571–1577, 2006 16908789

Park-Lee E, Jamal A, Cowan H, et al: Notes from the field: e-cigarette and nicotine pouch use among middle and high school students—United States, 2024. MMWR Morb Mortal Wkly Rep 73(35):774–778, 2024 39236021

Polosa R, Benowitz NL: Treatment of nicotine addiction: present therapeutic options and pipeline developments. Trends Pharmacol Sci 32(5):281–289, 2011 21256603

Pomerleau OF, Pomerleau CS: Neuroregulators and the reinforcement of smoking: towards a biobehavioral explanation. Neurosci Biobehav Rev 8(4):503–513, 1984 6151160

Pripfl J, Tomova L, Riecansky I, et al: Transcranial magnetic stimulation of the left dorsolateral prefrontal cortex decreases cue-induced nicotine craving and EEG delta power. Brain Stimul 7(2):226–233, 2014 24468092

Prochazka AV, Weaver MJ, Keller RT, et al: A randomized trial of nortriptyline for smoking cessation. Arch Intern Med 158(18):2035–2039, 1998 9778204

Ranpara A, Stefaniak AB, Williams K, et al: Modeled respiratory tract deposition of an aerosolized oil diluents used in delta-9 THC-based electronic cigarette liquid products. Front Public Health 9:744166, 2021 34805068

Rash CJ, Petry NM, Alessi SM: A randomized trial of contingency management for smoking cessation in the homeless. Psychol Addict Behav 32(2):141–148, 2018 29461070

Rigotti NA, Thorndike AN, Regan S, et al: Bupropion for smokers hospitalized with acute cardiovascular disease. Am J Med 119(12):1080–1087, 2006 17145253

Rigotti NA, Chang Y, Tindle HA, et al: E-cigarette use and subsequent tobacco use by adolescents: new evidence about the potential risk of e-cigarettes. JAMA 314(7):673–674, 2015 26284717

Rohsenow DJ, Monti PM, Colby SM, et al: Naltrexone treatment for alcoholics: effect on cigarette smoking rates. Nicotine Tob Res 5(2):231–236, 2003 12745496

Schroeder SA, Morris CD: Confronting a neglected epidemic: tobacco cessation for persons with mental illnesses and substance abuse problems. Annu Rev Public Health 31:297–314, 2010 20001818

Sheffer CE, Bickel WK, Brandon TH, et al: Preventing relapse to smoking with transcranial magnetic stimulation: feasibility and potential efficacy. Drug Alcohol Depend 182:8–18, 2018 29120861

Shiffman S, Dresler CM, Hajek P, et al: Efficacy of a nicotine lozenge for smoking cessation. Arch Intern Med 162(11):1267–1276, 2002 12038945

Soar KDL, Robson D, Cox S: Smoking amongst adults experiencing homelessness: a systematic review of prevalence rates, interventions, barriers and facilitators to quitting and staying quit. J Smok Cessat 15:94–108, 2020

Spector A, Alpert H, Karam-Hage M: Smoking cessation delivered by medical students is helpful to homeless population. Acad Psychiatry 31(5):402–405, 2007 17875625

Sutherland G, Stapleton JA, Russell MA, et al: Naltrexone, smoking behaviour and cigarette withdrawal. Psychopharmacol (Berl) 120(4):418–425, 1995 8539322

Sweeney CT, Fant RV, Fagerstrom KO, et al: Combination nicotine replacement therapy for smoking cessation: rationale, efficacy and tolerability. CNS Drugs 15(6):453–467, 2001 11524024

Tonstad S, Tønnesen P, Hajek P, et al: Effect of maintenance therapy with varenicline on smoking cessation: a randomized controlled trial. JAMA 296(1):64–71, 2006 16820548

Turner E, Jones M, Vaz LR, et al: Systematic review and meta-analysis to assess the safety of bupropion and varenicline in pregnancy. Nicotine Tob Res 21(8):1001–1010, 2019 29579233

Vijayaraghavan M, Pierce JP: Interest in smoking cessation related to a smoke-free policy among homeless adults. J Community Health 40(4):686–691, 2015 25559109

Vijayaraghavan M, Penko J, Vittinghoff E, et al: Smoking behaviors in a community-based cohort of HIV-infected indigent adults. AIDS Behav 18(3):535–543, 2014 23918243

Vijayaraghavan M, Hurst S, Pierce JP: Implementing tobacco control programs in homeless shelters: a mixed-methods study. Health Promot Pract 17(4):501–511, 2015 26678988

Vijayaraghavan M, Tieu L, Ponath C, et al: Tobacco cessation behaviors among older homeless adults: results from the HOPE HOME study. Nicotine Tob Res 18(8):1733–1739, 2016 26920648

Vijayaraghavan M, Olsen P, Weeks J, et al: Older African American homeless-experienced smokers' attitudes toward tobacco control policies—results from the HOPE HOME study. Am J Health Promot 32(2):381–391, 2018 28893086

Vijayaraghavan M, Elser H, Frazer K, et al: Interventions to reduce tobacco use in people experiencing homelessness. Cochrane Database Syst Rev 12(12):CD013413, 2020 33284989

Wasfi RA, Bang F, de Groh M, et al: Chronic health effects associated with electronic cigarette use: a systematic review. Front Public Health 10:959622, 2022 36276349

Weinberger AH, Reutenauer EL, Jatlow PI, et al: A double-blind, placebo-controlled, randomized clinical trial of oral selegiline hydrochloride for smoking cessation in nicotine-dependent cigarette smokers. Drug Alcohol Depend 107(2–3):188–195, 2010 19939587

Weiner E, Ball MP, Summerfelt A, et al: Effects of sustained-release bupropion and supportive group therapy on cigarette consumption in patients with schizophrenia. Am J Psychiatry 158(4):635–637, 2001 11282701

West R, Zatonski W, Cedzynska M, et al: Placebo-controlled trial of cytisine for smoking cessation. N Engl J Med 365(13):1193–1200, 2011 21991893

Williams JM, Anthenelli RM, Morris CD, et al: A randomized, double-blind, placebo-controlled study evaluating the safety and efficacy of varenicline for smoking cessation in patients with schizophrenia or schizoaffective disorder. J Clin Psychiatry 73(5):654–660, 2012 22697191

Wing VC, Barr MS, Wass CE, et al: Brain stimulation methods to treat tobacco addiction. Brain Stimul 6(3):221–230, 2013 22809824

Zhong J, Cao S, Gong W, et al: Electronic cigarettes use and intention to cigarette smoking among never-smoking adolescents and young adults: a meta-analysis. Int J Environ Res Public Health 13(5):E465, 2016 27153077

3

Alcohol Use Disorder

Henry R. Kranzler, M.D.
Clifford Knapp, Ph.D.
Emily E. Hartwell, Ph.D.

Alcohol affects multiple neurotransmitter systems, including virtually all the major systems associated with psychiatric symptoms (Lovinger and Roberto 2013). These diverse effects explain, at least in part, why chronic heavy drinking is commonly associated with many different co-occurring psychiatric symptoms and disorders (Castillo-Carniglia et al. 2019). Alcohol alters the absorption and metabolism of nutrients, and chronic heavy drinking can disturb intermediary metabolism and produce deficiency states. Heavy alcohol consumption can result in physiological dependence, with abrupt cessation causing withdrawal states. Although the most common effect of abrupt cessation of drinking is uncomplicated alcohol withdrawal syndrome (AWS), severe complications can also occur, particularly in patients who are medically compromised. Potential complications include tonic-clonic seizures and delirium tremens, which can be lethal.

Pharmacology of Ethanol and Its Relationship to Medication Development

Alcohol Pharmacokinetics

Alcohol (i.e., ethanol) differs from most chemical entities used as medications in that it is a small molecule with both polar and lipophilic characteristics and high water solubility but low lipid solubility. The effects of most medications are produced at concentrations in the micromolar range or lower, whereas the pharmacological actions of alcohol are seen only in the millimolar range. The behavioral effects of alcohol, such as relaxation and disinhibition, start to occur at blood alcohol concentrations (BACs) of 5–10 mM (Cui and Koob 2017). In many jurisdictions, drivers are considered impaired at a BAC of 17.8 mM (80 mg/dL). As BACs approach 50 mM, drinkers are at risk of coma or death. Tolerance to the effects of alcohol can develop with sustained consumption of large amounts of alcohol; therefore, chronic heavy drinkers are generally less sensitive to the detrimental effects of high BACs than individuals with no or limited histories of consuming large volumes of alcohol.

Alcohol is absorbed from the stomach and the small intestine and then readily diffuses into the body's water compartments. The rate of absorption of orally consumed alcohol is determined by the rate of gastric emptying and can be decreased by concurrent ingestion of food or increased when gastric emptying times shorten (e.g., with gastric bypass or other bariatric procedures). There is limited evidence that higher BAC peaks may occur after the ingestion of alcoholic beverages with higher concentrations of alcohol (such as vodka) compared with beer and wine (Mitchell et al. 2014).

Orally ingested alcohol is subject to a first-pass effect during which metabolism occurs mostly in the liver and to a lesser extent in the stomach. Alcohol dehydrogenases (ADHs) are the primary enzymes responsible for the first step in alcohol metabolism, in which alcohol undergoes conversion to acetaldehyde (Figure 3.1) (Zakhari 2006). Catalases and cytochrome P450 (CYP) enzymes (most notably, CYP2E) also play a role in the metabolism of alcohol by catalyzing its oxidation to acetaldehyde. Alcohol use can induce CYP2E by increasing its rate of synthesis (Jiang et al. 2020), thereby also increasing the rate at which other medications (e.g., warfarin) are metabolized.

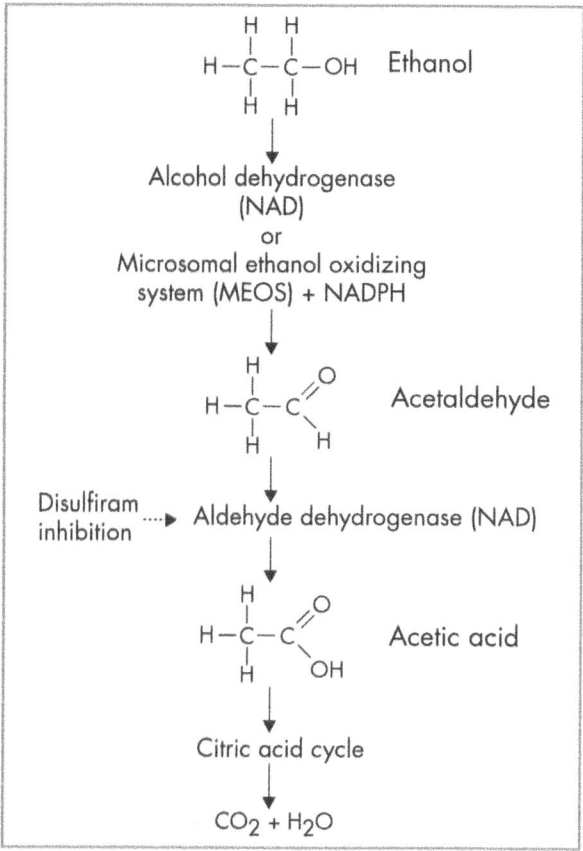

Figure 3.1 Primary route of ethanol metabolism. Ethanol is oxidized by alcohol dehydrogenase (in the presence of nicotinamide adenine dinucleotide [NAD]) or the microsomal ethanol oxidizing system (MEOS) (in the presence of reduced nicotinamide adenine dinucleotide phosphate [NADPH]). Acetaldehyde, the first product in ethanol oxidation, is metabolized to acetic acid by aldehyde dehydrogenase in the presence of NAD. Acetic acid is broken down through the citric acid cycle to carbon dioxide (CO_2) and water (H_2O). Impairment of the metabolism of acetaldehyde to acetic acid is the major mechanism of action of disulfiram for the treatment of alcoholism.

The alcohol metabolite acetaldehyde is converted to acetate by acetaldehyde dehydrogenases (ALDHs). Acetate can be transformed into acetyl-coenzyme A, which is an energy substrate. Volkow et al. (2013) reported that after the administration of alcohol to both social and heavy drinkers, brain glucose metabolism decreased and the uptake of radiolabeled acetate into the brain increased. This finding led to the hypothesis that acetate may become an important source of energy in the brain, particularly in brain glial cells, during periods of intoxication.

ADH becomes saturated at all but the lowest BACs (Cederbaum 2012). Once fully saturated, ADH metabolizes alcohol at a constant rate. Thus, from a practical point of view, alcohol can be considered to follow zero-order kinetics. This means that there are disproportionately large increases in BACs as greater amounts of alcohol are administered; BACs decline in a linear fashion over time after the discontinuation of alcohol intake. Clinically, this means that intoxication resolves at a steady rate and cannot be altered substantially, despite popular myths suggesting otherwise (e.g., drinking coffee, taking a cold shower).

Both sex and population group differences in alcohol pharmacokinetics have been reported. The first-pass effect for alcohol is lower in women than in men (Baraona et al. 2001; Frezza et al. 1990), which may reflect lower gastric ADH activity in women. Population group differences in alcohol pharmacokinetics have been linked to differences in the activity of isoenzymes encoded by allelic variants of genes *ADH* and *ALDH*. A prime example is the *ALDH*2* variant, which encodes an enzyme with very low levels of activity (Chen et al. 2021). This variant occurs with high frequency in East Asian populations, including those of Chinese, Japanese, and Korean ancestry. Individuals with the *ALDH*2* variant have higher blood concentrations of acetaldehyde after the ingestion of alcohol than do those homozygous for the wild-type allele. A higher concentration of this metabolite can produce aversive effects, which include flushing and tachycardia, similar to those produced by disulfiram when alcohol is consumed. These effects are thought to deter drinking and thereby protect individuals with one or two copies of the *ALDH*2* allele from developing alcohol use disorder (AUD).

Alcohol Pharmacodynamics

In social drinkers, the consumption of one to three standard drinks of alcohol causes mood elevation, stimulation, mild disinhibition, increased sociability, and decreased anxiety. These effects of alcohol positively reinforce alcohol consumption. The mood elevation and stimulant effects of a moderate dose of alcohol result from activation of the mesolimbic system, which includes the nucleus accumbens in the ventral striatum, a region innervated by dopamine neurons that project from the ventral tegmental area (VTA) located in the midbrain.

Another brain region, the dorsomedial striatum, may play a role in goal-directed behaviors involved in the repetitive seeking and consumption of alcohol (Koob and Volkow 2016). The regulation of alcohol consumption involves communication between the striatum and several other brain areas, including the prefrontal cortex, anterior cingulate cortex, and orbitofrontal cortex (Hernandez and Moorman 2020; Koob and Volkow 2016).

With an increase in BAC, there is increased sedation (Cui and Koob 2017). At very high BACs, there is a risk of severe CNS depression that can lead to coma and death. Chronic alcohol consumption results in tolerance to many of alcohol's behavioral effects; after sustained heavy drinking, a distinct pattern of withdrawal symptoms can appear as BAC declines. Withdrawal signs and symptoms include increased autonomic system activity, anxiety, dysphoria, and CNS excitability. These aversive effects may serve as negative reinforcers that motivate an individual to consume alcohol to provide symptomatic relief (Koob 2020). During abstinence following a protracted period of heavy drinking, individuals may experience persistent dysphoria and anxiety, which are risk factors for relapse (Heilig et al. 2010).

At its most severe, alcohol withdrawal may include delirium, psychosis, seizures, and death. Given the possibility of serious harm that can result from severe withdrawal, at-risk patients should receive careful evaluation, medications, and other forms of medical support.

GABAergic Receptor Systems

GABA type A ($GABA_A$) receptors are ligand-gated channels that are major mediators of alcohol-induced neuronal inhibition in the brain. This inhibition results from GABA-induced enhancement of neuronal chloride flux through channels formed by $GABA_A$ subunits, the result of which is the hyperpolarization of neurons. The intensity of these currents can be modulated by a variety of ligands that alter the frequency with which the chloride channels open. Alcohol, benzodiazepines, and barbiturates are examples of exogenous chemical entities that potentiate the effects of GABA through their effects on $GABA_A$ receptors.

A multitude of behavioral and electrophysiological studies indicate that many of alcohol's pharmacological effects may result from $GABA_A$ receptor activation. These effects include sedation, ataxia, decreased anxiety, and alcohol-induced reinforcement. The location of the receptors and sites as well as mechanisms of action of benzodiazepines and barbiturates involving $GABA_A$ receptors are well understood (Feng and Forman 2018; Kim et al. 2020; Zhu et al. 2018). In contrast, the mechanisms through which alcohol activates the same receptors remain uncertain. There is some electrophysiological evidence that in addition to its direct effects on brain $GABA_A$ receptors, alcohol may promote the presynaptic release of GABA in select areas of the brain, including the cerebellum (Criswell et al. 2008).

$GABA_A$ receptors in the brain most commonly are pentameric combinations of $\alpha 1-\alpha 6$, $\beta 1-\beta 3$, $\gamma 2$, and δ subunits. $GABA_A$ receptor subtypes often include one γ (or δ) subunit, two α subunits, and two β subunits (Olsen and Sieghart 2009). The distribution of $GABA_A$ receptor subtypes, each of which has a unique subunit composition, differs by both their brain regional distribution and their locations on neurons (Belelli et al. 2009; Jia et al. 2007). There has been an extensive effort to determine the role of different $GABA_A$ receptor subtypes in AUD (Jin et al. 2012), and several findings from animal studies suggest that treatments that target $GABA_A$ receptors composed of specific subunits could be useful in managing AUD (Chandler et al. 2019). Evidence that $GABA_A$ receptors composed of specific subunits are involved in regulating drinking includes findings of reduced alcohol consumption following interference with the expression of both $\alpha 4$ $GABA_A$ subunits and the δ subunit in the nucleus accumbens of rats (Nie et al. 2011; Rewal et al. 2012).

Glutamatergic Receptor Systems

Another major action of ethanol is the inhibition of the excitatory actions of the amino acid neurotransmitter glutamate on both the ionotropic glutamatergic receptors (GluRs) and metabotropic glutamatergic receptors (mGluRs). Ionotropic GluRs comprise several families of tetrameric ion channels that are opened by agonists to enhance cationic current flows. One such family, the N-methyl-D-aspartate (NMDA) receptors, comprises $GluN_1$, $GluN_{2A}-GluN_{2D}$, $GluN_{3A}$, and $GluN_{3B}$ subunits. These receptors mediate neurotransmission and can alter intracellular signaling and synaptic plasticity. Members of the 2-amino-3-hydroxy-5-methyl-4-isoxaz olepropionic acid (AMPA) family of ionotropic receptors are formed by the subunits $GLUA_1$–$GLUA_4$ and mediate fast synaptic transmission. Kainate receptors are a third family of ionotropic glutamatergic receptors and are composed of $GluK_1$–$GluK_5$ subunits.

Alcohol can suppress NMDA-mediated neurotransmission (Lovinger et al. 1989). These effects may underlie the impairment in cognitive function that follows alcohol consumption. They also appear to play a role in the regulation of alcohol self-administration. Exposure to alcohol can also inhibit AMPA receptors, but it acts with a lower potency on these receptors than on NMDA receptors (Ariwodola et al. 2003). There is some evidence that AMPA receptors regulate alcohol-seeking behaviors and consumption (Cannady et al. 2013; Sanchis-Segura et al. 2006).

Chronic ethanol-induced inhibition of NMDA receptor activity can produce changes that lead to hyperexcitable states, which emerge during alcohol withdrawal. These changes may involve both the activation and expression of NMDA receptors after prolonged exposure to high BACs (Hendricson et al. 2007). In hippocampal tissue, prolonged exposure to alcohol elevates the total amount of $GluN_1$, $GluN_{2A}$, and $GluN_{2B}$ subunit expression. One study reported that the expression of both NMDA and AMPA receptors was increased in rat cortical tissue by chronic alcohol exposure (Chandler et al. 1999). In human postmortem brain tissues, including those from the hippocampus and prefrontal cortex, levels of $GluN_{2B}$ mRNA were higher in tissues obtained from individuals with AUD than in those from control subjects (Farris and Mayfield 2014).

The role played by kainate receptors in AUD has not been extensively studied. In the basolateral amygdala, ethanol was found to reduce kainate receptor–mediated excitatory postsynaptic currents (Läck et al. 2008). Administration of LY466195, which selectively blocks activation of kainate receptors that contain the $GluK_1$ subunit, decreases the rewarding effects of alcohol and alcohol preference in animals (Quijano Cardé et al. 2021; Van Nest et al. 2017). The anticonvulsant topiramate is an antagonist of kainate receptors and has been shown to decrease alcohol consumption in clinical studies (Blodgett et al. 2014).

Glutamate also acts on mGluRs, which exert their actions through G protein–coupled receptors (GCPRs). Subtypes of GCPRs include the $mGluR_1$–$mGluR_5$ subtypes, which are divided into three groups: group 1 includes $mGluR_1$ and $mGluR_5$ receptors, group 2 includes $mGluR_2$ and mGluR$_3$, and group 3 includes mGluR$_4$ and mGluR$_6$–mGluR$_8$ (Goodwani et al. 2017). Studies suggest that the mGluR$_5$ receptors located primarily in the caudate nucleus, anterior cingulate cortex, and posterior cingulate cortex are involved in the development of alcohol dependence (Ceccarini et al. 2020; Leurquin-Sterk et al. 2018; Niswender and Conn 2010). Supporting this interpretation are rodent models of drinking in which negative allosteric modulators of mGluR$_5$ reduced alcohol consumption (Johnson and Lovinger 2020). Administration of the mGluR$_5$ antagonist 3-[(2-methyl-1,3-thiazol-4-yl)ethynyl]-pyridine decreased alcohol self-administration and the reinstatement of alcohol-seeking in alcohol-preferring rats (Cowen et al. 2005, 2007).

The expression of mGluR$_2$ autoreceptors is decreased in alcohol dependence (Meinhardt et al. 2013). These receptors act to negatively modulate glutamate release. Their downregulation in the infralimbic cortex may lead to increased glutamatergic signaling in the nucleus accumbens, which promotes alcohol-seeking behavior (Meinhardt et al. 2013). The administration of mGluR$_2$ selective agonists reduced alcohol consumption in animal studies, whereas antagonists of these receptors promoted alcohol self-administration in rats (Bäckström and Hyytiä 2005).

Adenosinergic Receptor Systems

Adenosine has been implicated in the mediation of several of the effects produced by alcohol administration. The administration of selective adenosine A$_1$ receptor antagonists blocks ethanol-induced loss of motor coordination (Connole et al. 2004). Treatment with adenosine A$_1$ agonists reduces the intensity of many adverse effects of ethanol withdrawal, including anxiety-related behaviors, tremors, and seizures (Concas et al. 1994).

Acute alcohol administration elevates extracellular concentrations of adenosine in cell culture systems (Clark and Dar 1989). Alcohol-induced increases in adenosine appear to mediate both the ataxic and sedative/hypnotic effects of alcohol (Dar 2015; El Yacoubi et al. 2003). Animal studies have indicated that alcohol-related increases in brain adenosine levels are related to its inhibitory effects on the nucleoside transporter equilibrative nucleoside transporter 1 (ENT1) (Ruby et al. 2010). Mice whose expression of *ENT1* was suppressed increased their consumption of alcohol and displayed decreased sensitivity to the effects of alcohol on motor coordination (Choi et al. 2004).

Dopaminergic Receptor Systems

Animal studies indicate that alcohol administration enhances the release of dopamine in the nucleus accumbens, a mesolimbic structure within the ventral striatum (Siciliano et al. 2018). The nucleus accumbens is implicated in mediation of the rewarding effects of many agents that are self-administered by animals and misused by humans (Di Chiara and Imperato 1988). Imaging studies of dopamine-induced displacement of the D_2/D_3 radioligand [^{11}C] raclopride demonstrated that alcohol can release dopamine in the ventral striatum of healthy adults, heavy drinkers, and social drinkers (Boileau et al. 2003; Oberlin et al. 2015; Urban et al. 2010; Yoder et al. 2015, 2016).

Several mechanisms may play a role in alcohol-induced increases in dopamine release from the nucleus accumbens. One such mechanism involves disinhibition and an increased rate of firing of dopamine neurons in the VTA, which project to the nucleus accumbens. Animal studies suggest that the effect results from activation of µ opioid receptors (MORs) that inhibit GABAergic interneurons that innervate VTA dopamine neurons (Spanagel 2009). As described later in "Serotonergic Systems," serotonin 3 (5-HT_3) receptors in the VTA may also act to modulate alcohol-induced dopamine release in the nucleus accumbens.

Interestingly, findings from rat studies suggest that the alcohol metabolite acetaldehyde contributes to the reinforcing effects of alcohol, which is at odds with the aversive effects of acetaldehyde (discussed later in "Alcohol-Sensitizing Agents"). Based on studies in which rats self-administer acetaldehyde directly into the VTA (Rodd et al. 2005, 2008), acetaldehyde may act to release dopamine in the nucleus accumbens, potentially contributing to this metabolite's reinforcing actions (Melis et al. 2007). In mice, chronic ethanol exposure may decrease ethanol-stimulated dopamine release in the nucleus accumbens (Karkhanis et al. 2016), potentially contributing to the genesis of AUD by augmenting the experience of AWS (particularly post-acute withdrawal anhedonia).

Opioidergic Receptor Systems

µ *Opioid Receptors*

MORs may play an important role in mediating the reinforcing effects of alcohol and producing alcohol craving. Animal studies demonstrated that chronic alcohol use may result in greater availability of MOR binding sites in the nucleus accumbens (Heinz et al. 2005) and that exposure to alcohol (in light and heavy alcohol use) may directly stimulate MOR binding sites in the nucleus accumbens and orbitofrontal cortex (Mitchell et al. 2012; Richard and Fields 2016).

The role of opioid receptors in the modulation of alcohol-induced dopamine release has been extensively investigated. Administration of the nonselective opioid receptor antagonist naltrexone to animals as they consumed alcohol blocked the elevation of brain dopamine levels (Gonzales and Weiss 1998). Furthermore, deletion of *OPRM1* (which encodes MOR type 1) reduced ethanol-induced elevations of striatal dopamine (Job et al. 2007); other studies have not replicated this finding (Ramachandra et al. 2011).

Variations in *OPRM1* may account for differences found in the release of striatal dopamine mediated through MORs. For example, in one study, alcohol-induced striatal dopamine release in social drinkers was detected only in carriers of the minor rs1799971 A118G allele of *OPRM1* (Ramachandra et al. 2011). Also, the association between *OPRM1* genotype and alcohol-induced stimulation, vigor, and positive mood appears to be related to its interaction with variation in the gene that encodes dopamine transporter 1 (*SLC6A3*) (Anton et al. 2012; Ray et al. 2014), which regulates dopamine levels in the synaptic cleft. A large-scale genetic study, however, showed that the *OPRM1* A118G single-nucleotide polymorphism (SNP) was not associated with levels of either alcohol consumption or sensitivity (Sloan et al. 2018).

κ *Opioid Receptors*

Whereas MORs are implicated in mediating alcohol's rewarding effects, κ opioid receptors (KORs) appear to play a different role in contributing to the risk of AUD. KORs are activated by the endogenous opioid peptide dynorphin, the stimulation of which can result in dysphoria, anhedonia, and other negative emotional states. These effects of KOR stimulation may play a role during alcohol withdrawal, including motivating individuals who experience withdrawal symptoms to continue drinking. Although one study of individuals with AUD showed significant associations between certain haplotypes of the preprodynorphin gene (*PDYN*) and both drinking and negative alcohol craving (Karpyak et al. 2013), the finding requires replication.

Chronic alcohol use can ultimately lead to decreased dopaminergic release in the nucleus accumbens, as mentioned earlier in "Dopaminergic Receptor Systems." This effect is reversed by the administration of KOR antagonists. Therefore, KOR-mediated reductions in striatal dopamine release may contribute to the anhedonia experienced by individuals with AUD, because chronic alcohol exposure increases the sensitivity of the KOR to agonists, according to research (Rose et al. 2016).

Postmortem studies have demonstrated significantly lower KOR availability in several brain regions, including the striatum, insula, amygdala, and frontal cortex, among alcohol-dependent subjects, suggesting a role for KORs in risk of AUD (Vijay et al. 2018). Moreover, reductions in alcohol consumption during drinking sessions with naltrexone administration were greater in subjects with lower KOR availability (de Laat et al. 2019). Greater KOR availability in the hippocampus, cingulate cortex, and prefrontal cortex measured during test drinking sessions was associated with higher levels of craving. Thus, the effectiveness of naltrexone in modulating alcohol consumption and craving may depend on the extent to which this opioid antagonist alters KOR availability.

In summary, the MOR and KOR systems play a role in both the reward and negative emotional states experienced by individuals who consume alcohol excessively. Not surprisingly, therefore, the administration of nonselective opioid receptor antagonists (most notably, naltrexone) can affect alcohol use patterns. Several preclinical studies have shown that opioid receptor antagonists reduce alcohol consumption (Altshuler et al. 1980; Boyle et al. 1998; Jimenez-Gomez et al. 2011). A meta-analysis of human laboratory studies showed that treatment with naltrexone can reduce craving for alcohol and alcohol's stimulant effects (Ray et al. 2019). Additionally, meta-analyses of clinical trials of naltrexone (e.g., Jonas et al. 2014) showed that naltrexone reduces alcohol consumption, and principally the likelihood of heavy drinking, in individuals with AUD.

Neuropeptides and Hypothalamic Hormones

Hypothalamic-Pituitary-Adrenal Axis and Alcohol: Corticotropin-Releasing Factor, Adrenocorticotropic Hormone, and Cortisol

Hypothalamic-pituitary-adrenal (HPA) axis dysfunction has been implicated in the development of AUD. The hypothalamic corticotropin-releasing factor (CRF) increases blood cortisol by inducing the release of adrenocorticotropic hormone from the anterior pituitary. Increases in plasma cortisol contribute to a heightened state of stress marked by anxiety and depressed mood. The emergence of this negative emotional state in relation to alcohol discontinuation in physiologically dependent individuals is believed to be a major driver of the negative reinforcement that drives relapse behaviors (Koob 2020).

The self-administration of alcohol initially results in increased blood cortisol levels (Richardson et al. 2008), an effect that is blunted in alcohol-dependent animals with prolonged alcohol consumption. This change in sensitivity to alcohol occurs in association with a decrease in CRF mRNA within the paraventricular nucleus of the hypothalamus. In a study, alcohol elicited less cortisol release in heavy social drinkers who engaged in binge drinking compared with light social drinkers, who showed a marked cortisol response (King et al. 2006). In individuals with alcohol dependence, hypercortisolism has been detected in the transition between periods of intoxication and withdrawal (Adinoff et al. 1998). Administration of mifepristone, a glucocorticoid receptor antagonist, decreased drinking and craving in subjects with AUD (Vendruscolo et al. 2015), suggesting that HPA dysfunction could contribute to the development or maintenance of AUD.

Several animal studies implicated signaling involving the CRF_1 receptor in the development of anxiety during withdrawal from alcohol (Kelly and Fudge 2018). Chronic alcohol administration can enhance CRF activity in several brain structures associated with the dysphoria and anxiety that accompany alcohol withdrawal. In animals, alcohol withdrawal was associated with increased release of CRF in the central amygdala (Gilpin et al. 2015), and withdrawal-induced increases in alcohol consumption were blocked by the administration of CFR_1 receptor antagonists (Funk et al. 2007). Notably, a CRF_1 antagonist infused into the central amygdala reduced alcohol self-administration during withdrawal in dependent animals but did not affect alcohol consumption in nondependent animals (Funk et al. 2006). Furthermore, a study reported that the occurrence of anxiety-like behavior seen after multiple episodes of alcohol withdrawal was blocked by the administration of a CRF_1 receptor antagonist (Overstreet et al. 2004). Taken together, these findings suggest that increases in CRF_1 receptor activity during alcohol withdrawal cause anxiety that increases alcohol intake.

Orexin System

Activation of orexin receptors by the neuropeptide orexin (hypocretin) released from neurons that project from the hypothalamus can produce arousal and play a role in stress responses and the development of anxiety (de Lecea et al. 1998; Sakurai et al. 1998). These neurons innervate the locus coeruleus, nucleus accumbens, thalamus, and many other brain areas (Peyron et al. 1998). Orexin's facilitation of alcohol consumption is evidenced in rodent models of drinking by reduced consumption following the infusion of orexin receptor antagonists into several brain areas, including the VTA (Srinivasan et al. 2012), the core of the nucleus accumbens (Brown et al. 2013), and the thalamus (Barson et al. 2015). In animal studies, antagonism of orexin receptors blocked cue-induced alcohol-seeking behavior (Lawrence et al. 2006) and reduced ethanol consumption in animals with extensive previous exposure to alcohol (Lopez et al. 2016). CRF can also stimulate hypothalamic orexin neurons that project to the ventral forebrain bed nucleus of the stria terminalis (BNST) and the amygdala (Winsky-Sommerer et al. 2004). Thus, given the role of orexin in the development of withdrawal-related anxiety, orexin could mediate some of the anxiety-inducing effects of CRF described in the previous paragraph.

Neuropeptide Y

Neuropeptide Y is a 36-amino-acid neuropeptide that is widely distributed in the nucleus accumbens, amygdala, striatum, locus coeruleus, and several other brain structures (Tanaka et al. 2021). Neuropeptide Y–containing interneurons are colocalized with GABA-containing neurons in the amygdala (Oberto et al. 2001); in addition, neuropeptide Y interacts with dopaminergic reward and emotion pathways, and its expression is inversely related to alcohol consumption (Robinson and Thiele 2017). Through its actions in the central amygdala, neuropeptide Y decreased alcohol consumption in dependent rats (Gilpin et al. 2008, 2011). When stimulated, the Y_1 receptor for neuropeptide Y, located in the BNST, inhibited binge alcohol drinking by increasing inhibitory synaptic transmission specifically in CRF neurons (Pleil et al. 2012).

Vasopressin and Oxytocin

The neuropeptides vasopressin and oxytocin are structurally related hormones that are released by the posterior pituitary and found in several brain areas. The behavioral effects of these two hormones differ in that vasopressin tends to promote anxiety, whereas oxytocin may have anxiolytic actions (Neumann and Landgraf 2012). Vasopressin is present in both the amygdala and the BNST, structures implicated in aversive emotional responses, particularly anxiety, in animals during withdrawal and periods of abstinence after long-term exposure to alcohol (de Vries and Miller 1998). Oxytocin is involved in social bonding, sexual activity, childbirth, and lactation. Its bidirectional interactions with the dopaminergic system and the HPA axis may account for its inverse relationship with addiction vulnerability (Buisman-Pijlman et al. 2014).

In one study, vasopressin infusion into the central amygdala led to anxiety-like behavior in rats that had undergone chronic intermittent exposure to alcohol (Harper et al. 2019). In contrast, intermittent alcohol use was decreased by the administration of an oxytocin receptor agonist and by a vasopressin V_{1b} receptor antagonist (Dannenhoffer et al. 2018). Other animal studies have shown similar effects (Edwards et al. 2012; Zhou et al. 2011).

Further evidence that vasopressin receptor activity regulates drinking in AUD was provided in a clinical trial by Ryan et al. (2017). Administration of the V_{1b} antagonist ABT-436 to men and women with alcohol dependence significantly increased the percentage of days that they abstained from alcohol but did not decrease the percentage of heavy drinking days (Ryan et al. 2017).

When administered by intracerebral infusion, oxytocin decreases alcohol self-administration (Peters et al. 2017) and alcohol cue-induced reinstatement of alcohol responding (Hansson et al. 2018). In alcohol-dependent animals and postmortem tissues from humans with AUD, oxytocin receptors were upregulated in both frontal and striatal areas (Hansson et al. 2018), implicating lower availability of oxytocin in those individuals as contributing to alcohol dependence. Supporting this relationship, oxytocin administration can reduce brain responses to alcohol-related cues (Hansson et al. 2018), decrease alcohol craving (Melby et al. 2021), and reduce symptoms of withdrawal in subjects with AUD (Pedersen et al. 2013). These findings suggest that oxytocin could play a role in the pharmacotherapy of AUD.

Noradrenergic, Serotonergic, and Nicotinic Receptor Systems

Noradrenergic Systems

Noradrenergic cell bodies are found in the brain stem and pons localized in discrete areas that include the locus coeruleus. These neurons innervate brain sites implicated in regulating alcohol consumption and in mediating the effects of alcohol withdrawal, which include the amygdala, BNST, paraventricular nucleus of the hypothalamus, and nucleus accumbens (Vazey et al. 2018). During alcohol withdrawal, the sympathetic nervous system becomes hyperactive (Heilig et al. 2010), with anxiety and heightened arousal resulting from the greatly increased activity of noradrenergic systems. This increased activity is also responsible for elevations in blood pressure and heart rate, sweating, and nausea and vomiting. Medications that counteract the increased sympathetic activity during alcohol withdrawal include the α_2-adrenergic receptor agonists clonidine and guanfacine (Haass-Koffler et al. 2018; Parale and Kulkarni 1986) and β-adrenergic blockers (Mirijello et al. 2015).

The regulation of CRF neurons by the noradrenergic system is implicated in stress-related increases in alcohol-seeking behaviors (Nobis et al. 2011; Smith and Aston-Jones 2008). In animal models, norepinephrine activated BSNT CRF neurons by stimulating β-adrenergic receptors (Broccoli et al. 2018; Snyder et al. 2019), and studies showed that the nonselective β-adrenergic antagonist propranolol reduced levels of responding for alcohol (Gilpin and Koob 2010).

Other evidence that noradrenergic neurons play a role in AUD includes the finding that treatment with prazosin, an adrenergic α_1-receptor antagonist, blocked both alcohol consumption and alcohol-seeking behavior in alcohol-preferring rats. Furthermore, the reinstatement of alcohol-seeking behavior by KOR agonists was reversed by the administration of prazosin (Funk et al. 2019; Verplaetse et al. 2012).

Clinical studies of the effects of prazosin on alcohol consumption in subjects with AUD have thus far yielded inconsistent results. In one trial in subjects with AUD, prazosin did not significantly alter alcohol consumption (Wilcox et al. 2018). However, another clinical trial showed that prazosin-treated subjects with AUD had a lower rate of heavy drinking than placebo-treated subjects (Simpson et al. 2018).

Serotonergic Systems

Serotonergic systems may play a role in the emergence of anxiety and craving in individuals with AUD. Serotonergic neurons project from the brain stem dorsal raphe to the forebrain and the BNST. Chronic alcohol exposure in mice resulted in the appearance of anxiety-related behaviors that occurred in association with increased sensitivity to the inhibitory effects of alcohol (Lowery-Gionta et al. 2015). The development of anxiety in animals chronically exposed to alcohol was blocked by the administration of a serotonin 5-HT$_{2C}$ receptor antagonist, SB-242084 (Marcinkiewcz et al. 2015). Evidence that serotonergic systems can influence craving among individuals with AUD includes the finding that the intravenous administration of *m*-chlorophenylpiperazine, a serotonin receptor agonist, to subjects with AUD increased their alcohol craving (Krystal et al. 1994; Umhau et al. 2011). In contrast, a lower dose of *m*-chlorophenylpiperazine administered orally decreased craving for alcohol in subjects with AUD (Buydens-Branchey et al. 1997).

Infusion of the 5-HT$_3$ antagonist zacopride into the shell of the nucleus accumbens blocks ethanol-induced dopamine release in this structure (Ding et al. 2015). In contrast, a study showed that dopamine release was enhanced by the infusion of the 5-HT$_3$ agonist 2-methyl-5-hydroxytryptamine in the nucleus accumbens, an effect that was greater in animals chronically exposed to ethanol (Yoshimoto et al. 1996). These studies suggest that 5-HT$_3$ receptors within the nucleus accumbens are involved in regulating the release of dopamine within that structure. Given the evidence that 5-HT$_3$ receptors are involved in regulating the reinforcing effects of alcohol, it has been hypothesized that 5-HT$_3$ antagonists block the rewarding effects of alcohol and could thus reduce drinking. In support of this hypothesis, in animals, systemic administration of zacopride decreased alcohol consumption during a 24-hour access period (Knapp and Pohorecky 1992).

Ondansetron, a 5-HT$_3$ antagonist that is approved clinically for treating nausea and vomiting, has been shown in alcohol-preferring rats and mice to decrease alcohol intake (Meert 1993; Tomkins et al. 1995). In clinical studies, ondansetron reduced both the number of drinks consumed per day and the number of drinks consumed per drinking day more than placebo in individuals with early-onset alcoholism (Johnson et al. 2000b). In an open-label trial, ondansetron administered as an oral solution decreased alcohol consumption to a greater degree in individuals with early-onset alcoholism than in those with late-onset alcoholism (Kranzler et al. 2003).

Nicotinic Receptor Systems

Nicotinic acetylcholine receptors are pentameric ligand-gated ion channels, composed of either combinations of α (2–4) and β (2–4) subunits or homomeric channels formed by α7, α9, or α10 subunits. Nicotinic receptors are expressed in brain regions that include the medial habenula, striatum, locus coeruleus, and VTA (Miller and Kamens 2020). Alcohol can stimulate nicotinic receptors within the VTA to increase the release of dopamine within the nucleus accumbens (Ericson et al. 2003; Gotti et al. 2010).

Evidence that the $\alpha_4\beta_2$-type nicotinic receptor plays a role in regulating alcohol consumption includes a reduction in ethanol consumption following the administration of both the full $\alpha_4\beta_2$ antagonist sazetidine A and the partial agonist varenicline (Hendrickson et al. 2010; Zwart et al. 2008). Clinically, studies of $\alpha_4\beta_2$ blockade by varenicline have shown reduced cue-induced craving (Roberts et al. 2017) and lower weekly percentages of heavy drinking days, drinks per day, and alcohol craving than in placebo-treated subjects (Litten et al. 2013). In a substudy, however, cue-induced craving was greater in subjects with AUD treated with varenicline for 3 and 6 weeks than in those who received placebo (Miranda et al. 2020).

Alcohol-dependent smokers treated with varenicline for nicotine dependence had higher rates of smoking abstinence at both 12 and 24 weeks, and they reported consuming fewer drinks per drinking day at 12 weeks than those treated with placebo (Hurt et al. 2018). However, the results of a meta-analysis of varenicline did not support its superiority over placebo in treating AUD (Gandhi et al. 2020; as reviewed later in "Partial Nicotinic Receptor Agonists").

Alcohol Treatment

General Considerations

Table 3.1 presents the four medications approved by the FDA for treating AUD: disulfiram, naltrexone, long-acting injectable naltrexone, and acamprosate. Table 3.2 presents the four most extensively investigated medications that are not approved in the United States for treating AUD but are being used off-label for that purpose: nalmefene (oral formulation), baclofen, gabapentin, and topiramate. Tables 3.1 and 3.2 provide information on the dosage range studied and both the effects on alcohol-related outcomes and the adverse effects associated with these medications.

Systematic efforts in the U.S. Veterans Health Administration to increase the use of medication-assisted treatment for AUD yielded a prescription rate of only 3.4% (Harris et al. 2012). Despite variation in the rates of medication prescribing for alcohol treatment over time and in different settings and surveys, pharmacotherapy for AUD remains one of the least utilized approaches to alcohol treatment.

Table 3.1 Medications approved by the FDA for treating alcohol use disorder

Characteristic	Disulfiram	Naltrexone	Long-acting injectable naltrexone	Acamprosate
Indication	Management of symptoms of selected patients with chronic alcohol use who want to remain in a state of enforced sobriety	Treatment of alcohol dependence	Treatment of alcohol dependence in outpatients who can abstain from alcohol	Maintenance of abstinence from alcohol in patients with alcohol dependence
FDA-approved dosage	250–500 mg/d	50 mg/d	380 mg IM/mo	1,998 mg/d (666 mg tid)
Dosage in clinical trials	125–500 mg/d	Initially 25–50 mg/d, with increases to 50–100 mg/d	190 or 380 mg IM/mo	1,000–3,000 mg/d
Efficacy	In meta-analysis (Skinner et al. 2014) (N = 2,414 subjects in 22 studies), open-label disulfiram treatment (15 studies) showed a medium to large effect on sustained abstinence from alcohol compared with control conditions. Blinded trials (7 studies) showed no effect of disulfiram. A large effect was observed compared with control conditions when medication compliance was supervised (13 studies), but effects were nonsignificant in 9 unsupervised studies.	Meta-analysis of placebo-controlled trials (Jonas et al. 2014) showed a small effect of naltrexone 50 mg/d on risk of any drinking (NNT = 20; 16 trials, N = 2,347) and a small effect on risk of binge drinking (NNT = 12; 19 trials, N = 2,875).	In the only published placebo-controlled trial of extended-release naltrexone (Garbutt et al. 2005), the median monthly number of binge drinking days declined from 19.3 d/mo at baseline to 6.0 d/mo in the placebo group, 4.5 d/mo in the 190-mg group, and 3.1 d/mo in the 380-mg group.	Meta-analysis of placebo-controlled trials (Jonas et al. 2014) showed a small effect on reducing the risk of any drinking among abstinent subjects (NNT = 12; 16 trials, N = 4,847) but no significant effect on the likelihood of binge drinking.

Table 3.1 Medications approved by the FDA for treating alcohol use disorder *(continued)*

Characteristic	Disulfiram	Naltrexone	Long-acting injectable naltrexone	Acamprosate
Most common adverse effects	Most common: moderate or severe drowsiness; severe adverse events (e.g., hepatitis, neuropathy, optic neuritis, psychosis, confusional states) are rare (Chick 1999)	Somnolence, nausea, vomiting, decreased appetite, abdominal pain, insomnia, and dizziness (Rösner et al. 2010b)	Same adverse events as oral naltrexone, plus injection site reactions (swelling, pain, induration)	Diarrhea was common and was the only adverse event that was more common with acamprosate than placebo (Rösner et al. 2010a)
Clinical notes	Should only be used in patients who are aware of the potential for adverse effects and who have a goal of complete abstinence from alcohol	Can block the effects of opioid analgesics and precipitate withdrawal in a patient physically dependent on opioids	Can block the effects of opioid analgesics and precipitate withdrawal in a patient physically dependent on opioids	Not metabolized (renally excreted), so can be used in patients with hepatic disease

Note. d = day; mo = month; NNT = number needed to treat for benefit to one person.
Source. Adapted from Kranzler and Soyka (2018).

Table 3.2 Non-FDA-approved medications for treating alcohol use disorder

Characteristic	Nalmefene (oral formulation)	Baclofen	Gabapentin	Topiramate
Indication	(EU) Helps reduce alcohol consumption in adults with alcohol dependence who consume ≥60 g/d (~4 drinks/d) for men or >40 g/d (~3 drinks/d) for women	To alleviate signs and symptoms of spasticity resulting from multiple sclerosis	Manage postherpetic neuralgia in adults and adjunctive therapy in treating partial seizures in patients age ≥3 y	Monotherapy for partial-onset or primary generalized tonic-clonic seizures; adjunctive therapy for partial-onset seizures or primary generalized tonic-clonic seizures and seizures associated with Lennox-Gastaut syndrome; migraine prophylaxis; weight loss and chronic weight management (combined with phentermine)
Dosage for AUD	(EU) 18 mg/d (oral tablet) prn; oral formulation not available in the United States; dosage in clinical trials: 5–80 mg/d qd or bid	Dosage in clinical trials: 30–180 mg/d in up to four divided doses	Dosage in clinical trials: 600–1,800 mg/d in three divided doses	Dosage in clinical trials: 75–300 mg/d in two divided doses

Table 3.2 Non-FDA-approved medications for treating alcohol use disorder *(continued)*

Characteristic	Nalmefene (oral formulation)	Baclofen	Gabapentin	Topiramate
Effects	Meta-analysis of five RCTs (N = 2,567) (Palpacuer et al. 2018) showed a small effect on binge drinking at both 6 mo and 1 y of treatment; nalmefene was associated with a reduction in total alcohol consumption by 20% at 6 mo	A Cochrane meta-analysis of 12 RCTs (N = 1,128) (Minozzi et al. 2018) showed no difference between baclofen and placebo for return to any drinking, % days abstinent, or % heavy drinking days; in a second meta-analysis of 13 RCTs (N = 1,492 participants) (Pierce et al. 2018), baclofen was associated with a small to moderate effect on both time to first drinking lapse and likelihood of abstinence during treatment; the effect was evident at a dosage of <60 mg/d, with no effect at higher dosage	Meta-analysis of seven RCTs (N = 751) (Kranzler et al. 2019a) showed that for all six outcome measures, effect estimates favored gabapentin over placebo, although only % heavy drinking days was significant	In a meta-analysis of seven RCTs (N = 1,125), there were small to medium effects of topiramate on abstinent days (Hedge's g = 0.468) and binge drinking days (Hedge's g = 0.406)
Most common adverse effects	Nausea (22.1%), dizziness (18.2%), insomnia (13.4%), headache (12.3%), vomiting (8.7%), fatigue (8.3%), somnolence (5.2%) (van den Brink et al. 2015)	With low-dose treatment (30 mg/day): drowsiness (39.1%), dizziness (26.4%), headache (25.3%), confusion (23.0%), muscle stiffness (16.1%), excessive perspiration (14.9%), itching or pruritus (14.9%), abnormal muscle movements (13.8%), numbness (12.6%), slurred speech (10.3%) (Hauser et al. 2017)	Dizziness (19.1%), somnolence (14.1%), ataxia or gait disorder (14.0%), peripheral edema (6.6%) (Wiffen et al. 2017)	Paresthesia (50.8%), dysgeusia (23.0%), anorexia (19.7%), difficulty with concentration/attention (14.8%), nervousness (14.2%), dizziness (11.5%), pruritus (10.4%) (Johnson et al. 2007); transient mental slowing and modest reductions in verbal fluency and working memory are generally dose related (Smith et al. 2016)

Table 3.2. Non-FDA-approved medications for treating alcohol use disorder (continued)

Characteristic	Nalmefene (oral formulation)	Baclofen	Gabapentin	Topiramate
Clinical notes	Not approved in U.S. for treating AUD	Approved in France for use in the management of alcohol dependence at a maximum recommended dosage of 80 mg/d	Additional studies needed to validate medication effects	To reduce risk and severity of adverse effects, begin treatment at 25–50 mg/d, with increases of 25–50 mg/d at weekly intervals to a maximum of 200 mg/d; contraindicated in patients with a predisposition or history of metabolic acidosis, renal calculi, or angle-closure glaucoma

Note. AUD = alcohol use disorder; d = day; EU = European Union; mo = month; NNT = number needed to treat; RCT = randomized controlled trial; y = year.
Source. Modified from Kranzler and Soyka (2018).

Pharmacotherapy of Heavy Drinking and Alcohol Use Disorder

Medications are most often used in the management of withdrawal symptoms (i.e., during detoxification) and to reduce alcohol consumption or promote abstinence. In the subsections that follow, we first discuss pharmacological approaches to alcohol detoxification. We then discuss the two major approaches to using medications to reduce drinking or promote abstinence: 1) the reduction or cessation of drinking through direct efforts to reduce either the positive or negative reinforcing effects of alcohol and 2) the treatment of co-occurring psychiatric symptoms and disorders, which are common among individuals with AUD and may impede their recovery. The reader is referred to reviews of alcohol treatment (e.g., Knox et al. 2019; Kranzler and Soyka 2018) and meta-analyses of multiple medications (e.g., Jonas et al. 2014; Minozzi et al. 2018; Palpacuer et al. 2018) or single medications (e.g., Blodgett et al. 2014; Kranzler et al. 2019a; Skinner et al. 2014), which are summarized in the subsections that follow.

Prevalence, Demographic and Clinical Correlates, and Treatment of Alcohol Withdrawal Syndrome

AWS, which is prevalent among individuals with unhealthy alcohol use, can have serious adverse outcomes. National surveys estimate that greater than one-third of the general U.S. population consumes alcohol at an unhealthy level. Among these individuals, 14.3% reported past-year AWS, providing a prevalence of AWS in the overall adult population of nearly 5% (Livne et al. 2022). Analysis also indicates that the prevalence of AWS is higher among males than females, among unmarried participants than married ones, and among those with the lowest versus highest income levels. Among individuals with unhealthy alcohol use, those with AWS had a greater likelihood of co-occurring psychiatric disorders, AUD, and other alcohol-related features (e.g., binge drinking) and greater health care utilization (Livne et al. 2022). Based on these findings, routine screening for unhealthy alcohol use is warranted to identify individuals with AWS whose treatment could prevent the development of serious adverse outcomes. An individual's risk of developing AWS can be assessed through validated tools, such as the Prediction of Alcohol Withdrawal Severity Scale (Maldonado et al. 2014).

The objectives in treating AWS are to relieve discomfort, prevent or treat complications, and prepare patients for rehabilitation. Effective management of withdrawal symptoms is often necessary for subsequent efforts at rehabilitation to be successful. However, treating withdrawal alone is not an adequate intervention, because relapse occurs commonly without ongoing treatment.

The identification of co-occurring medical problems is an important element in detoxification (Naranjo and Sellers 1986). Administration of thiamine (50–100 mg PO or PN) and multivitamins is a low-cost, low-risk intervention for the prophylaxis and treatment of alcohol-related neurological disturbances. The provision of good supportive care and the treatment of concurrent illness, including fluid and electrolyte repletion, are essential elements in caring for patients experiencing alcohol withdrawal (Naranjo and Sellers 1986).

It is important that patients experiencing AWS receive frequent reassurance, reality orientation, monitoring of vital signs, personal attention, and general nursing care (Naranjo and Sellers 1986). The medical problems commonly associated with AUD, which are reviewed in detail elsewhere (Schuckit 2018), may substantially complicate therapy, so patients should be referred for specialized medical evaluation and treatment when the severity of a medical disorder exceeds the capacity of the psychiatrist or general practitioner.

Controlling early withdrawal symptoms can prevent their progression to more serious ones. Treating alcohol withdrawal is the indication for which medications are most often prescribed in patients with AUD. Benzodiazepines are the major class of medications used to treat AWS; these agents act by positively modulating activity at the $GABA_A$ receptor complex, suppressing the hyperexcitability associated with the abrupt cessation of alcohol intake in individuals who are physically dependent on alcohol. Anticonvulsant medications, which can also decrease CNS hyperexcitability, are also commonly used in alcohol detoxification.

Detoxification is now most often done on an ambulatory basis, because it is much less costly and is not substantially less efficacious than inpatient detoxification (Hayashida et al. 1989). Inpatient detoxification is nonetheless indicated for patients with serious medical or surgical illness, a history of adverse withdrawal reactions, or current evidence of complicated withdrawal (e.g., delirium tremens).

In treating AWS, benzodiazepines are the most widely used medications. They are commonly prescribed using either fixed-dose or symptom-triggered regimens. In an inpatient setting, using a symptom-triggered regimen in which benzodiazepines were administered in response to escalating withdrawal signs and symptoms (assessed using a standardized tool) required less time and a lower benzodiazepine dosage than a fixed-dose approach (Saitz et al. 1994). Validated tools, such as the Clinical Institute Withdrawal Assessment for Alcohol—Revised (CIWA-Ar) (Sullivan et al. 1989), can be used by clinicians (e.g., nurses) who are trained in their administration.

In a meta-analysis of 149 controlled trials of medications to treat AWS, Bahji et al. (2022) found that chlordiazepoxide (n = 31), chlormethiazole (a medication used in Europe, but not available in the United States) (n = 25), diazepam (n = 23), lorazepam (n = 22), and carbamazepine (n = 14) were most studied. Most treatments were provided as monotherapy (n = 114), although some included adjunctive strategies (n = 23), combination treatments (n = 5), or comparisons of two formulations of the same benzodiazepine (n = 7). Medications that were superior to placebo in reducing incident alcohol withdrawal seizures were fixed-schedule chlormethiazole; fixed-schedule diazepam, lorazepam, or chlordiazepoxide; and divalproex. Only fixed-schedule diazepam reduced the incidence of delirium tremens. Oxcarbazepine, fixed-schedule oxazepam, and γ-hydroxybutyrate reduced end-point CIWA-Ar scores more than placebo. Although symptom-triggered approaches to treating AWS are now widely used, a fixed-dose schedule may be warranted among patients deemed to be at high risk of withdrawal complicated by seizures or delirium tremens.

Lai et al. (2022) conducted a systematic review and meta-analysis of randomized controlled trials (RCTs) that compared anticonvulsants with placebo or benzodiazepines to evaluate their relative efficacy and tolerability in treating AWS. They included 24 studies comprising a total of 2,223 patients. There was no evidence of significant differences on any of the efficacy outcomes (number of patients experiencing alcohol withdrawal–related seizures or delirium, CIWA-Ar score, or need for rescue medications) when comparing anticonvulsants with benzodiazepines. Anticonvulsants showed significantly greater odds of requiring rescue medications than benzodiazepines and significantly more dropouts attributable to adverse events than placebo. The authors concluded that their findings did not support the use of anticonvulsants as first-line treatments for AWS; thus, the best first-line treatments for AWS are benzodiazepines.

Although all benzodiazepines exert agonist effects on the $GABA_A$ receptor to suppress the neuronal hyperexcitability that underlies alcohol withdrawal, diazepam and chlordiazepoxide have traditionally been most widely used for treating AWS. Other key considerations in choosing between the benzodiazepines are their onset of action and duration of effect. More lipophilic agents (e.g., diazepam) have higher rates of absorption and faster onset of clinical effects, and less lipophilic agents (e.g., oxazepam) have a slower onset. However, long-acting agents, such as diazepam and chlordiazepoxide, are metabolized via hepatic oxidation to long-acting intermediate compounds with long half-lives and thus a long duration of effects. Once these long-acting agents reach steady state, they are, in essence, self-tapering. Their use is complicated by the impairment in liver function that is common in individuals with AUD. Oxazepam and lorazepam, which have an intermediate onset of action attributable to lower lipophilicity, are not metabolized to long-acting metabolites. Thus, these benzodiazepines carry less risk of accumulation than those that require oxidation before elimination.

In clinical practice, the selection of appropriate agents to treat AWS can be complicated by a range of real-world considerations that are not always addressed in clinical studies. These include co-occurring medical or psychiatric conditions, levels of staff training and experience, polypharmacy and polysubstance use, and patient-specific behavioral or cognitive factors. It is beyond the scope of this chapter to describe treatment approaches in these myriad clinical scenarios. Thus, the reader is referred to guidelines published by the American Society of Addiction Medicine (2020), which provide a useful overview of treatment protocols and detailed approaches to AWS pharmacotherapies and treatment options.

Medications to Reduce or Stop Drinking

The first approach to using medications to treat AUD involves promoting abstinence by producing adverse effects when alcohol is consumed or reducing drinking by modifying the neurotransmitter systems that mediate alcohol reinforcement. In the following subsections, we discuss these approaches, then we review medications for treating persistent psychiatric symptoms, which are aimed at reducing the motivation to self-medicate with alcohol.

Alcohol-Sensitizing Agents

The rationale behind prescribing alcohol-sensitizing medications is to promote an awareness in patients of the likely adverse reaction that would result from drinking alcohol and thereby deter drinking. This presumed indirect effect of the medication complicates controlled trials of the medication's efficacy, because a variety of environmental factors can interact with the medication effect.

Disulfiram

In the United States, the only alcohol-sensitizing medication approved to treat AUD is disulfiram (Antabuse), which inhibits the enzyme ALDH. Disulfiram was approved by the FDA for the treatment of AUD in 1949, before FDA approval required that medications demonstrate efficacy compared with placebo. Drinking alcohol after ingesting disulfiram substantially elevates the plasma concentration of aldehyde, resulting in the signs and symptoms characteristic of the disulfiram-ethanol reaction (DER). The intensity of the DER varies with both the dose of disulfiram and the volume of alcohol ingested.

The DER includes warmness and flushing of the skin, especially that of the upper chest and face, as well as increased heart rate, palpitations, and decreased blood pressure. The reaction can also include nausea, vomiting, shortness of breath, sweating, dizziness, blurred vision, and confusion. Although the DER generally lasts about 30 minutes and is self-limited, occasionally it includes marked tachycardia, hypotension, or bradycardia. Rarely, cardiovascular collapse, congestive heart failure, and seizures have occurred as part of the DER.

Pharmacology of disulfiram

Disulfiram is almost completely absorbed after oral administration. Because it binds irreversibly to ALDH, renewed enzyme activity depends on the synthesis of new enzyme. Thus, the risk of a DER can last for at least 2 weeks from the last ingestion of disulfiram, during which time alcohol should be avoided.

Disulfiram produces a variety of adverse effects independent of the DER, which commonly include drowsiness, lethargy, and fatigue (Chick 1999). More serious adverse effects, such as optic neuritis, peripheral neuropathy, and hepatotoxicity (including fulminant hepatic failure), occur rarely. Psychiatric effects of disulfiram principally occur at higher dosages and may result from the inhibition by disulfiram of a variety of enzymes in addition to ALDH, including dopamine β-hydroxylase (DBH). Inhibition of DBH increases dopamine levels, which can exacerbate psychotic symptoms in individuals with schizophrenia and occasionally may result in psychotic or depressive symptoms in other individuals.

Disulfiram is administered orally. Because there is an increased risk of side effects and toxic hazards as the dosage is increased, the dosage prescribed in the United States has been limited to 250–500 mg/day. However, titration of the dosage of disulfiram in association with a challenge dose of ethanol has shown that some patients require a disulfiram dosage greater than 1 g/day to produce a DER (Brewer 1984). The few studies that have examined the genetic moderators of disulfiram's effects have suggested that individuals carrying SNPs in *DBH* (which encodes a key enzyme in the conversion of dopamine to norepinephrine) and carriers of the null allele of *ALDH2* may experience more success with disulfiram treatment (Arias et al. 2014; Yoshimura et al. 2014). However, these studies were conducted exclusively in men and are yet to be replicated.

Clinical use of disulfiram

The largest and most methodologically rigorous study of disulfiram was a multicenter trial conducted by the Veterans Administration Cooperative Studies Group, in which more than 600 men with AUD were randomly assigned to receive disulfiram (either 1 or 250 mg/day) or an inactive placebo (Fuller et al. 1986). Patients assigned to the two disulfiram groups were told they were being given the medication and to avoid drinking because of the potential for a DER, but neither patients nor staff knew the dosage assigned to the individual participants. The results showed a direct relationship between adherence with the medication regimen (in all three groups) and abstinence but no advantage to the 250-mg/day dosage over either the 1-mg/day dosage or placebo. In a planned secondary analysis of data from patients who resumed drinking, the group who received disulfiram 250 mg/day had significantly fewer drinking days than either of the other two groups. Although these findings suggest that disulfiram could be helpful in reducing the frequency of drinking in men who cannot remain abstinent, this finding could have arisen by chance (Fuller et al. 1986). Furthermore, given the potential for disulfiram to produce serious adverse events with any drinking, it is not a good candidate for use in nonabstinent individuals or individuals not committed to abstinence (e.g., for harm reduction).

In a meta-analysis of 22 disulfiram studies for treating AUD (Skinner et al. 2014) in which the primary outcome was specific to each trial, disulfiram had a higher success rate than the control. However, when blinded ($n = 7$) and open-label ($n = 15$) RCTs were examined separately, only in open-label trials was disulfiram significantly more efficacious than the control; blinded RCTs did not show such an effect.

Consistent with this finding, the use of disulfiram has been proposed for treating selected groups of individuals with AUD in combination with special efforts to ensure treatment adherence. Specific behavioral efforts that have been suggested to enhance adherence with disulfiram (and other medications for treating AUD) include providing incentives to the patient for medication ingestion, contracting with the patient and a significant other to work together to ensure adherence ("Antabuse contract" [O'Farrell et al. 1995]), providing regular reminders and other information to the patient, and providing behavioral training and social support to reinforce adherence (Allen and Litten 1992). Chick et al. (1992) randomly assigned patients to receive disulfiram 200 mg/day or placebo for 6 months as an adjunct to outpatient alcohol treatment. Medication was ingested under the supervision of an individual nominated by the patient. The authors found that disulfiram treatment significantly increased abstinent days and decreased total drinks consumed, effects that were confirmed by parallel changes in levels of the hepatic enzyme γ-glutamyltransferase (GGT). Based on these findings, disulfiram is best suited for patients who are committed to abstinence from alcohol, cognitively and psychiatrically capable of adhering to the necessary dietary and environmental restrictions and cautions, and stably housed (ideally with a trusted partner, friend, or treatment provider who can participate in medication administration).

In summary, because disulfiram's effect on alcohol consumption is indirect and depends on creating the expectation of an adverse effect of drinking when combined with the agent, testing its efficacy has been methodologically challenging. If a clinician is considering prescribing disulfiram to a patient with AUD, the patient should be fully informed of the potential hazards of using the medication, including the need to avoid over-the-counter preparations with alcohol, foods prepared with alcohol, and medications that can interact with disulfiram. The DER can also occur with the use of alcohol-containing hand sanitizers. The decision whether to prescribe disulfiram should therefore be made jointly by the clinician and the patient after a thorough discussion of its potential risks and benefits. Given the risk of rare fulminant hepatic failure with disulfiram treatment, liver function tests are recommended before treatment, monthly for the first 3 months, and then every 3–6 months thereafter. Disulfiram should not be administered to anyone who does not agree to its use, who does not seek to be abstinent from alcohol, or who has any psychological or medical contraindications.

Agents That Reduce Alcohol Consumption Through Modification of the Neurotransmitter Systems That Mediate Alcohol Reinforcement

As reviewed in the first section of this chapter, several neurotransmitter systems influence the reinforcing or discriminative stimulus effects of ethanol. Although these systems often interact to influence drinking behavior, they will be discussed individually here for the sake of clarity.

Opioid Antagonists

Naltrexone and nalmefene are opioid antagonists with limited intrinsic agonist properties. Naltrexone has been studied more extensively than nalmefene as a treatment for AUD. Oral naltrexone was approved by the FDA to treat opioid dependence and AUD in 1984 and 1994, respectively. Extended-release naltrexone (XR-NTX) was approved in 2006 to treat AUD and in 2010 to treat opioid use disorder. Nalmefene is approved in the United States as a parenteral formulation to reverse the acute effects of opioids (e.g., following opioid overdose or analgesia), and it is approved in the European Union as an oral tablet to reduce heavy drinking on an as-needed basis.

Naltrexone

Naltrexone is an MOR antagonist that is converted in the liver into the metabolite 6β-naltrexol. The half-life of naltrexone is approximately 9 hours, and the half-life of 6β-naltrexol is approximately 8 hours (Wall et al. 1981). The FDA approval of naltrexone for treating AUD was based on the results of two single-site studies (O'Malley et al. 1992; Volpicelli et al. 1992) that showed it to be efficacious in preventing relapse to heavy drinking. In a 12-week placebo-controlled RCT, Volpicelli et al. (1992) evaluated naltrexone in a small sample of alcohol-dependent veterans as an adjunct to an intensive day treatment program. In that study, naltrexone was well tolerated and resulted in significantly less craving for alcohol and fewer drinking days than placebo. Naltrexone also limited the progression of drinking from the initial sampling of alcohol to a relapse to heavy drinking. Study subjects who drank while taking the medication reported less euphoria, suggesting that it blocked the endogenous opioid system's contribution to alcohol's "priming effect" (Volpicelli et al. 1995).

Most, but not all, subsequent studies of naltrexone have shown it to be efficacious for treating AUD, and a series of meta-analyses have shown it to be superior to placebo, principally in reducing the risk of heavy drinking (Jonas et al. 2014; Palpacuer et al. 2018; Rösner et al. 2010b; Srisurapanont and Jarusuraisin 2005). The most comprehensive meta-analysis of naltrexone (Jonas et al. 2014) included 53 RCTs with 9,140 participants. The investigators showed that for oral naltrexone (50 mg/day), the number needed to treat (NNT) to prevent one patient's return to heavy drinking was 12. For XR-NTX, there was no associated reduction in a return to either any drinking or heavy drinking, but the active medication was associated with a lower number of heavy drinking days than placebo.

Few randomized placebo-controlled naltrexone studies have exceeded 3 months in duration. The VA Cooperative Study (Krystal et al. 2001), a large multicenter study, included both 12-week and 52-week treatment durations, neither of which showed an advantage for naltrexone over placebo for any of the outcomes examined. In the pivotal study of XR-NTX for treating AUD (Garbutt et al. 2005), the treatment duration was 6 months. The treatment duration in the COMBINE study (Anton et al. 2006), which included oral naltrexone, was 4 months. These studies are discussed in detail in the following paragraphs.

In follow-up studies of patients treated with naltrexone or placebo for 12 weeks (Anton et al. 2001, 2006; O'Malley et al. 1996), the relapse rate, number of drinking days, and number of heavy drinking days among naltrexone-treated participants all increased gradually after the cessation of therapy. A posttreatment reduction in the effects of XR-NTX on drinking outcomes was also seen in a study of individuals experiencing homelessness and AUD (Collins et al. 2021). An exception to this pattern of findings was seen in a 24-week RCT in which individuals with AUD and PTSD were randomly assigned to receive oral naltrexone or placebo combined with either prolonged-exposure therapy or supportive counseling (Foa et al. 2013). In the study by Foa et al., naltrexone treatment was associated with a significantly lower percentage of drinking days than placebo, an effect that persisted at 6 months after treatment. The optimal duration of treatment of AUD with naltrexone remains to be determined, although it is likely greater than 12 weeks.

An alternative approach to the daily use of naltrexone is to "target" the medication to high-risk drinking situations (Kranzler et al. 1997). Kranzler et al. (2003) compared the effects of naltrexone 50 mg with those of placebo in an 8-week study of problem drinkers, most of whom met criteria for an AUD. Patients were randomly assigned to receive study medication either daily or targeted to situations identified by them as having a high risk for heavy drinking. Irrespective of whether they received naltrexone or placebo, patients in the targeted condition showed a reduced likelihood of any drinking, and overall naltrexone was associated with a 19% greater reduction in the likelihood of heavy drinking than placebo.

In a subsequent study, Kranzler et al. (2009) compared 12 weeks of daily or targeted naltrexone or placebo in a sample of 163 problem drinkers, the majority of whom met criteria for AUD, but whose goal was to reduce their drinking to safe limits. On the primary outcome measure of mean drinks per day, men in the targeted naltrexone group drank significantly less at week 12 than those in the other groups. On a secondary outcome measure, drinks per drinking day, the targeted naltrexone group drank significantly less than the other groups during week 12, with no effect of sex. These results suggest that naltrexone may be useful in reducing heavy drinking and support the use of a targeted approach to treating heavy drinking with an opioid antagonist. A similar approach to prescribing nalmefene, whose targeted use is approved by the European Medicines Agency to treat AUD in the European Union, is described later in this subsection.

The COMBINE study, a large placebo-controlled trial, compared naltrexone, acamprosate, and both medications in combination with either medical management or intensive psychotherapy (Anton et al. 2006). The combination of naltrexone with medical management, compared with medical management alone, produced a modest reduction in days of heavy drinking and a modest increase in the percentage of days abstinent. The efficacy of naltrexone was not enhanced by the addition of an intensive psychosocial intervention.

Because poor compliance with oral naltrexone may reduce its beneficial effects, long-acting injectable formulations have been developed. In a pilot study (Kranzler et al. 1998), participants with AUD who received a subcutaneous XR-NTX formulation showed a greater reduction in the frequency of heavy drinking compared with those who received placebo. Two XR-NTX formulations developed for intramuscular injection have also been tested as treatments for AUD. The first of these formulations was evaluated in a 12-week placebo-controlled trial in 315 patients who also received motivational enhancement therapy (Kranzler et al. 2004). Although XR-NTX did not reduce the risk of heavy drinking in that study, it delayed the onset of any drinking following initial abstinence, increased the total number of days abstinent, and doubled the likelihood that subjects remained abstinent throughout the study period (Kranzler et al. 2004). A second intramuscular XR-NTX formulation was studied in 624 individuals with AUD who were randomly assigned to receive six monthly injections of XR-NTX 380 mg, XR-NTX 190 mg, or matching placebo (Garbutt et al. 2005). The 380-mg formulation was associated with a 25% greater reduction in the rate of heavy drinking than placebo. Although the 190-mg formulation was associated with a 17% greater reduction in heavy drinking than placebo, the difference was not significant after controlling for multiple comparisons. Thus, only the 380-mg formulation of XR-NTX was approved by the FDA for treating AUD; the same formulation was subsequently approved for treating opioid use disorder. A secondary analysis of data from that study (O'Malley et al. 2007) showed that in the subgroup of participants with 4 or more days of voluntary abstinence before treatment was initiated (~13% of the total sample), those treated with XR-NTX (n = 28) had significantly better outcomes than those treated with placebo (n = 26) on a variety of self-reported drinking measures and also had a greater reduction in γ-glutamyl transpeptidase levels. These findings suggest that the beneficial effects of 380 mg XR-NTX may be limited to participants who were abstinent at treatment initiation, consistent with the medication label required by the FDA.

In a pilot study that compared oral naltrexone and XR-NTX, 23 male veterans received a 30-day prescription of naltrexone 50 mg PO, and 22 received a single intramuscular injection of 380 mg XR-NTX before discharge (Busch et al. 2017). Days without binge drinking increased from 13.6% during pretreatment to 75.0% at 45 days posttreatment in the oral naltrexone group and from 13.6% to 77.8% in the XR-NTX group. The small sample size and short study duration did not provide an adequate comparison of the two formulations, so a longer study in a larger sample is required.

The adverse effects commonly associated with XR-NTX formulations are the same as those associated with the oral formulation and include nausea, headache, and fatigue. However, because the approved XR-NTX formulation is delivered via deep gluteal injection, it is associated with local reactions at the injection site, which commonly include swelling, pain, and induration.

Another approach to improving the response to treatment with naltrexone has been to combine it with other medications. Kiefer et al. (2003) randomly assigned 160 detoxified patients with AUD to receive naltrexone, acamprosate, naltrexone plus acamprosate, or placebo for 12 weeks under double-blind conditions. They found that naltrexone, acamprosate, and the two medications combined were significantly more efficacious than placebo. In addition, the naltrexone group showed a tendency to have a longer time to the first drink and time to relapse than did the acamprosate group. The combined medication group had a significantly lower relapse rate than groups who received either placebo or acamprosate but was not statistically superior to naltrexone alone. A single-blind study by Rubio et al. (2001) compared naltrexone (50 mg/day) with acamprosate ($\leq$1,998 mg/day) over a 12-month treatment period. These investigators found a significant advantage for naltrexone over placebo for the following outcomes: rates of abstinence and relapse, cumulative abstinence, time to relapse, number of drinks per drinking day, severity of craving, and retention rate.

Altogether, the available data show that oral naltrexone and XR-NTX are both well tolerated and may be particularly efficacious in reducing relapse to heavy drinking, using either continuous administration or a targeted approach to address identified high-risk situations. The optimal duration of treatment is still uncertain but appears to be longer than 12 weeks; the benefits of combining behavioral treatments with naltrexone and XR-NTX also remain uncertain. Finally, combinations of naltrexone with acamprosate have not demonstrated superiority over naltrexone alone, and some evidence supports greater efficacy if the patient can achieve abstinence before initiation of naltrexone treatment, especially with XR-NTX.

Early pharmacogenetic studies of naltrexone investigated whether carriers of the 118G allele of *OPRM1*, which encodes the MOR, have a better clinical response to naltrexone than individuals homozygous for the more common A118 allele. This area of study was based on the hypothesis that changes in the receptor associated with the polymorphism affected the binding or efficacy of the opioid antagonist. In a secondary analysis of 141 European-ancestry participants from three completed 12-week RCTs of naltrexone (Oslin et al. 2003), 118G-allele carriers treated with naltrexone had lower rates of relapse to heavy drinking and longer time to relapse than those treated with placebo. A secondary analysis of the COMBINE study (n = 604 European-ancestry participants) also showed a strong moderating effect of the A118G SNP, with 118G-allele carriers treated with naltrexone reporting a lower percentage of heavy drinking days, a higher percentage of abstinent days, and a greater likelihood of a good clinical outcome than the naltrexone-treated A118-allele homozygotes or either placebo group (Anton et al. 2008). However, subsequent studies (Arias et al. 2014; Gelernter et al. 2007), including two prospectively designed trials (Oslin et al. 2015; Schacht et al. 2017), failed to support the moderating effect of the A118G SNP on naltrexone treatment response.

It must be noted that the studies investigating the moderating effect of the A118G SNP have been conducted in relatively small samples and predominantly in individuals of European descent. One way to mitigate the small sample size and risk of falsely rejecting an association is to aggregate the effects from multiple studies using meta-analysis. A 2020 meta-analysis of the effect of the A118G SNP on response to naltrexone treatment of AUD (Hartwell et al. 2020) failed to show an interaction effect, arguing against the clinical use of this pharmacogenetic approach in treating patients with AUD with naltrexone.

Nalmefene

The opioid antagonist nalmefene has also been evaluated as a treatment for AUD. A pilot study showed that nalmefene 40 mg/day was superior to both nalmefene 10 mg/day and placebo in preventing relapse to heavy drinking in a small sample of individuals with AUD (Mason et al. 1994). A subsequent study showed no difference between nalmefene at 20 and 80 mg/day, although the nalmefene-treated subjects combined had significantly better outcomes on measures of heavy drinking than the placebo group (Mason et al. 1999). A 12-week multisite dose-ranging study that compared placebo with nalmefene at 5, 20, and 40 mg/day was conducted in recently abstinent outpatients with AUD (Anton et al. 2004). During treatment, all subjects showed a reduction in self-reported heavy drinking days and on biological measures of drinking, but the active medication and placebo groups did not differ on these measures.

Three European multicenter trials of nalmefene up to 12 months in duration that used the medication on an as-needed basis provided more consistent evidence of its efficacy in treating AUD (Gual et al. 2012; Mann et al. 2012; van den Brink et al. 2014). These studies showed that nalmefene reduced heavy drinking days by 1.6–2.3 days per month and total drinking volume by 0.5–1 standard drink per day compared with placebo. In addition, nalmefene significantly reduced GGT serum concentrations in two of the three studies and alanine aminotransferase serum concentrations in all three studies. Based on these findings, the European Medicines Agency approved nalmefene 18 mg for use on an as-needed basis to reduce heavy drinking in alcohol-dependent individuals.

A secondary analysis of an RCT conducted in Finland, in which patients with alcohol dependence received nalmefene 10–40 mg or placebo on an as-needed basis for 28 weeks (Karhuvaara et al. 2007), examined the moderating effect of SNPs in *OPRM1*, *OPRD1* (which encodes the δ opioid receptor), and *OPRK1* (which encodes the KOR) on treatment response in 272 study participants. Despite an effect of nalmefene on drinking outcomes in the overall study (Karhuvaara et al. 2007), the secondary analysis showed no main or moderating effects of the genotypes on drinking outcomes (Arias et al. 2008).

Summary of the use of opioid antagonists to treat alcohol use disorder
There is abundant evidence supporting the use of naltrexone to treat AUD. In unselected samples of patients, however, this medication has only a small effect size (Rösner et al. 2010b). Evidence is growing that naltrexone may be of utility in subgroups of patients. The ready identification of these individuals is of great clinical interest, as is the potential utility of combining naltrexone with other medications and with specific kinds of psychotherapy. The optimal dosage and duration of treatment are two important clinical questions that remain to be adequately addressed. New approaches to the use of naltrexone, including targeted administration and extended-release formulations, promise to enhance the clinical utility of the medication. The literature supporting three large multicenter trials that demonstrated the efficacy of nalmefene was the basis for its approval in Europe as a treatment for AUD.

Acamprosate

Acamprosate (calcium acetyl homotaurine) is an amino acid derivative with a mechanism of action that is yet to be clearly defined. It acts as a weak antagonist of NMDA receptors and inhibits mGluR$_5$ (Blednov and Harris 2008; Mann et al. 2008). Thus, acamprosate appears to reduce the excitability of glutamatergic systems during withdrawal from alcohol, a hypothesis supported by the finding that it reduces anxiety in animals during ethanol withdrawal (Kotlinska and Bochenski 2008). In treatment-seeking patients with AUD, acamprosate administration reduced craving induced by alcohol priming (Hammarberg et al. 2009). This effect may involve acamprosate-induced modulation of dopamine release within the nucleus accumbens. However, there is evidence that in alcohol-dependent individuals with high levels of craving, naltrexone is more effective than acamprosate in reducing drinking (Richardson et al. 2008).

Initially evaluated in a single-center trial in France, acamprosate was shown to be twice as effective as placebo in reducing the rate at which individuals with AUD returned to drinking (Lhuintre et al. 1985). The safety and efficacy of the medication have been studied most widely in Europe, with three studies serving as the basis for its FDA approval for clinical use in the United States (Paille et al. 1995; Pelc et al. 1997; Sass et al. 1996).

As with naltrexone, meta-analytic studies (Bouza et al. 2004; Chick et al. 2003; Kranzler and Van Kirk 2001; Mann et al. 2008; Rösner et al. 2010a) provide consistent evidence of acamprosate's efficacy in the treatment of AUD. A Cochrane Review of 24 RCTs with 6,915 participants showed that acamprosate significantly reduced the risk of any drinking and increased the total number of abstinent days (Rösner et al. 2010a). The likelihood of beneficial effects in industry-sponsored trials did not differ significantly from that of publicly funded trials. The authors concluded that acamprosate appeared to be a safe and effective treatment to support continuous abstinence after detoxification in patients with AUD, although the size of the treatment effect was modest (Rösner et al. 2010a).

Nonetheless, two large multicenter trials in the United States (Anton et al. 2006; Mason et al. 2006), a large European study (Mann et al. 2009), and a large Australian study (Morley et al. 2006) failed to detect beneficial effects of acamprosate in placebo-controlled trials for treating alcohol dependence. In the COMBINE trial (Anton et al. 2006), acamprosate treatment did not significantly alter measures of alcohol consumption irrespective of the intensity of the concomitant psychosocial treatment provided. Combining naltrexone with acamprosate also failed to decrease drinking outcomes significantly.

Substantial differences in the results of the published studies have been attributed to the greater severity of alcohol dependence in the studies showing efficacy and the high prevalence of co-occurring drug misuse in the studies. The small therapeutic effect of acamprosate can be difficult to detect in heterogeneous samples that are typically recruited to participate in multicenter studies.

One study has implications for the use of acamprosate in combination with disulfiram. Besson et al. (1998) randomly assigned patients to receive acamprosate or placebo. Because some participants were taking disulfiram when they entered the study, they were randomized separately from those not taking disulfiram. Acamprosate was superior to placebo on measures of total abstinence and on cumulative abstinent days. Interestingly, the group receiving both acamprosate and disulfiram showed a significantly greater percentage of abstinent days than any of the other three groups. However, because the design was not fully randomized, one cannot conclude that the combination would be more efficacious if initiated together or in an otherwise unselected patient group.

In summary, although meta-analyses provide evidence of a beneficial effect of acamprosate in relapse prevention, they fail to demonstrate superior efficacy to placebo in several large clinical trials. Additional research is needed to identify the patient characteristics and therapeutic approaches that can be used to identify individuals with AUD whose symptoms are most likely to respond to acamprosate.

In a study comparing the effects of 21 days of treatment with acamprosate or naltrexone on cue-induced craving, Ooteman et al. (2009) examined the moderating effect of SNPs in seven genes: *OPRM1*, *DRD1* and *DRD2*, *GRIN2B*, and *GABRA6*, *GABRB2*, and *GABRG2*. These encode the μ opioid receptor, dopamine 1 and 2 receptors, an NMDA glutamate receptor, and 3 GABA receptors, respectively. Although the authors found that variants in *DRD2*, *GABRA6*, and *GABRB2* moderated the response to acamprosate, the analysis used a significance level of 0.10 without correction for multiple comparisons. Thus, these results should be taken as preliminary, and replication in larger samples with a longer period of medication administration, as well as additional response measures, is necessary. Other studies have shown preliminary evidence of a moderating effect on acamprosate's reduction of relapse risk by variants in two other genes: *GRIN2B*, which encodes the glutamatergic (NMDA) receptor subunit (Karpyak et al. 2014), and *GATA4* (Kiefer et al. 2011), which encodes a protein that regulates the transcription of the atrial natriuretic peptide, implicated in the pathophysiology of alcohol dependence.

Anticonvulsants

Carbamazepine and valproate

The potential utility of anticonvulsants for the treatment of AUD was demonstrated initially in placebo-controlled studies of carbamazepine (Mueller et al. 1997), valproate (Salloum et al. 2005), and topiramate (Johnson et al. 2003, 2007). In a 12-month pilot study, Mueller et al. (1997) found an early advantage to carbamazepine on number of drinks per drinking day, time to first heavy drinking day, and consecutive days of heavy drinking. Although Salloum et al. (2005) reported a significant decrease in alcohol consumption in patients with bipolar disorder and AUD treated with valproate, a 12-week double-blind, placebo-controlled pilot study of divalproex in alcohol-dependent individuals without bipolar disorder found no difference in outcomes by medication group (Brady et al. 2002).

Topiramate

A meta-analysis of seven RCTs (including a total of 1,125 participants with AUD) showed that topiramate at up to 300 mg/day in two divided doses yielded small to moderate effects on drinking, with the largest effect on abstinence, followed by heavy drinking, GGT concentration, and craving (the only outcome for which there was not a statistically significant advantage to the active medication) (Blodgett et al. 2014).

Topiramate treatment is associated with a variety of adverse events, the most frequent of which are paresthesia, anorexia (with weight loss), difficulty with memory or concentration, and taste disturbances. These effects are generally mild to moderate in severity. Uncommonly, topiramate causes visual adverse events, including myopia, angle-closure glaucoma, and increased intraocular pressure, which require discontinuation of the medication. To minimize topiramate's adverse effects, a slow titration to the maximal tolerated dosage (e.g., ≤300 mg/day over a period of 6 weeks) is recommended. Finding the optimal dosage of topiramate that is efficacious for treating AUD while minimizing the likelihood of treatment discontinuation attributable to adverse effects is a challenge.

An SNP (rs2832407) in the gene encoding the kainate receptor GluK1 subunit, to which topiramate preferentially binds (Kranzler et al. 2009), has been investigated for its potential moderating effects on alcohol consumption as well as the variability seen in topiramate-related adverse effects experienced by heavy drinkers taking this medication (Kranzler et al. 2014; Ray et al. 2009). Although an initial study (Kranzler et al. 2014) demonstrated the moderating effect of rs2832407 on topiramate's reduction in heavy drinking days and increase in abstinent days, a subsequent prospective study (Kranzler et al. 2021b) and a combined analysis of both datasets (Kranzler et al. 2021a) failed to demonstrate a moderating effect of the SNP.

Zonisamide

The anticonvulsant zonisamide has structural similarities to topiramate and similar effects on behavior, most notably in promoting weight loss. Zonisamide showed promise in the treatment of AUDs in a laboratory-based study after a single 100-mg dose (Sarid-Segal et al. 2009) and in small open-label (Knapp et al. 2010; Rubio et al. 2010) and placebo-controlled (Arias et al. 2010) clinical trials, in which the maximal dosage was 600 mg/day. A double-blind, placebo-controlled clinical trial (Knapp et al. 2015) compared the effects of zonisamide (400 mg/day) with those of topiramate (300 mg/day) and a third anticonvulsant, levetiracetam (2,000 mg/day). Zonisamide and topiramate both were associated with significantly greater reductions in drinks per day, percentage of drinking days, and percentage of heavy drinking days than placebo. In the levetiracetam group, only the reduction in percentage of heavy drinking days was significantly greater than placebo. Topiramate was associated with significantly greater evidence of mental slowing than placebo at study weeks 11 and 12. Treatment with both topiramate and zonisamide was associated with modest reductions in verbal fluency and working memory. Thus, zonisamide may have effects on drinking that are similar in magnitude to those of topiramate, but with fewer cognitive adverse effects.

Gabapentin

Because it is approved by the FDA to treat partial-onset seizures, postherpetic neuralgia, and restless legs syndrome, gabapentin is widely prescribed; in addition, its use, especially off-label to treat a variety of psychiatric symptoms (including anxiety and insomnia), is increasing (Goodman and Brett 2017). Studies of the efficacy of gabapentin monotherapy for treating AUD have yielded mixed findings. Kranzler et al. (2019a) conducted a meta-analysis of seven placebo-controlled RCTs that estimated the effects of gabapentin at dosages that ranged from 600 to 3,600 mg/day on six alcohol-related outcomes in a total of 751 individuals with AUD (Kranzler et al. 2019a). All effect estimates were in a direction that favored gabapentin over placebo; however, only for the percentage of heavy drinking days was there significant evidence of a benefit, where the size of the effect was medium to large.

Gabapentin has also been studied in combination with naltrexone. Anton et al. (2011) conducted an RCT in a sample of 150 individuals who received 16 weeks of treatment with naltrexone only (50 mg/day), naltrexone (50 mg/day) with gabapentin (≤1,200 mg/day) added for the first 6 weeks, or double placebo. The naltrexone-gabapentin group had a significantly longer time to first heavy drinking day, fewer heavy drinking days, and fewer drinks per drinking day than the other two groups—differences that diminished over the last 10 weeks of the study. The study also showed that a history of alcohol withdrawal was associated with better outcomes in the naltrexone-gabapentin group.

A subsequent 16-week, placebo-controlled RCT of gabapentin (at a dosage of ≤1,200 mg/day) was conducted in 96 treatment-seeking individuals with AUD and recent alcohol withdrawal (Anton et al. 2020). Of the 90 evaluable participants, 12 of 44 (27%) in the gabapentin group had no heavy drinking days, compared with 4 of 46 (9%) who received placebo, an NNT of 5.4. The gabapentin group was also more likely to report total abstinence (18%) than the placebo group (4%), an NNT of 6.2. When differentiated by the level of pretreatment alcohol withdrawal, only the high-withdrawal-severity group had greater reductions in no heavy drinking days (NNT = 3.1) and total abstinence (NNT = 2.7) than the placebo group; the low-alcohol-withdrawal group showed no significant differences. These findings were similar for other drinking variables, where gabapentin was more efficacious than placebo in the high-alcohol-withdrawal group only. Thus, the utility of gabapentin for treating AUD may be limited to individuals with a high level of withdrawal severity.

The tolerability of gabapentin in AUD trials has generally been good; however, at dosages greater than 1,800 mg/day (Wang and Zhu 2017), gabapentin is associated with clinically important adverse effects, including dizziness, somnolence, ataxia or gait disorder, and peripheral edema (Wiffen et al. 2017). Furthermore, it was estimated that 1% of the U.S. general population misuses gabapentin for recreational purposes, self-medication, or intentional self-harm, either alone or in combination with other substances (including alcohol) (Smith et al. 2016). The use of gabapentin to treat AUD may best be limited to patients experiencing acute alcohol withdrawal, although further research on its role in alcohol treatment is needed. Dosages greater than 1,800 mg/day should probably be avoided to reduce the risk of adverse effects.

Baclofen

Baclofen is a $GABA_B$ agonist widely used for its antispasmodic effects. Over the past two decades, baclofen has been evaluated as a treatment for AUD, owing to the implication of $GABA_B$ in reward signaling and various psychiatric and neurological disorders (e.g., schizophrenia, substance use disorders, epilepsy) (D'Souza and Markou 2011; Fatemi et al. 2011; Heaney and Kinney 2016). In 2018, baclofen was approved in France for treating AUD. However, two meta-analyses published that same year came to different conclusions concerning its efficacy (Minozzi et al. 2018; Pierce et al. 2018).

A Cochrane meta-analysis (Minozzi et al. 2018) of 12 RCTs of baclofen comprised 1,128 participants with a diagnosis of alcohol dependence who were currently drinking. The dosage of baclofen tested was 10–150 mg/day. Analyses showed no difference between baclofen and placebo for the primary outcomes of return to any drinking, percentage of days abstinent, or percentage of heavy drinking days at the end of treatment. There were also no differences in the number of participants with at least one adverse event or in dropout rates. Baclofen treatment was associated with more drinks per drinking day and greater depression severity. The adverse events that were significantly more common with baclofen therapy included vertigo, somnolence/sedation, paresthesia, and muscle spasms/rigidity. The authors concluded that based on these findings, baclofen should not be considered a first-line treatment for AUD.

In contrast, a meta-analysis of 13 RCTs comprising 1,492 individuals with AUD (Pierce et al. 2018) showed that baclofen was associated with significant, small to medium effects on the time to first lapse to drinking and likelihood of abstinence during treatment. There was a significant difference based on baclofen dosage; studies of dosages up to 60 mg/day showed an association of the agent with a medium effect on the time to a first lapse in drinking, whereas studies of dosages greater than 60 mg/day did not. Higher daily alcohol consumption at baseline was associated with a larger

Alcohol Use Disorder 113

baclofen treatment effect. The basis for the discrepancy between these meta-analyses is unclear.

Given the lack of consensus regarding the efficacy of baclofen, it is not recommended for use as a first-line treatment for AUD. If baclofen is prescribed to treat AUD, the dosage should be 60 mg/day or lower, both because of the lack of demonstrated efficacy at the higher dosage and because of a dosage-related increase in the risk of sedation (Reynaud et al. 2017), which can be particularly problematic in combination with alcohol.

To our knowledge, the only pharmacogenetic study of baclofen conducted is a secondary analysis of data from a subset of 72 participants with AUD who were randomly assigned to treatment with baclofen (30 or 75 mg/day) or placebo (Morley et al. 2018). The authors examined the moderating effect of rs29220 in *GABBR1*, a subunit of the $GABA_B$ receptor gene. The study showed that baclofen therapy in rs29220*C allele homozygotes was associated with a longer time to relapse and a greater proportion of abstinent days than placebo treatment or baclofen treatment in participants with one or two rs29220*G alleles. No significant moderating effects were found for rs29230 in *GABBR1* or rs7865648 in *GABBR2* (which encodes a second $GABA_B$ receptor subunit). The authors concluded that variation in rs29220 allele frequency in different populations may help to explain the lack of efficacy of baclofen in some studies, although further research is needed.

Serotonergic Medications

Selective serotonin reuptake inhibitors
A variety of antidepressants, including selective serotonin reuptake inhibitors (SSRIs), have been tested in humans to determine their effects on alcohol consumption. Findings on the effects of these medications for treating AUD are inconsistent. Naranjo et al. (1990) first reported that fluoxetine 60 mg/day reduced average daily alcohol consumption by approximately 17% from baseline levels, whereas treatment with fluoxetine 40 mg/day or placebo had no effect. Using a crossover design, Gerra et al. (1992) compared the effects of fluoxetine, acamprosate, and placebo in individuals with AUD and a positive or negative family history of the disorder. Although both active medications were superior to placebo in reducing the number of drinks consumed, the effect of fluoxetine was significant only in patients with a positive family history of AUD, whereas acamprosate produced a significant reduction only in patients with a negative family history of

AUD. Subsequent studies showed no advantage for fluoxetine over placebo on drinking behavior among individuals with severe AUD recruited from an alcohol treatment program at a Veterans Affairs Medical Center (Kabel and Petty 1996) or in combination with coping skills psychotherapy in a 12-week placebo-controlled trial (Kranzler et al. 1995).

Naranjo et al. (1987) found that citalopram 40 mg/day, but not 20 mg/day, reduced the number of drinks per day and increased the number of abstinent days from baseline in nondepressed, early-stage problem drinkers, a finding that was subsequently replicated (Naranjo et al. 1992). In another study, however, in which citalopram 40 mg/day was combined with a brief psychosocial intervention in a 12-week treatment trial, only during the first week of treatment did the active medication show an advantage over placebo (Naranjo et al. 1995). Balldin et al. (1994) found no overall advantage to citalopram compared with placebo; however, when the data were reanalyzed based on the pretreatment level of alcohol consumption, the lighter-drinking subgroup had lower daily alcohol intake on active treatment. Tiihonen et al. (1996) found a significant advantage for citalopram over placebo on study retention and on collateral informants' reports of the patients' condition, with a trend for decreased alcohol consumption and GGT levels in the active treatment group.

In a secondary analysis of their fluoxetine trial, Kranzler et al. (1996) found that individuals with high-risk or high-severity alcoholism (Type B; characterized by an earlier age at alcoholism onset) experienced a poorer symptom response to the active medication than to placebo. Pettinati et al. (2000) found that patients with low-risk or low-severity alcoholism (Type A; characterized by a later age at alcoholism onset) drank on fewer days and were more likely to be abstinent in the 12-week treatment trial when treated with sertraline than with placebo. In a 6-month posttreatment follow-up of these subjects (Dundon et al. 2004), the Type A/Type I subgroup (later onset, more environmentally mediated, and low impulsivity and novelty seeking) treated with sertraline maintained the beneficial effects seen during treatment. In contrast, subjects with AUD in the Type B/Type II subgroup (earlier onset, male predominance, and high impulsivity and novelty seeking) who were initially treated with sertraline were more likely to increase their heavy drinking during the follow-up period than those treated with placebo.

In clinical practice, depression and anxiety often are bidirectionally related to alcohol use. In a 2022 meta-analysis, Fluyau et al. (2022) analyzed the effects of SSRIs on substance use patterns in individuals with

Alcohol Use Disorder 115

co-occurring depression, anxiety, and PTSD. They found that SSRIs (particularly fluoxetine) reduced depression and anxiety symptoms in individuals with AUD and concomitantly decreased alcohol use and craving.

Ondansetron

The 5-HT$_3$ antagonist ondansetron was shown by Johnson et al. (2000b) to reduce drinking behavior only among patients with early-onset alcoholism (onset of problem drinking before age 25). At a dosage of 4 µg/kg bid (substantially lower than the dosage used for its antiemetic effects), ondansetron was superior to placebo on the proportion of days abstinent and the intensity of alcohol intake. In contrast, in patients with late-onset alcoholism, the effects of ondansetron on drinking behavior were in nearly all respects comparable to those of placebo.

A pilot clinical trial (Johnson et al. 2000a) and a functional MRI study (Myrick et al. 2008) showed that ondansetron combined with naltrexone may provide additional benefits. These benefits include decreases in drinks per drinking day, craving for alcohol, and alcohol cue-induced activation of the ventral striatum.

Pharmacogenetics of serotonergic medications

A placebo-controlled RCT of sertraline (Kranzler et al. 2011) showed that its effects on drinking and heavy drinking in alcohol-dependent individuals were moderated by both age at onset of alcohol dependence and the 5-HTTLPR polymorphism in the serotonin transporter gene. Specifically, sertraline decreased drinking significantly in individuals with late-onset AUD with the L'L' genotype (an effect that persisted during a 3-month follow-up period; Kranzler et al. 2012), whereas individuals with early-onset AUD with the L'L' genotype had fewer drinking and heavy drinking days when treated with placebo. These findings have yet to be replicated.

Johnson et al. (2011) showed that ondansetron reduced drinking only in alcohol-dependent participants with the 5-HTTLPR LL genotype. Furthermore, an SNP in the 3' untranslated region (3'-UTR) of the serotonin transporter gene (Seneviratne et al. 2009) interacted with the 5-HTTLPR polymorphism in the same gene to moderate the response to ondansetron. Thus, drinking was reduced by ondansetron most in individuals with the L'L' genotype at 5-HTTLPR and the TT genotype of the 3'-UTR SNP. Further analysis found an additional three variants in 5-HT$_3$ receptor genes that moderated the ondansetron response (Johnson et al. 2013).

Antipsychotic Medications

Quetiapine

A placebo-controlled trial of the atypical antipsychotic quetiapine in patients differentiated by AUD subtype (Kampman et al. 2007) showed a significant effect on drinking and heavy drinking days among individuals with earlier-onset, higher-severity AUD (n = 28), but not among individuals with later-onset, lower-severity AUD (n = 33). However, a placebo-controlled multisite trial in a total sample of 224 participants with AUD showed no efficacy of the medication for any alcohol-related outcome (Litten et al. 2012).

Aripiprazole

Aripiprazole is an atypical antipsychotic agent that acts as a partial agonist at dopamine D_2 and serotonin 5-HT_{1A} receptors. A human laboratory study in healthy subjects showed that aripiprazole significantly and dose-dependently increased the sedative effects of alcohol and, to a lesser degree, decreased the euphoric effects of alcohol (Kranzler et al. 2008). The administration of aripiprazole over a 6-day period reduced drinking by alcohol-dependent subjects both before and during a human laboratory session (Voronin et al. 2008). Alcohol-dependent subjects pretreated with aripiprazole showed less activation in the ventral striatum in response to alcohol-related cue exposure than those who received placebo (Myrick et al. 2010). Despite these findings suggesting that aripiprazole has value in treating AUD, a 12-week multisite placebo-controlled RCT (Anton et al. 2008) showed no difference between treatment groups in the percentage of days abstinent, percentage of subjects' no drinking days, and time to first drinking day, although the aripiprazole group reported fewer drinks per drinking day than the placebo group.

Based on the findings just described and a meta-analysis of 13 RCTs of antipsychotic treatment of individuals with primary AUD without schizophrenia or bipolar disorder (Kishi et al. 2013), there does not seem to be a role for antipsychotic medications in treating AUD alone. The meta-analysis, aside from one isolated outcome, showed no increases in abstinence or reductions in drinking or craving in this population (Kishi et al. 2013). Like depression and anxiety, however, the relationship between heavy alcohol use and co-occurring bipolar or psychotic disorders (for which antipsychotics are often prescribed) can be complex in clinical practice. Another meta-analysis demonstrated benefits of pharmacological treatment (quetiapine) of bipolar mania and improved abstinence from alcohol, but not bipolar depression in individuals with bipolar disorder (Stokes et al. 2020). For individuals with schizophrenia, co-occurring AUD has been associated with a poorer course of schizophrenia, with antipsychotic treatment possibly delaying the first or recurrent schizophrenic episodes in this challenging population (Pathak et al. 2020). Therefore, although antipsychotics may not be efficacious for treating AUD alone, they may have a beneficial role in treating serious psychopathology among individuals who drink heavily.

Partial Nicotinic Receptor Agonists

Varenicline, a partial nicotinic receptor agonist, is approved for treating tobacco use disorder. Although some studies have shown that it reduces drinking more than placebo in individuals with AUD, a meta-analysis of 10 studies (Gandhi et al. 2020) that included 731 individuals, 55.1% of whom were smokers, showed no significant differences in the percentage of heavy drinking days, number of drinks per drinking day, or percentage of days abstinent between the active and placebo groups. The only measure on which varenicline was superior to placebo was craving, in which varenicline-treated participants showed significantly greater reductions than those receiving placebo.

Summary of Medications to Reduce or Stop Drinking

A practice guideline published by the U.S. Department of Veterans Affairs and the U.S. Department of Defense (2015) recommended topiramate, disulfiram, acamprosate, and naltrexone as first-line treatments for AUD. A practice guideline published by the American Psychiatric Association recommended offering the FDA-approved medications (disulfiram, naltrexone, and acamprosate) to patients with moderate to severe AUD and gabapentin or topiramate to patients who prefer one of these agents or whose symptoms are intolerant of or have not responded to the FDA-approved medications (Reus et al. 2018).

As reviewed here, the medications for which there is the most consistent evidence of efficacy in treating AUD are the opioid antagonists and topiramate. Opioid antagonists are associated with a small, but generally consistent, effect on reducing heavy drinking. Topiramate is associated with a small to medium effect on reducing the frequency of both any drinking and heavy drinking. The clinical utility of disulfiram seems to depend on the availability of a mechanism to ensure adherence with the oral formulation. Evidence supporting the use of acamprosate is consistent only for studies conducted in Europe, which show a small effect on reducing drinking frequency. In contrast, U.S. studies of acamprosate have not shown it to be efficacious. Although gabapentin showed a medium to large effect on reducing heavy drinking in a meta-analysis, the finding was driven largely by a single study (Mason et al. 2014). There are similar inconsistent findings with baclofen. Thus, the body of evidence for gabapentin and baclofen appears not to support their use as first-line treatments for AUD.

Further research is needed to determine which patient groups, dosage schedules, routes and durations of therapy, and concomitant psychosocial treatments are optimal for use with these medications. The literature on genetic variation as a moderator of the response to naltrexone and topiramate has not been replicated and cannot be recommended at this time. Although a pharmacogenetic approach is one avenue by which the treatment of AUD could be enhanced, treatment response is a complex trait influenced by multiple genetic variants of small effect (Manolio et al. 2009). Although the effect sizes seen with treatment-relevant variants were larger than disease-related ones (Maranville and Cox 2016), suggesting that pharmacogenetic variants have large effects compared with variants contributing to etiology, it is unlikely that a single SNP, even one that encodes an amino acid substitution, could be clinically useful in personalizing treatment. The use of polygenic risk scores (PRSs), an overall measure of genetic risk for a trait, are more likely to provide clinically actionable predictors of treatment response. However, the calculation of PRSs requires the availability of large genome-wide association studies of a trait in a base sample and genome-wide genotyping in a target sample (Wray et al. 2021). To date, the largest genome-wide association study of an AUD pharmacotherapy sample that can be used as a base sample for calculating PRSs (Biernacka et al. 2021) comprises only about 1,000 individuals, a fraction of the number required for the generation of PRSs that are likely to be powerful enough to predict treatment outcomes in independent RCTs.

In selecting a medication to prescribe to a patient with AUD, there should be an initial discussion with the patient regarding their goal for treatment. For patients with a goal of reducing heavy drinking, we recommend naltrexone as a first-line treatment. An initial trial of 50 mg/day can be followed by a doubling of the dosage (i.e., 50 mg bid) in patients who do not show a substantial reduction in heavy drinking after a month of treatment.

Long-acting naltrexone, an alternative to oral treatment, could improve treatment adherence, although it is much more costly than the oral formulation. Patients who wish to stop drinking and can achieve an initial period of abstinence can be prescribed acamprosate 666 mg tid. Disulfiram is recommended only for patients who can achieve initial abstinence and have previously benefited from treatment with that medication. For patients whose symptoms do not respond satisfactorily to these treatments, topiramate can be helpful in reducing the frequency of both drinking and heavy drinking. Topiramate treatment should be initiated at a low dosage (25–50 mg/day), with a gradual increase (by 25–50 mg/day at weekly intervals) to a maximum of 150 mg bid to minimize adverse effects. There is little evidence to guide combination therapy with these medications, but such an approach can be used clinically with little potential for adverse pharmacokinetic interactions. The approach should be used carefully nonetheless in patients with serious medical or psychiatric disorders or in the context of polypharmacy.

Agents to Treat Psychiatric Symptoms or Disorders That Co-occur With Alcohol Use Disorder

Epidemiological studies have shown high rates of drug dependence and psychiatric disorders in community samples of individuals with AUD. For example, the NESARC-III trial (Grant et al. 2015) showed significant associations between 12-month and lifetime AUD and other substance use disorders, major depressive disorder, bipolar I disorder, antisocial personality disorder, and borderline personality disorder across all levels of AUD severity. It also showed modest associations between AUD and panic disorder, specific phobia, and generalized anxiety disorder across most levels of AUD severity.

In general, the indications for using psychotropic medications to treat disorders that co-occur with AUD are the same as those for individuals with psychiatric illness without AUD. However, the choice of medication should account for the increased potential for adverse effects in individuals with AUD. For example, adverse effects can result from interactions of alcohol pharmacotherapy with medical disorders that are commonly associated with AUD and from pharmacokinetic interactions with medications prescribed to treat those disorders (Sullivan and O'Connor 2004).

Although mood symptoms commonly co-occur with AUD and often diminish with abstinence (Brown et al. 1995), some symptoms, including insomnia, can persist for weeks or months despite reduced drinking or abstinence. Even in the absence of classic symptoms of alcohol withdrawal, persistent, low-level symptoms, which have been called *subacute withdrawal*, may be present.

Antidepressants

A methodological limitation of early studies of the efficacy of antidepressant medications to treat these symptoms was that they enrolled unselected groups of detoxified patients. The heterogeneity among participants and other study limitations (e.g., small sample sizes yielding inadequate statistical power) contributed to the absence of evidence of efficacy of these medications, with respect to both reductions in psychiatric symptoms and drinking behavior (Ciraulo and Jaffe 1981).

In a meta-analysis of 14 RCTs of antidepressants in patients with a co-occurring substance use disorder and unipolar depression (Nunes and Levin 2004), 8 studies (6 of which were studies of patients with AUD) showed a significant or near-significant advantage for the active medication over placebo. The pooled effect size on this measure was in the small to moderate range. There was a trend for the medication effect to be larger in studies of AUD than for other substance use disorders, and the effect size for substance use outcomes was proportional to that for the treatment of depression. The predictors of medication response included the magnitude of the placebo response (the greater the placebo response, the smaller the medication advantage), presence of a diagnosis of depression after a week of abstinence (better antidepressant response), and female gender (poorer medication response). Nunes and Levin (2004) concluded that antidepressants exert a modest beneficial effect for patients with combined depression and substance use disorders and that it is necessary to treat both disorders.

In a subsequent 14-week study of patients with depression and AUD, Pettinati et al. (2010) compared sertraline (200 mg/day), naltrexone (100 mg/day), sertraline plus naltrexone, and double placebo. The combined treatment group had a significantly higher abstinence rate (53.7%) and longer time before experiencing relapse to heavy alcohol use (median = 98 days) than the other three groups. The naltrexone-only, sertraline-only, and placebo groups did not differ from one another. Although the serious adverse event rate in the combined treatment group was about half that in the other treatment groups, the potential for drug–drug interactions should be considered when combining medications (Guerzoni et al. 2018). Although the study by Pettinati et al. (2010) remains to be replicated, it provides clear support for the efficacy of combined medication therapy for co-occurring AUD and depression or any co-occurring psychiatric disorder.

Antidepressants have also been evaluated as treatments for co-occurring AUD and anxiety symptoms or disorders. In two studies, anxiety symptoms were significantly decreased in subjects with co-occurring AUD and social anxiety disorder who were treated with the SSRI paroxetine, although in neither study was alcohol consumption markedly altered (Book et al. 2008; Thomas et al. 2008). In abstinent subjects with co-occurring agoraphobia or social anxiety disorder, adding the SSRI fluvoxamine to an intensive psychosocial relapse prevention program did not lead to greater reductions in either alcohol intake or anxiety symptoms than psychosocial treatment alone (Schadé et al. 2005).

In summary, despite evidence that most instances of postwithdrawal depression and anxiety will spontaneously remit within a few days to several weeks of abstinence from alcohol (Brown and Schuckit 1988; Brown et al. 1995; Schuckit 1983), pharmacological treatment of patients with persistent symptoms is warranted. SSRIs are the first-line treatment for depression and some anxiety disorders because they have a favorable side-effect profile and they do not have the anticholinergic, hypotensive, sedative, or cardiovascular effects of tricyclic antidepressants. However, SSRIs can exacerbate the tremor, anxiety, and insomnia often experienced by individuals recently detoxified from alcohol. Although the findings of Nunes and Levin (2004) showed that SSRIs may be less efficacious than other antidepressants for the treatment of depression among patients with a substance use disorder, combining an SSRI with naltrexone is a promising strategy for treating co-occurring depression and AUD.

Benzodiazepines and Buspirone

Other medications that have been used to treat anxiety and depression in the postwithdrawal state include benzodiazepines and buspirone. Although benzodiazepines are widely used in the treatment of acute alcohol withdrawal and are prescribed by some clinicians to treat the anxiety, depression, and sleep disturbances that can persist for months afterward, their use in individuals with AUD is controversial given their potential for misuse and dependence. The benzodiazepines currently available for clinical use vary substantially in their pharmacokinetics, acute euphoriant effects, and frequency of reported dependence. Because of its rapid onset of action, diazepam may have greater abuse potential than benzodiazepines with an intermediate or slow speed of onset, including oxazepam and lorazepam. Irrespective of variation in abuse potential, the use of benzodiazepines in individuals with AUD and other substance use disorders during the postwithdrawal period for the management of anxiety or insomnia should be avoided because of the risk of misuse, dependence, and overdose. Although benzodiazepines alone are comparatively safe, even in overdose, their combination with other brain depressants (including alcohol) can be lethal. Furthermore, dependence on both alcohol and benzodiazepines may increase depressive symptoms (Schuckit 1983), and co-occurring AUD and benzodiazepine use disorder may be more difficult to treat than AUD alone (Sokolow et al. 1981).

Buspirone, a nonbenzodiazepine anxiolytic, acts to reduce anxiety largely via its partial agonist activity at serotonergic (5-HT_{1A}) autoreceptors. Buspirone is approved for the management of anxiety disorders or the short-term relief of anxiety symptoms, is less sedating than diazepam or clorazepate, does not interact with alcohol to impair psychomotor skills, and does not appear to have abuse liability (Griffith et al. 1986; Mattila et al. 1982; Seppälä et al. 1982). Thus, buspirone is more suitable than benzodiazepines to treat anxiety symptoms among individuals with AUD. In contrast to benzodiazepines, however, buspirone does not have acute anxiolytic effects, nor is it useful in the treatment of alcohol withdrawal.

There have been four placebo-controlled, double-blind trials of buspirone to treat anxiety symptoms among individuals with AUD. An early double-blind, placebo-controlled trial of buspirone in such patients (Bruno 1989) showed significantly greater retention in treatment and greater decreases in alcohol craving, anxiety, and depression scores in buspirone-treated patients. Both groups showed significant declines in alcohol consumption during the study, with no greater effect observed among buspirone-treated patients. In a placebo-controlled trial in abstinent individuals with AUD and co-occurring generalized anxiety disorder, Tollefson et al. (1992) found that buspirone resulted in greater treatment retention and greater reductions in anxiety. Although buspirone-treated patients also showed greater improvement on a subjective, global measure of drinking outcome, measures of alcohol consumption were not reported in this study. Kranzler et al. (1994) also found that buspirone was more effective than placebo in retaining anxious patients with AUD in treatment. Buspirone also delayed relapse to heavy drinking and reduced the number of drinking days during a 6-month posttreatment follow-up period. The beneficial effects of buspirone on both anxiety and drinking were most evident among patients with the highest baseline anxiety scores. (However, a study of an anxious, severely alcohol-dependent patient sample [Malcolm et al. 1992] showed that buspirone was no better than placebo in reducing either anxiety or drinking.) Thus, there appears to be a role for buspirone in the treatment of anxiety symptoms in patients with AUD.

Lithium

Although early studies of lithium, including some that were placebo controlled (Kline et al. 1974; Merry et al. 1976), showed that its use was associated with fewer days of problematic drinking, attrition rates were high. Notably, in a placebo-controlled study of individuals with AUD who were not selected for co-occurring depression (Fawcett et al. 1987), adherence to the medication regimen, irrespective of medication group, was associated with abstinence. In that study, adherent patients taking active medication who had therapeutic serum levels (≥ 0.4 mEq/L) were abstinent more often than were compliant subjects with subtherapeutic lithium levels. After the first 6 months, however, even subjects who were adherent early in the study tended to stop taking the medication. Nevertheless, the association between early adherence and sobriety persisted, suggesting that the beneficial effects of lithium are greatest in the early months after detoxification. However, Dorus and colleagues (1989) conducted a multicenter RCT in 457 veterans with AUD, of whom approximately one-third were depressed. Participants were randomly assigned to receive either lithium (600–1,200 mg/day) or matching placebo. There were no significant differences between lithium-treated and placebo-treated patients in either the depressed or nondepressed groups on any drinking or depression outcome measures. A subsequent study showed that lithium was not superior to placebo in individuals with AUD who were not selected for a co-occurring psychiatric disorder (Fawcett et al. 2000). Thus, lithium should probably be reserved for treating AUD that co-occurs with bipolar disorder.

Key Points

- Alcohol has widespread physiological effects, affecting the GABAergic, glutamatergic, adenosinergic, dopaminergic, opioidergic, noradrenergic, serotonergic, and nicotinic receptor systems as well as other neuropeptides and hormonal systems. Pharmacotherapies targeting the myriad systems impacted by alcohol consumption have been tested as potential treatments for alcohol use disorder (AUD), with varying degrees of success.
- Alcohol withdrawal syndrome is potentially life-threatening. Benzodiazepines remain the mainstay pharmacotherapy to treat alcohol withdrawal syndrome, although anticonvulsants also appear to be beneficial.
- Pharmacotherapies for AUD fall into two categories: alcohol-sensitizing agents (e.g., disulfiram) and medications that reduce alcohol consumption by modifying the neurotransmitter systems that mediate alcohol reinforcement (e.g., naltrexone, acamprosate, topiramate, and gabapentin). Disulfiram, naltrexone, and acamprosate are the only FDA-approved AUD pharmacotherapies in the United States; naltrexone and topiramate show the most robust evidence base to support their efficacy.
- In general, except for the central role that benzodiazepines play in the treatment of alcohol withdrawal, medications approved for treating AUD continue to be underutilized despite a near doubling in the last 20 years of addiction clinicians' endorsement of the use of naltrexone for treating AUD (Ehrie et al. 2020; Mark et al. 2003).
- A key consideration in promoting effective pharmacotherapy is the development of data-driven guidelines on the optimal dosing and duration of treatment. There is also a need for well-powered studies of the safety and efficacy of medications in women, specific populations (in terms of ethnicity, race, sexual orientation, and gender identity), and adolescents and older adults. In addition, studies of cost-effectiveness and cost benefit are needed to support the routine coverage of pharmacotherapies for AUD by medical insurance plans.
- There are ongoing efforts to personalize the pharmacotherapy of AUD based on clinical or genetic characteristics. These efforts are informed by novel phenotyping and genetic approaches, including the use of polygenic risk scores, made possible by the widespread availability of data from genome-wide association studies in large populations (e.g.,

Kranzler et al. 2019b; Zhou et al. 2020). Although this is an area of intense clinical interest, it has yet to bear fruit. Advances will depend on the availability of large datasets that include reliable measures of treatment outcomes and are linked to genomic data from biobanks.
- It has long been recognized that the relationship between AUD and psychiatric symptomatology is complex (Kranzler and Tinsley 2004; Meyer 1986). Despite ameliorating persistent mood and anxiety symptoms, medications that are prescribed to individuals with AUD and co-occurring disorders will not necessarily reduce alcohol consumption, even when pathological mood states contribute to the initiation of heavy drinking. The neuroadaptive changes and complex learning that constitute the alcohol dependence syndrome (Edwards and Gross 1976) may not resolve when just one major contributing factor is brought under control.
- An additional challenge for the treatment of individuals with AUD is combining efficacious medications with empirically based psychological interventions and, when feasible, self-help group participation. Abstinence-oriented groups (e.g., Alcoholics Anonymous) may be willing to work with physicians around the issue of proper dosage, compliance, and early detection of side effects of disulfiram, the use of which is supportive of their goal of total abstinence. However, these groups may be less supportive of pharmacotherapies that focus on harm reduction through reduced heavy drinking rather than abstinence as a primary goal.
- To date, most studies of medications to treat AUD have focused on monotherapy. As the research literature on the use of medications to treat AUD grows, it will be possible to assess the utility of different medication combinations and a variety of psychotherapies.
- With pharmacotherapeutic options increasing, efforts should be directed to the alcohol treatment community writ large to promote their use as a standard ingredient in alcohol rehabilitation.

References

Adinoff B, Iranmanesh A, Veldhuis J, et al: Disturbances of the stress response: the role of the HPA axis during alcohol withdrawal and abstinence. Alcohol Health Res World 22(1):67–72, 1998 15706736

Allen JP, Litten RZ: Techniques to enhance compliance with disulfiram. Alcohol Clin Exp Res 16(6):1035–1041, 1992 1471757

Altshuler HL, Phillips PE, Feinhandler DA: Alteration of ethanol self-administration by naltrexone. Life Sci 26(9):679–688, 1980 6767889

American Society of Addiction Medicine: The ASAM Clinical Practice Guideline on Alcohol Withdrawal Management. J Addict Med 14(3 Suppl 1):1–72, 2020 32511109

Anton RF, Moak DH, Latham PK, et al: Posttreatment results of combining naltrexone with cognitive-behavior therapy for the treatment of alcoholism. J Clin Psychopharmacol 21(1):72–77, 2001 11199951

Anton RF, Pettinati H, Zweben A, et al: A multi-site dose ranging study of nalmefene in the treatment of alcohol dependence. J Clin Psychopharmacol 24(4):421–428, 2004 15232334

Anton RF, O'Malley SS, Ciraulo DA, et al: Combined pharmacotherapies and behavioral interventions for alcohol dependence: the COMBINE study: a randomized controlled trial. JAMA 295(17):2003–2017, 2006 16670409

Anton RF, Oroszi G, O'Malley S, et al: An evaluation of mu-opioid receptor (OPRM1) as a predictor of naltrexone response in the treatment of alcohol dependence: results from the Combined Pharmacotherapies and Behavioral Interventions for Alcohol Dependence (COMBINE) study. Arch Gen Psychiatry 65(2):135–144, 2008 18250251

Anton RF, Myrick H, Wright TM, et al: Gabapentin combined with naltrexone for the treatment of alcohol dependence. Am J Psychiatry 168(7):709–717, 2011 21454917

Anton RF, Voronin KK, Randall PK, et al: Naltrexone modification of drinking effects in a subacute treatment and bar-lab paradigm: influence of OPRM1 and dopamine transporter (SLC6A3) genes. Alcohol Clin Exp Res 36(11):2000–2007, 2012 22551036

Anton RF, Latham P, Voronin K, et al: Efficacy of gabapentin for the treatment of alcohol use disorder in patients with alcohol withdrawal symptoms: a randomized clinical trial. JAMA Intern Med 180(5):728–736, 2020 32150232

Arias AJ, Armeli S, Gelernter J, et al: Effects of opioid receptor gene variation on targeted nalmefene treatment in heavy drinkers. Alcohol Clin Exp Res 32(7):1159–1166, 2008 18537939

Arias AJ, Feinn R, Oncken C, et al: Placebo-controlled trial of zonisamide for the treatment of alcohol dependence. J Clin Psychopharmacol 30(3):318–322, 2010 20473070

Arias AJ, Gelernter J, Gueorguieva R, et al: Pharmacogenetics of naltrexone and disulfiram in alcohol dependent, dually diagnosed veterans. Am J Addict 23(3):288–293, 2014 24724887

Ariwodola OJ, Crowder TL, Grant KA, et al: Ethanol modulation of excitatory and inhibitory synaptic transmission in rat and monkey dentate granule neurons. Alcohol Clin Exp Res 27(10):1632–1639, 2003 14574234

Bäckström P, Hyytiä P: Suppression of alcohol self-administration and cue-induced reinstatement of alcohol seeking by the mGlu2/3 receptor agonist LY379268 and the mGlu8 receptor agonist (S)-3,4-DCPG. Eur J Pharmacol 528(1–3):110–118, 2005 16324694

Bahji A, Bach P, Danilewitz M, et al: Comparative efficacy and safety of pharmacotherapies for alcohol withdrawal: a systematic review and network meta-analysis. Addiction 117(10):2591–2601, 2022 35194860

Balldin J, Berggren U, Engel J, et al: Effect of citalopram on alcohol intake in heavy drinkers. Alcohol Clin Exp Res 18(5):1133–1136, 1994 7847595

Baraona E, Abittan CS, Dohmen K, et al: Gender differences in pharmacokinetics of alcohol. Alcohol Clin Exp Res 25(4):502–507, 2001 11329488

Barson JR, Ho HT, Leibowitz SF: Anterior thalamic paraventricular nucleus is involved in intermittent access ethanol drinking: role of orexin receptor 2. Addict Biol 20(3):469–481, 2015 24712379

Belelli D, Harrison NL, Maguire J, et al: Extrasynaptic GABAA receptors: form, pharmacology, and function. J Neurosci 29(41):12757–12763, 2009 19828786

Besson J, Aeby F, Kasas A, et al: Combined efficacy of acamprosate and disulfiram in the treatment of alcoholism: a controlled study. Alcohol Clin Exp Res 22(3):573–579, 1998 9622434

Biernacka JM, Coombes BJ, Batzler A, et al: Genetic contributions to alcohol use disorder treatment outcomes: a genome-wide pharmacogenomics study. Neuropsychopharmacology 46(12):2132–2139, 2021 34302059

Blednov YA, Harris RA: Metabotropic glutamate receptor 5 (mGluR5) regulation of ethanol sedation, dependence and consumption: relationship to acamprosate actions. Int J Neuropsychopharmacol 11(6):775–793, 2008 18377703

Blodgett JC, Del Re AC, Maisel NC, et al: A meta-analysis of topiramate's effects for individuals with alcohol use disorders. Alcohol Clin Exp Res 38(6):1481–1488, 2014 24796492

Boileau I, Assaad JM, Pihl RO, et al: Alcohol promotes dopamine release in the human nucleus accumbens. Synapse 49(4):226–231, 2003 12827641

Book SW, Thomas SE, Randall PK, et al: Paroxetine reduces social anxiety in individuals with a co-occurring alcohol use disorder. J Anxiety Disord 22(2):310–318, 2008 17448631

Bouza C, Angeles M, Muñoz A, et al: Efficacy and safety of naltrexone and acamprosate in the treatment of alcohol dependence: a systematic review. Addiction 99(7):811–828, 2004 15200577

Boyle AE, Stewart RB, Macenski MJ, et al: Effects of acute and chronic doses of naltrexone on ethanol self-administration in rhesus monkeys. Alcohol Clin Exp Res 22(2):359–366, 1998 9581641

Brady KT, Myrick H, Henderson S, et al: The use of divalproex in alcohol relapse prevention: a pilot study. Drug Alcohol Depend 67(3):323–330, 2002 12127203

Brewer C: How effective is the standard dose of disulfiram? A review of the alcohol-disulfiram reaction in practice. Br J Psychiatry 144:200–202, 1984 6704608

Broccoli L, Uhrig S, von Jonquieres G, et al: Targeted overexpression of CRH receptor subtype 1 in central amygdala neurons: effect on alcohol-seeking behavior. Psychopharmacology (Berl) 235(6):1821–1833, 2018 29700576

Brown RM, Khoo SY, Lawrence AJ: Central orexin (hypocretin) 2 receptor antagonism reduces ethanol self-administration, but not cue-conditioned ethanol-seeking, in ethanol-preferring rats. Int J Neuropsychopharmacol 16(9):2067–2079, 2013 23601187

Brown SA, Schuckit MA: Changes in depression among abstinent alcoholics. J Stud Alcohol 49(5):412–417, 1988 3216643

Brown SA, Inaba RK, Gillin JC, et al: Alcoholism and affective disorder: clinical course of depressive symptoms. Am J Psychiatry 152(1):45–52, 1995 7802119

Bruno F: Buspirone in the treatment of alcoholic patients. Psychopathology 22(Suppl 1):49–59, 1989 2657838

Buisman-Pijlman FT, Sumracki NM, Gordon JJ, et al: Individual differences underlying susceptibility to addiction: role for the endogenous oxytocin system. Pharmacol Biochem Behav 119:22–38, 2014 24056025

Busch AC, Denduluri M, Glass J, et al: Pre-discharge injectable vs. oral naltrexone to improve post-discharge treatment engagement among hospitalized veterans with alcohol use disorder: a randomized pilot proof-of-concept study. Alcohol Clin Exp Res 41(7):1352–1360, 2017 28605827

Buydens-Branchey L, Branchey M, Fergeson P, et al: Hormonal, psychological, and alcohol craving changes after m-chlorophenylpiperazine administration in alcoholics. Alcohol Clin Exp Res 21(2):220–226, 1997 9113256

Cannady R, Fisher KR, Durant B, et al: Enhanced AMPA receptor activity increases operant alcohol self-administration and cue-induced reinstatement. Addict Biol 18(1):54–65, 2013 23126443

Castillo-Carniglia A, Keyes KM, Hasin DS, et al: Psychiatric comorbidities in alcohol use disorder. Lancet Psychiatry 6(12):1068–1080, 2019 31630984

Ceccarini J, Leurquin-Sterk G, Crunelle CL, et al: Recovery of decreased metabotropic glutamate receptor 5 availability in abstinent alcohol-dependent patients. J Nucl Med 61(2):256–262, 2020 31481578

Cederbaum AI: Alcohol metabolism. Clin Liver Dis 16(4):667–685, 2012 23101976

Chandler CM, Reeves-Darby J, Jones SA, et al: α5GABAA subunit-containing receptors and sweetened alcohol cue-induced reinstatement and active sweetened alcohol self-administration in male rats. Psychopharmacology (Berl) 236(6):1797–1806, 2019 30637435

Chandler LJ, Norwood D, Sutton G: Chronic ethanol upregulates NMDA and AMPA, but not kainate receptor subunit proteins in rat primary cortical cultures. Alcohol Clin Exp Res 23(2):363–370, 1999 10069569

Chen YC, Yang LF, Lai CL, et al: Acetaldehyde enhances alcohol sensitivity and protects against alcoholism: evidence from alcohol metabolism in subjects with variant ALDH2*2 gene allele. Biomolecules 11(8):1183, 2021 34439848

Chick J: Safety issues concerning the use of disulfiram in treating alcohol dependence. Drug Saf 20(5):427–435, 1999 10348093

Chick J, Gough K, Falkowski W, et al: Disulfiram treatment of alcoholism. Br J Psychiatry 161:84–89, 1992 1638335

Chick J, Lehert P, Landron F, et al: Does acamprosate improve reduction of drinking as well as aiding abstinence? J Psychopharmacol 17(4):397–402, 2003 14870951

Choi DS, Cascini MG, Mailliard W, et al: The type 1 equilibrative nucleoside transporter regulates ethanol intoxication and preference. Nat Neurosci 7(8):855–861, 2004 15258586

Ciraulo DA, Jaffe JH: Tricyclic antidepressants in the treatment of depression associated with alcoholism. J Clin Psychopharmacol 1(3):146–150, 1981 7298891

Clark M, Dar MS: Effect of acute ethanol on release of endogenous adenosine from rat cerebellar synaptosomes. J Neurochem 52(6):1859–1865, 1989 2498462

Collins SE, Duncan MH, Saxon AJ, et al: Combining behavioral harm-reduction treatment and extended-release naltrexone for people experiencing homelessness and alcohol use disorder in the USA: a randomised clinical trial. Lancet Psychiatry 8(4):287–300, 2021 33713622

Concas A, Cuccheddu T, Floris S, et al: 2-Chloro-N6-cyclopentyladenosine (CCPA), an adenosine A1 receptor agonist, suppresses ethanol withdrawal syndrome in rats. Alcohol Cucchi'd 29(3):261–264, 1994 7945566

Connole L, Harkin A, Maginn M: Adenosine A1 receptor blockade mimics caffeine's attenuation of ethanol-induced motor incoordination. Basic Clin Pharmacol Toxicol 95(6):299–304, 2004 15569276

Cowen MS, Djouma E, Lawrence AJ: The metabotropic glutamate 5 receptor antagonist 3-[(2-methyl-1,3-thiazol-4-yl)ethynyl]-pyridine reduces ethanol self-administration in multiple strains of alcohol-preferring rats and regulates olfactory glutamatergic systems. J Pharmacol Exp Ther 315(2):590–600, 2005 16014750

Cowen MS, Krstew E, Lawrence AJ: Assessing appetitive and consummatory phases of ethanol self-administration in C57BL/6J mice under operant conditions: regulation by mGlu5 receptor antagonism. Psychopharmacology (Berl) 190(1):21–29, 2007 17096086

Criswell HE, Ming Z, Kelm MK, et al: Brain regional differences in the effect of ethanol on GABA release from presynaptic terminals. J Pharmacol Exp Ther 326(2):596–603, 2008 18502983

Cui C, Koob GF: Titrating tipsy targets: the neurobiology of low-dose alcohol. Trends Pharmacol Sci 38(6):556–568, 2017 28372826

Dannenhoffer CA, Kim EU, Saalfield J, et al: Oxytocin and vasopressin modulation of social anxiety following adolescent intermittent ethanol exposure. Psychopharmacology (Berl) 235(10):3065–3077, 2018 30141056

Dar MS: Ethanol-induced cerebellar ataxia: cellular and molecular mechanisms. Cerebellum 14(4):447–465, 2015 25578036

de Laat B, Goldberg A, Shi J, et al: The kappa opioid receptor is associated with naltrexone-induced reduction of drinking and craving. Biol Psychiatry 86(11):864–871, 2019 31399255

de Lecea L, Kilduff TS, Peyron C, et al: The hypocretins: hypothalamus-specific peptides with neuroexcitatory activity. Proc Natl Acad Sci U S A 95(1):322–327, 1998 9419374

de Vries GJ, Miller MA: Anatomy and function of extrahypothalamic vasopressin systems in the brain. Prog Brain Res 119:3–20, 1998 10074777

Di Chiara G, Imperato A: Drugs abused by humans preferentially increase synaptic dopamine concentrations in the mesolimbic system of freely moving rats. Proc Natl Acad Sci U S A 85(14):5274–5278, 1988 2899326

Ding Z-M, Ingraham CM, Rodd ZA, et al: The reinforcing effects of ethanol within the nucleus accumbens shell involve activation of local GABA and serotonin receptors. J Psychopharmacol 29(6):725–733, 2015 25922425

Dorus W, Ostrow DG, Anton R, et al: Lithium treatment of depressed and nondepressed alcoholics. JAMA 262(12):1646–1652, 1989 2504944

D'Souza MS, Markou A: Neuronal mechanisms underlying development of nicotine dependence: implications for novel smoking-cessation treatments. Addict Sci Clin Pract 6(1):4–16, 2011 22003417

Dundon W, Lynch KG, Pettinati HM, et al: Treatment outcomes in type A and B alcohol dependence 6 months after serotonergic pharmacotherapy. Alcohol Clin Exp Res 28(7):1065–1073, 2004 15252293

Edwards G, Gross MM: Alcohol dependence: provisional description of a clinical syndrome. BMJ 1(6017):1058–1061, 1976 773501

Edwards S, Guerrero M, Ghoneim OM, et al: Evidence that vasopressin V1b receptors mediate the transition to excessive drinking in ethanol-dependent rats. Addict Biol 17(1):76–85, 2012 21309953

Ehrie J, Hartwell EE, Morris PE, et al: Survey of addiction specialists' use of medications to treat alcohol use disorder. Front Psychiatry 11:47, 2020 32116860

El Yacoubi M, Ledent C, Parmentier M, et al: Caffeine reduces hypnotic effects of alcohol through adenosine A2A receptor blockade. Neuropharmacology 45(7):977–985, 2003 14573390

Ericson M, Molander A, Löf E, et al: Ethanol elevates accumbal dopamine levels via indirect activation of ventral tegmental nicotinic acetylcholine receptors. Eur J Pharmacol 467(1–3):85–93, 2003 12706460

Farris SP, Mayfield RD: RNA-Seq reveals novel transcriptional reorganization in human alcoholic brain. Int Rev Neurobiol 116:275–300, 2014 25172479

Fatemi SH, Folsom TD, Thuras PD: Deficits in GABA(B) receptor system in schizophrenia and mood disorders: a postmortem study. Schizophr Res 128(1–3):37–43, 2011 21303731

Fawcett J, Clark DC, Aagesen CA, et al: A double-blind, placebo-controlled trial of lithium carbonate therapy for alcoholism. Arch Gen Psychiatry 44(3):248–256, 1987 3103580

Fawcett J, Kravitz HM, McGuire M, et al: Pharmacological treatments for alcoholism: revisiting lithium and considering buspirone. Alcohol Clin Exp Res 24(5):666–674, 2000 10832908

Feng HJ, Forman SA: Comparison of αβδ and αβγ GABAA receptors: allosteric modulation and identification of subunit arrangement by site-selective general anesthetics. Pharmacol Res 133:289–300, 2018 29294355

Fluyau D, Mitra P, Jain A, et al: Selective serotonin reuptake inhibitors in the treatment of depression, anxiety, and post-traumatic stress disorder in substance use disorders: a Bayesian meta-analysis. Eur J Clin Pharmacol 78(6):931–942, 2022 35246699

Foa EB, Yusko DA, McLean CP, et al: Concurrent naltrexone and prolonged exposure therapy for patients with comorbid alcohol dependence and PTSD: a randomized clinical trial. JAMA 310(5):488–495, 2013 23925619

Frezza M, di Padova C, Pozzato G, et al: High blood alcohol levels in women: the role of decreased gastric alcohol dehydrogenase activity and first-pass metabolism. N Engl J Med 322(2):95–99, 1990 2248624

Fuller RK, Branchey L, Brightwell DR, et al: Disulfiram treatment of alcoholism: a Veterans Administration cooperative study. JAMA 256(11):1449–1455, 1986 3528541

Funk CK, O'Dell LE, Crawford EF, et al: Corticotropin-releasing factor within the central nucleus of the amygdala mediates enhanced ethanol self-administration in withdrawn, ethanol-dependent rats. J Neurosci 26(44):11324–11332, 2006 17079660

Funk CK, Zorrilla EP, Lee MJ, et al: Corticotropin-releasing factor 1 antagonists selectively reduce ethanol self-administration in ethanol-dependent rats. Biol Psychiatry 61(1):78–86, 2007 16876134

Funk D, Coen K, Tamadon S, et al: Effects of the alpha-1 antagonist prazosin on KOR agonist-induced reinstatement of alcohol seeking. Int J Neuropsychopharmacol 22(11):724–734, 2019 31556948

Gandhi KD, Mansukhani MP, Karpyak VM, et al: The impact of varenicline on alcohol consumption in subjects with alcohol use disorders: systematic review and meta-analyses. J Clin Psychiatry 81(2):19r12924, 2020 32097546

Garbutt JC, Kranzler HR, O'Malley SS, et al: Efficacy and tolerability of long-acting injectable naltrexone for alcohol dependence. JAMA 293:1617–1625, 2005 15811981

Gelernter J, Gueorguieva R, Kranzler HR, et al: Opioid receptor gene (OPRM1, OPRK1, and OPRD1) variants and response to naltrexone treatment for alcohol dependence: results from the VA Cooperative Study. Alcohol Clin Exp Res 31(4):555–563, 2007 17374034

Gerra G, Caccavari R, Delsignore R, et al: Effects of fluoxetine and Ca-acetyl-homotaurinate on alcohol intake in familial and non-familial alcoholic patients. Curr Ther Res Clin Exp 52(2):291–295, 1992

Gilpin NW, Koob GF: Effects of β-adrenoceptor antagonists on alcohol drinking by alcohol-dependent rats. Psychopharmacology (Berl) 212(3):431–439, 2010 20676608

Gilpin NW, Misra K, Koob GF: Neuropeptide Y in the central nucleus of the amygdala suppresses dependence-induced increases in alcohol drinking. Pharmacol Biochem Behav 90(3):475–480, 2008 18501411

Gilpin NW, Misra K, Herman MA, et al: Neuropeptide Y opposes alcohol effects on gamma-aminobutyric acid release in amygdala and blocks the transition to alcohol dependence. Biol Psychiatry 69(11):1091–1099, 2011 21459365

Gilpin NW, Herman MA, Roberto M: The central amygdala as an integrative hub for anxiety and alcohol use disorders. Biol Psychiatry 77(10):859–869, 2015 25433901

Gonzales RA, Weiss F: Suppression of ethanol-reinforced behavior by naltrexone is associated with attenuation of the ethanol-induced increase in dialysate dopamine levels in the nucleus accumbens. J Neurosci 18(24):10663–10671, 1998 9852601

Goodman CW, Brett AS: Gabapentin and pregabalin for pain: is increased prescribing a cause for concern? N Engl J Med 377(5):411–414, 2017 28767350

Goodwani S, Saternos H, Alasmari F, et al: Metabotropic and ionotropic glutamate receptors as potential targets for the treatment of alcohol use disorder. Neurosci Biobehav Rev 77:14–31, 2017 28242339

Gotti C, Guiducci S, Tedesco V, et al: Nicotinic acetylcholine receptors in the mesolimbic pathway: primary role of ventral tegmental area alpha6beta2* receptors in mediating systemic nicotine effects on dopamine release, locomotion, and reinforcement. J Neurosci 30(15):5311–5325, 2010 20392953

Grant BF, Goldstein RB, Saha TD, et al: Epidemiology of DSM-5 alcohol use disorder: results from the National Epidemiologic Survey on Alcohol and Related Conditions III. JAMA Psychiatry 72(8):757–766, 2015 26039070

Griffith JD, Jasinski DR, Casten GP, et al: Investigation of the abuse liability of buspirone in alcohol-dependent patients. Am J Med 80(3B):30–35, 1986 3963032

Gual A, He Y, Torup L, et al: ESENSE 2: a randomized, double-blind, placebo-controlled study of nalmefene, as-needed use in alcohol dependent patients. Alcohol Clin Exp Res 36(S1):246A, 2012

Guerzoni S, Pellesi L, Pini LA, et al: Drug-drug interactions in the treatment for alcohol use disorders: a comprehensive review. Pharmacol Res 133:65–76, 2018 29719204

Haass-Koffler CL, Swift RM, Leggio L: Noradrenergic targets for the treatment of alcohol use disorder. Psychopharmacology (Berl) 235(6):1625–1634, 2018 29460163

Hammarberg A, Jayaram-Lindström N, Beck O, et al: The effects of acamprosate on alcohol-cue reactivity and alcohol priming in dependent patients: a randomized controlled trial. Psychopharmacology (Berl) 205(1):53–62, 2009 19319508

Hansson AC, Koopmann A, Uhrig S, et al: Oxytocin reduces alcohol cue-reactivity in alcohol-dependent rats and humans. Neuropsychopharmacology 43(6):1235–1246, 2018 29090683

Harper KM, Knapp DJ, Butler RK, et al: Amygdala arginine vasopressin modulates chronic ethanol withdrawal anxiety-like behavior in the social interaction task. Alcohol Clin Exp Res 43(10):2134–2143, 2019 31386210

Harris AH, Oliva E, Bowe T, et al: Pharmacotherapy of alcohol use disorders by the Veterans Health Administration: patterns of receipt and persistence. Psychiatr Serv 63(7):679–685, 2012 22549276

Hartwell EE, Feinn R, Morris PE, et al: Systematic review and meta-analysis of the moderating effect of rs1799971 in OPRM1, the mu-opioid receptor gene, on response to naltrexone treatment of alcohol use disorder. Addiction 115(8):1426–1437, 2020 31961981

Hauser P, Fuller B, Ho SB, et al: The safety and efficacy of baclofen to reduce alcohol use in veterans with chronic hepatitis C: a randomized controlled trial. Addiction 112(7):1173–1183, 2017 28192622

Hayashida M, Alterman AI, McLellan AT, et al: Comparative effectiveness and costs of inpatient and outpatient detoxification of patients with mild-to-moderate alcohol withdrawal syndrome. N Engl J Med 320(6):358–365, 1989 2913493

Heaney CF, Kinney JW: Role of GABA(B) receptors in learning and memory and neurological disorders. Neurosci Biobehav Rev 63:1–28, 2016 26814961

Heilig M, Egli M, Crabbe JC, et al: Acute withdrawal, protracted abstinence and negative affect in alcoholism: are they linked? Addict Biol 15(2):169–184, 2010 20148778

Heinz A, Reimold M, Wrase J, et al: Correlation of stable elevations in striatal mu-opioid receptor availability in detoxified alcoholic patients with alcohol craving: a positron emission tomography study using carbon 11-labeled carfentanil. Arch Gen Psychiatry 62(1):57–64, 2005 15630073

Hendricson AW, Maldve RE, Salinas AG, et al: Aberrant synaptic activation of N-methyl-D-aspartate receptors underlies ethanol withdrawal hyperexcitability. J Pharmacol Exp Ther 321(1):60–72, 2007 17229881

Hendrickson LM, Zhao-Shea R, Pang X, et al: Activation of alpha4* nAChRs is necessary and sufficient for varenicline-induced reduction of alcohol consumption. J Neurosci 30(30):10169–10176, 2010 20668200

Hernandez JS, Moorman DE: Orbitofrontal cortex encodes preference for alcohol. eNeuro 7(4):ENEURO.0402-19.2020, 2020 32661066

Hurt RT, Ebbert JO, Croghan IT, et al: Varenicline for tobacco-dependence treatment in alcohol-dependent smokers: a randomized controlled trial. Drug Alcohol Depend 184:12–17, 2018 29324248

Jia F, Pignataro L, Harrison NL: GABAA receptors in the thalamus: alpha4 subunit expression and alcohol sensitivity. Alcohol 41(3):177–185, 2007 17521848

Jiang Y, Zhang T, Kusumanchi P, et al: Alcohol metabolizing enzymes, microsomal ethanol oxidizing system, cytochrome P450 2E1, catalase, and aldehyde dehydrogenase in alcohol-associated liver disease. Biomedicines 8(3):50, 2020 32143280

Jimenez-Gomez C, Winger G, Dean RL, et al: Naltrexone decreases D-amphetamine and ethanol self-administration in rhesus monkeys. Behav Pharmacol 22(1):87–90, 2011 21160425

Jin Z, Bazov I, Kononenko O, et al: Selective changes of GABA(A) channel subunit mRNAs in the hippocampus and orbitofrontal cortex but not in prefrontal cortex of human alcoholics. Front Cell Neurosci 5:30, 2012 22319468

Job MO, Tang A, Hall FS, et al: Mu (µ) opioid receptor regulation of ethanol-induced dopamine response in the ventral striatum: evidence of genotype specific sexual dimorphic epistasis. Biol Psychiatry 62(6):627–634, 2007 17336938

Johnson BA, Ait-Daoud N, Prihoda TJ: Combining ondansetron and naltrexone effectively treats biologically predisposed alcoholics: from hypotheses to preliminary clinical evidence. Alcohol Clin Exp Res 24(5):737–742, 2000a 10832917

Johnson BA, Roache JD, Javors MA, et al: Ondansetron for reduction of drinking among biologically predisposed alcoholic patients: a randomized controlled trial. JAMA 284(8):963–971, 2000b 10944641

Johnson BA, Ait-Daoud N, Bowden CL, et al: Oral topiramate for treatment of alcohol dependence: a randomised controlled trial. Lancet 361(9370):1677–1685, 2003 12767733

Johnson BA, Rosenthal N, Capece JA, et al: Topiramate for treating alcohol dependence: a randomized controlled trial. JAMA 298(14):1641–1651, 2007 17925516

Johnson BA, Ait-Daoud N, Seneviratne C, et al: Pharmacogenetic approach at the serotonin transporter gene as a method of reducing the severity of alcohol drinking. Am J Psychiatry 168(3):265–275, 2011 21247998

Johnson BA, Seneviratne C, Wang X-Q, et al: Determination of genotype combinations that can predict the outcome of the treatment of alcohol dependence using the 5-HT(3) antagonist ondansetron. Am J Psychiatry 170(9):1020–1031, 2013 23897038

Johnson KA, Lovinger DM: Allosteric modulation of metabotropic glutamate receptors in alcohol use disorder: insights from preclinical investigations. Adv Pharmacol 88:193–232, 2020 32416868

Jonas DE, Amick HR, Feltner C, et al: Pharmacotherapy for adults with alcohol use disorders in outpatient settings: a systematic review and meta-analysis. JAMA 311(18):1889–1900, 2014 24825644

Kabel DI, Petty F: A double blind study of fluoxetine in severe alcohol dependence: adjunctive therapy during and after inpatient treatment. Alcohol Clin Exp Res 20:780–784, 1996 8800399

Kampman KM, Pettinati HM, Lynch KG, et al: A double-blind, placebo-controlled pilot trial of quetiapine for the treatment of Type A and Type B alcoholism. J Clin Psychopharmacol 27(4):344–351, 2007 17632217

Karhuvaara S, Simojoki K, Virta A, et al: Targeted nalmefene with simple medical management in the treatment of heavy drinkers: a randomized double-blind placebo-controlled multicenter study. Alcohol Clin Exp Res 31(7):1179–1187, 2007 17451401
Karkhanis AN, Huggins KN, Rose JH, et al: Switch from excitatory to inhibitory actions of ethanol on dopamine levels after chronic exposure: role of kappa opioid receptors. Neuropharmacology 110(Pt A):190–197, 2016 27450094
Karpyak VM, Winham SJ, Preuss UW, et al: Association of the PDYN gene with alcohol dependence and the propensity to drink in negative emotional states. Int J Neuropsychopharmacol 16(5):975–985, 2013 23101464
Karpyak VM, Biernacka JM, Geske JR, et al: Genetic markers associated with abstinence length in alcohol-dependent subjects treated with acamprosate. Transl Psychiatry 4(10):e462, 2014 25290263
Kelly EA, Fudge JL: The neuroanatomic complexity of the CRF and DA systems and their interface: what we still don't know. Neurosci Biobehav Rev 90:247–259, 2018 29704516
Kiefer F, Jahn H, Tarnaske T, et al: Comparing and combining naltrexone and acamprosate in relapse prevention of alcoholism: a double-blind, placebo-controlled study. Arch Gen Psychiatry 60(1):92–99, 2003 12511176
Kiefer F, Witt SH, Frank J, et al: Involvement of the atrial natriuretic peptide transcription factor GATA4 in alcohol dependence, relapse risk and treatment response to acamprosate. Pharmacogenomics J 11(5):368–374, 2011 20585342
Kim JJ, Gharpure A, Teng J, et al: Shared structural mechanisms of general anaesthetics and benzodiazepines. Nature 585(7824):303–308, 2020 32879488
King A, Munisamy G, de Wit H, et al: Attenuated cortisol response to alcohol in heavy social drinkers. Int J Psychophysiol 59(3):203–209, 2006 16359745
Kishi T, Sevy S, Chekuri R, et al: Antipsychotics for primary alcohol dependence: a systematic review and meta-analysis of placebo-controlled trials. J Clin Psychiatry 74(7):e642–e654, 2013 23945459
Kline NS, Wren JC, Cooper TB, et al: Evaluation of lithium therapy in chronic and periodic alcoholism. Am J Med Sci 268(1):15–22, 1974 4606532
Knapp CM, Sarid-Segal O, Richardson MA, et al: Open label trial of the tolerability and efficacy of zonisamide in the treatment of alcohol dependence. Am J Drug Alcohol Abuse 36(2):102–105, 2010 20337506
Knapp CM, Ciraulo DA, Sarid-Segal O, et al: Zonisamide, topiramate, and levetiracetam: efficacy and neuropsychological effects in alcohol use disorders. J Clin Psychopharmacol 35(1):34–42, 2015 25427171

Knapp DJ, Pohorecky LA: Zacopride, a 5-HT3 receptor antagonist, reduces voluntary ethanol consumption in rats. Pharmacol Biochem Behav 41(4):847–850, 1992 1594653

Knox J, Hasin DS, Larson FRR, et al: Prevention, screening, and treatment for heavy drinking and alcohol use disorder. Lancet Psychiatry 6(12):1054–1067, 2019 31630982

Koob GF: Neurobiology of opioid addiction: opponent process, hyperkatifeia, and negative reinforcement. Biol Psychiatry 87(1):44–53, 2020 31400808

Koob GF, Volkow ND: Neurobiology of addiction: a neurocircuitry analysis. Lancet Psychiatry 3(8):760–773, 2016 27475769

Kotlinska J, Bochenski M: The influence of various glutamate receptors antagonists on anxiety-like effect of ethanol withdrawal in a plus-maze test in rats. Eur J Pharmacol 598(1–3):57–63, 2008 18838071

Kranzler HR, Soyka M: Diagnosis and pharmacotherapy of alcohol use disorder: a review. JAMA 320(8):815–824, 2018 30167705

Kranzler H, Tinsley J (eds): Dual Diagnosis and Psychiatric Treatment: Substance Abuse and Comorbid Disorders, 2nd Edition. New York, Marcel Dekker, 2004

Kranzler HR, Van Kirk J: Efficacy of naltrexone and acamprosate for alcoholism treatment: a meta-analysis. Alcohol Clin Exp Res 25(9):1335–1341, 2001 11584154

Kranzler HR, Burleson JA, Del Boca FK, et al: Buspirone treatment of anxious alcoholics: a placebo-controlled trial. Arch Gen Psychiatry 51(9):720–731, 1994 8080349

Kranzler HR, Burleson JA, Korner P, et al: Placebo-controlled trial of fluoxetine as an adjunct to relapse prevention in alcoholics. Am J Psychiatry 152(3):391–397, 1995 7864265

Kranzler HR, Burleson JA, Brown J, et al: Fluoxetine treatment seems to reduce the beneficial effects of cognitive-behavioral therapy in type B alcoholics. Alcohol Clin Exp Res 20(9):1534–1541, 1996 8986200

Kranzler HR, Tennen H, Penta C, et al: Targeted naltrexone treatment of early problem drinkers. Addict Behav 22(3):431–436, 1997 9183513

Kranzler HR, Modesto-Lowe V, Nuwayser ES: Sustained-release naltrexone for alcoholism treatment: a preliminary study. Alcohol Clin Exp Res 22(5):1074–1079, 1998 9726277

Kranzler HR, Pierucci-Lagha A, Feinn R, et al: Effects of ondansetron in early- versus late-onset alcoholics: a prospective, open-label study. Alcohol Clin Exp Res 27(7):1150–1155, 2003 12878921

Kranzler HR, Wesson DR, Billot L: Naltrexone depot for treatment of alcohol dependence: a multicenter, randomized, placebo-controlled clinical trial. Alcohol Clin Exp Res 28(7):1051–1059, 2004 15252291

Kranzler HR, Covault J, Pierucci-Lagha A, et al: Effects of aripiprazole on subjective and physiological responses to alcohol. Alcohol Clin Exp Res 32(4):573–579, 2008 18261195

Kranzler HR, Tennen H, Armeli S, et al: Targeted naltrexone for problem drinkers. J Clin Psychopharmacol 29(4):350–357, 2009 19593174

Kranzler HR, Armeli S, Tennen H, et al: A double-blind, randomized trial of sertraline for alcohol dependence: moderation by age of onset [corrected] and 5-hydroxytryptamine transporter-linked promoter region genotype. J Clin Psychopharmacol 31(1):22–30, 2011 21192139

Kranzler HR, Armeli S, Tennen H: Post-treatment outcomes in a double-blind, randomized trial of sertraline for alcohol dependence. Alcohol Clin Exp Res 36(4):739–744, 2012 21981418

Kranzler HR, Covault J, Feinn R, et al: Topiramate treatment for heavy drinkers: moderation by a GRIK1 polymorphism. Am J Psychiatry 171(4):445–452, 2014 24525690

Kranzler HR, Feinn R, Morris P, et al: A meta-analysis of the efficacy of gabapentin for treating alcohol use disorder. Addiction 114(9):1547–1555, 2019a 31077485

Kranzler HR, Zhou H, Kember RL, et al: Genome-wide association study of alcohol consumption and use disorder in 274,424 individuals from multiple populations. Nat Commun 10(1):1499, 2019b 30940813

Kranzler HR, Hartwell EE, Feinn R, et al: Combined analysis of the moderating effect of a GRIK1 polymorphism on the effects of topiramate for treating alcohol use disorder. Drug Alcohol Depend 225:108762, 2021a 34049101

Kranzler HR, Morris PE, Pond T, et al: Prospective randomized pharmacogenetic study of topiramate for treating alcohol use disorder. Neuropsychopharmacology 46(8):1407–1413, 2021b 33568796

Krystal JH, Webb E, Cooney N, et al: Specificity of ethanol-like effects elicited by serotonergic and noradrenergic mechanisms. Arch Gen Psychiatry 51(11):898–911, 1994 7944878

Krystal JH, Cramer JA, Krol WF, et al: Naltrexone in the treatment of alcohol dependence. N Engl J Med 345(24):1734–1739, 2001 11742047

Läck AK, Ariwodola OJ, Chappell AM, et al: Ethanol inhibition of kainate receptor-mediated excitatory neurotransmission in the rat basolateral nucleus of the amygdala. Neuropharmacology 55(5):661–668, 2008 18617194

Lai JY, Kalk N, Roberts E: The effectiveness and tolerability of anti-seizure medication in alcohol withdrawal syndrome: a systematic review, meta-analysis and GRADE of the evidence. Addiction 117(1):5–18, 2022 33822427

Lawrence AJ, Cowen MS, Yang HJ, et al: The orexin system regulates alcohol-seeking in rats. Br J Pharmacol 148(6):752–759, 2006 16751790

Leurquin-Sterk G, Ceccarini J, Crunelle CL, et al: Lower limbic metabotropic glutamate receptor 5 availability in alcohol dependence. J Nucl Med 59(4):682–690, 2018 29348321

Lhuintre JP, Daoust M, Moore ND, et al: Ability of calcium bis acetyl homotaurine, a GABA agonist, to prevent relapse in weaned alcoholics. Lancet 1(8436):1014–1016, 1985 2859465

Litten RZ, Fertig JB, Falk DE, et al: A double-blind, placebo-controlled trial to assess the efficacy of quetiapine fumarate XR in very heavy-drinking alcohol-dependent patients. Alcohol Clin Exp Res 36(3):406–416, 2012 21950727

Litten RZ, Ryan ML, Fertig JB, et al: A double-blind, placebo-controlled trial assessing the efficacy of varenicline tartrate for alcohol dependence. J Addict Med 7(4):277–286, 2013 23728065

Livne O, Feinn R, Knox J, et al: Alcohol withdrawal in past-year drinkers with unhealthy alcohol use: prevalence, characteristics, and correlates in a national epidemiologic survey. Alcohol Clin Exp Res 46(3):422–433, 2022 35275407

Lopez MF, Moorman DE, Aston-Jones G, et al: The highly selective orexin/hypocretin 1 receptor antagonist GSK1059865 potently reduces ethanol drinking in ethanol dependent mice. Brain Res 1636:74–80, 2016 26851547

Lovinger DM, Roberto M: Synaptic effects induced by alcohol. Curr Top Behav Neurosci 13:31–86, 2013 21786203

Lovinger DM, White G, Weight FF: Ethanol inhibits NMDA-activated ion current in hippocampal neurons. Science 243(4899):1721–1724, 1989 2467382

Lowery-Gionta EG, Marcinkiewcz CA, Kash TL: Functional alterations in the dorsal raphe nucleus following acute and chronic ethanol exposure. Neuropsychopharmacology 40(3):590–600, 2015 25120075

Malcolm R, Anton RF, Randall CL, et al: A placebo-controlled trial of buspirone in anxious inpatient alcoholics. Alcohol Clin Exp Res 16(6):1007–1013, 1992 1335217

Maldonado JR, Sher Y, Ashouri JF, et al: The "Prediction of Alcohol Withdrawal Severity Scale" (PAWSS): systematic literature review and pilot study of a new scale for the prediction of complicated alcohol withdrawal syndrome. Alcohol 48(4):375–390, 2014 24657098

Mann K, Kiefer F, Spanagel R, et al: Acamprosate: recent findings and future research directions. Alcohol Clin Exp Res 32(7):1105–1110, 2008 18540918

Mann K, Kiefer F, Smolka M, et al: Searching for responders to acamprosate and naltrexone in alcoholism treatment: rationale and design of the PREDICT study. Alcohol Clin Exp Res 33(4):674–683, 2009 19170666

Mann K, Bladstrom A, Torup L, et al: Shifting the paradigm: ESENSE1: a randomized, double-blind, placebo controlled study of nalmefene, as-needed use in alcohol dependent patients. Alcohol Clin Exp Res 36(S1):246A, 2012

Manolio TA, Collins FS, Cox NJ, et al: Finding the missing heritability of complex diseases. Nature 461(7265):747–753, 2009 19812666

Maranville JC, Cox NJ: Pharmacogenomic variants have larger effect sizes than genetic variants associated with other dichotomous complex traits. Pharmacogenomics J 16(4):388–392, 2016 26149738

Marcinkiewcz CA, Dorrier CE, Lopez AJ, et al: Ethanol induced adaptations in 5-HT2c receptor signaling in the bed nucleus of the stria terminalis: implications for anxiety during ethanol withdrawal. Neuropharmacology 89:157–167, 2015 25229718

Mark TL, Kranzler HR, Song X, et al: Physicians' opinions about medications to treat alcoholism. Addiction 98(5):617–626, 2003 12751979

Mason BJ, Ritvo EC, Morgan RO, et al: A double-blind, placebo-controlled pilot study to evaluate the efficacy and safety of oral nalmefene HCl for alcohol dependence. Alcohol Clin Exp Res 18(5):1162–1167, 1994 7847600

Mason BJ, Salvato FR, Williams LD, et al: A double-blind, placebo-controlled study of oral nalmefene for alcohol dependence. Arch Gen Psychiatry 56(8):719–724, 1999 10435606

Mason BJ, Goodman AM, Chabac S, et al: Effect of oral acamprosate on abstinence in patients with alcohol dependence in a double-blind, placebo-controlled trial: the role of patient motivation. J Psychiatr Res 40(5):383–393, 2006 16546214

Mason BJ, Quello S, Goodell V, et al: Gabapentin treatment for alcohol dependence: a randomized clinical trial. JAMA Intern Med 174(1):70–77, 2014 24190578

Mattila MJ, Aranko K, Seppala T: Acute effects of buspirone and alcohol on psychomotor skills. J Clin Psychiatry 43(12 Pt 2):56–61, 1982 6130074

Meert TF: Effects of various serotonergic agents on alcohol intake and alcohol preference in Wistar rats selected at two different levels of alcohol preference. Alcohol Alcohol 28(2):157–170, 1993 8517886

Meinhardt MW, Hansson AC, Perreau-Lenz S, et al: Rescue of infralimbic mGluR2 deficit restores control over drug-seeking behavior in alcohol dependence. J Neurosci 33(7):2794–2806, 2013 23407939

Melby K, Gråwe RW, Aamo TO, et al: Efficacy of self-administered intranasal oxytocin on alcohol use and craving after detoxification in patients with alcohol dependence: a double-blind placebo-controlled trial. Alcohol Alcohol 56(5):565–572, 2021 33352584

Melis M, Enrico P, Peana AT, et al: Acetaldehyde mediates alcohol activation of the mesolimbic dopamine system. Eur J Neurosci 26(10):2824–2833, 2007 18001279

Merry J, Reynolds CM, Bailey J, et al: Prophylactic treatment of alcoholism by lithium carbonate: a controlled study. Lancet 1(7984):481–482, 1976 74457

Meyer R: How to understand the relationship between psychopathology and addictive disorders: another example of the chicken and the egg, in Psychopathology and Addictive Disorders. Edited by Meyer R. New York, Guilford, 1986, pp 3–16

Miller CN, Kamens HM: The role of nicotinic acetylcholine receptors in alcohol-related behaviors. Brain Res Bull 163:135–142, 2020 32707263

Minozzi S, Saulle R, Rösner S: Baclofen for alcohol use disorder. Cochrane Database Syst Rev 11(11):CD012557, 2018 30484285

Miranda R Jr, O'Malley SS, Treloar Padovano H, et al: Effects of alcohol cue reactivity on subsequent treatment outcomes among treatment-seeking individuals with alcohol use disorder: a multisite randomized, double-blind, placebo-controlled clinical trial of varenicline. Alcohol Clin Exp Res 44(7):1431–1443, 2020 32363592

Mirijello A, D'Angelo C, Ferrulli A, et al: Identification and management of alcohol withdrawal syndrome. Drugs 75(4):353–365, 2015 25666543

Mitchell JM, O'Neil JP, Janabi M, et al: Alcohol consumption induces endogenous opioid release in the human orbitofrontal cortex and nucleus accumbens. Sci Transl Med 4(116):116ra6, 2012 22238334

Mitchell MC Jr, Teigen EL, Ramchandani VA: Absorption and peak blood alcohol concentration after drinking beer, wine, or spirits. Alcohol Clin Exp Res 38(5):1200–1204, 2014 24655007

Morley KC, Teesson M, Reid SC, et al: Naltrexone versus acamprosate in the treatment of alcohol dependence: a multi-centre, randomized, double-blind, placebo-controlled trial. Addiction 101(10):1451–1462, 2006 16968347

Morley KC, Luquin N, Baillie A, et al: Moderation of baclofen response by a GABAB receptor polymorphism: results from the BacALD randomized controlled trial. Addiction 113(12):2205–2213, 2018 29968397

Mueller TI, Stout RL, Rudden S, et al: A double-blind, placebo-controlled pilot study of carbamazepine for the treatment of alcohol dependence. Alcohol Clin Exp Res 21(1):86–92, 1997 9046378

Myrick H, Anton RF, Li X, et al: Effect of naltrexone and ondansetron on alcohol cue-induced activation of the ventral striatum in alcohol-dependent people. Arch Gen Psychiatry 65(4):466–475, 2008 18391135

Myrick H, Li X, Randall PK, et al: The effect of aripiprazole on cue-induced brain activation and drinking parameters in alcoholics. J Clin Psychopharmacol 30(4):365–372, 2010 20571434

Naranjo C, Sellers E: Clinical assessment and pharmacotherapy of the alcohol withdrawal syndrome, in Recent Developments in Alcoholism, Vol 4. Edited by Galanter M. New York, Plenum, 1986, pp 265–281

Naranjo CA, Sellers EM, Sullivan JT, et al: The serotonin uptake inhibitor citalopram attenuates ethanol intake. Clin Pharmacol Ther 41(3):266–274, 1987 3469057

Naranjo CA, Kadlec KE, Sanhueza P, et al: Fluoxetine differentially alters alcohol intake and other consummatory behaviors in problem drinkers. Clin Pharmacol Ther 47(4):490–498, 1990 2328557

Naranjo CA, Poulos CX, Bremner KE, et al: Citalopram decreases desirability, liking, and consumption of alcohol in alcohol-dependent drinkers. Clin Pharmacol Ther 51(6):729–739, 1992 1535302

Naranjo CA, Bremner KE, Lanctôt KL: Effects of citalopram and a brief psychosocial intervention on alcohol intake, dependence and problems. Addiction 90(1):87–99, 1995 7888983

Neumann ID, Landgraf R: Balance of brain oxytocin and vasopressin: implications for anxiety, depression, and social behaviors. Trends Neurosci 35(11):649–659, 2012 22974560

Nie H, Rewal M, Gill TM, et al: Extrasynaptic delta-containing GABAA receptors in the nucleus accumbens dorsomedial shell contribute to alcohol intake. Proc Natl Acad Sci USA 108(11):4459–4464, 2011 21368141

Niswender CM, Conn PJ: Metabotropic glutamate receptors: physiology, pharmacology, and disease. Annu Rev Pharmacol Toxicol 50:295–322, 2010 20055706

Nobis WP, Kash TL, Silberman Y, et al: β-Adrenergic receptors enhance excitatory transmission in the bed nucleus of the stria terminalis through a corticotrophin-releasing factor receptor-dependent and cocaine-regulated mechanism. Biol Psychiatry 69(11):1083–1090, 2011 21334600

Nunes EV, Levin FR: Treatment of depression in patients with alcohol or other drug dependence: a meta-analysis. JAMA 291(15):1887–1896, 2004 15100209

Oberlin BG, Dzemidzic M, Tran SM, et al: Beer self-administration provokes lateralized nucleus accumbens dopamine release in male heavy drinkers. Psychopharmacology (Berl) 232(5):861–870, 2015 25163422

Oberto A, Panzica GC, Altruda F, et al: GABAergic and NPY-Y(1) network in the medial amygdala: a neuroanatomical basis for their functional interaction. Neuropharmacology 41(5):639–642, 2001 11587719

O'Farrell TJ, Allen JP, Litten RZ: Disulfiram (Antabuse) contracts in treatment of alcoholism. NIDA Res Monogr 150:65–91, 1995 8742773

Olsen RW, Sieghart W: GABA-A receptors: subtypes provide diversity of function and pharmacology. Neuropharmacology 56(1):141–148, 2009 18760291

O'Malley SS, Jaffe AJ, Chang G, et al: Naltrexone and coping skills therapy for alcohol dependence: a controlled study. Arch Gen Psychiatry 49(11):881–887, 1992 1444726

O'Malley SS, Jaffe AJ, Chang G, et al: Six-month follow-up of naltrexone and psychotherapy for alcohol dependence. Arch Gen Psychiatry 53(3):217–224, 1996 8611058

O'Malley SS, Garbutt JC, Gastfriend DR, et al: Efficacy of extended-release naltrexone in alcohol-dependent patients who are abstinent before treatment. J Clin Psychopharmacol 27(5):507–512, 2007 17873686

Ooteman W, Naassila M, Koeter MWJ, et al: Predicting the effect of naltrexone and acamprosate in alcohol-dependent patients using genetic indicators. Addict Biol 14(3):328–337, 2009 19523047

Oslin DW, Berrettini W, Kranzler HR, et al: A functional polymorphism of the mu-opioid receptor gene is associated with naltrexone response in alcohol-dependent patients. Neuropsychopharmacology 28(8):1546–1552, 2003 12813472

Oslin DW, Leong SH, Lynch KG, et al: Naltrexone vs placebo for the treatment of alcohol dependence: a randomized clinical trial. JAMA Psychiatry 72(5):430–437, 2015 25760804

Overstreet DH, Knapp DJ, Breese GR: Modulation of multiple ethanol withdrawal-induced anxiety-like behavior by CRF and CRF1 receptors. Pharmacol Biochem Behav 77(2):405–413, 2004 14751471

Paille FM, Guelfi JD, Perkins AC, et al: Double-blind randomized multicentre trial of acamprosate in maintaining abstinence from alcohol. Alcohol Alcohol 30(2):239–247, 1995 7662044

Palpacuer C, Duprez R, Huneau A, et al: Pharmacologically controlled drinking in the treatment of alcohol dependence or alcohol use disorders: a systematic review with direct and network meta-analyses on nalmefene, naltrexone, acamprosate, baclofen and topiramate. Addiction 113(2):220–237, 2018 28940866

Parale MP, Kulkarni SK: Studies with alpha 2-adrenoceptor agonists and alcohol abstinence syndrome in rats. Psychopharmacology (Berl) 88(2):237–239, 1986 2869542

Pathak S, Jiang Y, DiPetrillo L, et al: Course of psychosis in schizophrenia with alcohol use disorder: a post hoc analysis of the Clinical Antipsychotic Trials of Intervention Effectiveness in Schizophrenia Phase 1 study. J Clin Psychiatry 81(2):19m12731, 2020 32220153

Pedersen CA, Smedley KL, Leserman J, et al: Intranasal oxytocin blocks alcohol withdrawal in human subjects. Alcohol Clin Exp Res 37(3):484–489, 2013 23025690

Pelc I, Verbanck P, Le Bon O, et al: Efficacy and safety of acamprosate in the treatment of detoxified alcohol-dependent patients: a 90-day placebo-controlled dose-finding study. Br J Psychiatry 171:73–77, 1997 9328500

Peters ST, Bowen MT, Bohrer K, et al: Oxytocin inhibits ethanol consumption and ethanol-induced dopamine release in the nucleus accumbens. Addict Biol 22(3):702–711, 2017 26810371

Pettinati HM, Volpicelli JR, Kranzler HR, et al: Sertraline treatment for alcohol dependence: interactive effects of medication and alcoholic subtype. Alcohol Clin Exp Res 24(7):1041–1049, 2000 10924008

Pettinati HM, Oslin DW, Kampman KM, et al: A double-blind, placebo-controlled trial combining sertraline and naltrexone for treating co-occurring depression and alcohol dependence. Am J Psychiatry 167(6):668–675, 2010 20231324

Peyron C, Tighe DK, van den Pol AN, et al: Neurons containing hypocretin (orexin) project to multiple neuronal systems. J Neurosci 18(23):9996–10015, 1998 9822755

Pierce M, Sutterland A, Beraha EM, et al: Efficacy, tolerability, and safety of low-dose and high-dose baclofen in the treatment of alcohol dependence: a systematic review and meta-analysis. Eur Neuropsychopharmacol 28(7):795–806, 2018 29934090

Pleil KE, Lopez A, McCall N, et al: Chronic stress alters neuropeptide Y signaling in the bed nucleus of the stria terminalis in DBA/2J but not C57BL/6J mice. Neuropharmacology 62(4):1777–1786, 2012 22182779

Quijano Cardé NA, Perez EE, Feinn R, et al: Antagonism of GluK1-containing kainate receptors reduces ethanol consumption by modulating ethanol reward and withdrawal. Neuropharmacology 199:108783, 2021 34509497

Ramachandra V, Kang F, Kim C, et al: The μ opioid receptor is not involved in ethanol-stimulated dopamine release in the ventral striatum of C57BL/6J mice. Alcohol Clin Exp Res 35(5):929–938, 2011 21294756

Ray LA, Miranda R Jr, MacKillop J, et al: A preliminary pharmacogenetic investigation of adverse events from topiramate in heavy drinkers. Exp Clin Psychopharmacol 17(2):122–129, 2009 19331489

Ray LA, Bujarski S, Squeglia LM, et al: Interactive effects of OPRM1 and DAT1 genetic variation on subjective responses to alcohol. Alcohol Alcohol 49(3):261–270, 2014 24421289

Ray LA, Green R, Roche DJO, et al: Naltrexone effects on subjective responses to alcohol in the human laboratory: a systematic review and meta-analysis. Addict Biol 24(6):1138–1152, 2019 31148304

Reus VI, Fochtmann LJ, Bukstein O, et al: The American Psychiatric Association Practice Guideline for the Pharmacological Treatment of Patients With Alcohol Use Disorder. Am J Psychiatry 175(1):86–90, 2018 29301420

Rewal M, Donahue R, Gill TM, et al: Alpha4 subunit-containing GABAA receptors in the accumbens shell contribute to the reinforcing effects of alcohol. Addict Biol 17(2):309–321, 2012 21507158

Reynaud M, Aubin HJ, Trinquet F, et al: A randomized, placebo-controlled study of high-dose baclofen in alcohol-dependent patients: the ALPADIR Study. Alcohol Alcohol 52(4):439–446, 2017 28525555

Richard JM, Fields HL: Mu-opioid receptor activation in the medial shell of nucleus accumbens promotes alcohol consumption, self-administration and cue-induced reinstatement. Neuropharmacology 108:14–23, 2016 27089981

Richardson K, Baillie A, Reid S, et al: Do acamprosate or naltrexone have an effect on daily drinking by reducing craving for alcohol? Addiction 103(6):953–959, 2008 18482418

Roberts W, Harrison ELR, McKee SA: Effects of varenicline on alcohol cue reactivity in heavy drinkers. Psychopharmacology (Berl) 234(18):2737–2745, 2017 28600734

Robinson SL, Thiele TE: The role of neuropeptide Y (NPY) in alcohol and drug abuse disorders. Int Rev Neurobiol 136:177–197, 2017 29056151

Rodd ZA, Bell RL, Zhang Y, et al: Regional heterogeneity for the intracranial self-administration of ethanol and acetaldehyde within the ventral tegmental area of alcohol-preferring (P) rats: involvement of dopamine and serotonin. Neuropsychopharmacology 30(2):330–338, 2005 15383830

Rodd ZA, Oster SM, Ding ZM, et al: The reinforcing properties of salsolinol in the ventral tegmental area: evidence for regional heterogeneity and the involvement of serotonin and dopamine. Alcohol Clin Exp Res 32(2):230–239, 2008 18162075

Rose JH, Karkhanis AN, Chen R, et al: Supersensitive kappa opioid receptors promotes ethanol withdrawal-related behaviors and reduce dopamine signaling in the nucleus accumbens. Int J Neuropsychopharmacol 19(5):pyv127, 2016 26625893

Rösner S, Hackl-Herrwerth A, Leucht S, et al: Acamprosate for alcohol dependence. Cochrane Database Syst Rev 2010(9):CD004332, 2010a 20824837

Rösner S, Hackl-Herrwerth A, Leucht S, et al: Opioid antagonists for alcohol dependence. Cochrane Database Syst Rev (12):CD001867, 2010b 21154349

Rubio G, Jiménez-Arriero MA, Ponce G, et al: Naltrexone versus acamprosate: one year follow-up of alcohol dependence treatment. Alcohol Alcohol 36(5):419–425, 2001 11524308

Rubio G, López-Muñoz F, Ponce G, et al: Zonisamide versus diazepam in the treatment of alcohol withdrawal syndrome. Pharmacopsychiatry 43(7):257–262, 2010 20927698

Ruby CL, Adams CA, Knight EJ, et al: An essential role for adenosine signaling in alcohol abuse. Curr Drug Abuse Rev 3(3):163–174, 2010 21054262

Ryan ML, Falk DE, Fertig JB, et al: A Phase 2, double-blind, placebo-controlled randomized trial assessing the efficacy of ABT-436, a novel V1b receptor antagonist, for alcohol dependence. Neuropsychopharmacology 42(5):1012–1023, 2017 27658483

Saitz R, Mayo-Smith MF, Roberts MS, et al: Individualized treatment for alcohol withdrawal: a randomized double-blind controlled trial. JAMA 272(7):519–523, 1994 8046805

Sakurai T, Amemiya A, Ishii M, et al: Orexins and orexin receptors: a family of hypothalamic neuropeptides and G protein-coupled receptors that regulate feeding behavior. Cell 92(4):573–585, 1998 9491897

Salloum IM, Cornelius JR, Daley DC, et al: Efficacy of valproate maintenance in patients with bipolar disorder and alcoholism: a double-blind placebo-controlled study. Arch Gen Psychiatry 62(1):37–45, 2005 15630071

Sanchis-Segura C, Borchardt T, Vengeliene V, et al: Involvement of the AMPA receptor GluR-C subunit in alcohol-seeking behavior and relapse. J Neurosci 26(4):1231–1238, 2006 16436610

Sarid-Segal O, Knapp CM, Burch W, et al: The anticonvulsant zonisamide reduces ethanol self-administration by risky drinkers. Am J Drug Alcohol Abuse 35(5):316–319, 2009 19637104

Sass H, Soyka M, Mann K, et al: Relapse prevention by acamprosate: results from a placebo-controlled study on alcohol dependence. Arch Gen Psychiatry 53(8):673–680, 1996; erratum: Arch Gen Psychiatry 53(12):1097, 1996 8694680

Schacht JP, Randall PK, Latham PK, et al: Predictors of naltrexone response in a randomized trial: reward-related brain activation, OPRM1 genotype, and smoking status. Neuropsychopharmacology 42(13):2640–2653, 2017 28409564

Schadé A, Marquenie LA, van Balkom AJ, et al: The effectiveness of anxiety treatment on alcohol-dependent patients with a comorbid phobic disorder: a randomized controlled trial. Alcohol Clin Exp Res 29(5):794–800, 2005 15897725

Schuckit M: Alcoholic patients with secondary depression. Am J Psychiatry 140(6):711–714, 1983 6846629

Schuckit MA: Alcohol and alcohol use disorders, in Harrison's Principles of Internal Medicine, 20th Edition. Edited by Jameson J, Fauci AS, Kasper DL, et al. New York, McGraw Hill, 2018

Seneviratne C, Huang W, Ait-Daoud N, et al: Characterization of a functional polymorphism in the 3' UTR of SLC6A4 and its association with drinking intensity. Alcohol Clin Exp Res 33(2):332–339, 2009 19032574

Seppälä T, Aranko K, Mattila MJ, et al: Effects of alcohol on buspirone and lorazepam actions. Clin Pharmacol Ther 32(2):201–207, 1982 6124334

Siciliano CAN, Karkhanis AN, Holleran KM, et al: Cross-species alterations in synaptic dopamine regulation after chronic alcohol exposure. Handb Exp Pharmacol 248:213–238, 2018 29675581

Simpson TL, Saxon AJ, Stappenbeck C, et al: Double-blind randomized clinical trial of prazosin for alcohol use disorder. Am J Psychiatry 175(12):1216–1224, 2018 30153753

Skinner MD, Lahmek P, Pham H, et al: Disulfiram efficacy in the treatment of alcohol dependence: a meta-analysis. PLoS One 9(2):e87366, 2014 24520330

Sloan ME, Klepp TD, Gowin JL, et al: The OPRM1 A118G polymorphism: converging evidence against associations with alcohol sensitivity and consumption. Neuropsychopharmacology 43(7):1530–1538, 2018 29497164

Smith RJ, Aston-Jones G: Noradrenergic transmission in the extended amygdala: role in increased drug-seeking and relapse during protracted drug abstinence. Brain Struct Funct 213(1–2):43–61, 2008 18651175

Smith RV, Havens JR, Walsh SL: Gabapentin misuse, abuse and diversion: a systematic review. Addiction 111(7):1160–1174, 2016 27265421

Snyder AE, Salimando GJ, Winder DG, et al: Chronic intermittent ethanol and acute stress similarly modulate BNST CRF neuron activity via noradrenergic signaling. Alcohol Clin Exp Res 43(8):1695–1701, 2019 31141179

Sokolow L, Welte J, Hynes G, et al: Multiple substance use by alcoholics. Br J Addict 76(2):147–158, 1981 6944083

Spanagel R: Alcoholism: a systems approach from molecular physiology to addictive behavior. Physiol Rev 89(2):649–705, 2009 19342616

Srinivasan S, Simms JA, Nielsen CK, et al: The dual orexin/hypocretin receptor antagonist, almorexant, in the ventral tegmental area attenuates ethanol self-administration. PLoS One 7(9):e44726, 2012 23028593

Srisurapanont M, Jarusuraisin N: Naltrexone for the treatment of alcoholism: a meta-analysis of randomized controlled trials. Int J Neuropsychopharmacol 8(2):267–280, 2005 15850502

Stokes PRA, Jokinen T, Amawi S, et al: Pharmacological treatment of mood disorders and comorbid addictions: a systematic review and meta-analysis. Can J Psychiatry 65(11):749–769, 2020 32302221

Sullivan JT, Sykora K, Schneiderman J, et al: Assessment of alcohol withdrawal: the revised Clinical Institute Withdrawal Assessment for Alcohol Scale (CIWA-Ar). Br J Addict 84(11):1353–1357, 1989 2597811

Sullivan L, O'Connor P: Medical disorders in substance abuse patients, in Dual Diagnosis and Psychiatric Treatment: Substance Abuse and Comorbid

Disorders, 2nd Edition. Edited by Kranzler H, Tinsley J. New York, Marcel Dekker, 2004, pp 515–554

Tanaka M, Yamada S, Watanabe Y: The role of neuropeptide Y in the nucleus accumbens. Int J Mol Sci 22(14):7287, 2021 34298907

Thomas SE, Randall PK, Book SW, et al: A complex relationship between co-occurring social anxiety and alcohol use disorders: what effect does treating social anxiety have on drinking? Alcohol Clin Exp Res 32(1):77–84, 2008 18028529

Tiihonen J, Ryynänen OP, Kauhanen J, et al: Citalopram in the treatment of alcoholism: a double-blind placebo-controlled study. Pharmacopsychiatry 29(1):27–29, 1996 8852531

Tollefson GD, Montague-Clouse J, Tollefson SL: Treatment of comorbid generalized anxiety in a recently detoxified alcoholic population with a selective serotonergic drug (buspirone). J Clin Psychopharmacol 12(1):19–26, 1992 1552035

Tomkins DM, Le AD, Sellers EM: Effect of the 5-HT3 antagonist ondansetron on voluntary ethanol intake in rats and mice maintained on a limited access procedure. Psychopharmacology (Berl) 117(4):479–485, 1995 7604151

Umhau JC, Schwandt ML, Usala J, et al: Pharmacologically induced alcohol craving in treatment seeking alcoholics correlates with alcoholism severity, but is insensitive to acamprosate. Neuropsychopharmacology 36(6):1178–1186, 2011 21289601

Urban NB, Kegeles LS, Slifstein M, et al: Sex differences in striatal dopamine release in young adults after oral alcohol challenge: a positron emission tomography imaging study with [11C]raclopride. Biol Psychiatry 68(8):689–696, 2010 20678752

U.S. Department of Veterans Affairs, U.S. Department of Defense: VA/DoD Clinical Practice Guideline for the Management of Substance Use Disorders. Washington, DC, Department of Veterans Affairs, Department of Defense, 2015. Available at: https://www.healthquality.va.gov/guidelines/MH/sud/VADoDSUDCPGFinal1.pdf. Accessed March 26, 2022.

van den Brink W, Sørensen P, Torup L, et al: Long-term efficacy, tolerability and safety of nalmefene as-needed in patients with alcohol dependence: a 1-year, randomised controlled study. J Psychopharmacol 28(8):733–744, 2014 24671340

van den Brink W, Strang J, Gual A, et al: Safety and tolerability of as-needed nalmefene in the treatment of alcohol dependence: results from the Phase III clinical programme. Expert Opin Drug Saf 14(4):495–504, 2015 25652768

Van Nest D, Hernandez NS, Kranzler HR, et al: Effects of LY466195, a selective kainate receptor antagonist, on ethanol preference and drinking in rats. Neurosci Lett 639:8–12, 2017 28013091

Vazey EM, den Hartog CR, Moorman DE: Central noradrenergic interactions with alcohol and regulation of alcohol-related behaviors. Handb Exp Pharmacol 248:239–260, 2018 29687164

Vendruscolo LF, Estey D, Goodell V, et al: Glucocorticoid receptor antagonism decreases alcohol seeking in alcohol-dependent individuals. J Clin Invest 125(8):3193–3197, 2015 26121746

Verplaetse TL, Rasmussen DD, Froehlich JC, et al: Effects of prazosin, an α1-adrenergic receptor antagonist, on the seeking and intake of alcohol and sucrose in alcohol-preferring (P) rats. Alcohol Clin Exp Res 36(5):881–886, 2012 21981346

Vijay A, Cavallo D, Goldberg A, et al: PET imaging reveals lower kappa opioid receptor availability in alcoholics but no effect of age. Neuropsychopharmacology 43(13):2539–2547, 2018 30188515

Volkow ND, Kim SW, Wang GJ, et al: Acute alcohol intoxication decreases glucose metabolism but increases acetate uptake in the human brain. Neuroimage 64:277–283, 2013 22947541

Volpicelli JR, Alterman AI, Hayashida M, et al: Naltrexone in the treatment of alcohol dependence. Arch Gen Psychiatry 49(11):876–880, 1992 1345133

Volpicelli JR, Watson NT, King AC, et al: Effect of naltrexone on alcohol "high" in alcoholics. Am J Psychiatry 152(4):613–615, 1995 7694913

Voronin K, Randall P, Myrick H, et al: Aripiprazole effects on alcohol consumption and subjective reports in a clinical laboratory paradigm: possible influence of self-control. Alcohol Clin Exp Res 32(11):1954–1961, 2008 18782344

Wall ME, Brine DR, Perez-Reyes M: Metabolism and disposition of naltrexone in man after oral and intravenous administration. Drug Metab Dispos 9(4):369–375, 1981 6114837

Wang J, Zhu Y: Different doses of gabapentin formulations for postherpetic neuralgia: a systematical review and meta-analysis of randomized controlled trials. J Dermatolog Treat 28(1):65–77, 2017 27798973

Wiffen PJ, Derry S, Bell RF, et al: Gabapentin for chronic neuropathic pain in adults. Cochrane Database Syst Rev 6(6):CD007938, 2017 28597471

Wilcox CE, Tonigan JS, Bogenschutz MP, et al: A randomized, placebo-controlled, clinical trial of prazosin for the treatment of alcohol use disorder. J Addict Med 12(5):339–345, 2018 29664896

Winsky-Sommerer R, Yamanaka A, Diano S, et al: Interaction between the corticotropin-releasing factor system and hypocretins (orexins): a novel circuit mediating stress response. J Neurosci 24(50):11439–11448, 2004 15601950

Wray NR, Lin T, Austin J, et al: From basic science to clinical application of polygenic risk scores: a primer. JAMA Psychiatry 78(1):101–109, 2021 32997097

Yoder KK, Kareken DA, Regat A, et al: Dopamine D(2) receptor availability is associated with subjective responses to alcohol. J Neurosci 35:15523–15538, 2015

Yoder KK, Albrecht DS, Dzemidzic M, et al: Differences in IV alcohol-induced dopamine release in the ventral striatum of social drinkers and nontreatment-seeking alcoholics. Drug Alcohol Depend 160:163–169, 2016 26832934

Yoshimoto K, Yayama K, Sorimachi Y, et al: Possibility of 5-HT3 receptor involvement in alcohol dependence: a microdialysis study of nucleus accumbens dopamine and serotonin release in rats with chronic alcohol consumption. Alcohol Clin Exp Res 20(9 Suppl):311A–319A, 1996 8986229

Yoshimura A, Kimura M, Nakayama H, et al: Efficacy of disulfiram for the treatment of alcohol dependence assessed with a multicenter randomized controlled trial. Alcohol Clin Exp Res 38(2):572–578, 2014 24117666

Zakhari S: Overview: how is alcohol metabolized by the body? Alcohol Res Health 29(4):245–254, 2006 17718403

Zhou H, Sealock JM, Sanchez-Roige S, et al: Genome-wide meta-analysis of problematic alcohol use in 435,563 individuals yields insights into biology and relationships with other traits. Nat Neurosci 23(7):809–818, 2020 32451486

Zhou Y, Colombo G, Carai MA, et al: Involvement of arginine vasopressin and V1b receptor in alcohol drinking in Sardinian alcohol-preferring rats. Alcohol Clin Exp Res 35(10):1876–1883, 2011 21575018

Zhu S, Noviello CM, Teng J, et al: Structure of a human synaptic GABAA receptor. Nature 559(7712):67–72, 2018 29950725

Zwart R, Carbone AL, Moroni M, et al: Sazetidine-A is a potent and selective agonist at native and recombinant alpha 4beta 2 nicotinic acetylcholine receptors. Mol Pharmacol 73(6):1838–1843, 2008 18367540

4

Cannabis and Cannabinoids

Thanos Rossopoulos, M.D.
Carla Marienfeld, M.D.

The cannabis plant contains various cannabinoid chemicals, which primarily act through the endocannabinoid system but also have effects on other neurotransmitter systems. Cannabinoids can be further classified by their origination as phytocannabinoids (e.g., derived from the cannabis plant), synthetic cannabinoids, and endogenous cannabinoids. The most common phytocannabinoids are tetrahydrocannabinol (THC), which is most responsible for the psychoactive effects, and cannabidiol (CBD), which has minimal psychoactive effects and is increasingly available in a multitude of cosmetic and nutritional products marketed for the treatment of a wide range of conditions. Intoxication can present with a self-described "high," along with several clinically significant and impairing symptoms; this can be treated with nonpharmacological support or aided with the use of anxiolytics and, in some cases, antipsychotics, particularly if cannabis-induced psychosis (CIP) is present. Cessation of chronic use of cannabis can lead to a withdrawal syndrome with significant effects on mood and sleep, which can last up to 2 weeks.

Cannabis use disorder (CUD) includes all the diagnostic features of a substance use disorder but may be missed without adequate screening by clinicians. There are no FDA-approved medications for the treatment of CUD or cannabis withdrawal, but several agents have demonstrated potential benefit in research studies and clinical practice. Several cannabinoid system–based treatments (namely, CBD, fatty-acid amide hydrolase [FAAH] inhibitors, and nabiximols), along with the antiepileptic medication gabapentin, demonstrate some weak evidence for reduction in cannabis use and amelioration of withdrawal symptoms that support their potential clinical use. Certain antipsychotics have demonstrated benefits in reducing cannabis use, whereas some antidepressants, lithium, and lofexidine have demonstrated reductions in withdrawal symptoms. Some studies support the use of naltrexone and varenicline as potential CUD treatment options. N-acetylcysteine (NAC) may be of benefit in the treatment of CUD in adolescents and young adults. In cannabinoid hyperemesis syndrome (CHS), which can present with impairing cycles of vomiting in the setting of cannabis use, conventional antiemetics may largely be ineffective. Hot-water hydrotherapy, topical capsaicin, certain first-generation antipsychotics (namely, haloperidol and droperidol), and some benzodiazepines appear to be most effective for CHS; more studies are needed for all these modalities. Further research is needed for the use of pharmacotherapies for CUD in patients with psychiatric comorbidities and those who are pregnant or breastfeeding. Because there are no FDA-approved medications for CUD, further studies are required for nearly all these drug classes to establish sound clinical recommendations.

Pharmacology and Neurobiology

Cannabis shares characteristics with other addictive substances—that is, reinforcement is mediated via the nucleus accumbens (part of the ventral striatum) (Bossong et al. 2009) and cessation is associated with a withdrawal syndrome (Budney et al. 1999; Haney et al. 1999). THC, the main psychoactive component of cannabis, interacts with cannabinoid receptors (CB_1 and CB_2). In both animal and human self-administration studies, THC was shown to have reinforcing properties (Hart et al. 2005; Justinova et al. 2003). PET data in humans indicated that THC facilitates dopamine release in the striatum (Bossong et al. 2009), thereby sharing a key feature of all agents with a confirmed misuse liability.

The endocannabinoid neurotransmitter system is one of the most widespread systems in the CNS, consisting of two known cannabinoid receptor types (CB_1 and CB_2) and endogenous ligands (endocannabinoids). In mammals, CB_1 receptors are most highly concentrated in the hippocampus, neocortex, basal ganglia, cerebellum, and anterior olfactory nucleus (Glass et al. 1997; Herkenham et al. 1991; Matsuda et al. 1993). This distribution is consistent with the psychoactive effects of cannabis, along with its effects on pain, mood, motivation, and cognition (Piomelli 2003; Viveros et al. 2005). CB_2 receptors, in contrast, are mostly expressed peripherally in immune cells (mediating anti-inflammatory effects), the gastrointestinal tract, and the peripheral nervous system (Gong et al. 2006; Van Sickle et al. 2005).

Cannabinoids—chemicals that interact with cannabinoid receptors—are structurally diverse. They can be classified into three groups: 1) phytocannabinoids, which are produced in the cannabis plant; 2) synthetic cannabinoids, which do not occur in nature but interact with cannabinoid receptors; and 3) endocannabinoids, which are endogenous ligands that interact with cannabinoid receptors (Sun and Bennett 2007). Cannabis plants produce approximately 70 known phytocannabinoids (Radwan et al. 2009). The most important known phytocannabinoids include CBD (a CB_1 and CB_2 antagonist), FAAH inhibitors (FAAH is an endogenous integral membrane enzyme that degrades endocannabinoids), and THC (a CB_1 and CB_2 receptor partial agonist) (Pertwee 2008). The psychotropic effects of cannabis are produced mainly by THC, although other cannabinoids and plant components may modify its effects (Elsohly and Slade 2005). CBD, in contrast, does not appear to produce psychoactive effects. There are many synthetic cannabinoids; the most widely known is the naphthoylindole JWH-018. The best characterized endocannabinoids are 2-arachidonoylglycerol and anandamide, both of which are synthesized and degraded by endogenous enzymes.

In a previous study, chronic THC administration in rats was associated with CB_1 receptor downregulation and desensitization (Breivogel et al. 2003), suggesting a potential mechanism for the development of the withdrawal syndrome in humans. It is hypothesized that following chronic exposure and downregulation of the endocannabinoid system, abstinence leads to an abrupt decrease in endocannabinoid system activity.

Pharmacological strategies using THC or CBD may offer benefit in treatment for CUD, with mechanisms similar to those that have demonstrated efficacy in other substance use disorders (e.g., with nicotine or opioids). An additional strategy is to modulate endocannabinoid concentration. As mentioned earlier in this section, endocannabinoids are degraded by various enzymes; anandamide is degraded by FAAH, and reversal of this may offer a pharmacological target by increasing concentrations of anandamide and opposing the downregulation of the endocannabinoid system that follows chronic THC exposure (D'Souza et al. 2019). Additionally, CB_1 receptors are highly present on γ-aminobutyric acid (GABA)-ergic interneurons and glutamatergic neurons, which may also contribute to the euphoric, anxiolytic, and psychoactive effects (Moreira and Lutz 2008). Modulation of GABA or glutamate systems (via anticonvulsants) is therefore also a potential pharmacological target (Mason et al. 2012; Miranda et al. 2017).

CB_1 is coexpressed with serotonin and dopamine receptors and interacts with the serotonin and dopamine neurotransmitter systems (Best and Regehr 2008; Melis et al. 2004). As such, these systems are potential pharmacological targets for CUD, driving investigation of many of the existing psychotropic medications that modulate these systems.

THC potency varies widely among different samples of cannabis (McLaren et al. 2008), and the ratios of other plant compounds to THC vary as well (Hillig and Mahlberg 2004). Potency is commonly measured by THC content, but the psychoactive effect may also depend on levels of other cannabinoids or plant chemicals (e.g., CBD or terpenes), which may interact with one another to impact the potency, effect, and experience of cannabis.

Synthetic cannabinoid receptor agonists are a large family of chemically unrelated molecules that act on cannabinoid receptors, often with greater potency than that of THC. Synthetic cannabinoids can be found in over-the-counter products marketed as "incense" or "potpourri" ("not intended for human consumption") and sold under labels such as "Spice" and "K2" (U.S. Drug Enforcement Administration 2020). In contrast to THC, which is a partial agonist, many of the synthetic cannabinoids act as full agonists at cannabinoid receptors; this can make them up to 800 times more potent than plant-based cannabinoids, which may yield a higher potential for adverse behavioral effects (Vardakou et al. 2010).

Intoxication and Acute Presentations

Cannabis intoxication can be clinically significant and impairing. Patients describe experiencing a "high feeling" (a sensation of euphoria) as well as sedation, lethargy, impairment in short-term memory, impaired judgment, impaired motor performance, and the sensation that time is passing slowly. Occasionally, anxiety, dysphoria, or social withdrawal occurs. Perceptual disturbances, such as hallucinations or auditory, visual, or tactile illusions, can be present (American Psychiatric Association 2022). Within 2 hours of cannabis use, physiological manifestations occur, including conjunctival injection, increased appetite, dry mouth, and tachycardia (American Psychiatric Association 2022). Onset of cannabis symptoms depends on the route of administration; effects can begin within a few minutes (when smoked) or within 30–90 minutes (when orally ingested). Effects can last for 2–3 hours (when inhaled) to 4–12 hours (when orally ingested) (American Psychiatric Association 2022; Grotenhermen 2003). The intensity and severity of symptoms are more pronounced with higher doses, with a higher THC/CBD ratio, and with some synthetic cannabinoid use (owing to a full agonist effect) (American Psychiatric Association 2022; Martinotti et al. 2017).

Urine drug testing is a standard tool to detect THC metabolites. The immunoassay is the most common test performed and is sensitive to several THC metabolites. Single-exposure users can have marijuana detected in the urine for up to 72 hours, whereas THC can be detected in the urine of chronic users for more than 30 days after cessation. The long detection window is attributable to the highly lipophilic nature of cannabinoids and storage in lipid compartments throughout the body. Synthetic cannabinoids are difficult to detect in urine because of their rapid metabolization and structural differences from THC. In some immunoassay urine drug screens, the antiretroviral agent efavirenz and (rarely) certain nonsteroidal anti-inflammatory drugs can trigger false-positive results (Moeller et al. 2017; Saitman et al. 2014). Confirmation tests using gas or liquid chromatography and mass spectrometry can identify and differentiate a larger number of synthetic compounds.

Withdrawal Presentation

An acute withdrawal syndrome, usually lasting approximately 1–2 weeks, can develop within 24–72 hours of cessation or significant reduction in heavy or prolonged cannabis use. Criteria for cannabis withdrawal are outlined in DSM-5 (American Psychiatric Association 2022) and require three or more of the following signs and symptoms within 1 week of cessation of heavy and prolonged use: irritability, anger, or aggression; nervousness or anxiety; sleep difficulty (e.g., insomnia, disturbing dreams); decreased appetite or weight loss; restlessness; depressed mood; and/or one of the following physical symptoms causing significant discomfort: abdominal pain, shakiness/tremors, sweating, fever, chills, or headache (American Psychiatric Association 2022). Additionally, fatigue, yawning, and difficulty concentrating are also common. These signs and symptoms can manifest with significant functional impairment and cause significant distress. They can contribute to difficulty quitting or increase risk of return to cannabis use (American Psychiatric Association 2022). Patients describe emergence or reemergence of primary psychiatric symptoms (e.g., anxiety, insomnia, dysphoria) after discontinuation of or decreases in cannabis use. Occasionally, patients do not attribute these symptoms to cannabis withdrawal, providing a potential opportunity for patient education.

Pharmacological Management of Intoxication

First-line management for nonsevere acute cannabis intoxication is nonpharmacological, including providing supportive care with hydration, monitoring vital signs, and placing the patient in a quiet room with minimal stimuli (Williams and Hill 2020). In more moderate or severe cases with behavioral or psychiatric symptoms, there are pharmacological options. To manage anxiety, sedative-hypnotics (e.g., clonazepam, lorazepam, oxazepam) or nonbenzodiazepine anxiolytics (e.g., hydroxyzine) may offer benefit. Second-generation antipsychotics (e.g., risperidone or quetiapine) can also be helpful in the presence of perceptual disturbances. More severe cases, such as with agitation or psychotic symptoms, may require more powerful antipsychotics, such as haloperidol, chlorpromazine, or olanzapine (Crippa et al. 2012; Williams and Hill 2020).

Cannabis Use Disorder Presentation

Patients with CUD present to health care settings in a variety of ways, and providers should be aware of the possible different symptom presentations. Common presenting concerns in patients with an underlying CUD include depression and anxiety, psychotic symptoms, respiratory infection and chronic cough, sleep disturbances, relationship difficulties, poor school or work performance, and nausea or vomiting (Turner et al. 2014).

Further information should be gathered from patients who acknowledge past-year cannabis use, which may help differentiate between low-risk and problematic use or a CUD (Turner et al. 2014). Patients who use cannabis may often experience their use as a method to cope with mood, sleep, pain, or other physiological or psychological problems (American Psychiatric Association 2022). Patients who use cannabis to seek relaxation and alleviate anxiety may find it difficult to reduce use because of rebound anxiety or withdrawal symptoms. Any presenting symptoms may hint at problematic use and should trigger clinical review of the criteria for CUD (Turner et al. 2014). Only one-fourth of people perceive great risk from smoking cannabis once or twice weekly, in contrast with other substances (Substance Abuse and Mental Health Services Administration 2022), making CUD an often-overlooked diagnosis. Nonetheless, the criteria for CUD (outlined earlier) include all the diagnostic features of a substance use disorder.

Pharmacological Management Approaches for Cannabis Use Disorder and Cannabis Withdrawal

At present, there is no FDA-approved medication for treating CUD or cannabis withdrawal. Several pharmacotherapies have been investigated, but no studies demonstrate robust benefit, indicating a need for further research.

The most promising pharmacotherapies include treatments that target specific cannabinoid systems (e.g., CBD, nabiximols, and FAAH inhibitors) as well as non-cannabinoid-related pharmacotherapies (e.g., gabapentin). Other pharmacotherapies show some possible benefit and are summarized in Table 4.1. Medications that have not shown benefit are presented in Table 4.2. Medications with more potential benefit, along with dosing recommendations, are presented in Table 4.3. The remainder of this section is organized by medication class where appropriate.

Antidepressants

Currently, no studies robustly support the use of antidepressants for promoting abstinence or reducing cannabis use (Kondo et al. 2020; Nielsen et

Table 4.1 Pharmacological treatment of cannabis use: outcomes, direction of effect, and level of evidence

Class	Medication[a]	Abstinence	Reduction	Retention	Withdrawal	Adverse effect	Evidence quality
Antidepressant	Bupropion	None	None	None	Possibly	None	Insufficient
	Escitalopram	None	—	None	None	None	Insufficient/low
	Fluoxetine	—	None	None	None	None	Insufficient/low
	Mirtazapine	None	None	—	Possibly	—	Insufficient
	Nefazodone	None	None	Worse	None	Present	Insufficient
	Venlafaxine XR	Harm	Harm	None	—	—	Insufficient
	Vilazodone	—	None	None	Possibly	—	Insufficient/low
Antipsychotic	Clozapine	—	—	—	—	—	Insufficient
	Quetiapine	None	Possibly	None	Possibly	None	Insufficient/low
	Ziprasidone	—	—	Possibly	—	—	Insufficient

Table 4.1 Pharmacological treatment of cannabis use: outcomes, direction of effect, and level of evidence *(continued)*

Class	Medication[a]	Abstinence	Reduction	Retention	Withdrawal	Adverse effect	Evidence quality
Anticonvulsant or mood stabilizer	Divalproex sodium	None	None	—	None	Present	Insufficient
	Gabapentin	None	Possibly	None	Yes	None	Insufficient
	Lithium	None	None	None	Possibly	None	Insufficient
	Pregabalin	—	None	—	—	—	Insufficient
	Topiramate	None	Yes	Worse	—	Present	Insufficient
Cognitive enhancer	Atomoxetine	—	None	None	None	None	Insufficient
	Lofexidine	—	—	—	Yes	—	Insufficient

Table 4.1 Pharmacological treatment of cannabis use: outcomes, direction of effect, and level of evidence *(continued)*

Class	Medication[a]	Abstinence	Reduction	Retention	Withdrawal	Adverse effect	Evidence quality
Cannabinoid based	Cannabidiol	Possibly	Yes	None	Possibly	None	Low
	Dronabinol	None	None	Yes	Yes	None	Low/moderate
	Dronabinol/ lofexidine	None	—	None	None	None	Low/moderate
	FAAH inhibitor	—	Yes	None	Yes	None	Insufficient
	Nabilone	—	Possibly	None	Possibly	—	Insufficient
	Nabiximols	Possibly	Possibly	None	Possibly	None	Low/moderate

Table 4.1 Pharmacological treatment of cannabis use: outcomes, direction of effect, and level of evidence (continued)

Class	Medication[a]	Abstinence	Reduction	Retention	Withdrawal	Adverse effect	Evidence quality
Other	Buspirone	—	None	Worse?	None	None	Low
	Naltrexone	—	Possibly	—	—	None	Low
	Oxytocin	—	None	—	—	—	Insufficient
	Progesterone	—	—	—	None	—	Insufficient
	Varenicline	Possibly	Possibly	—	Possibly	—	Insufficient
	N-acetylcysteine	None	Possibly	None	None	None	Insufficient/low

Source. Data compiled from a variety of clinical studies.
Note. FAAH = fatty-acid amide hydrolase; XR = extended release; — = no data.
[a]Medications are organized by class and direction of effect for the following outcomes: abstinence (participants' self-report and/or as verified by urine test results), reduction in cannabis use (frequency or amount), retention (likelihood of remaining in a clinical study or treatment setting), withdrawal symptoms, adverse effects, and evidence quality.

Table 4.2 Ineffective treatments for cannabis use

Class	Medication[a]
Antidepressant	Escitalopram
	Fluoxetine
	Nefazodone
	Extended-release venlafaxine
Mood stabilizer	Divalproex sodium
Anticonvulsant	Pregabalin
Cognitive enhancer	Atomoxetine
Other	Buspirone
	Galantamine
	Oxytocin
	Progesterone

[a]Medications that have been studied and showed no evidence of improvement or harm in the following outcomes: abstinence, reduction in use, retention, and withdrawal symptoms.

al. 2019). Some antidepressants may nonetheless have utility in the treatment of CUD and cannabis withdrawal and can be considered for specific individuals.

Limited evidence supports a possible beneficial effect in reduction of some symptoms associated with cannabis use with vilazodone, bupropion, and mirtazapine. Vilazodone, titrated to 20–40 mg/day, demonstrated a 30% reduction in one aspect of craving in males but not females, but total craving scores were not different from placebo (McRae-Clark et al. 2016). Extended-release (XL) bupropion, dosed at 150–300 mg/day, outperformed placebo both in craving scores (magnitude of effect not reported) and in study or treatment retention (improvement by 17%) (Penetar et al. 2012). Mirtazapine improved sleep duration in cannabis users (Frewen et al. 2008). Conversely, venlafaxine may lead to an increase in cannabis use (Levin et al. 2013), and nefazodone can cause significant side effects (e.g., diarrhea), resulting in challenges with adherence and making determination of efficacy difficult (Carpenter et al. 2009).

Table 4.3 Dosing and use: treatments with some or limited benefit for the treatment of cannabis use and withdrawal

Medication	Cannabis use reduction	Withdrawal symptoms	Dosing	Comments (when to use, special populations)
Gabapentin	X	X	300–600 mg tid	—
Cannabidiol	X	X	400–800 mg/d	May only see marginal benefit
FAAH inhibitor	X	X	4 mg/d[a]	Not clinically available
Nabiximols	X		2.7 mg THC/2.5 mg CBD/100 μL spray; 5–30 sprays/d	—
N-acetylcysteine	X		1,200 mg bid	Benefit only shown in adolescents and young adults (ages 15–21)
Dronabinol		X	20–40 mg bid or tid; maximum of 120 mg	Can use in conjunction with lofexidine

Table 4.3 Dosing and use: treatments with some or limited benefit for the treatment of cannabis use and withdrawal *(continued)*

Medication	Cannabis use reduction	Withdrawal symptoms	Dosing	Comments (when to use, special populations)
Can consider the following medications (some limited benefit)				
Quetiapine	X	X	Titrate from 25 to 300 mg/d over 4 wk	—
Ziprasidone	X		80–400 mg/d	—
Clozapine	X		50–425 mg/d	—
Topiramate	X		Titrate to 200 mg/d over 4 wk	Monitor closely for poor tolerance or adverse effects; may be useful in adolescents
Vilazodone		X	20–40 mg/d	Reduces purposefulness or intent to use; did not show benefit in females
Bupropion		X	150–300 mg/d	Reduction in cravings
Mirtazapine		X	15–45 mg/d[b]	Improvement in sleep, appetite

Table 4.3 Dosing and use: treatments with some or limited benefit for the treatment of cannabis use and withdrawal *(continued)*

Medication	Cannabis use reduction	Withdrawal symptoms	Dosing	Comments (when to use, special populations)
Lithium		X	500 mg bid	Improvements in sleep, appetite, stomachaches
Lofexidine		X	0.6 mg tid	When used in conjunction with dronabinol
Naltrexone	X	X	380 mg IM every 4 wk	—
Varenicline	X		0.5–1 mg bid	—

Note. CBD = cannabidiol; d = day; FAAH = fatty-acid amide hydrolase; THC = tetrahydrocannabinol; wk = weeks.
[a]Dosing for specific FAAH inhibitor PF-04457845.
[b]Dosing not reported in study; this represents standard dosing.

Antipsychotics

There is insufficient research examining most antipsychotics used to treat CUD (Kondo et al. 2020). Nonetheless, quetiapine (titrated from 25 to 300 mg/day over 4 weeks) demonstrated some, albeit limited, effectiveness in the reduction of cannabis use (17% increase in the odds of moderate use compared with heavy use) and withdrawal symptoms (10% decrease in a composite withdrawal score weekly over 12 weeks) (Mariani et al. 2021). In a comparison study without a placebo control, both clozapine and ziprasidone reduced the frequency of cannabis use (magnitude of benefit was not reported), but there was no benefit to one over the other (Schnell et al. 2014).

Anticonvulsants and Mood Stabilizers

Gabapentin, which is approved by the FDA for postherpetic neuralgia and as an adjunct for partial seizures, is a structural analog of GABA. It acts by inhibiting the $\alpha_2\delta$ subunit of presynaptic voltage-gated calcium channels, thereby reducing excitatory neurotransmission (Sills 2006); this is thought to normalize corticotropin-releasing factor–induced GABA activation in the amygdala that is seen with alcohol dependence and withdrawal (Koob 2008; Roberto et al. 2008) and thus acts similarly for cannabis (Mason et al. 2012). Additionally, there is a hypothesis for a common pathway through which cannabinoids or gabapentin modulates pain and other physiological processes (Eckard and Kinsey 2021), given that CB_1 agonism also reduces synaptic transmission by inhibiting presynaptic voltage-gated calcium channels (Howlett et al. 2010).

Data suggest that when paired with individual counseling, gabapentin (dosed at 1,200 mg/day, which can be divided) can be helpful with reduction in cannabis use (decrease in number of days using marijuana per week) and withdrawal symptoms. In a previous study, gabapentin was associated with improvements in sleep, cravings, and cannabis-related problems (marijuana-related psychological and physical problems), along with benefits for depressive symptoms, neurocognitive performance, and adherence (Mason et al. 2012). A small pilot study with a related medication, pregabalin, showed less promise (Lile et al. 2022).

Miranda et al. (2017) reported that topiramate (titrated to 200 mg/day over 4 weeks) may have some promise for reducing cannabis use in users ages 15–24 (magnitude unreported, but a modest effect size was noted for reduction in grams used per day). However, the benefit in reduction of use was largely overshadowed by its adverse effects (worse neurocognitive performance and worse depressive symptoms), side effects, and poor adherence (Miranda et al. 2017).

There is no evidence to suggest that valproic acid or lithium has any role in abstinence or reduction in cannabis use (Kondo et al. 2020; Nielsen et al. 2019). Lithium (dosed at 500 mg bid) may nonetheless have some benefit for certain withdrawal symptoms (sleep disturbances, loss of appetite, and stomachache) (Johnston et al. 2014).

Cognitive Enhancers

Although a small early study of atomoxetine suggested possible cannabis reduction, albeit with unwelcome gastrointestinal side effects (Tirado et al. 2008), a larger study did not show a reduction in cannabis use despite improvement in some ADHD symptoms (McRae-Clark et al. 2010). Lofexidine, an α_2-agonist approved by the FDA to treat opioid withdrawal, has been shown (at 0.6 mg tid) to decrease symptoms of cannabis withdrawal, particularly in conjunction with dronabinol (20 mg tid), although further study is needed (Haney et al. 2008; Levin et al. 2016). Human laboratory studies suggested that modafinil may favorably affect intoxication symptoms (Sugarman et al. 2011), whereas clonidine may not (Cone et al. 1988). Galantamine, a cholinesterase inhibitor, did not appear to have any benefit for withdrawal symptoms (Sugarman et al. 2019).

Cannabinoid-Based Treatments

Three THC-based potential treatments have been studied: dronabinol, nabilone, and nabiximols. Dronabinol (approved by the FDA for treatment of anorexia in patients with AIDS and for nausea/vomiting in patients receiving chemotherapy for cancer) is a synthetic form of THC (a partial agonist at CB_1 and CB_2) that demonstrated improvement in withdrawal symptoms (magnitude not reported). Dosing is 20 mg bid for 8 weeks, followed by a 2-week taper. Additionally, dronabinol demonstrated a 15% improvement in study retention over 8 weeks; however, it was not apparent that it helps with abstinence or reduction in use (Levin et al. 2011). Nabilone, a similar synthetic form of THC that is also approved by the FDA as an antiemetic for patients receiving chemotherapy, did not seem to have any benefit in reducing cannabis use (Hill et al. 2017).

Nabiximols, currently an investigational non-FDA-approved agent in the United States but approved in Canada for treatment of multiple sclerosis spasticity, may be helpful. The buccal spray, which is a combination of CBD and THC in a near 1:1 ratio (or more specifically, THC 2.7 mg and CBD 2.5 mg per spray), is administered four times a day in self-titrated doses up to a daily maximum of 32 or 42 sprays. Several studies have shown a reduction in cannabis use with nabiximols, including 22% fewer days of cannabis use (Lintzeris et al. 2019), a 28% greater reduction in grams used per week (Trigo et al. 2018), or approximately four times greater odds of reducing use by 50% or more (Mills et al. 2022) compared with placebo. Evidence is mixed regarding whether there is a reduction in cannabis withdrawal symptoms with nabiximols. Although one clinical trial suggested promise in the reduction of the withdrawal course from 4.9 to 3.1 days, along with a 66% reduction in withdrawal scores (Allsop et al. 2014), and another trial showed improvement in craving measures (Trigo et al. 2018), some results were equivocal (Lintzeris et al. 2019; Trigo et al. 2018) or not reported (Mills et al. 2022).

Non-THC-based treatments include CBD alone and FAAH inhibitors, which indirectly increase the concentration of endocannabinoids by preventing their enzymatic degradation. CBD is currently approved by the FDA for the treatment of seizures associated with Lennox-Gastaut syndrome or Dravet syndrome, typically found in pediatric populations. At a dosage of 400–800 mg/day (considerably higher than dosing in commercially available products), CBD has shown a small effect in reducing cannabis use, as measured by lower urinary concentrations and an increase in abstinence by up to an additional half-day per week. Furthermore, CBD was also demonstrated to reduce cannabis withdrawal symptoms (Freeman et al. 2020). Interestingly, CBD also has been shown to inhibit hydrolysis and reuptake of endocannabinoids (similar to FAAH inhibitors, described in the next paragraph), which may contribute to these effects (Freeman et al. 2020).

Cannabinoid degradative enzyme inhibitors (FAAH inhibitors) have been promising. Specifically, a novel FAAH inhibitor PF-04457845 (which is not commercially available in the United States at the time of this writing) improved self-reported cannabis use, as measured by number of joints smoked per day, with a reduction of almost one joint per day at 4 weeks compared with placebo. Additionally, withdrawal symptoms as measured by a composite scale improved during the first 2 days of use, with the effect not significant beyond that time frame; more studies are needed to assess this further (D'Souza et al. 2019).

Other Medications

N-Acetylcysteine

NAC, a glutamatergic modulator approved by the FDA for acetaminophen overdose and as an adjuvant inhalant for bronchopulmonary conditions, is commonly sold as a dietary supplement for its antioxidant properties. Its action upregulating the cystine-glutamate exchanger in the nucleus accumbens is hypothesized to reduce drug-seeking behavior (Kalivas et al. 2009; Moussawi et al. 2009).

Studies have shown that NAC dosed at 1,200 mg bid is effective in reducing cannabis use in non-treatment-seeking adolescent populations (ages 15–21), with twice the odds of having negative urine cannabinoid test results (Gray et al. 2012). Unfortunately, this effect was not demonstrated in an adult population (Gray et al. 2017). Differences in neurodevelopment, cannabis use profiles, engagement in behavioral treatment, and medication adherence may contribute to this discrepancy, but further studies are needed to build on these findings and determine which populations may most benefit from NAC treatment (Gray et al. 2012, 2017).

Naltrexone

Naltrexone has the potential to decrease cannabis use, with a small 8-week trial of naltrexone 380 mg IM every 4 weeks demonstrating that participants reduced the number of cannabis using days per week by 1–2 days (Haney et al. 2015; Notzon et al. 2018). More studies are needed to investigate this effect further.

Varenicline

Varenicline, a selective nicotinic acetylcholine receptor partial agonist, is effective in tobacco cessation (dosed to a maximum of 2 mg/day) and demonstrated a reduction in cannabis use, withdrawal symptoms, and abstinence in a pilot study (McRae-Clark et al. 2021). Given the small, preliminary nature of that study, the magnitude of the effects was not characterized. The results are not generalizable currently, requiring further studies to characterize the validity of the observed effect.

Buspirone

Buspirone has little role in treating cannabis dependence, with no evidence of reduction in use or improvement in withdrawal symptoms (McRae-Clark et al. 2009, 2015; Nielsen et al. 2019).

Hormones

There is insufficient evidence to suggest the efficacy of hormone therapy. Oxytocin requires further study; an underpowered study showed a potential reduction in cannabis use when oxytocin was combined with motivational enhancement therapy (Sherman et al. 2017). Progesterone does not appear to have any benefit for withdrawal symptoms in women (Sherman et al. 2019).

Pharmacology for Significant Medical or Physiological Considerations Related to Cannabis Use

Cannabis-Induced Psychosis

Cannabis intoxication can produce transient psychosis-like effects, including the following symptoms: depersonalization, derealization, ideas of reference, grandiosity, paranoid delusions, flight of ideas, disorganized thinking, and auditory and visual hallucinations. These effects are more commonly reported with high-THC-content cannabis (Moore et al. 2007).

Although no causal relationship has been demonstrated, chronic cannabis use, especially during adolescence, has been associated with later development of schizophrenia in populations with an increased vulnerability to this disorder. Both CIP and eventual diagnosis with schizophrenia are more strongly associated with earlier age of use, more frequent cannabis use, and use of high-THC-content products (Di Forti et al. 2015; Gage et al. 2016, 2017).

Treatment of intoxication that manifests as psychosis is mostly supportive, with pharmacotherapy for severe symptoms or behavioral dysregulation. Second-generation antipsychotics should be tried first to reduce the risk of adverse effects (e.g., extrapyramidal symptoms) seen more commonly in first-generation antipsychotics (Grewal and George 2017). There were no differences in outcomes of olanzapine (Berk et al. 1999) or risperidone (Berk et al. 2000) during controlled trials comparing them to haloperidol for treatment of CIP. Aripiprazole also showed benefit (Rolland et al. 2013). If antipsychotics fail to abate symptoms of CIP, use of antiepileptic medications such as valproate sodium or carbamazepine can be considered, although further studies of these medications are needed (Grewal and George 2017). One may want to consider adjunctive anxiolytics such as benzodiazepines in CIP, particularly if accompanied by agitation or panic. Benzodiazepines such as lorazepam and alprazolam can be used as part of acute symptom management (Crippa et al. 2012; Pauselli 2018).

Cannabinoid Hyperemesis Syndrome

CHS can be seen in chronic use of cannabis, particularly in older adolescents and adults. It presents as episodic vomiting, abdominal pain, and nausea that patients often report is temporarily relieved by hot showers. Cannabis use is commonly perceived to offer antiemetic and appetite stimulatory effects (as an example, dronabinol is approved by the FDA for chemotherapy-related nausea and vomiting), and this condition can often go unrecognized and undiagnosed. CHS typically consists of three phases: 1) a prodromal phase, characterized by nausea, abdominal pain, and fear of vomiting; 2) a hyperemetic phase, in which multiple intense episodes of vomiting can occur and may result in seeking medical attention; and 3) a recovery phase, in which symptoms resolve and normal eating resumes. Rome IV diagnostic criteria were developed to provide objective diagnostic criteria for CHS and are as follows: symptoms being present for the past 3 months, with an onset greater than 6 months prior; stereotypical episodes typically lasting less than 1 week; at least three episodes in the last year and two episodes in the last 6 months; and no vomiting between episodes (Stanghellini et al. 2016). All of the Rome IV criteria must be associated with chronic use of cannabis (a pattern of use that is not specifically defined) and must cease upon stopping cannabis use (Perisetti et al. 2020).

How chronic cannabis use can lead to CHS is not well understood (Perisetti et al. 2020). Hypotheses include overstimulation of gastrointestinal CB_1 receptors (in contrast with the antiemetic CB_1 receptors located in the chemoreceptor trigger zone in the brain), cannabinoid buildup in lipids, and genetic polymorphisms in the cytochrome P450 system resulting in slower THC metabolism; all of these potentially contribute to the development of CHS (Senderovich et al. 2022).

The best method to alleviate CHS is undoubtedly discontinuation of cannabinoid use (Senderovich et al. 2022). Although there are no FDA-approved medications for treatment of CHS, several supportive measures can be used. Typical antiemetics (e.g., ondansetron, prochlorperazine, and promethazine) may not be as effective as the other interventions described here (Richards et al. 2017).

Hot bathing, or hot-water hydrotherapy, has anecdotally been an effective therapeutic modality for CHS, but it has not been rigorously researched. Hot baths may also be helpful in other functional nausea and vomiting disorders (Perisetti et al. 2020; Senderovich et al. 2022). Hot bathing is proposed to improve symptoms by redirecting blood flow from the enteric system to the skin, in addition to modulating substance P, a pain and inflammatory neuropeptide found in nerve endings (Senderovich et al. 2022).

A similar mechanism of action has been proposed for topical capsaicin. When applied abdominally at a concentration of 0.1%–0.25% up to three times a day, capsaicin has demonstrated effectiveness in studies. For example, it has demonstrated a 21% greater reduction in nausea (by visual analog scale) compared with placebo (Dean et al. 2020), as well as shorter length of hospital or emergency department stays. However, larger studies are required to better assess this treatment's efficacy.

Several case studies have supported the use of benzodiazepines (e.g., lorazepam and clonazepam). Both systematic reviews for adult and pediatric CHS found that benzodiazepines were most frequently reported for acute treatment in a number of case studies and case reports; however, there is a lack of high-quality studies that measure the impact of these medications specifically (Reinert et al. 2021; Richards et al. 2017). An early prospective report demonstrated the effectiveness of cannabis abstinence; patients with CHS were offered benzodiazepines over the first 2 weeks, but the authors did not detail the response (Allen et al. 2004). A study of patients with cyclical vomiting syndrome (CVS) reported that lorazepam was most effective during the acute phase, although the authors did not comment on dosing (Namin et al. 2007). A case series demonstrated effective acute cessation of symptoms in the hospital, with clonazepam given twice at a dose of 0.5 mg (Kheifets et al. 2019). In the pediatric literature, case studies reported that clonazepam dosed at 0.25–0.5 mg nightly (Gammeter et al. 2016) or a single dose of lorazepam 1 mg IV may be effective (Cox et al. 2012; Mahmad et al. 2015).

The first-generation antipsychotics haloperidol and droperidol have shown some promise in treating CHS. Haloperidol (dosing of 0.05–0.1 mg/kg IV) has shown improvement in nausea and vomiting superior to that of ondansetron, along with shorter emergency department stays (Ruberto et al. 2021). Droperidol, administered intravenously at 0.625–2.5 mg, has demonstrated improvement in nausea scores as well as reduction in length of stay, largely through retrospective data (Senderovich et al. 2022). Both of these medications need further study, and the risks of extrapyramidal symptoms (i.e., acute dystonia) and QTc prolongation should be considered.

CVS presents with symptoms similar to those of CHS but is idiopathic in nature. Treatment options for CVS may therefore offer potential options for pharmacotherapy of CHS. Tricyclic antidepressants (TCAs) have demonstrated efficacy in CVS in the long term. It is likely for this reason that TCAs have been most commonly studied for long-term treatment in CHS as well (Richards et al. 2017), but further studies are needed. For CVS, amitriptyline can be started at 25 mg and titrated to 1 mg/kg/day, which demonstrated efficacy in a prospective cohort of patients with CVS (93% improvement at 3 months; 88% improvement at 2 years). Although a number of patients in the prospective study used cannabis, the impact of active use (or cessation of use) on their symptoms or the resolution of their symptoms, respectively, was not characterized (Hejazi et al. 2010; Namin et al. 2007).

Other case studies have supported possible use of propranolol (Richards and Dutczak 2017) and the neurokinin-1 receptor antagonist aprepitant (Parvataneni et al. 2019); further studies of these medications will be needed to characterize the benefit.

Population Considerations

Adolescents

Cannabis use peaks during adolescence and emerging adulthood. This timing is particularly concerning in this population, because the developing brain may be especially vulnerable to the effects of cannabis use. The endocannabinoid system is active in the developing brain and neural development from prenatal life, during adolescence, and even into adulthood (Lubman et al. 2015; Trezza et al. 2012).

During adolescence, critical development is affected by extensive pruning of cortical synapses and increased myelination in areas such as the cerebral cortex, hippocampus, basal ganglia, and cerebellum. It is not surprising, then, that many of these areas tend to have a high density of presynaptic CB_1 receptors, and activation by endocannabinoids can inhibit transmission of both GABAergic and glutamatergic synapses. Glutamate transmission is important to synaptic pruning. It is thought primarily for this reason that exogenous cannabinoid use during adolescence may be detrimental, because it has the potential to disrupt these processes during a critical time. It has also been suggested that these same mechanisms are affected or disrupted in the pathogenesis of schizophrenia. Exogenous cannabinoids may significantly affect and potentially disrupt the synaptic pruning process during a critical development period (adolescence) through effects on this physiology (Lubman et al. 2015).

CB_1 receptors are also important in white matter development, because white matter areas tend to have higher CB_1 receptor expression, but this difference diminishes into adulthood. With exogenous cannabis use, downregulation of these CB_1 receptors can occur, which may impair white matter development (Lubman et al. 2015).

The most common clinical pharmacological approach for treatment in adolescents and young adults is to use the currently over-the-counter supplement NAC, dosed at 1,200 mg bid. NAC has been demonstrated to be most effective in patients ages 15–21 (Gray et al. 2012). The role of NAC in modulating glutamatergic processes implicated in the endocannabinoid system during adolescence may explain the favorable findings in adolescents and not adults.

Additionally, one study (with a high dropout rate due to tolerability) of topiramate in adolescents, which employed slow titration up to 200 mg/day over 4 weeks (provided the individual did not develop significant side effects), showed some potential benefit (Miranda et al. 2017). However, the degree of benefit of topiramate was not well characterized (Miranda et al. 2017).

Psychiatric Comorbidities

In general, it is important to treat both CUD and comorbid psychiatric diagnoses at the same time, instead of sequentially as in past approaches. Patients with unrecognized or untreated psychiatric symptoms have been repeatedly shown to do less well in substance treatment (Kranzler et al. 1996; Rooke et al. 2011). It has been hypothesized that when the underlying psychiatric illness is effectively treated, patients with dual diagnoses may be more likely to respond to substance treatment. One approach to maximize pharmacology is to consider the use of medications outlined in this chapter as having potential benefit for cannabis withdrawal or CUD that also may have some benefit for a particular patient's co-occurring psychiatric diagnoses.

Research on pharmacotherapy for CUD in patients with co-occurring psychiatric conditions is sparse. Most clinical trials, including those discussed earlier in this section, tend to exclude individuals with psychiatric comorbidities. Moreover, trials that do evaluate pharmacotherapy in patients with dual diagnoses tend to include polysubstance populations or focus on drugs other than cannabis. Nevertheless, a strong body of literature suggests that associations exist between cannabis use and higher rates of co-occurring psychiatric disorders, such as mood disorder, ADHD, PTSD, anxiety disorder, personality disorders, other substance use disorders, and psychosis (Hasin and Walsh 2020).

With co-occurring depression and CUD, fluoxetine was shown previously to help with depressive symptoms but did not illustrate any benefit for cannabis use (Cornelius et al. 1999, 2000, 2010). Adjuvant gabapentin used in co-occurring bipolar disorder demonstrated favorable MRI changes that may be consistent with lower manic/mixed and depressive symptoms and lower cannabis use, demonstrating that this therapy is worth exploring further (Prisciandaro et al. 2022). A single study did not demonstrate any efficacy for improving depressive symptoms with NAC in adults with CUD (Tomko et al. 2020).

For co-occurring ADHD and CUD, as discussed earlier in "Cognitive Enhancers," atomoxetine does not appear to be helpful in cannabis use reduction, although its use does show improvement in some ADHD symptoms (McRae-Clark et al. 2010). Although no studies exist exploring therapeutics for dually diagnosed PTSD and CUD, there has been a suggestion for further exploration of FAAH inhibitors given some potentially complementary physiology through increasing the endocannabinoid anandamide, which may be deficient in PTSD (Kondev et al. 2021). As stated previously, gabapentin may be helpful for withdrawal symptoms and reduction of cannabis use (Mason et al. 2012). Furthermore, there is evidence suggesting that gabapentin has efficacy in various forms of anxiety disorders and has applicability to other CUDs (Ahmed et al. 2019).

A strong association and possible bidirectional link exists between cannabis and psychosis. Individuals with schizophrenia are reported to be two to three times more likely to develop CUD than those without schizophrenia (Lev-Ran et al. 2013; Martins and Gorelick 2011). Additionally, some experts believe that early cannabis use is a causal factor in developing psychosis (Hasin and Walsh 2020). To differentiate cannabis-induced psychiatric disorders from primary psychiatric disorders likely worsened by cannabis use, we use the history of exposures and resultant symptoms as well as the timeline of symptom development.

Based on the findings of a systematic review of treatment of CUD in patients with psychotic disorders, treatment with antipsychotic medication does not appear to be associated with a worsening of cannabis craving or use and may improve cannabis use, but further studies are needed (Baker et al. 2012). Although the literature is lacking regarding studies of CUD with psychotic disorders, there are studies examining general substance use disorders that may be important to mention. A review of patients with dually diagnosed substance use disorder and psychotic disorders from several case reports, open trials, and retrospective studies (no clinical trials) reported that the majority of the studies suggest second-generation antipsychotics are effective for psychotic symptom control in patients with co-occurring substance use disorder, particularly clozapine, although the authors focused on substances as a broad term and did not specify only cannabis. The review hypothesized that compared with first-generation antipsychotics, second-generation antipsychotics may afford more cognitive resources to avoid substance use, given that first-generation antipsychotics may have more cognitive side effects. Additionally, the broader receptor affinity and mesolimbic selectivity of some second-generation antipsychotics may also suggest benefit for patients with schizophrenia and substance use disorders (San et al. 2007).

Regarding specific antipsychotics, there is little evidence to suggest one agent over another. A case report of eight patients with bipolar disorder or schizophrenia cited reduction of cannabis use with quetiapine (Potvin et al. 2004). As discussed earlier in "Antipsychotics," ziprasidone and clozapine were shown to help reduce cannabis use (Schnell et al. 2014). Although one study found that clozapine and olanzapine improved cannabis craving scores more than risperidone (although there was no placebo arm) (Machielsen et al. 2012), the authors of a Cochrane Review found that the quality of evidence was too poor to determine any conclusion (Temmingh et al. 2018).

Efforts and expert opinions have suggested CBD as a potential non-antipsychotic pharmacotherapy for psychosis (Davies and Bhattacharyya 2019; Hahn 2018; McLoughlin et al. 2014; Schubart et al. 2014). The proposed mechanism is that CBD attenuates the effects of THC on CB_1 receptors, in addition to increasing endocannabinoid anandamide levels (Davies and Bhattacharyya 2019). And, as discussed earlier in "Cannabinoid-Based Treatments," CBD dosed at 400–800 mg/day may have benefit in reducing cannabis use and aid in ameliorating withdrawal symptoms (Freeman et al. 2020). Some short clinical studies demonstrated that CBD dosing of up to 800 mg/day as monotherapy (Leweke et al. 2012) or 1,000 mg/day as an adjunct to antipsychotics (McGuire et al. 2018) reduced psychotic symptoms (particularly positive ones) in patients with schizophrenia. However, other studies have failed to corroborate this beneficial effect (Boggs et al. 2018).

Too few studies have examined CBD as a potential treatment for patients who have received dual diagnoses or even for patients with either CUD or psychotic disorder separately, preventing conclusions about the most effective pharmacotherapies for this subpopulation (McLoughlin et al. 2014). In a case series examining medical cannabis (Bedrolite) with a low THC-to-CBD ratio, it did not appear to have utility in the treatment of inpatients with psychotic disorder and comorbid CUD (Schipper et al. 2018). Nonetheless, studies have shown that CBD alone is safe and well tolerated; in addition to potential for its antipsychotic effects (Davies and Bhattacharyya 2019), preliminary findings suggest anxiolytic and antidepressant effects (García-Gutiérrez et al. 2020). These findings support the development of further research to explore the potential use of CBD for patients with CUD and psychiatric comorbidities.

Pregnant and Breastfeeding Individuals

Marijuana is the most used substance in pregnancy. THC crosses the placenta and is passed in breast milk (DeJong et al. 2022). Although many of the studies on neonatal and childhood development have a number of limitations, which may explain their inconsistent results, cannabis may be harmful during pregnancy, with potential for adverse effects on maternal, fetal, and long-term neurobehavioral development (Joseph and Vettraino 2020; Metz and Borgelt 2018; Ryan et al. 2018). Evidence suggests that cannabis use is associated with increased risks of preterm and very preterm birth

(1.4 times), small for gestational age (1.4 times), neonatal ICU admission, and select structural malformations (gastrointestinal and CNS) (Bandoli et al. 2021).

The endocannabinoid system is detectable from the early stages of embryonic development and plays a critical role in early stages of neuronal development and cell survival. By binding to CB_1 receptors during fetal development, THC indirectly reduces endogenous endocannabinoid synthesis and further CB_1 expression, which is hypothesized to disrupt the signaling during this formative time period (Wang et al. 2004). Because CB_1 receptors are more highly concentrated in mesocorticolimbic structures during fetal development, this may have downstream consequences on emotional regulation, cognition, and memory (Keimpema et al. 2011).

As such, the American College of Obstetricians and Gynecologists recommends that individuals who are attempting pregnancy, currently pregnant, or breastfeeding should be encouraged to discontinue marijuana use (Committee on Obstetric Practice 2017). These positions are also supported by the American Academy of Pediatrics (Ryan et al. 2018). Because of a paucity of data in humans and adverse outcomes in animal studies, experts, including the FDA, strongly discourage use of cannabis products in any form (including CBD) during pregnancy and lactation (Joseph and Vettraino 2020).

Another important consideration is CHS, which can be challenging to differentiate from hyperemesis gravidarum, a condition that typically presents in the first trimester with associated ketonuria, weight loss, and electrolyte disturbances. Helpful symptoms to differentiate CHS from hyperemesis gravidarum may include onset of symptoms before pregnancy, a history consistent with recent or active cannabis use, and symptomatic relief with hot showers. In a case report, haloperidol was helpful in relieving symptoms of CHS during pregnancy, and its use may outweigh potential risks to the mother or the fetus (La Sala et al. 2022).

No studies support the use of pharmacotherapies for pregnant or lactating people with CUD. Per World Health Organization (2014) recommendations and corroboration by other experts (DeJong et al. 2022), psychosocial interventions (e.g., cognitive-behavioral therapy, contingency management) are favored for CUD. It may be reasonable to consider gabapentin, which is safe in lactation and pregnancy, for withdrawal symptoms, provided adequate folate supplementation is taking place. As mentioned in the previous paragraph, use of any of the cannabinoid products (e.g., CBD, dronabinol, nabiximols) is not recommended for pregnant or lactating people.

Key Points

- Cannabis, an addictive substance, largely modulates its effects through the endocannabinoid system but also has effects on other neurotransmitter systems. Several of these systems are targets for medications for cannabis use disorder (CUD), cannabis withdrawal, or both.
- Intoxication can present with a self-described "high," along with several clinically significant and impairing symptoms that can be targets for supportive or symptom-driven medication management.
- Treatment of cannabis intoxication is largely supportive, but pharmacological aid with anxiolytics (e.g., benzodiazepines) and, in some cases, antipsychotics can be helpful.
- Cannabis withdrawal syndrome commonly presents with effects on mood, anxiety, and sleep. Gabapentin, cannabidiol, fatty-acid amide hydrolase inhibitors, and dronabinol may alleviate some of these withdrawal symptoms.
- There is limited benefit in treatment of withdrawal symptoms with certain antidepressants (vilazodone, bupropion, and mirtazapine), lithium, and lofexidine.
- There are no FDA-approved medications for treatment of CUD or withdrawal, but several agents have demonstrated potential benefit from a variety of classes.
- Gabapentin, cannabidiol, fatty-acid amide hydrolase (FAAH) inhibitors, nabiximols, and dronabinol may help with a small reduction in cannabis use.
- *N*-acetylcysteine may increase the reduction in cannabis use in young adult and adolescent populations.
- Cannabis-induced psychosis (CIP) can be treated with antipsychotic medications. Consider adjunctive benzodiazepine use if cannabis-induced psychosis is accompanied by agitation or panic.
- Cannabis hyperemesis syndrome (CHS) can be treated with hot water therapy, topical capsaicin, certain first-generation antipsychotics

(namely, haloperidol and droperidol), and benzodiazepines (namely, clonazepam); conventional antiemetics may largely be ineffective.
- Further research is needed on medications for treatment of CUD for individuals with co-occurring psychiatric disorders and for pregnant and breastfeeding patients.
- Further studies are needed to demonstrate any robust effect for all medications for CUD, cannabis withdrawal, and co-occurring conditions.

References

Ahmed S, Bachu R, Kotapati P, et al: Use of gabapentin in the treatment of substance use and psychiatric disorders: a systematic review. Front Psychiatry 10:228, 2019 31133886

Allen JH, de Moore GM, Heddle R, et al: Cannabinoid hyperemesis: cyclical hyperemesis in association with chronic cannabis abuse. Gut 53(11):1566–1570, 2004 15479672

Allsop DJ, Copeland J, Lintzeris N, et al: Nabiximols as an agonist replacement therapy during cannabis withdrawal: a randomized clinical trial. JAMA Psychiatry 71(3):281–291, 2014 24430917

American Psychiatric Association: Diagnostic and Statistical Manual of Mental Disorders, 5th Edition. Arlington, VA, American Psychiatric Association, 2013

American Psychiatric Association: Diagnostic and Statistical Manual of Mental Disorders, 5th Edition, Text Revision. Washington, DC, American Psychiatric Association, 2022

Baker AL, Thornton LK, Hides L, et al: Treatment of cannabis use among people with psychotic disorders: a critical review of randomised controlled trials. Curr Pharm Des 18(32):4923–4937, 2012 22716135

Bandoli G, Jelliffe-Pawlowski L, Schumacher B, et al: Cannabis-related diagnosis in pregnancy and adverse maternal and infant outcomes. Drug Alcohol Depend 225:108757, 2021 34049105

Berk M, Brook S, Trandafir AI: A comparison of olanzapine with haloperidol in cannabis-induced psychotic disorder: a double-blind randomized controlled trial. Int Clin Psychopharmacol 14(3):177–180, 1999 10435771

Berk M, Brook S, Nur F, et al: Risperidone compared to haloperidol in cannabis-induced psychotic disorder: a double blind randomized controlled trial. Int J Psychiatry Clin Pract 4(2):139–142, 2000 24921450

Best AR, Regehr WG: Serotonin evokes endocannabinoid release and retrogradely suppresses excitatory synapses. J Neurosci 28(25):6508–6515, 2008 18562622

Boggs DL, Surti T, Gupta A, et al: The effects of cannabidiol (CBD) on cognition and symptoms in outpatients with chronic schizophrenia a randomized placebo controlled trial. Psychopharmacology (Berl) 235(7):1923–1932, 2018 29619533

Bossong MG, van Berckel BN, Boellaard R, et al: Delta 9-tetrahydrocannabinol induces dopamine release in the human striatum. Neuropsychopharmacology 34(3):759–766, 2009 18754005

Breivogel CS, Scates SM, Beletskaya IO, et al: The effects of delta9-tetrahydrocannabinol physical dependence on brain cannabinoid receptors. Eur J Pharmacol 459(2–3):139–150, 2003 12524139

Budney AJ, Novy PL, Hughes JR: Marijuana withdrawal among adults seeking treatment for marijuana dependence. Addiction 94(9):1311–1322, 1999 10615717

Carpenter KM, McDowell D, Brooks DJ, et al: A preliminary trial: double-blind comparison of nefazodone, bupropion-SR, and placebo in the treatment of cannabis dependence. Am J Addict 18(1):53–64, 2009 19219666

Committee on Obstetric Practice: Committee Opinion No. 722: marijuana use during pregnancy and lactation. Obstet Gynecol 130(4):e205–e209, 2017 28937574

Cone EJ, Welch P, Lange WR: Clonidine partially blocks the physiologic effects but not the subjective effects produced by smoking marijuana in male human subjects. Pharmacol Biochem Behav 29(3):649–652, 1988 2834758

Cornelius JR, Salloum IM, Haskett RF, et al: Fluoxetine versus placebo for the marijuana use of depressed alcoholics. Addict Behav 24(1):111–114, 1999 10189977

Cornelius JR, Salloum IM, Haskett RF, et al: Fluoxetine versus placebo in depressed alcoholics: a 1-year follow-up study. Addict Behav 25(2):307–310, 2000 10795957

Cornelius JR, Bukstein OG, Douaihy AB, et al: Double-blind fluoxetine trial in comorbid MDD-CUD youth and young adults. Drug Alcohol Depend 112(1–2):39–45, 2010 20576364

Cox B, Chhabra A, Adler M, et al: Cannabinoid hyperemesis syndrome: case report of a paradoxical reaction with heavy marijuana use. Case Rep Med 2012:757696, 2012 22685471

Crippa JA, Derenusson GN, Chagas MH, et al: Pharmacological interventions in the treatment of the acute effects of cannabis: a systematic review of literature. Harm Reduct J 9:7, 2012 22273390

Davies C, Bhattacharyya S: Cannabidiol as a potential treatment for psychosis. Ther Adv Psychopharmacol 9:2045125319881916, 2019 31741731

Dean DJ, Sabagha N, Rose K, et al: A pilot trial of topical capsaicin cream for treatment of cannabinoid hyperemesis syndrome. Acad Emerg Med 27(11):1166–1172, 2020 32569429

DeJong KN, Choby B, Valent AM: Strategies for prevention or treatment of tobacco and cannabis use disorder. Clin Obstet Gynecol 65(2):397–419, 2022 35318983

Di Forti M, Marconi A, Carra E, et al: Proportion of patients in South London with first-episode psychosis attributable to use of high potency cannabis: a case-control study. Lancet Psychiatry 2(3):233–238, 2015 26359901

D'Souza DC, Cortes-Briones J, Creatura G, et al: Efficacy and safety of a fatty acid amide hydrolase inhibitor (PF-04457845) in the treatment of cannabis withdrawal and dependence in men: a double-blind, placebo-controlled, parallel group, phase 2a single-site randomised controlled trial. Lancet Psychiatry 6(1):35–45, 2019 30528676

Eckard ML, Kinsey SG: Gabapentin attenuates somatic signs of precipitated THC withdrawal in mice. Neuropharmacology 190:108554, 2021 33845073

Elsohly MA, Slade D: Chemical constituents of marijuana: the complex mixture of natural cannabinoids. Life Sci 78(5):539–548, 2005 16199061

Freeman TP, Hindocha C, Baio G, et al: Cannabidiol for the treatment of cannabis use disorder: a phase 2a, double-blind, placebo-controlled, randomised, adaptive Bayesian trial. Lancet Psychiatry 7(10):865–874, 2020 32735782

Frewen A, Montebello M, Baillie A, et al: The role of mirtazapine in cannabis withdrawal, in College on Problems of Drug Dependence. Annual Meeting, Quebec City, Quebec, Canada, The College on Problems of Drug Dependence, 2008

Gage SH, Hickman M, Zammit S: Association between cannabis and psychosis: epidemiologic evidence. Biol Psychiatry 79(7):549–556, 2016 26386480

Gage SH, Jones HJ, Burgess S, et al: Assessing causality in associations between cannabis use and schizophrenia risk: a two-sample Mendelian randomization study. Psychol Med 47(5):971–980, 2017 27928975

Gammeter WB, Duke KA, Soundy TJ: Case report of intractable vomiting and abdominal pain related to heavy daily cannabis use. S D Med 60–63, 2016 28817852

García-Gutiérrez MS, Navarrete F, Gasparyan A, et al: Cannabidiol: a potential new alternative for the treatment of anxiety, depression, and psychotic disorders. Biomolecules 10(11):1575, 2020 33228239

Glass M, Dragunow M, Faull RL: Cannabinoid receptors in the human brain: a detailed anatomical and quantitative autoradiographic study in the fetal, neonatal and adult human brain. Neuroscience 77(2):299–318, 1997 9472392

Gong JP, Onaivi ES, Ishiguro H, et al: Cannabinoid CB2 receptors: immunohistochemical localization in rat brain. Brain Res 1071(1):10–23, 2006 16472786

Gray KM, Carpenter MJ, Baker NL, et al: A double-blind randomized controlled trial of N-acetylcysteine in cannabis-dependent adolescents. Am J Psychiatry 169(8):805–812, 2012 22706327

Gray KM, Sonne SC, McClure EA, et al: A randomized placebo-controlled trial of N-acetylcysteine for cannabis use disorder in adults. Drug Alcohol Depend 177:249–257, 2017 28623823

Grewal RS, George TP: Cannabis-induced psychosis: a review. Psychiatric Times, July 14, 2017. Available at: https://www.psychiatrictimes.com/view/cannabis-induced-psychosis-review. Accessed February 3, 2025.

Grotenhermen F: Pharmacokinetics and pharmacodynamics of cannabinoids. Clin Pharmacokinet 42(4):327–360, 2003 12648025

Hahn B: The potential of cannabidiol treatment for cannabis users with recent-onset psychosis. Schizophr Bull 44(1):46–53, 2018 29083450

Haney M, Ward AS, Comer SD, et al: Abstinence symptoms following oral THC administration to humans. Psychopharmacology (Berl) 141(4):385–394, 1999 10090646

Haney M, Hart CL, Vosburg SK, et al: Effects of THC and lofexidine in a human laboratory model of marijuana withdrawal and relapse. Psychopharmacology (Berl) 197(1):157–168, 2008 18161012

Haney M, Ramesh D, Glass A, et al: Naltrexone maintenance decreases cannabis self-administration and subjective effects in daily cannabis smokers. Neuropsychopharmacology 40(11):2489–2498, 2015 25881117

Hart CL, Haney M, Vosburg SK, et al: Reinforcing effects of oral delta9-THC in male marijuana smokers in a laboratory choice procedure. Psychopharmacology (Berl) 181(2):237–243, 2005 15830233

Hasin D, Walsh C: Cannabis use, cannabis use disorder, and comorbid psychiatric illness: a narrative review. J Clin Med 10(1):15, 2020 33374666

Hejazi RA, Reddymasu SC, Namin F, et al: Efficacy of tricyclic antidepressant therapy in adults with cyclic vomiting syndrome: a two-year follow-up study. J Clin Gastroenterol 44(1):18–21, 2010 20027010

Herkenham M, Lynn AB, Johnson MR, et al: Characterization and localization of cannabinoid receptors in rat brain: a quantitative in vitro autoradiographic study. J Neurosci 11(2):563–583, 1991 1992016

Hill KP, Palastro MD, Gruber SA, et al: Nabilone pharmacotherapy for cannabis dependence: a randomized, controlled pilot study. Am J Addict 26(8):795–801, 2017 28921814

Hillig KW, Mahlberg PG: A chemotaxonomic analysis of cannabinoid variation in Cannabis (Cannabaceae). Am J Bot 91(6):966–975, 2004 21653452

Howlett AC, Blume LC, Dalton GD: CB(1) cannabinoid receptors and their associated proteins. Curr Med Chem 17(14):1382–1393, 2010 20166926

Johnston J, Lintzeris N, Allsop DJ, et al: Lithium carbonate in the management of cannabis withdrawal: a randomized placebo-controlled trial in an inpatient setting. Psychopharmacology (Berl) 231(24):4623–4636, 2014 24880749

Joseph P, Vettraino IM: Cannabis in pregnancy and lactation: a review. Mo Med 117(5):400–405, 2020 33311738

Justinova Z, Tanda G, Redhi GH, et al: Self-administration of delta9-tetrahydrocannabinol (THC) by drug naive squirrel monkeys. Psychopharmacology (Berl) 169(2):135–140, 2003 12827345

Kalivas PW, Lalumiere RT, Knackstedt L, et al: Glutamate transmission in addiction. Neuropharmacology 56(Suppl 1):169–173, 2009 18675832

Keimpema E, Mackie K, Harkany T: Molecular model of cannabis sensitivity in developing neuronal circuits. Trends Pharmacol Sci 32(9):551–561, 2011 21757242

Kheifets M, Karniel E, Landa D, et al: Resolution of cannabinoid hyperemesis syndrome with benzodiazepines: a case series. Isr Med Assoc J 21(6):404–407, 2019 31280510

Kondev V, Winters N, Patel S: Cannabis use and posttraumatic stress disorder comorbidity: epidemiology, biology and the potential for novel treatment approaches. Int Rev Neurobiol 157:143–193, 2021 33648669

Kondo KK, Morasco BJ, Nugent SM, et al: Pharmacotherapy for the treatment of cannabis use disorder: a systematic review. Ann Intern Med 172(6):398–412, 2020 32120384

Koob GF: A role for brain stress systems in addiction. Neuron 59(1):11–34, 2008 18614026

Kranzler HR, Del Boca FK, Rounsaville BJ: Comorbid psychiatric diagnosis predicts three-year outcomes in alcoholics: a posttreatment natural history study. J Stud Alcohol 57(6):619–626, 1996 8913993

La Sala MS, Constantino E, Koola MM, et al: Treatment of cannabis hyperemesis syndrome using haloperidol in a pregnant patient: case report. J Clin Psychopharmacol 42(5):506–508, 2022 35943399

Lev-Ran S, Imtiaz S, Rehm J, et al: Exploring the association between lifetime prevalence of mental illness and transition from substance use to substance use disorders: results from the National Epidemiologic Survey of Alcohol and Related Conditions (NESARC). Am J Addict 22(2):93–98, 2013 23414492

Levin FR, Mariani JJ, Brooks DJ, et al: Dronabinol for the treatment of cannabis dependence: a randomized, double-blind, placebo-controlled trial. Drug Alcohol Depend 116(1–3):142–150, 2011 21310551

Levin FR, Mariani J, Brooks DJ, et al: A randomized double-blind, placebo-controlled trial of venlafaxine-extended release for co-occurring cannabis dependence and depressive disorders. Addiction 108(6):1084–1094, 2013 23297841

Levin FR, Mariani JJ, Pavlicova M, et al: Dronabinol and lofexidine for cannabis use disorder: a randomized, double-blind, placebo-controlled trial. Drug Alcohol Depend 159:53–60, 2016 26711160

Leweke FM, Piomelli D, Pahlisch F, et al: Cannabidiol enhances anandamide signaling and alleviates psychotic symptoms of schizophrenia. Transl Psychiatry 2(3):e94, 2012 22832859

Lile JA, Alcorn JL, Hays LR, et al: Influence of pregabalin maintenance on cannabis effects and related behaviors in daily cannabis users. Exp Clin Psychopharmacol 30(5):560–574, 2022 33983765

Lintzeris N, Bhardwaj A, Mills L, et al: Nabiximols for the treatment of cannabis dependence: a randomized clinical trial. JAMA Intern Med 179(9):1242–1253, 2019 31305874

Lubman DI, Cheetham A, Yücel M: Cannabis and adolescent brain development. Pharmacol Ther 148:1–16, 2015 25460036

Machielsen M, Beduin AS, Dekker N, et al: Differences in craving for cannabis between schizophrenia patients using risperidone, olanzapine or clozapine. J Psychopharmacol 26(1):189–195, 2012 21768161

Mahmad AI, Jehangir W, Littlefield JM II, et al: Cannabis hyperemesis syndrome: a case report review of treatment. Toxicol Rep 2:889–890, 2015 28962425

Mariani JJ, Pavlicova M, Jean Choi C, et al: Quetiapine treatment for cannabis use disorder. Drug Alcohol Depend 218:108366, 2021 33153828

Martinotti G, Santacroce R, Papanti D, et al: Synthetic cannabinoids: psychopharmacology, clinical aspects, psychotic onset. CNS Neurol Disord Drug Targets 16(5):567–575, 2017 28412921

Martins SS, Gorelick DA: Conditional substance abuse and dependence by diagnosis of mood or anxiety disorder or schizophrenia in the U.S. population. Drug Alcohol Depend 119(1–2):28–36, 2011 21641123

Mason BJ, Crean R, Goodell V, et al: A proof-of-concept randomized controlled study of gabapentin: effects on cannabis use, withdrawal and executive function deficits in cannabis-dependent adults. Neuropsychopharmacology 37(7):1689–1698, 2012 22373942

Matsuda LA, Bonner TI, Lolait SJ: Localization of cannabinoid receptor mRNA in rat brain. J Comp Neurol 327(4):535–550, 1993 8440779

McGuire P, Robson P, Cubala WJ, et al: Cannabidiol (CBD) as an adjunctive therapy in schizophrenia: a multicenter randomized controlled trial. Am J Psychiatry 175(3):225–231, 2018 29241357

McLaren J, Swift W, Dillon P, et al: Cannabis potency and contamination: a review of the literature. Addiction 103(7):1100–1109, 2008 18494838

McLoughlin BC, Pushpa-Rajah JA, Gillies D, et al: Cannabis and schizophrenia. Cochrane Database Syst Rev 2014(10):CD004837, 2014 25314586

McRae-Clark AL, Carter RE, Killeen TK, et al: A placebo-controlled trial of buspirone for the treatment of marijuana dependence. Drug Alcohol Depend 105(1–2):132–138, 2009 19699593

McRae-Clark AL, Carter RE, Killeen TK, et al: A placebo-controlled trial of atomoxetine in marijuana-dependent individuals with attention deficit hyperactivity disorder. Am J Addict 19(6):481–489, 2010 20958842

McRae-Clark AL, Baker NL, Gray KM, et al: Buspirone treatment of cannabis dependence: a randomized, placebo-controlled trial. Drug Alcohol Depend 156:29–37, 2015 26386827

McRae-Clark AL, Baker NL, Gray KM, et al: Vilazodone for cannabis dependence: a randomized, controlled pilot trial. Am J Addict 25(1):69–75, 2016 26685701

McRae-Clark AL, Gray KM, Baker NL, et al: Varenicline as a treatment for cannabis use disorder: a placebo-controlled pilot trial. Drug Alcohol Depend 229(Pt B):109111, 2021 34655945

Melis M, Pistis M, Perra S, et al: Endocannabinoids mediate presynaptic inhibition of glutamatergic transmission in rat ventral tegmental area dopamine neurons through activation of CB1 receptors. J Neurosci 24(1):53–62, 2004 14715937

Metz TD, Borgelt LM: Marijuana use in pregnancy and while breastfeeding. Obstet Gynecol 132(5):1198–1210, 2018 30234728

Mills L, Dunlop A, Montebello M, et al: Correlates of treatment engagement and client outcomes: results of a randomised controlled trial of nabiximols for the treatment of cannabis use disorder. Subst Abuse Treat Prev Policy 17(1):67, 2022 36209081

Miranda R Jr, Treloar H, Blanchard A, et al: Topiramate and motivational enhancement therapy for cannabis use among youth: a randomized placebo-controlled pilot study. Addict Biol 22(3):779–790, 2017 26752416

Moeller KE, Kissack JC, Atayee RS, et al: Clinical interpretation of urine drug tests: what clinicians need to know about urine drug screens. Mayo Clin Proc 92(5):774–796, 2017 28325505

Moore TH, Zammit S, Lingford-Hughes A, et al: Cannabis use and risk of psychotic or affective mental health outcomes: a systematic review. Lancet 370(9584):319–328, 2007 17662880

Moreira FA, Lutz B: The endocannabinoid system: emotion, learning and addiction. Addict Biol 13(2):196–212, 2008 18422832

Moussawi K, Pacchioni A, Moran M, et al: N-acetylcysteine reverses cocaine-induced metaplasticity. Nat Neurosci 12(2):182–189, 2009 19136971

Namin F, Patel J, Lin Z, et al: Clinical, psychiatric and manometric profile of cyclic vomiting syndrome in adults and response to tricyclic therapy. Neurogastroenterol Motil 19(3):196–202, 2007 17300289

Nielsen S, Gowing L, Sabioni P, et al: Pharmacotherapies for cannabis dependence. Cochrane Database Syst Rev 1(1):CD008940, 2019 30687936

Notzon DP, Kelly MA, Choi CJ, et al: Open-label pilot study of injectable naltrexone for cannabis dependence. Am J Drug Alcohol Abuse 44(6):619–627, 2018 29420073

Parvataneni S, Varela L, Vemuri-Reddy SM, et al: Emerging role of aprepitant in cannabis hyperemesis syndrome. Cureus 11(6):e4825, 2019 31403013

Pauselli L: Cannabis-induced psychotic disorders, in The Complex Connection Between Cannabis and Schizophrenia. Edited by Compton MT, Manseau MW. San Diego, CA, Academic Press, 2018, pp 183–197

Penetar DM, Looby AR, Ryan ET, et al: Bupropion reduces some of the symptoms of marihuana withdrawal in chronic marihuana users: a pilot study. Subst Abuse 6:63–71, 2012 22879754

Perisetti A, Gajendran M, Dasari CS, et al: Cannabis hyperemesis syndrome: an update on the pathophysiology and management. Ann Gastroenterol 33(6):571–578, 2020 33162734

Pertwee RG: The diverse CB1 and CB2 receptor pharmacology of three plant cannabinoids: delta9-tetrahydrocannabinol, cannabidiol and delta9-tetrahydrocannabivarin. Br J Pharmacol 153(2):199–215, 2008 17828291

Piomelli D: The molecular logic of endocannabinoid signalling. Nat Rev Neurosci 4(11):873–884, 2003 14595399

Potvin S, Stip E, Roy JY: The effect of quetiapine on cannabis use in 8 psychosis patients with drug dependency. Can J Psychiatry 49(10):711, 2004 15560324

Prisciandaro JJ, Mellick W, Squeglia LM, et al: Results from a randomized, double-blind, placebo-controlled, crossover, multimodal-MRI pilot study of gabapentin for co-occurring bipolar and cannabis use disorders. Addict Biol 27(1):e13085, 2022 34390300

Radwan MM, Elsohly MA, Slade D, et al: Biologically active cannabinoids from high-potency Cannabis sativa. J Nat Prod 72(5):906–911, 2009 19344127

Reinert JP, Niyamugabo O, Harmon KS, et al: Management of pediatric cannabinoid hyperemesis syndrome: a review. J Pediatr Pharmacol Ther 26(4):339–345, 2021 34035677

Richards JR, Dutczak O: Propranolol treatment of cannabinoid hyperemesis syndrome: a case report. J Clin Psychopharmacol 37(4):482–484, 2017 28604421

Richards JR, Gordon BK, Danielson AR, et al: Pharmacologic treatment of cannabinoid hyperemesis syndrome: a systematic review. Pharmacotherapy 37(6):725–734, 2017 28370228

Roberto M, Gilpin NW, O'Dell LE, et al: Cellular and behavioral interactions of gabapentin with alcohol dependence. J Neurosci 28(22):5762–5771, 2008 18509038

Rolland B, Geoffroy PA, Jardri R, et al: Aripiprazole for treating cannabis-induced psychotic symptoms in ultrahigh-risk individuals. Clin Neuropharmacol 36(3):98–99, 2013 23673914

Rooke SE, Norberg MM, Copeland J: Successful and unsuccessful cannabis quitters: comparing group characteristics and quitting strategies. Subst Abuse Treat Prev Policy 6:30, 2011 22074446

Ruberto AJ, Sivilotti MLA, Forrester S, et al: Intravenous haloperidol versus ondansetron for cannabis hyperemesis syndrome (HaVOC): a randomized, controlled trial. Ann Emerg Med 77(6):613–619, 2021 33160719

Ryan SA, Ammerman SD, O'Connor ME: Marijuana use during pregnancy and breastfeeding: implications for neonatal and childhood outcomes. Pediatrics 142(3):e20181889, 2018 30150209

Saitman A, Park HD, Fitzgerald RL: False-positive interferences of common urine drug screen immunoassays: a review. J Anal Toxicol 38(7):387–396, 2014 24986836

San L, Arranz B, Martinez-Raga J: Antipsychotic drug treatment of schizophrenic patients with substance abuse disorders. Eur Addict Res 13(4):230–243, 2007 17851245

Schipper R, Dekker M, de Haan L, et al: Medicinal cannabis (Bedrolite) substitution therapy in inpatients with a psychotic disorder and a comorbid cannabis use disorder: a case series. J Psychopharmacol 32(3):353–356, 2018 29039260

Schnell T, Koethe D, Krasnianski A, et al: Ziprasidone versus clozapine in the treatment of dually diagnosed (DD) patients with schizophrenia and cannabis use disorders: a randomized study. Am J Addict 23(3):308–312, 2014 24628830

Schubart CD, Sommer IE, Fusar-Poli P, et al: Cannabidiol as a potential treatment for psychosis. Eur Neuropsychopharmacol 24(1):51–64, 2014 24309088

Senderovich H, Patel P, Jimenez Lopez B, et al: A systematic review on cannabis hyperemesis syndrome and its management options. Med Princ Pract 31(1):29–38, 2022 34724666

Sherman BJ, Baker NL, McRae-Clark AL: Effect of oxytocin pretreatment on cannabis outcomes in a brief motivational intervention. Psychiatry Res 249:318–320, 2017 28152465

Sherman BJ, Caruso MA, McRae-Clark AL: Exogenous progesterone for cannabis withdrawal in women: feasibility trial of a novel multimodal methodology. Pharmacol Biochem Behav 179:22–26, 2019 30711528

Sills GJ: The mechanisms of action of gabapentin and pregabalin. Curr Opin Pharmacol 6(1):108–113, 2006 16376147

Stanghellini V, Chan FK, Hasler WL, et al: Gastroduodenal disorders. Gastroenterology 150(6):1380–1392, 2016 27147122

Substance Abuse and Mental Health Services Administration: Key Substance Use and Mental Health Indicators in the United States: Results From the 2021 National Survey on Drug Use and Health (HHS Publ No PEP22-07-01-005, NSDUH Series H-57). Rockville, MD, Center for Behavioral Health Statistics and Quality, Substance Abuse and Mental Health Services Administration, 2022. Available at: https://www.samhsa.gov/data/sites/default/files/reports/rpt42731/2022-nsduh-nnr.pdf. Accessed February 3, 2025.

Sugarman DE, Poling J, Sofuoglu M: The safety of modafinil in combination with oral Δ9-tetrahydrocannabinol in humans. Pharmacol Biochem Behav 98(1):94–100, 2011 21176784

Sugarman DE, De Aquino JP, Poling J, et al: Feasibility and effects of galantamine on cognition in humans with cannabis use disorder. Pharmacol Biochem Behav 181:86–92, 2019 31082417

Sun Y, Bennett A: Cannabinoids: a new group of agonists of PPARs. PPAR Res 2007:023513, 2007 18288264

Temmingh HS, Williams T, Siegfried N, et al: Risperidone versus other antipsychotics for people with severe mental illness and co-occurring substance misuse. Cochrane Database Syst Rev 1(1):CD011057, 2018 29355909

Tirado CF, Goldman M, Lynch K, et al: Atomoxetine for treatment of marijuana dependence: a report on the efficacy and high incidence of gastrointestinal adverse events in a pilot study. Drug Alcohol Depend 94(1–3):254–257, 2008 18182254

Tomko RL, Baker NL, Hood CO, et al: Depressive symptoms and cannabis use in a placebo-controlled trial of N-acetylcysteine for adult cannabis use disorder. Psychopharmacology (Berl) 237(2):479–490, 2020 31712969

Trezza V, Campolongo P, Manduca A, et al: Altering endocannabinoid neurotransmission at critical developmental ages: impact on rodent emotionality and cognitive performance. Front Behav Neurosci 6:2, 2012 22291624

Trigo JM, Soliman A, Quilty LC, et al: Nabiximols combined with motivational enhancement/cognitive behavioral therapy for the treatment of cannabis dependence: a pilot randomized clinical trial. PLoS One 13(1):e0190768, 2018 29385147

Turner SD, Spithoff S, Kahan M: Approach to cannabis use disorder in primary care: focus on youth and other high-risk users. Can Fam Physician 60(9):801–808, e423–e432, 2014 25217674

U.S. Drug Enforcement Administration: K2/Spice. April 2020. Available at: https://www.dea.gov/sites/default/files/2020-06/K2-spice-2020.pdf. Accessed February 3, 2025.

Van Sickle MD, Duncan M, Kingsley PJ, et al: Identification and functional characterization of brainstem cannabinoid CB2 receptors. Science 310(5746):329–332, 2005 16224028

Vardakou I, Pistos C, Spiliopoulou Ch: Spice drugs as a new trend: mode of action, identification and legislation. Toxicol Lett 197(3):157–162, 2010 20566335

Viveros MP, Marco EM, File SE: Endocannabinoid system and stress and anxiety responses. Pharmacol Biochem Behav 81(2):331–342, 2005 15927244

Wang X, Dow-Edwards D, Anderson V, et al: In utero marijuana exposure associated with abnormal amygdala dopamine D2 gene expression in the human fetus. Biol Psychiatry 56(12):909–915, 2004 15601599

Williams AR, Hill KP: Care of the patient using cannabis. Ann Intern Med 173(9):ITC65–ITC80, 2020 33127270

World Health Organization: Guidelines for the Identification and Management of Substance Use and Substance Use Disorders in Pregnancy. Geneva, World Health Organization, 2014

Opioids

John A. Renner, Jr., M.D.
Jeffrey DeVido, M.D., M.T.S.
Kendra Kobrin, M.D., Ph.D.

Opioids are common analgesics but are high-risk medications because they can cause dysregulation of sex hormones, hyperalgesia, opioid use disorder (OUD), and, at worst, lethal overdose.[1] Opioids act mainly on the μ opioid receptor (MOR) to influence intracellular and neurotransmitter signaling and, on a broader scale, the regulation of mesocorticolimbic brain pathways. Opioids produce strong tolerance, dependence, and withdrawal effects. Tolerance to analgesic and mood effects develops more rapidly than tolerance to respiratory depression, leading to a heightened risk of overdose death when escalating doses are used to overcome tolerance.

Medically supervised withdrawal (MSW) can be accomplished with an array of different medications, including those that similarly target MORs (e.g., methadone, buprenorphine) or target symptoms of withdrawal (e.g., clonidine, lofexidine, acetaminophen, loperamide). However, MSW alone is not a treatment for OUD and is often followed by opioid relapse. Therefore,

---

[1] Technically, the term *opioid* refers to all substances that primarily activate the opioid receptors and includes natural, semisynthetic, and synthetic opioids; the term *opiate* includes only the naturally occurring opioids, such as morphine and heroin. For simplicity, in this chapter, we use *opioid* throughout.

patients should be advised to follow MSW with long-term treatment that can include long-term opioid agonist or naltrexone therapy to promote treatment retention and harm reduction. Patients chronically taking opioids for pain can develop complex opioid dependence, necessitating gradual cessation of opioids or, if that is not tolerated, treatment with long-term methadone or buprenorphine. Classically, methadone may be started immediately; buprenorphine requires the patient to be experiencing withdrawal, whereas naltrexone requires the patient to abstain from opioids for 7 days before initiation (an often clinically challenging expectation). To reduce barriers to initiation of treatment and to reduce the risk of precipitated withdrawal, novel buprenorphine low-dose, high-dose, and full agonist crossover protocols are emerging, in addition to alternative naltrexone initiation protocols; however, large-scale studies on these approaches are currently lacking.

Pharmacology and Neurobiology of Opioids

Koob (2020) conceptualized the development of OUD as a three-stage process characterized as follows: 1) binge/intoxication, 2) withdrawal/negative affect, and 3) preoccupation/anticipation. This pattern is driven by the hedonic effects of the opioids, coupled with neuroadaptations that favor learned associations between use and previously neutral environmental stimuli. Additional physiological adaptations support the development of dependence and withdrawal states when access to opioid use is discontinued, further compelling return to use. Finally, executive top-down cognitive control mechanisms erode in conjunction with the emergence of strong cravings, still further favoring continued use. The body's adaptations to opioids, therefore, favor increasing drug intake and link intake to cues and contexts that can trigger craving and relapse (Koob 2020). These adaptations are thought to be mediated by alterations of neuronal signaling in functional brain circuits, most prominently in the mesocorticolimbic system. Changes ultimately can be traced also to the cellular level, where opioids interact with their receptors to alter neuronal activity and intracellular signaling cascades that can affect cellular functioning and gene expression.

Pharmacology

Opioids have long been used for their analgesic effects. After rapid intravenous injection of an opioid, individuals may experience warm skin flushing and a "rush" consisting of pleasure, relaxation, and satisfaction, which lasts about 45 seconds (Seecof and Tennant 1986). Unfortunately, opioids can also cause nausea, vomiting, apathy, poor concentration, sedation, delirium, and lethal respiratory depression, and their use may result in the development of OUD. Respiratory depression is a potentially lethal effect of opioids and is often the cause of death resulting from opioid overdose (for further discussion, see sections "Intoxication Presentation" and "Pharmacological Management of Intoxication"). Opioids may cause vagus nerve–mediated bradycardia, vasodilation, and decreased sympathetic tone; morphine, hydromorphone, hydrocodone, and meperidine can lead to histamine release, which can lower blood pressure (Chen and Ashburn 2015). Opioids inhibit secretion of gonadotropin-releasing hormone and corticotropin-releasing hormone, which can cause hypogonadism with chronic use (de Vries et al. 2020). Major gastrointestinal effects include constipation resulting from decreased gut motility and changes in secretion of gastric and intestinal fluids. Opioids also cause pupillary constriction (miosis).

Repeated administration of opioids predictably results in the development of tolerance to these medications, manifested as the need to administer a larger dose to produce a given level of effect. Tolerance maintains homeostasis, because the body counteracts the effects of continued opioids by activating opposing processes. In the individual who has developed tolerance, discontinuation of opioid use results in a withdrawal syndrome, which the individual experiences as an array of unpleasant symptoms such as diarrhea, myalgia, diaphoresis, anxiety, and nausea/vomiting. However, different individuals can exhibit a wide array of withdrawal symptoms of varying severity. Tolerance largely resets after withdrawal, creating a highly dangerous situation if an individual returns to using opioids at the previous dose, which can result in fatal opioid overdose.

Tolerance to analgesic and mood effects appears to develop more rapidly (in 1–2 weeks) than tolerance to respiratory depression, which can result in accidental overdose when a larger than previous dose of opioid is taken to achieve a given level of analgesia or euphoria (Camí and Farré 2003; Hayhurst and Durieux 2016). Tolerance in the gastrointestinal tract also appears to occur much more slowly; therefore, constipation can be a chronic side effect that does not remit (Hayhurst and Durieux 2016). Some tolerance to miosis may occur, but it is likely to remain apparent on physical examination of intoxicated patients (Chang et al. 2007). Some tolerance to the inhibition of growth hormone-releasing hormone and corticotropin-releasing hormone release occurs; however, chronic opioid use can still lead to hypogonadotropic hypogonadism with central (decreased attention, decreased libido, fatigue, depressive state) and peripheral (muscle hypotrophy, osteoporosis, anemia, erectile dysfunction, delayed ejaculation) effects (O'Rourke and Wosnitzer 2016).

Opioids can be absorbed from the gastrointestinal tract (including the rectum), nasal mucosa, and lung, and some can be absorbed through the skin and oral mucosa (Lam et al. 2020). After absorption from the gastrointestinal tract, many opioids undergo substantial first-pass metabolism; thus they are more potent when administered by injection. The plasma half-life of opioids is 2–3 hours for morphine, oxycodone, and hydromorphone; 3–4 hours for fentanyl,[2] meperidine, and codeine; 3–5 hours for buprenorphine; and up to 24 hours for methadone (Trescot et al. 2008). Table 5.1 provides a list of some common opioids and their pharmacodynamics and unique features.

Pharmacokinetic features distinguish some of the commonly used opioids. Codeine must undergo biotransformation into morphine by the liver enzyme CYP2D6 to exert its full therapeutic effects. Approximately 90% of the excretion of morphine occurs during the first 24 hours, but traces are detectable in urine for more than 48 hours. Heroin (diacetylmorphine) is hydrolyzed to 6-monoacetylmorphine (6-MAM), which is then hydrolyzed to morphine. Morphine and 6-MAM are responsible for the pharmacological effects of heroin. Heroin produces effects more rapidly than morphine because it is more lipid soluble and therefore crosses the blood–brain barrier faster. Because heroin is rapidly metabolized, within minutes, only its metabolites are tested for in the urine and can be found up to 48 hours after heroin administration (Gutstein and Akil 2001; Jaffe et al. 2004).

Fentanyl is a synthetic opioid that is 50–100 times more potent than morphine or heroin. Fentanyl is active without metabolism and crosses the

---

[2] As is discussed in this chapter, emerging clinical experience with individuals chronically using high-potency opioids (e.g., fentanyl and fentanyl analogs) paints a clinical picture consistent with long-acting opioid pharmacokinetics. This phenomenon is proposed to be attributable to fentanyl's high lipophilicity (accumulation in body fat stores and consequent slow release), which maintains blood levels higher than would be expected relative to the known pharmacokinetics of fentanyl when not used chronically.

Table 5.1 Characteristics of some common opioids

Opioid	Half-life	Notable features	Urine toxicology window (days)[a]
Heroin (diacetylmorphine)	3–15 min	Semisynthetic opioid synthesized via acetylation of opium	3
		Traverses the BBB rapidly	
		Metabolized quickly to 6-MAM and morphine	
Morphine	2–3 h	Natural opioid (extracted from opium)	3
		90% excreted in urine in 24 h	
Oxycodone	2–3 h	Semisynthetic opioid	1–1.5 (immediate release)
		Available in immediate-release and controlled-release formulations	1.5–3 (controlled release)
Hydromorphone	2–3 h	Semisynthetic opioid	1–2
		Immediate-release and extended-release formulations, along with parenteral formulations	
Fentanyl	3–14 h	Synthetic opioid	2–3
		Highly lipophilic	

Table 5.1 Characteristics of some common opioids *(continued)*

Opioid	Half-life	Notable features	Urine toxicology window (days)[a]
		100 times more potent than morphine	
		High risk of overdose or poisoning, given the low therapeutic window	
		Quickly crosses the BBB	
		Wide volume of distribution	
Meperidine	3–4 h	Synthetic opioid	1–2
		Anticholinergic, so no miosis observed	
		Convulsive seizures seen in high doses	
		Serotonin syndrome seen with concurrent MAOI and SSRI medication use	
Codeine	3–4 h	Natural opioid	1–2
		Antitussive and analgesic effects	
		Metabolite important for effect: morphine and hydrocodone	
Buprenorphine	3–5 h	Semisynthetic opioid	1–14
		Poor oral bioavailability	

Opioids 197

Table 5.1 Characteristics of some common opioids *(continued)*

Opioid	Half-life	Notable features	Urine toxicology window (days)[a]
		Used for analgesia, treatment of OUD	
		Treatment for OUD does not require an OTP; as of 2023, no special DEA registration (X-waiver) is required	
		Ceiling effect for respiratory depression but no ceiling effect for analgesia	
Methadone	24 h	Synthetic opioid	1–14
		Used for analgesia, treatment of OUD	
		Treatment for OUD requires administration through an OTP, although can be initiated in acute care hospital settings	
		Can take up to 5 days at consistent dosing to reach steady state; too-rapid up-titrations can lead to overdose	

Source. Adapted from DePriest AZ et al. 2015; Kale 2019.

[a]Detection windows listed here are in reference to immunoassays. The detection windows are variable depending on the nature of the immunoassay (e.g., detection cutoff levels) and amount and duration of exposure (generally opioids are detectable for longer periods if the use of that opioid has been of greater duration and in greater amounts).

Note. 6-MAM = 6-monoacetylmorphine; BBB = blood–brain barrier; DEA = U.S. Drug Enforcement Administration; h = hour; MAOI = monoamine oxidase inhibitor; OTP = opioid treatment program; OUD = opioid use disorder; SSRI = selective serotonin reuptake inhibitor.

blood–brain barrier rapidly because of its high lipophilicity, so it has almost instantaneous effects when given intravenously. It has a short duration of action of up to 10 minutes, but it has a highly variable half-life (≤14 hours) and a wide volume of distribution, meaning it can stay stored in muscle and fat for much longer than its duration of action. Fentanyl is metabolized in the liver, mainly by cytochrome P450 (CYP) 3A4 and CYP3A5, to inactive metabolites, including norfentanyl (Kuip et al. 2017; Moss and Carlo 2019; Saiz-Rodríguez et al. 2019).

Specific urine tests for synthetic and semisynthetic opioids, such as buprenorphine, methadone, and fentanyl, may need to be ordered separately, because many routine urine immunoassay toxicology screens assess only for the presence of those opiates that are metabolized with morphine as the metabolite (Moeller et al. 2017). It may often be difficult to identify the exact opioid a patient with OUD is using, because the illicit opioid supply has increasingly been composed of nonpharmaceutical fentanyl, fentanyl analogs, and novel synthetic opioids (Armenian et al. 2018). Therefore, it may be impossible to know the exact pharmacokinetic or characteristic features of an illicit opioid in a particular patient.

Increasingly, as part of a comprehensive public health approach to addressing illicit drug use, authorities have been advocating for the use of consumer-based drug supply testing for fentanyl. The harm-reduction principle behind this approach proposes that if individuals know that fentanyl is present in the drugs they are about to use, they may alter their behavior (i.e., use around others, ensure a supply of naloxone is at hand, or not use that supply at all). These fentanyl immunoassay test strips were originally designed for use in urine samples but have been repurposed to be used off-label for consumer-based testing. Local and national authorities have supported the use of fentanyl test strips (Centers for Disease Control and Prevention 2024a; Substance Abuse and Mental Health Services Administration 2024) and have provided guidance on the proper use of these strips in practice. Typically, individuals are instructed to set aside about 10 mg of the drug, mix it with approximately 0.5–1 teaspoon of water, place the test strip in the liquid, and wait for the liquid to be absorbed for 15 seconds (Centers for Disease Control and Prevention 2024a). Although this strategy has been demonstrated to be highly sensitive and specific for point-of-care testing, further research is needed to assess the impact of fentanyl test strip use on overdose prevention (Kutscher et al. 2024).

Mechanisms of Action

The effects of opioids are mediated mainly through the three classic opioid receptors, including (most prominently) the MOR and, to a lesser extent and with some variability, the κ opioid receptor (KOR) and the δ opioid receptor (DOR) (Zhang et al. 1998). The binding of an opioid to an opioid receptor classically activates an inhibitory G protein, triggering a complex intracellular signaling cascade that involves inhibition of adenylyl cyclase, ultimately resulting in decreased neuronal excitability (Williams et al. 2001). Additionally, opioid receptors have been found to signal through G protein–independent cascades mediated by scaffolding proteins such as arrestin (Darcq and Kieffer 2018).

Most medicinal opioids are full agonists at the MOR, meaning they produce a high amount of G protein activation. High densities of MORs in the nervous system are found in the dorsal horn of the spinal cord, the brain stem, the thalamus, and the cortex, where they can modulate the intensity of incoming pain signals. MORs in the brain stem respiratory centers are involved in respiratory drive and, when overly agonized, can lead to respiratory depression. Full agonists produce a dose–response effect on respiratory depression that has no ceiling (Selley et al. 1998, 2003; Spahn et al. 2018). The rewarding effect of opioids is mediated in part by activation of MORs in the ventral tegmental area, causing increased dopamine release in the nucleus accumbens (Nestler et al. 2001).

Full MOR agonists include poppy plant derivatives (e.g., morphine and codeine), morphine-related semisynthetic agents (e.g., heroin and oxycodone), synthetic agents (e.g., fentanyl, methadone, and meperidine), and endogenous opioids (e.g., endorphins, enkephalins, and endomorphins). A minority of opioids are partial MOR agonists (i.e., buprenorphine) that activate the MOR to a lesser extent. Buprenorphine, for example, additionally demonstrates a ceiling effect in regard to respiratory depression (i.e., beyond a certain dosage level, additional buprenorphine will not cause additional respiratory depression), which adds to its utility as a pharmacological treatment for OUD by mitigating some of the risk of fatal opioid overdose (Ciraulo et al. 2006). Other partial agonists include pentazocine and butorphanol, but they are not used in OUD treatment. The opioid antagonists (e.g., naloxone, naltrexone, nalmefene) bind to MORs and effectively block the actions of opioid agonists, but they do not alter the activity of the receptors directly.

Opioids can have varying activity at the KOR and the DOR. A few opioid analgesics, including butorphanol and nalbuphine, may produce analgesia by stimulating KORs, but dysphoria and hallucinations also may occur in response to the activation of these receptors. Nalbuphine is also an MOR antagonist that may induce withdrawal in opioid-dependent individuals.

The mechanisms that mediate opioid tolerance are not entirely known. However, research does demonstrate that chronic opioid exposure suppresses release of norepinephrine from the locus coeruleus and increases release of dopamine into the nucleus accumbens, which then causes upregulation of norepinephrine release and downregulation of dopamine signaling to compensate (Kosten and George 2002; Kreek et al. 2012). Other processes implicated in the development of tolerance include desensitization (uncoupling of a receptor from its G protein due to phosphorylation), internalization of the receptor by endocytosis, changes in the affinity of the receptor for β-arrestin, and downregulation of the signaling pathways downstream from the receptor (Cao et al. 2010; Christie 2008; Dang and Christie 2012; Groer et al. 2011; Nestler et al. 2001). These biological changes can persist past discontinuation of opioids and then, consequently, result in withdrawal, possibly through increases in extracellular levels of the excitatory neurotransmitters glutamate and aspartate (Aghajanian et al. 1994).

Even if the acute biological changes of withdrawal normalize with abstinence, chronic changes remain, as evidenced by the increased risk of relapse even after withdrawal symptoms cease. Chronic changes may involve sensitivity to opioid-associated environmental cues that can trigger craving and relapse (Kosten and George 2002). The mechanism may involve activation of glutamatergic neurons in the prefrontal cortex, which can then stimulate the release of dopamine in the nucleus accumbens (mimicking opioid effects) and norepinephrine release from the locus coeruleus (mimicking opioid withdrawal) (Kosten and George 2002).

Intoxication Presentation

Opioids can produce reduced levels of consciousness (including coma) in a dose-dependent fashion. A euphoric effect on mood may be reported if the patient is alert enough to communicate. More specific effects on the CNS include miosis and respiratory depression, with the latter causing most opioid overdose deaths (Donroe and Tetrault 2017). Hypoxia resulting from respiratory depression can result in pulmonary edema, which is often noted in opioid overdose deaths. Furthermore, cerebral edema occurs in about half of all opioid overdose deaths, which is also linked to systemic hypoxia (Pelletier and Andrew 2017).

Opioids can also cause delirium, hypotension, bradycardia, low body temperature, nausea, constipation, and urinary retention. Many opioid agonists, including fentanyl, meperidine, tramadol, and methadone, are also serotonergic and therefore could contribute to the development of serotonin syndrome, especially if given with other serotonergic medications. Serotonin syndrome manifests as a combination of neuromuscular and autonomic hyperactivity and altered mental status (Baldo and Rose 2020). The diagnosis of serotonin syndrome is often made based on the presence of three of the five Hunter criteria: "spontaneous clonus, inducible clonus AND agitation OR diaphoresis, ocular clonus AND agitation OR diaphoresis, tremor AND hyperreflexia, and hypertonic AND temperature over 100.4 Fahrenheit AND ocular clonus OR inducible clonus" (Talton 2020, p. 456).

Withdrawal Presentation

Opioid withdrawal (sometimes abbreviated OW) is a syndrome of uncomfortable symptoms that spontaneously occur on cessation (or marked decrease) of opioid administration in an individual who has become physiologically dependent on an opioid agonist. Opioid dependence, the prerequisite for opioid withdrawal, can develop after just a few days of regular opioid use. Precipitated opioid withdrawal (sometimes abbreviated POW) is a subset of opioid withdrawal that is caused by administration of an opioid antagonist or high-affinity partial agonist to an individual while there is an opioid agonist active in the body. Opioid withdrawal symptoms can occur after a marked reduction in opioid intake or after opioid discontinuation. Precipitated opioid withdrawal can occur after a single dose of an opioid antagonist or high-affinity partial agonist (Bickel et al. 1987; Heishman et al. 1989; Jones 1979). Withdrawal is clinically significant, in part, because it is a significant risk factor for relapse.

The intensity of withdrawal depends on several factors. These factors include the dose and potency of the opioid being used before withdrawal, duration of use of that opioid, rate of removal or displacement of opioids from receptors, extent of continuous use, and even personality and psychological variables, such as state of mind at the time of withdrawal or expectations of the severity of symptoms (Kleber 1981).

Generally, the characteristics of withdrawal symptoms are opposite those of the acute agonist effects. For example, whereas constipation occurs during use of opioids, bowel hypermotility often occurs in withdrawal, and individuals tend to experience diarrhea, along with other symptoms such as diaphoresis, lacrimation, and rhinorrhea, prompting a phrase that may be helpful for diagnosis: "everything is runny." In addition, myalgias, piloerection, anxiety, insomnia, and abdominal cramping may be prominent. Generally, the shorter the duration of action of the drug, the more severe the withdrawal syndrome after discontinuation or reduction. Conventionally, the more rapidly the symptoms emerge, the shorter the total duration of the symptoms. With short-acting opioid agonists such as heroin and morphine, early symptoms may occur 8–12 hours after the last dose, and severe syndromes peak in 48–72 hours. Untreated, the acute phase of morphine or heroin withdrawal lasts 7–10 days. Withdrawal from fentanyl starts 8–16 hours after the last administration and lasts up to 8 days (with wide variation, depending on chronicity and level of fentanyl use, as noted earlier in this section), whereas withdrawal from the longer-acting methadone starts 30 hours after the last administration and can last for more than 2 weeks (Pergolizzi et al. 2020). Codeine withdrawal is generally less severe than that for the more potent opioid agonists, which tracks with its lower potency relative to other agonists.

Buprenorphine withdrawal syndrome has been characterized as relatively mild, with a peak in self-reported symptoms 3 days after the last buprenorphine intake (Fudala et al. 1990; Jasinski et al. 1978; Kosten and Kleber 1988; Mello and Mendelson 1980). However, clinical experience with patients after long-term buprenorphine administration has identified a wide range of symptomatology, with some patients reporting a prolonged and significant opioid withdrawal state. Withdrawal from κ-agonists (e.g., nalorphine) is generally mild and qualitatively distinct. Meperidine withdrawal develops within 3 hours after the last dose, peaks in 5–12 hours, and generally ends in 4–5 days. With meperidine, subjective symptoms, such as craving and restlessness, may be much more severe than the autonomic changes.

An often-underappreciated protracted abstinence syndrome may follow the acute opioid withdrawal syndrome and last for many weeks (Martin et al. 1973). In one study of individuals with heroin use disorder given methadone for MSW, withdrawal distress peaked at day 20 after the final day of methadone dosing, and it was not until day 40 that symptom scores reached normal levels (Gossop et al. 1987). During this protracted abstinence phase, there may be excessive somatic concerns, decreased stress tolerance, poor self-image, and disturbed sleep. Opioid effects are especially reinforcing during this protracted withdrawal phase, perhaps providing one explanation for early relapse (Cushman and Dole 1973; Martin et al. 1973).

Previously, ratings of withdrawal severity from agents such as heroin, morphine, and methadone were made with the Himmelsbach scale (Himmelsbach 1941), which emphasized objective or measurable signs over subjective reports (Table 5.2). Work giving greater weight to subjective aspects of withdrawal distress, however, has shown that individuals using opioids experience subjective mood changes, fatigue, dysphoria, and vague discomfort many hours before objective signs, such as lacrimation or yawning, can be detected. A useful and commonly used scale that combines both objective and subjective measures is the Clinical Opiate Withdrawal Scale (COWS; Wesson and Ling 2003). COWS is available through a number of nonproprietary online sources, including the National Institute on Drug Abuse (2025) and the American Society of Addiction Medicine (2025).

Pharmacological Management of Intoxication

Opioids in overdose can result in respiratory depression and death. Overdose effects and respiratory depression can be reversed with opioid antagonists, such as naloxone. Historically, naloxone has been administered in increments of 0.4 mg intravenously or intramuscularly and repeated until effective in reversing respiratory depression (Fareed et al. 2011). In some instances, continuous naloxone intravenous infusions may be needed to reverse and maintain individuals until systemic opioids are sufficiently metabolized.

Naloxone has also long been used off-label intranasally, often through repurposing of the intravenous formulation into aerosolizing devices. In 2015, a self-contained naloxone nasal spray delivery device gained FDA approval, consisting of a 4-mg single-dose spray unit. It is dispensed as two individual administration units to allow for the multiple dosing that may be required in some overdose situations. Additional generic naloxone nasal spray devices were approved by the FDA in 2019. Naloxone nasal sprays were

Table 5.2 Signs and symptoms of opioid withdrawal

Early	Middle	Late
Lacrimation	Restless sleep	Increased severity of earlier symptoms
Yawning	Dilated pupils	Tachycardia
Rhinorrhea	Anorexia	Nausea
Sweating	Gooseflesh	Vomiting
	Restlessness	Diarrhea
	Irritability	Abdominal cramps
	Tremor	Increased blood pressure
		Mood lability
		Depression
		Muscle spasms
		Weakness
		Bone pain

Source. Adapted from Ciraulo and Ciraulo (1988).

approved by the FDA for over-the-counter sales (i.e., without a prescription) in 2023.

With the increasing frequency of overdoses due to nonpharmaceutical fentanyl, fentanyl analogs, and novel high-potency synthetic opioids (HPSOs), higher initial naloxone doses have been suggested. After 2015, median cumulative naloxone doses given to patients whose symptoms responded to treatment were 3.4 mg for overdose due to fentanyl or other potent opioids and 2 mg for overdose due to heroin (Moe et al. 2020). In 2021, devices delivering naloxone 8 mg intranasally (IN) were approved by the FDA to help address the higher doses often needed to reverse fentanyl and related synthetic opioid overdoses (discussed later in this section). However, it is not clear whether a single higher-dose intranasal spray is more clinically effective in reversing opioid overdoses than consecutive 4-mg intranasal administrations. There are concerns about the possibility of a more significant opioid withdrawal experience after 8-mg versus 4-mg IN administration of naloxone, which might unfortunately discourage use of the product (Bell et al. 2019; Carpenter et al. 2020; Hill et al. 2022; Krotulski et al. 2022). What seems to be most significant in determining the success of naloxone opioid overdose reversal, especially in fentanyl-involved overdoses, is how quickly naloxone is administered in relation to opioid ingestion.

Widespread efforts to distribute intranasal naloxone in the community have increased access to overdose treatment in the field, and these efforts have become a cornerstone of many community-based responses to the opioid overdose crisis. Concerns that widespread availability of naloxone would lead to riskier use of opioids have not been borne out, with one study showing that opioid overdose rates were lower in counties that had widespread community naloxone distribution than in counties without (Naumann et al. 2019).

Naloxone has a short half-life (~30–45 minutes) and is most bioavailable via intranasal, intramuscular, and intravenous routes of administration. Naloxone is poorly bioavailable orally. When administered to treat an overdose in an individual physiologically dependent on opioids, naloxone rapidly displaces agonist opioids from MORs, thereby restoring consciousness and respiration. However, the rapidity and extent of displacement in the absence of any replacement receptor agonism induces a severe withdrawal syndrome (within seconds intravenously; within <5 minutes intranasally). The withdrawal syndrome lasts for the duration of naloxone action and may be ameliorated with nonopioid symptomatic medications (discussed later in "Symptomatic Treatment").

In individuals who are physically dependent on or who have experienced overdose with long-acting opioids such as methadone, naloxone may be effectively metabolized before the long-acting opioids, resulting in reoverdose or reintoxication after naloxone reversal despite no new opioid ingestion. Therefore, after a patient recovers adequate ventilation after a naloxone reversal of opioid overdose, they should still be monitored for return of respiratory depression ($\leq$48 hours if long-acting opioid exposure is suspected), and providers should be prepared to readminister naloxone if necessary. In some instances, patients may also require intubation and admission to the ICU for fully supportive care, including possible intravenous naloxone drips. If respiratory depression does not resolve with naloxone administration, then other causes of respiratory difficulties and impaired consciousness should be explored. In addition, if a patient has signs of opioid intoxication without respiratory depression, supportive care and monitoring would be the appropriate treatment to ensure that respiratory depression does not develop (Wishik et al. 2021).

Furthermore, overdoses with fentanyl and other HPSOs may present idiosyncratic reactions not seen with other opioids. For example, rapid complete vocal cord closure (VCC) and chest wall rigidity (also known as wooden chest syndrome) in response to fentanyl administration have been noted in both the anesthesia literature and animal research models. The mechanism for these unique reactions—which are not encountered with other opioids—is not well understood but appears to be via noradrenergic and cholinergic pathways independent of the MOR (Bennett et al. 1997; Miner et al. 2021; Torralva and Janowsky 2019). Therefore, naloxone may not be effective in reversing these distinct overdose reactions, and mechanical ventilation and even muscle paralytic medications may be required; however, administration of naloxone before onset of VCC or wooden chest syndrome may prevent the development of these idiosyncratic reactions.

Finally, because fentanyl has such a rapid time of onset, and because respiratory depression, chest wall rigidity, or VCC may occur within 2 minutes after ingestion, the window for possible successful naloxone reversal or initiation of mechanical ventilation may be much shorter than the window for such interventions with other opioids (i.e., upward of 30 minutes in a heroin overdose).

Pharmacological Management of Withdrawal

It is important to treat withdrawal because it can cause significant distress and is a major risk factor for relapse. However, treatment of withdrawal alone is ineffective for promoting remission of OUD. Two-thirds of patients who receive treatment for opioid withdrawal but do not receive ongoing treatment for OUD (e.g., buprenorphine, methadone, or naltrexone pharmacotherapies) will experience relapse to opioid use within the first few months following treatment (Bailey et al. 2013). This finding was reinforced in a study in which inpatients started on buprenorphine for OUD had reduced illicit opioid use in the following 6 months compared with those who received short-term treatment for withdrawal alone without initiation of a long-term medication (Stein et al. 2020). Strong efforts must be made to interest the patient in long-term treatment that continues after withdrawal symptoms subside (see "Maintenance Pharmacological Management of Opioid Use Disorder").

The two most common pharmacological approaches to the treatment of opioid withdrawal are 1) symptomatic management and 2) agonist opioid replacement followed by taper. In symptomatic management, the individual's specific opioid withdrawal symptoms are targeted with pharmacotherapies for those symptoms, without the use of opioids (e.g., ibuprofen for myalgias or loperamide for diarrhea; these specific pharmacotherapies are discussed in greater detail in "Other Symptomatic Medications"). An agonist opioid replacement strategy would, conversely, utilize opioid medications to address opioid withdrawal symptoms. In agonist opioid replacement, the goal may be either to gradually taper off the replacement opioids (MSW, more colloquially referred to as *detoxification*) or to establish a maintenance opioid medication (i.e., methadone or buprenorphine) that would then be continued indefinitely. In some instances, a patient may require symptomatic management pharmacotherapies while opioid agonist replacement treatment is being undertaken, because some opioid withdrawal symptoms may emerge before initiation or during titration of agonist opioid replacement treatment.

As discussed earlier, maintenance treatments provide the best chance for long-term success in treating OUD, and a patient seeking treatment for opioid withdrawal can be in an ideal motivational situation to consider maintenance treatment. MSW alone, however—whether using methadone or buprenorphine protocols—is often followed by relapse if maintenance treatment is not provided (Dunn et al. 2011) (discussed later in "Maintenance Pharmacological Management of Opioid Use Disorder"). Nonetheless, after a careful conversation about the treatment options and likelihood of long-term success, in conjunction with an exploration of a patient's individual goals and priorities, a patient may opt for a medication-free approach to treating OUD once acute opioid withdrawal has been managed. However, if a patient decides to pursue maintenance treatment, symptomatic management presents a viable strategy for segueing into antagonist maintenance treatment (i.e., naltrexone), whereas MSW can present an excellent opportunity for segueing into opioid maintenance treatment because the MSW can be initiated using buprenorphine or methadone.

Agonist Opioid Taper Approach

Methadone

In the United States, methadone has long been used to treat acute opioid withdrawal symptoms. The process of using methadone to treat acute withdrawal symptoms followed by taper is often a part of MSW and can be accomplished over a period as long as 6 months in an ambulatory methadone program or as brief as several days in a hospital setting. In brief MSW, the goal is to make the experience less distressing, but the suppression of all withdrawal symptoms may not be possible. If the daily opioid dose is known, one could, in theory, begin with a gradual taper using a pharmacologically equivalent methadone dose. The drawback to this approach is that the published equivalencies of oral methadone vary markedly. For example, one source cited reported equivalencies of oral morphine to oral methadone ranging from 4:1 to 14:1 (Gordon et al. 1999), although the equivalency may be as low as 2.5:1 (Ripamonti et al. 1998). In addition, for individuals taking illicitly produced opioids (which may be mixtures of various opioids), it may be difficult or impossible to accurately determine their daily dose. Thus, caution should be used when dosing is guided by equivalency tables.

Because of methadone's increased duration of action and oral efficacy, withdrawal may be suppressed with lower doses of oral methadone than would be predicted from the published analgesic equivalency ratios. For patients taking street heroin, the initial dose of methadone is usually 30 mg PO. If withdrawal symptoms or signs persist, one may add an additional 10-mg dose in a few hours. Overshooting the methadone dose by escalating doses beyond these amounts too quickly or by using equivalency tables is a serious concern because methadone takes 4–5 days to reach steady state. As a result, blood levels of methadone may continue to rise for 4–5 days despite consistent dosing levels. If the initial dose is escalated too quickly, individuals can experience opioid overdose 4–5 days later despite no evidence of overdose on day 1.

Now that fentanyl use has become more commonplace, doses of methadone higher than 30–40 mg may be required to quell withdrawal, but the risks of sedation and respiratory depression from increasing doses must be balanced against the benefit for withdrawal. Once a stabilizing dosage has been found, methadone can be tapered off by approximately 5 mg/day within 5–8 days (American Psychiatric Association 2006). To facilitate adherence in outpatient MSW, the treatment period may need to be prolonged. Reasonable tapering schedules are 10% per week from high doses and 3% per week from dosages less than 20 mg/day (Senay et al. 1977).

Buprenorphine

Since the 1990s, buprenorphine has been recognized as an effective agent for treatment of opioid withdrawal. In one study, sublingual buprenorphine appeared to be as effective as methadone in a 7-week taper (Bickel et al. 1987). Sublingual buprenorphine, available for the office-based treatment of OUD, has become one of the standard options for withdrawal treatment. However, the optimal withdrawal protocol is still under study, and clinically there is wide variability in buprenorphine MSW protocols. Nonetheless, the principle with buprenorphine MSW is similar to that described with methadone: establish a starting dose that quells withdrawal, then taper at a clinically tolerable rate. Currently, many clinicians follow the guidelines for buprenorphine initiation outlined in "Maintenance Pharmacological Management of Opioid Use Disorder," Table 5.5, followed by a 2–5-day medication taper (Cheskin et al. 1994; Horspool et al. 2008).

One important distinction between methadone and buprenorphine for MSW is that traditional protocols require the individual to demonstrate withdrawal before the initial buprenorphine dose is administered (to avoid precipitated opioid withdrawal), whereas methadone initiation requires no withdrawal symptoms to be present. For some individuals, the experience of any withdrawal symptoms may be highly destabilizing; therefore, the provider embarking on a traditional buprenorphine initiation protocol should be ready to provide adjunctive symptomatic treatment options if needed.

Symptomatic Treatment

Clonidine and Lofexidine

Clonidine and lofexidine are both α_2-agonists commonly used to treat opioid withdrawal. Although clonidine has been used in this manner for decades, it does not carry FDA approval for this indication, whereas lofexidine has FDA approval for the treatment of opioid withdrawal. α_2-Agonists have been shown to suppress many of the uncomfortable autonomic symptoms of the withdrawal syndrome (Gold et al. 1978; Kleber et al. 1985).

Patients taking opioids can be transitioned to taking oral clonidine at dosages starting at 0.1–0.2 mg tid (≤0.6 mg/day in inpatient settings). Clonidine can be given for approximately 7–10 days for patients stopping shorter-acting opioids and for up to 14 days for those stopping long-acting opioids. Lofexidine is dosed at 0.54 mg (three 0.18-mg tablets) qid for 7–14 days, followed by a 2-day to 4-day taper (reducing by one tablet per dose every 1–2 days). Limiting the outpatient use of α_2-agonists are three major side effects: hypotension (which may be marked), sedation, and rebound hypertension. For this reason, dosages greater than 1.0 mg/day clonidine and 2.88 mg/day lofexidine are not recommended in outpatient settings, and treatment duration should be limited to the amount of time necessary to successfully minimize acute opioid withdrawal symptoms. Another important limitation of α_2-agonists is that although they suppress autonomic signs of withdrawal, symptoms such as lethargy, restlessness, insomnia, and craving are not well relieved (Charney et al. 1981; Jasinski et al. 1985). Compared with clonidine, lofexidine is less likely to produce hypotension or sedation; however, lofexidine is significantly more expensive (Kuszmaul et al. 2020; Strang et al. 1999).

Other Symptomatic Medications

Individuals experiencing opioid withdrawal may report a wide range of physiological and psychological symptoms, and pharmacological interventions targeted to ameliorate these experiences can be beneficial. Because of interindividual differences, the authors recommend asking the patient for descriptions of their most bothersome symptoms and targeting those specifically, rather than giving all patients the same combination of symptomatic medications. Refer to Table 5.3 for further specific information on commonly used nonopioid pharmacological symptomatic medications.

Opioid Use Disorder Presentation

The diagnosis of OUD can be made using DSM-5 (American Psychiatric Association 2013) and DSM-5-TR (American Psychiatric Association 2022) criteria. It is important to highlight that 9 of the 11 diagnostic criteria are behavioral in nature, whereas the two physiological criteria (tolerance and withdrawal) are neither necessary nor sufficient to make an OUD diagnosis. (For further information, see the discussion of substance use disorder [SUD] diagnostic criteria in the Preface of this book.)

The progression from initial use of opioids to OUD may take different pathways and may start with use of either prescribed or illicit opioids.

Table 5.3 Commonly used symptomatic nonopioid medications to treat opioid withdrawal

Medication	Use	As-needed dosing (all PO formulations)	Notes
Hydroxyzine	Anxiety and insomnia	25 mg tid	May need dose decrease in renal/hepatic compromise
Loperamide	Diarrhea	2 mg tid	Monitor for dehydration
Dicyclomine	Abdominal cramps	10 mg tid	May need dose decrease in renal/hepatic compromise
Diphenhydramine	Anxiety and insomnia	50 mg tid	IV and IM formulations available; dose decrease needed in hepatic compromise
Ibuprofen	Pain	400 mg every 4–6 h	Caution in patients with kidney disease; good hydration necessary
Acetaminophen	Pain	650–1,000 mg every 4–6 h	May need dose decrease in severe hepatic compromise; IV formulation available
Benzodiazepines (lorazepam)[a]	Anxiety	0.5–1 mg every 4–6 h	IV and IM formulations available
Ondansetron	Nausea/vomiting	4 mg bid	Rare risk of QT prolongation/cardiac arrhythmias; dose decrease in hepatic compromise may be needed

Table 5.3 Commonly used symptomatic nonopioid medications to treat opioid withdrawal *(continued)*

Medication	Use	As-needed dosing (all PO formulations)	Notes
Promethazine	Nausea/vomiting	12.5–25 mg PO every 4–6 h	IM and rectal formulations available
Clonidine	Decrease sympathetic tone often increased in withdrawal state	0.1 mg tid	Hypotension; rebound hypertension possible after long-term use; concurrent use of tricyclic antidepressants not advised
Lofexidine[b]	Decrease sympathetic tone often increased in withdrawal state	0.54 mg qid for 7–14 d, followed by a 2–4-d taper	Hypotension; rebound hypertension possible after long-term use; concurrent use of tricyclic antidepressants not advised
Trazodone	Insomnia	25–100 mg at bedtime	May need dose decrease in renal/hepatic compromise; rare priapism
Doxepin	Insomnia	6–50 mg at bedtime	May need dose decrease in hepatic compromise

Note. IM = intramuscular; IV = intravenous; PO = per os.

[a]Given the misuse potential of benzodiazepines, the high concurrence of opioid and benzodiazepine misuse, and the additive risk potential for respiratory depression with benzodiazepines and opioids, care should be taken when using benzodiazepines as an adjunctive medication for treating opioid withdrawal.

[b]Approved by the FDA for the treatment of opioid withdrawal.

In vulnerable individuals, brief experimentation with opioids may lead to OUD through neuroadaptive changes resulting from the initially rewarding experience that favor continued use (see the Volkow-Koob three-part model of addiction development described in section "Pharmacology and Neurobiology of Opioids"). Opioids can be reinforcing by directly inducing pleasurable effects (positive reinforcement) or by reducing aversive affects or the experience of noxious stimuli, such as those experienced in withdrawal, or relief of anxiety or pain (negative reinforcement). Repeated reinforcement associated with opioid use, whether positive or negative, leads to erosion of control over intake, drives continued use despite negative consequences, and enhances craving, all of which form the behavioral basis of OUD. Certain reinforcers, such as relief of withdrawal symptoms (which may occur several times a day when an individual is using short-acting opioids), can strongly reinforce opioid use behavior patterns. Furthermore, the rituals, paraphernalia, and environmental setting of using opioids often become associated with the positive experience of use, thereby becoming cues favoring or triggering further use. This process of previously neutral environmental stimuli becoming imbued with powerfully motivating associations is termed *incentive salience.*

OUD can be conceptualized as a chronic illness, akin to diabetes, asthma, or hypertension, that has a relapsing and remitting course and can carry significant risk of morbidity and mortality. Compared with diabetes, hypertension, and asthma, SUDs have similar rates of genetic heritability and similar treatment adherence and relapse rates (McLellan et al. 2000). OUD and opioid misuse have been associated with high mortality rates related to factors such as overdose, suicide, homicide/violence, trauma, and medical sequalae (e.g., infection, cardiovascular and hepatic failure). A Swedish study reported a 20% mortality rate during a 1-year period in a group of patients with OUD who served as the control group in a double-blind, placebo-controlled long-term buprenorphine study (Kakko et al. 2003). Since the study's publication, the increasing availability of fentanyl and other high-potency synthetic opioids has likely also affected mortality rates in those with OUD, the impact of which is yet to be fully characterized.

Currently, no reliable means are available to predict long-term prognosis of OUD as measured by drug use, work, crime, or psychological adjustment. Although the achievement of temporary abstinence is associated with improvement in several factors (legal problems, in particular), simply achieving abstinence does not ensure an adequate psychosocial adjustment (Kosten et al. 1987a; Rounsaville et al. 1987). Therefore, full recovery from OUD often requires not just cessation of substance use but also exploration of (and commitment to) life changes that favor long-standing improvements in quality of life (e.g., meaningful work, healthy relationships, awareness and avoidance of high-risk situations) that mitigate the behavioral aspects of OUD described earlier in this section. Mutual help groups and various behavioral treatments can assist in achieving this recovery from OUD (Humphreys et al. 2020).

Maintenance Pharmacological Management of Opioid Use Disorder

In line with the conceptualization of OUD as a chronic relapsing illness akin to diabetes, it is not surprising that one of the most effective treatments for OUD remains maintenance treatment with medications: methadone, buprenorphine, or naltrexone. This is not unlike chronic management of diabetes or hypertension through long-term use of insulin or antihypertensive agents, respectively. The duration of maintenance OUD medication treatment is often debated, but clinical experience and empirical evidence support the notion that the longer an individual is in treatment with medications for OUD, the better they do overall; that is, there are fewer relapses and overdoses, as well as reductions in transmission of HIV and hepatitis, hospital utilization, and criminal activity (Anderson and Kearney 2000; Cornish et al. 2010; Gomes et al. 2022; Jarlenski et al. 2022). For this reason, clinical guidelines recommend that medications for OUD be continued indefinitely (Anderson and Kearney 2000; Bruneau et al. 2018; Mancher and Leshner 2019).

Maintenance pharmacological management begins with a comprehensive evaluation of the patient. The purpose of the evaluation is 1) to establish accurate diagnoses and map motivation and preferences for particular types of treatment; 2) to determine the presence of co-occurring psychopathology, other SUDs, or other misuse; and 3) to identify medical conditions, as well as other psychosocial factors, that may affect treatment choice. History of prior treatment engagements and outcomes, as well as logistic and treatment access factors, is also important to define in the assessment process. After a diagnosis of OUD is established, it is essential to lay out the various treatment options alongside the benefits, risks, and alternatives of these options, including each of the medication options available for treatment of OUD. Although many factors can contribute to the recommendation of one medication option over another, some general considerations include the following: the need for a highly structured treatment environment (methadone as opposed to buprenorphine or naltrexone), owing to disorganization or prior difficulties with less structured treatment programs; the inability to tolerate brief abstinent periods prior to medication initiation (methadone and buprenorphine as opposed to naltrexone or nonclassic initiation of buprenorphine); employment or other logistical barriers that preclude daily dosing (buprenorphine or naltrexone as opposed to methadone); and employment in safety-sensitive occupations that forbid agonist treatment (naltrexone as opposed to methadone or buprenorphine). Medication-specific factors are explored in further detail in the following sections.

Research on the efficacy of medication for OUD suggests that counseling or psychotherapy plays a critical role in patient success, but that extra counseling beyond close prescriber monitoring may not be necessary for patients with a multitude of positive prognostic factors, such as no additional co-occurring substance use or psychiatric conditions and no history of intravenous use, among other factors (Ball and Ross 1991; Fiellin et al. 2006; O'Brien et al. 1995; Weiss and Rao 2017; Weiss et al. 2011; Woody et al. 1995).

Methadone

Dole and Nyswander (1965) first introduced long-term methadone treatment for OUD in 1964. This approach should be distinguished from the use of methadone for the treatment of pain, which is typically of short duration in an acute setting. Methadone for the treatment of pain does not require connection to an opioid treatment program (OTP), as opposed to methadone for the treatment of OUD. The effectiveness of long-term methadone for OUD has been well documented (Ball and Ross 1991; Ling et al. 1998). Methadone can alleviate craving and withdrawal and induce cross-tolerance to other opioids so that euphoria is diminished. Effects were less dramatic in studies with less motivated patients with more mental health problems than those treated by Dole and Nyswander (Sells 1979). Nevertheless, long-term methadone reduces opioid and nonopioid substance use, health problems (including HIV rates), and crime (e.g., Ball and Ross 1991; Ball et al. 1988a,

1988b; Gerstein and Harwood 1990; Sees et al. 2000; Senay 1985; Sullivan et al. 2005). Despite these benefits, some patients have a negative attitude toward this treatment approach. In particular, many individuals have difficulty with the controls mandated in a methadone clinic and are often misinformed about methadone itself, factors that may make them reluctant to enter into this form of treatment (Hunt et al. 1985). In addition, some health professionals and members of the general public consider it a controversial treatment. Even with the extensive research documenting the efficacy of long-term methadone, some believe its primary purpose is crime reduction; others confuse physiological dependence on methadone with addiction and see it as merely a substitution of one addiction for another. Despite these reservations, opioid agonist treatment has been adopted independently in at least 77 countries (Dhawan et al. 2014).

Methadone is an MOR agonist with unique properties that make it particularly useful as a long-term maintenance pharmacotherapy. Methadone is reliably absorbed orally, does not reach a peak concentration until about 4 hours after administration, and maintains a large extravascular reservoir (Kreek 1979). Together, these properties minimize acute euphoric effects. The reservoir results in a plasma half-life of 1–2 days, so there are usually no rapid blood level drops that could lead to withdrawal syndromes between daily doses. Because of the long half-life, the steady-state methadone blood level is not achieved until 4–5 days after a stable dose is given. The methadone dose must be increased slowly (in an outpatient setting every 5 days or so) to avoid an accidental overdose that might occur were the dose rapidly increased without waiting 5 days for the full effect of a dose change to present itself (Baxter et al. 2013). There is wide variability in blood levels with identical doses (Kreek 1979), and the patient requires an individualized dose to achieve the desired effect of methadone, which is twofold: easing withdrawal from, and reducing craving for, the opioid of misuse. Because of the need to increase the methadone dose slowly over days, it may take some time to achieve the ideal dose that reduces withdrawal and craving. These beneficial effects of methadone have to be weighed against the adverse effects, especially while a patient's dose is in the process of being increased. Indications that a methadone dose is too high include the emergence of adverse effects such as sedation, confusion, and especially respiratory depression, which is the cause of death in most opioid overdoses. Patients require close monitoring for adverse effects while the methadone dose is being increased, and these effects will likely be strongest at 4 hours postdose (when levels are at peak) and 4–5 days after a dose increase when the blood level has stabilized at its height (see the next paragraph for further discussion of adverse effects).

Because of the aforementioned concerns about dosing, methadone is typically started at a low dosage of 10–30 mg/day and usually does not exceed 40 mg on the first day of dosing. In the outpatient setting during initiation, guidelines have recommended increasing the dose every 5 days in increments of 5 mg or less (Baxter et al. 2013). Indications that the dose should be started on the lower end include patient characteristics of advanced age, liver dysfunction, any health condition that interferes with breathing or wakefulness, cardiac risk factors, and taking interacting medications. The inpatient level of care has intensive monitoring, allowing faster methadone dose increases; the outpatient level of care has the least intensive monitoring, necessitating slower dose increases. Once an individual has tolerated methadone for an initial 2 weeks or so, the dose can be increased slightly faster: every 3–5 days by 5–10 mg. If doses are missed for 3 days or more, dosing may need to be restarted at a lower dose to avoid adverse effects, including overdose.

Because dosing is so individualized, serum levels of methadone are not usually followed as an indication of effectiveness; rather, the focus is reduction of craving and withdrawal. Some individuals' symptoms unexpectedly respond inadequately to methadone even at dosages as high as 200 mg/day (Leavitt 2003; Tennant 1987). In this case, serum methadone levels drawn at 4 hours after dosing (peak) and at 24 hours after dosing (trough) can be compared to identify rapid metabolizers, in whom the ratio of peak-to-trough methadone levels is 2 or higher. Rapid metabolizers may have better symptom response on another treatment such as buprenorphine, or they may require higher-than-typical dosing or even split dosing. Others have proposed identification of individual metabolic differences through measurement of the serum methadone/metabolite ratio (MMR) shortly after dosing, thereby potentially eliminating the need for peak/trough measurements (McCarthy et al. 2020).

Additionally, numerous medication and diet interactions can profoundly influence methadone blood levels. Methadone is metabolized by hepatic enzymes in the CYP system, primarily by CYP3A4 (Shinderman et al. 2003). In addition, hepatic enzyme-inducing medications, such as phenobarbital, phenytoin, carbamazepine, isoniazid, rifampin, nevirapine, and large doses of vitamin C, may markedly reduce serum methadone concentrations (Bell et al. 1988; Kreek 1979). Agents that raise methadone levels include ketoconazole, fluconazole, sertraline, amitriptyline, paroxetine, fluvoxamine, fluoxetine, diazepam, alprazolam, and zidovudine, which implies that enzymes that metabolize these medications, including CYP2D6, CYP2C9, and CYP2C19, may also contribute to methadone metabolism (Table 5.4).

Even with adequate methadone plasma levels, some patients continue to misuse medications, such as sedatives, possibly because they are seeking a form of intoxication rather than relief of opioid craving (Bell et al. 1990).

Although tolerance develops to methadone, as with all opioids, some pharmacological effects of methadone may persist (Kreek 1983; also see earlier discussion in "Pharmacology and Neurobiology of Opioids"). Euphoria and drowsiness are generally more pronounced in the first weeks of treatment. Slight but measurable mood elevation occurs concurrently with peak plasma levels in patients whose symptoms are stabilized with methadone and may be one reason that some patients stay in treatment (McCaul et al. 1982). Full tolerance may not develop to constipation, perspiration, decreased libido, pupillary constriction, and sexual dysfunction. Opioid-induced endocrine effects of methadone usually resolve after a few months, but chronic use of opioids may lower testosterone and follicle-stimulating hormone levels. However, no strong correlation exists between these levels and sexual dysfunction. During the early months of treatment, patients may have altered electroencephalographic sleep patterns and insomnia. Although electroencephalographic results appear to normalize, sleep disturbance may persist. At higher doses (generally >100 mg), methadone may induce prolongation of the QTc interval that could lead to torsades de pointes (Kornick et al. 2003; Krantz et al. 2002, 2003), especially when individuals receiving methadone maintenance are coadministered other known QTc-prolonging medications. Patients at risk may require dose reductions and careful electrocardiographic monitoring. There is no evidence for long-term organ damage with methadone.

Federal, state, and sometimes local regulations govern OTPs, which are the only facilities licensed to provide long-term methadone for treatment of OUD. Federal standards exist for admission, frequency of urine testing, methadone dosage, quantity of take-home medication, and treatment of OUD in pregnant people. Historically, regulations stipulated that patients must be at least 18 years old (with some exceptions, such as emancipated

Table 5.4 Methadone metabolism and interacting medications

Reduces serum methadone levels	Increases serum methadone levels
Phenobarbital	Ketoconazole
Phenytoin	Fluconazole
Carbamazepine	Sertraline
Isoniazid	Amitriptyline
Rifampin	Paroxetine
Nevirapine	Fluvoxamine
Vitamin C in large doses	Fluoxetine
Risperidone	Diazepam
	Alprazolam
	Zidovudine
	Erythromycin

Source. Ferrari A et al. 2004.

minors 16–18 years old) and that "the person became addicted at least 1 year before admission for treatment" and "is currently addicted," although the comparable terminology for "addiction" is now *opioid use disorder* (Substance Abuse and Mental Health Services Administration 2015, p. 21). The 1-year history has not been a requirement for people recently released from prison or a chronic care institution (provided that they would have been eligible for methadone before incarceration or institutionalization), for pregnant people, or for selected patients who have previously received methadone (Substance Abuse and Mental Health Services Administration 2015).

In March 2020, some of the rules governing methadone were relaxed because of the COVID-19 pandemic, in which duration of take-home doses increased and telemedicine monitoring was allowed for existing patients receiving methadone but not for induction onto methadone (Substance Abuse and Mental Health Services Administration 2020). Despite loosening of restrictions on methadone, access to methadone for new patients may have declined during the COVID-19 pandemic (Joudrey et al. 2021). Nonetheless, as of passage of the Consolidated Appropriations Act of 2023, several key changes were made to OTP regulations. One such change was the elimination of the X-waiver requirement to prescribe buprenorphine (discussed later in "Legal and Regulatory Considerations for Buprenorphine for the Treatment of Opioid Use Disorder"). Additional COVID-19-era public health emergency regulations were made permanent and included the following: 1) up to 28 days of take-home methadone doses for patients deemed to have stable symptoms and up to 14 days of take-home doses for patients deemed to have less stable symptoms, with greater discretion given to OTPs to assess stability; 2) expansion of the definition of *practitioner* to include nonphysician prescribers (e.g., nurse practitioners, physician assistants); and 3) elimination of the requirement of documented 1 year of opioid use to qualify for methadone treatment (Medications for the Treatment of Opioid Use Disorder 2022).

Traditionally, the maximum first-day methadone dose is 30 mg, with an additional 10 mg permitted if withdrawal symptoms persist after the initial dose. Patients initially return daily for each dose of methadone. Because patients may underreport their drug use, random urine testing is required (Magura et al. 1987). Until 2023, after 90 days of methadone treatment, patients who had been free from nonprescribed opioids for 30 days were eligible for weekend take-home doses. Eventually, patients who had been drug free for the previous 9 months could qualify for up to six take-home doses per week. After 2 years of treatment, patients who remained drug free could earn up to a 30-day supply of take-home doses. As noted in the previous paragraph, these strict regulations have loosened with the passage of the Consolidated Appropriations Act of 2023, giving OTPs greater flexibility for determining take-home medication procedures.

Reasons for discharge from a methadone program include persistent substance use, sporadic attendance, in-clinic drug dealing, and aggressive behavior at the clinic. Although patients who behave in these ways may undermine the treatment milieu, some clinicians are reluctant to discharge them because of concerns that they would do worse without treatment.

Although standard regulations and a common underlying philosophy result in many similarities among methadone programs, there are also several differences. Programs based on the original model of Dole and Nyswander (1965) tend to use a high methadone dosage ($\geq$80–120 mg/day) or more flexible dosing to ensure cross-tolerance and suppression of craving. In that model, illicit opioid use is seen as a response to a metabolic deficiency; indefinite continuation of methadone is thought to be the only way to preclude relapse. In these programs, response to continued opioid use may be met with increases in methadone dosing rather than dose decreases or termination from treatment. For this reason, it may not be uncommon for some individuals' symptoms to stabilize (sometimes for decades or longer) with daily methadone dosing of 200 mg or greater.

An alternative medical methadone program involves monthly visits at a physician's office to get a take-home supply of methadone tablets at a dosage of up to 100 mg/day. In patients with highly stable symptoms, the medical model has led to increased patient satisfaction and initiation of more new employment and social activities (King et al. 2002). The percentage of patients who experienced relapse, got into legal difficulty, or dropped out of treatment was very low (Novick et al. 1988). The medical model has not been successful for patients with unstable symptoms or those newly started on methadone, and there are concerns about the potential for diversion and overdose (Wesson 1988). This model is not currently an approved model of care in the United States.

Other programs use a methadone dosage in the range of 20–60 mg/day and less flexible dosing. Patients are viewed not as having a biological illness but rather as being responsible people who will do best if methadone is eventually tapered off. These programs are thus less tolerant of continued drug use and are more likely to discharge patients for problem behavior. The dosages of methadone used in these programs are often not high enough to prevent euphoria from illicit opioids. These programs generally have lower rates of retention in treatment (Brown et al. 1982). In a study of six methadone clinics believed to be operating effectively, the percentage of patients who had used illicit injection drugs during the month before the interview ranged from 9% to 57% (Ball and Ross 1991; Ball et al. 1988a, 1988b). Even after adjustment for differences among patients, the factors associated with less injection drug use (in addition to a higher methadone dosage) were the quality of program leadership and services provided. Another important factor is variability within programs; some counselors are demonstrably more effective than others. There are also demographic and psychological correlates of retention. Retention is better for patients who are employed, married, Black, and older. People with criminal histories and higher levels of psychopathology tend to leave treatment sooner. However, patients who receive case management and psychiatric services show significant improvement and retention in treatment comparable to that of patients without significant psychiatric comorbidity (Cacciola et al. 2001; Grella et al. 1997).

Treatment outcome is, of course, determined by multiple factors. Many of the factors contributing to retention rates also affect treatment outcome. There is no formula to determine how likely a person is to remain in remission from OUD while receiving treatment, but certain factors have been correlated with greater success. For example, patients without serious psychopathology or criminal backgrounds tend to have good treatment outcomes. This is not to say, however, that patients with these issues never improve. In one 2.5-year follow-up study, patients with criminal backgrounds showed significant improvement in substance use and in family, legal, and psychological problems (Kosten et al. 1987b). For patients with severe psychopathology, long-term methadone programs appear to be more helpful than therapeutic communities (see McLellan et al. 1986). Patients with more criminality and less psychopathology appear to prefer MSW to long-term medication for OUD (Kosten et al. 1986). Duration and severity of opioid use do not correlate with treatment outcome. Certain program factors can also enhance treatment outcomes; for example, among successful primary care–run programs, a common theme was having "integrated clinical teams with support staff who were often advanced practice clinicians (nurses and pharmacists) as clinical case managers" (Lagisetty et al. 2017, p. 2).

The factors that correlate with treatment success do not clearly apply to continued remission after tapering off a long-term medication for OUD. Greater success is correlated with less criminal behavior, a more stable family relationship, more stable employment, a shorter drug history, long-term methadone at a lower dosage before cessation, and discharge status, with patient and staff consensus being more favorable than unilateral discharge from treatment (Dole and Joseph 1978). In one study, individuals were followed for an average of 2 years after their long-term methadone was tapered off (Stimmel et al. 1977). Although only 28% of the total sample remained abstinent, 83% of those who had completed treatment remained abstinent. Treatment completion meant urine was persistently negative for nonprescribed medication, insight and coping skills were healthy, long-term planning was present, good social functioning was present, and stability or improvement in job functioning was present, among other things. In the study by Stimmel et al. (1977), before tapering off, patients who remained abstinent received methadone for an average of about 2 years, whereas those who experienced relapse received methadone for an average of 1 year. In another study of 105 patients for whom long-term methadone was tapered off, investigators documented an 82% relapse rate within 12 months (Ball and Ross 1991). These studies suggest that clinicians should exercise caution when recommending gradual discontinuation of long-term opioid agonists, even for successful patients. Other research has failed to identify patient characteristics or clinical approaches associated with long-term abstinence after the termination of long-term opioid agonist treatment (Calsyn et al. 2006). When patients elect to discontinue long-term opioid agonist treatment, a very gradual reduction of dosage over 3–6 months is preferred, with careful monitoring of drug craving and withdrawal symptoms.

Patients who need to reenter treatment at a later date often do much better than they did during their original treatment, showing less dependence, criminality, and physical disability (Kosten et al. 1986). Such findings suggest that intermittent treatment appears to be beneficial. Therefore, reentry does not necessarily indicate failure and may instead be a step toward eventual recovery. On the other hand, there is a high probability that those who discontinue opioid agonist therapy will resume injection drug use, with attendant risks for hepatitis and HIV infection (Ball et al. 1988a,; 1988b).

It is also important to note that dosing of methadone for pain is significantly different from that for maintenance treatment of OUD. The analgesic effect of methadone lasts approximately 4–6 hours; therefore, for chronic or acute analgesic dosing, methadone may be dosed 3–4 times daily. Therefore, methadone maintenance dosing (once a day) does not provide appropriate analgesia by itself, despite what may be seemingly high doses. Individuals receiving methadone maintenance who have acute analgesia needs should receive their daily maintenance dosing in addition to other full-agonist opioid or nonopioid analgesic medications. In some instances, in the setting of acute analgesia needs, individuals may receive their daily maintenance dosing in divided doses throughout the day to maximize methadone analgesia; however, this should be undertaken in a hospital setting with close collaboration alongside the patient's OTP.

The authors also suggest that providers outside of OTP settings become acquainted with their local OTP to better understand the local OTP's treatment approaches, policies, and procedures. This can prove invaluable when working to co-manage the care of individuals simultaneously receiving services in these treatment environments.

Buprenorphine

Buprenorphine is a semisynthetic opioid that was first synthesized in 1966 by chemists working with the British home products company Reckitt and Colman, who were seeking to create compounds that preserved the advantageous properties of opioids while minimizing the deleterious side effects (Campbell and Lovell 2012). Buprenorphine acts primarily as an MOR partial agonist and a strong antagonist at the KOR. Buprenorphine has a very high affinity for the μ receptor and can precipitate withdrawal by displacing other opioids from the receptor. However, buprenorphine also dissociates very slowly from the MOR, it has high lipophilicity, it is highly protein bound, and its metabolite (buprenorphine-3-glucuronide) enters enterohepatic circulation, all of which likely account for its long duration of action (24–48 hours). An additional benefit of buprenorphine is that risk of overdose-induced respiratory depression may be low. As a partial agonist, buprenorphine has a ceiling effect on respiratory depression as the dose is increased (Ciraulo et al. 2006; Walsh et al. 1994). Although buprenorphine was initially believed to produce a less severe withdrawal syndrome than full-agonist opioids because of its unique pharmacodynamics, clinical experience has demonstrated that individuals physically dependent on buprenorphine may experience a wide range of withdrawal severities when buprenorphine is discontinued (Derbel et al. 2016).

Buprenorphine for the Treatment of Pain

Injectable buprenorphine was first approved by the FDA for the treatment of moderate to severe pain in 1981 (0.3–0.6 mg IM or slow IV [over 2 minutes] every 6 hours prn) (Indivior 2023). A long-acting transdermal patch formulation of buprenorphine was approved in 2010 for the treatment of pain severe enough to require daily, around-the-clock, long-term opioid treatment and for which alternative options are inadequate (available in per-hour strengths of 5, 7.5, 10, 15, and 20 μg, typically placed every 7 days prn) (Purdue Pharma 2014). Similarly, a buccal film formulation of buprenorphine was approved in 2015 for the treatment of pain severe enough to require daily, around-the-clock, long-term opioid treatment and for which alternative options are inadequate (available in strengths of 75,

150, 300, 450, 600, 750, and 900 µg, administered every 12 hours prn) (Endo Pharmaceuticals 2016).

Buprenorphine for the Treatment of Opioid Use Disorder

In 1978, Jasinski et al. originally suggested the potential value of buprenorphine for the treatment of OUD (Campbell and Lovell 2012). The efficacy of long-term buprenorphine for the treatment of opioid dependence was established in a large multicenter randomized clinical trial (Ling et al. 1998). In this study, individuals taking buprenorphine 16 mg/day sublingually had fewer opioid-positive urine drug screen results and lower self-reported craving scores than individuals taking buprenorphine dosages of 1, 4, or 8 mg/day sublingually. In another study, buprenorphine (16–24 mg sublingually three times a week) and high-dose methadone (60–100 mg/day) were effective in treating OUD and superior to low-dose methadone (20 mg/day) in clinic retention and suppression of opioid use (Johnson et al. 2000). In a study comparing maintenance treatment versus tapering after 4 weeks of stabilization with buprenorphine, far superior treatment retention was observed in the maintenance group, supporting the benefits of long-term maintenance treatment over brief stabilization followed by MSW (Fiellin et al. 2014).

In 2002, the FDA approved a sublingual buprenorphine tablet and a combination sublingual buprenorphine/naloxone tablet for office-based treatment of OUD (although the buprenorphine monoproduct had been used outside of the United States, including in France since 1995, for the treatment of OUD prior to this). A comparable film formulation of combination buprenorphine/naloxone was approved in 2010. An intradermal implant 6-month formulation of buprenorphine (74.2 mg) and a subcutaneous 30-day, long-acting injectable (LAI) formulation (100 and 300 mg/5 mL) gained FDA approval for the treatment of OUD in 2016 and 2017, respectively. Manufacturing of the intradermal implant was discontinued by the manufacturer in 2020.

As of 2022, the sublingual formulations of buprenorphine come in various dosages and forms. A generic buprenorphine monoproduct tablet is available in 2- and 8-mg strengths, and its use is primarily reserved for individuals with known adverse reactions to naloxone and for pregnant individuals (discussed later in this section).

The preferred first-line sublingual buprenorphine-containing product for the treatment of OUD is the combination buprenorphine/naloxone formulation, which comes in both generic and branded forms. The addition of naloxone is intended to discourage intravenous misuse of the buprenorphine medication by taking advantage of differences between the bioavailability of naloxone and buprenorphine: naloxone is most bioavailable via intranasal, intramuscular, and intravenous routes of administration and is comparatively poorly bioavailable via sublingual and oral routes of ingestion. Conversely, buprenorphine is most bioavailable via sublingual, intravenous, and intramuscular routes of administration. Therefore, if a product containing both buprenorphine and naloxone is taken as directed (i.e., sublingually), then buprenorphine will be bioavailable, whereas the naloxone component will be only minimally bioavailable, if it all. However, if the individual dissolves this combination product and injects it, then both the naloxone and buprenorphine components will be readily bioavailable; thereby the likelihood will increase of precipitating a clinically significant withdrawal syndrome if the individual also has full agonists active in their system at the time of injection and is physically dependent on opioids.

Of note, studies have demonstrated that despite the relatively poor bioavailability of naloxone via the sublingual and oral routes of administration, some naloxone still enters the systemic circulation and can therefore potentially blunt some of the potential reinforcing opioid agonist effects of the buprenorphine (Mendelson et al. 1997). However, the clinical importance of this phenomenon is uncertain. Nonetheless, clinical studies have demonstrated that the buprenorphine monoproduct is misused to a greater extent than the buprenorphine/naloxone combination product, further supporting the recommendation for preferential treatment utilizing the combination product (Hakansson et al. 2007; Jones et al. 2015; Nielsen et al. 2007; Nordmann et al. 2012).

Buprenorphine/naloxone is available in both tablet and rapidly dissolving film formulations. A generic buprenorphine/naloxone tablet formulation comes in strengths of 2/0.5 mg and 8/2 mg. Three different film formulations of buprenorphine/naloxone are approved by the FDA for the treatment of OUD. Suboxone film is available in strengths of 2/0.5 mg, 4/1 mg, 8/2 mg, and 12/3 mg. Zubsolv film is available in strengths of 0.7/0.18 mg, 1.4/0.38 mg, 2.9/0.71 mg, 5.7/1.4 mg, 8.6/2.1 mg, and 11.4/2.9 mg. According to the manufacturer Orexo US (2016), the proprietary Zubsolv formulation has higher buprenorphine bioavailability than Suboxone or generic buprenorphine/naloxone tablets, allowing for the patient to take a lower dose of the buprenorphine-containing product (per the manufacturer: one Zubsolv tablet 5.7/1.4 mg sublingually provides buprenorphine exposure equivalent to one Suboxone tablet 8/2 mg sublingually). In addition, the greater number of dosage strength options offered by Zubsolv can reputedly allow for more nuanced dosing (Orexo US 2016). In clinical practice, however, the authors note that these differences may be of utility in only a small number of patients. Finally, Cassipa is a buprenorphine/naloxone sublingual film that is available in one strength (16/4 mg). Cassipa is bioequivalent to two Suboxone 8/2 mg films (Teva Pharmaceuticals USA 2018).

Administered at typical dosages of 2–24 mg/day sublingually, buprenorphine attenuates or blocks opioid-induced euphoria. It is not clear whether this effect is a result of cross-tolerance or some other action at the receptor. It is important to note that the rate of transmucosal absorption of buprenorphine is similar regardless of formulation and the rapidity with which those formulations dissolve in oral fluid. Practically, this results in the clinical recommendation that patients keep their saliva in their mouth for at least 5 minutes following the buprenorphine product being fully dissolved (whether film or tablet) to ensure maximal absorption.

Two extended-release buprenorphine (XR-BUP) formulations for the treatment of OUD in the United States have been approved by the FDA: Brixadi and Sublocade. Brixadi is available in weekly and monthly subcutaneous injection formulations, at strengths of 8 mg/0.16 mL, 16 mg/0.32 mL, 24 mg/0.48 mL, and 32 mg/0.64 mL (weekly) and 64 mg/0.18 mL, 96 mg/0.27 mL, and 128 mg/0.36 mL (monthly). The Brixadi initiation protocol used in the trial leading to FDA approval was a standard buprenorphine induction approach in which participants experiencing withdrawal received a sublingual dose of buprenorphine 4 mg, followed by buprenorphine 16 mg subcutaneously in a weekly injection (estimated equivalent of 8 mg/day). Originally, the FDA-approved prescribing information for Sublocade indicated that a standard sublingual buprenorphine induction should be performed with a maintenance dosage of at least 8 mg/day for 1 week, followed by a subcutaneous injection of 300 mg (estimated equivalent of 12–16 mg/day), followed by monthly 100-mg injections thereafter. In February 2025, the FDA approved a more rapid injection protocol that involves only a single dose of transmucosal buprenorphine followed by a 1-hour observation period prior to the initial Sublocade injection (Indivior 2025). Therefore, one noteworthy difference between these two XR-BUP formulations is that Brixadi has more potential dosing options, whereas Sublocade has only a single target dose. The clinical implications of this difference are not yet certain. The injection procedures are also different. Sublocade is typically administered low on the anterior abdomen, where the matrix in which it is suspended solidifies and slowly dissolves over the course of the following month (although alternative injection site locations—e.g., thigh, upper arm, buttock—were FDA approved in February 2025). Brixadi is administered via subcutaneous injection to either the buttock, thigh, upper arm, or abdomen. Data show that LAI buprenorphine is noninferior to sublingual buprenorphine and may even lead to a greater number of patients with no reported opioid use at all (Lofwall et al. 2018). In addition, emerging research supports additional potential positive effects of LAI buprenorphine outside of abstinence from illicit opioids alone, such as improvements in employment, medication satisfaction, decreased health care utilization, and improved overall perceptions of quality of life (Ling et al. 2019, 2020). Emerging research also suggests the possibility that XR-BUP may be particularly beneficial for individuals who are using fentanyl, perhaps in association with the comparatively higher serum buprenorphine levels achieved with XR-BUP treatment relative to sublingual buprenorphine treatment (Mariani et al. 2021; Nunes et al. 2024).

Legal and Regulatory Considerations for Buprenorphine for the Treatment of Opioid Use Disorder

Much has changed in the regulatory landscape of buprenorphine prescribing in recent years. Previously, prescribing buprenorphine required obtaining a waiver from the U.S. Department of Health and Human Services (HHS), commonly known as the *X-waiver*. Obtaining this waiver required prescribers to undergo specialized training for 8–24 hours in duration (depending on professional licensure). In addition, prescribers who had obtained their X-waiver and who wanted to prescribe buprenorphine to their patients with OUD were subject to regulatory limits on the number of patients they could concurrently treat.

With the passage of the Consolidated Appropriations Act of 2023, the X-waiver and all associated patient limit regulations were discontinued. Therefore, any prescriber with U.S. Drug Enforcement Administration (DEA) certification to prescribe controlled substances (Schedule II–V) may also now prescribe buprenorphine for the treatment of OUD without any caps on the number of patients that they can simultaneously treat, and the prescriber need not undergo any additional training specific to buprenorphine to prescribe buprenorphine for this purpose (H.R. 2617–117th Congress [2021–2022] 2022). However, the Substance Abuse and Mental Health Services Administration (SAMHSA) and the DEA have indicated that all DEA certificate holders will need to attest to having completed training in addiction assessment and management as part of their new certification application or renewal process. More information on training programs that satisfy these new requirements is available through the Department of Justice website (see: https://www.deadiversion.usdoj.gov/faq/MATE_Act_faq.html).

Nonetheless, some regulatory nuances persist for some of the different buprenorphine formulations. For example, prescribing and administering LAI buprenorphine requires completion of a product-specific Risk Evaluation and Mitigation Strategy (REMS) training program.

A final regulatory and legal consideration involves the treatment of youth with OUD using buprenorphine or buprenorphine/naloxone. Although these products carry FDA approval for individuals 16 or older, treatment of individuals ages 16–18 may be subject to state-specific laws and regulations regarding parental consent. Prescribers considering treatment of youth, therefore, should avail themselves of either pediatric or adolescent medicine specialists or other legal or risk management counsel to determine the legal and regulatory landscape in which they intend to undertake this treatment.

During the COVID-19 pandemic public health emergency, SAMHSA loosened restrictions and allowed buprenorphine initiation and follow-up to be done via telemedicine instead of in person (Substance Abuse and Mental Health Services Administration 2020). Before that, prescribers were required to assess a patient in person to prescribe buprenorphine, because buprenorphine is a Schedule III controlled substance and is therefore subject to the terms and conditions of the Ryan Haight Online Pharmacy Consumer Protection Act of 2008.

In January 2025, DEA and HHS permanently ruled that providers can initiate buprenorphine via telemedicine (audio or visual) and prescribe up to a 6-month supply without seeing the patient in person. After the 6-month period or once the patient is seen in person, providers need to follow DEA and state regulations for prescription of controlled substances on further follow-up care (Substance Abuse and Mental Health Services Administration 2025).

Buprenorphine Initiations

In a traditional buprenorphine initiation, patients should show clear evidence of opioid withdrawal (as determined by a withdrawal scale such as COWS [Wesson and Ling 2003]) before being given the first dose of buprenorphine, to avoid precipitating severe withdrawal. The initial dose of buprenorphine should be given at least 12–24 hours after the last dose of heroin and 36 hours after the last dose of methadone (Gunderson et al. 2011; McNicholas and Howell 2000). In individuals transitioning from methadone to buprenorphine, standard teaching is that the methadone dosage should be slowly tapered to 30 mg/day, and the patient's symptoms should be stabilized at that dosage for at least 1–2 weeks before the transfer to buprenorphine is attempted.

On the first day, a sublingual buprenorphine/naloxone dose of 2/0.5 mg to 4/1 mg can be given every 2–4 hours, up to a maximum total of 8/2 mg/day. On the following days, the dosage can be increased by 2/0.5 mg/day to 4/1 mg/day until the initial target of 12/3 to 16/4 mg/day is reached (see Table 5.5). Many patients' symptoms will be stabilized at a dosage of 16/4 mg/day or less. As noted earlier in this section, the combination buprenorphine/naloxone tablet or film should be used for both initiation and long-term treatment, as opposed to the buprenorphine monoproduct. The buprenorphine-only tablet has classically been reserved for individuals with well-established intolerance to the combination product and for pregnant people (because the effects of low-dose exposure to systemic naloxone on fetal development are not well understood). Nonetheless, more recent studies have supported the use of the combined tablet in pregnant people as well (Link et al. 2020).

Buprenorphine has proved to be an acceptable treatment for a wide range of individuals with OUD—especially younger individuals, those without access to methadone treatment, and those with life constraints that preclude them from participating in daily dosing and other constraints of methadone treatment (Mariolis et al. 2019). Buprenorphine also offers significant advantages for patients taking multiple other medications, such as those taking antiretroviral therapy. Although most antiretrovirals can either decrease or increase methadone levels, they do not appear to affect the pharmacodynamic properties of buprenorphine, even if they may alter buprenorphine levels. A notable exception is atazanavir and ritonavir, both of which elevate buprenorphine levels and alter its pharmacodynamics. Nonetheless, buprenorphine can be safely prescribed with appropriate observation (Gruber and McCance-Katz 2010).

Alternative Buprenorphine Initiation Protocols

Other buprenorphine initiation protocols have been developed that offer some alternatives to the traditional initiation approach. These alternative strategies emerge from clinical experience in which certain individuals did not tolerate traditional initiation protocols (sometimes attributed to the rise in chronic fentanyl and other HPSO exposure), from logistical constraints that made the traditional approach impractical (i.e., repeated multiday in-office dosing), and from attempts to increase access (i.e., greater observation and access to medications in an emergency department setting). Currently, these protocols fall into three general categories: low-dose, high-dose, and crossover protocols. The traditional initiation protocol remains the most researched and widely practiced method of initiating buprenorphine, especially in the outpatient setting, where the majority of initiations are undertaken.

For a review of a proposed foundational neuropharmacological working model to explain the possible reason for differential successes with alternative initiation protocols, please refer to Greenwald et al. (2022). In short, Greenwald et al. posited that success of buprenorphine initiation is a function of the opioid balance at the time of buprenorphine initiation, which is dependent on the MOR affinity, lipophilicity, and intrinsic MOR efficacy of the prior opioid (referred to as the *ALE value*), establishing the opioid imbalance that must be accounted for during initiation of buprenorphine to restore balance. As a result, individuals with negative opioid balance at the time of initiation (in withdrawal) may benefit from a higher-dose buprenorphine initiation protocol that capitalizes on buprenorphine's agonist properties regardless of the ALE value of the previously used opioid. In contrast, as the balance shifts positive (more intrinsic agonist activity with higher-ALE-value opioids), the low-dose or crossover protocols become potentially more beneficial. Next, we describe these alternative buprenorphine initiation protocols in greater detail.

Low-Dose Buprenorphine Initiation

In this protocol, the first step is a 24-hour washout period from the opioid of choice, until the individual reaches mild to moderate withdrawal symptom

Table 5.5 Traditional initiation on sublingual buprenorphine/naloxone tablets

Patient status	Day 1		Day 2
	First buprenorphine/naloxone dose	Supplemental buprenorphine/naloxone dose	
Not currently dependent	2/0.5 mg		4/1 mg
Dependent on heroin or opioid pain medication	2/0.5 to 4/1 mg[a]	Redose every 1–2 h, if withdrawal continues, up to a total of 8/2 mg	If the patient is still experiencing withdrawal, give first-day dosage plus 2/0.5 to 4/1 mg
Dependent on methadone ≤30 mg/d	2/0.5 mg[a]	Redose every 1–2 h, if withdrawal continues, up to a total of 8/2 mg	If the patient is still experiencing withdrawal, give first-day dosage plus 2/0.5 to 4/1 mg; if oversedated, give <8/2 mg

Source. Adapted from McNicholas and Howell (2000).
[a]Do not begin buprenorphine until patient shows evidence of opioid withdrawal.

severity (COWS score of 8–12). Adjunctive medications may be used to help manage emerging withdrawal symptoms. Buprenorphine dosing is then initiated in atypically small doses (0.5 mg) over the initial day of treatment until a total of 2 mg has been administered. After that, dosing is switched to 2-mg increments every 2–3 hours until a total of 6–8 mg has been given on day 1. Subsequent days are handled similarly to the traditional initiation protocol. The goal with the low-dose initiation protocol is to only gingerly displace residual full-agonist opioids, preventing precipitated withdrawal, and to help potentially reverse the receptor adaptations that maintain physiological dependence/tolerance.

High-Dose Buprenorphine Initiation

In distinction from traditional buprenorphine initiations, another emerging approach is rapid high-dose initiation (*macrodosing*) in which individuals are administered up to 32 mg buprenorphine/naloxone in the first few hours of presentation. Case reports and series describe the effectiveness of this approach in both inpatients who received naloxone in the setting of opioid overdose and individuals who did not receive naloxone but were experiencing opioid withdrawal (Antoine et al. 2021; Edwards et al. 2020; Herring et al. 2019; LeSaint et al. 2020; Phillips et al. 2019). As with the low-dose approach, the literature describes a number of different dosing strategies that involve initial doses of 4 or 8 mg that are rapidly titrated up to total doses ranging from 16 to 32 mg/day; in one protocol, initial dosing was 4–8 mg, with reassessment after 30–60 minutes and repeat dosing (8–24 mg) every 30–60 minutes for individuals with a COWS score of 8 or greater (total buprenorphine dose ≤32 mg) (Herring et al. 2019). There are currently no universally accepted guidelines standardizing the high-dose/macrodosing approach. Nonetheless, several specialty-specific guidelines or position statements support consideration of high-dose buprenorphine/naloxone initiations, especially in the emergency department setting (Cao et al. 2020; Hawk et al. 2021).

Crossover Buprenorphine Initiation

The crossover initiation strategy (alternatively known as *microdosing* or the *Bernese method*) involves introducing very small doses of buprenorphine on the first day of treatment, often while the individual continues to take full-agonist opioids. In this technique, the dose of buprenorphine builds up more slowly over a number of days rather than in a single day as in traditional induction (De Aquino et al. 2021), thereby potentially minimizing the possibility of precipitated withdrawal. Although it was first proposed for patients with chronic pain who were taking high-dose full-agonist opioids, there has been increasing interest in (and publication about) utilizing this method in patients with OUD, especially with the increasing use of fentanyl in the population (Azar et al. 2018; Hämmig et al. 2016; Klaire et al. 2019; Kornfeld and Reetz 2015; Miller et al. 2023; Moe et al. 2021; Raheemullah and Lembke 2019; Rozylo et al. 2020). There is significant procedural variation cited in the literature, and there are currently no universally accepted guidelines to guide crossover buprenorphine procedure selection.

In hospitalized patients, one approach involves converting patients to estimated equivalents of opioids available on a hospital formulary, such as transdermal fentanyl or intravenous hydrocodone, then slowly introducing sublingual buprenorphine concurrently in doses starting as low as 0.25 mg and titrating up to buprenorphine/naloxone 12/3–16/4 mg over the course of 1–5 days (Azar et al. 2018; Klaire et al. 2019). One case series described *microinduction* (microdosing initiation) beginning with buprenorphine 0.5 mg on the first day, with the previous day's dose doubled on each consecutive day until 8 mg/day was reached (Terasaki et al. 2019). Other published reports described the use of transdermal buprenorphine (20 µg/hour, not approved by the FDA for this indication) with a transition to sublingual buprenorphine/naloxone while tapering the prior opioids (Raheemullah and Lembke 2019). Furthermore, a 2023 report described success in transitioning a hospitalized individual from unregulated fentanyl to sublingual buprenorphine/naloxone utilizing a 48-hour transdermal buprenorphine bridge (Azar et al. 2023).

In outpatient settings, this approach can be challenging because of concerns of concomitant use of illicit opioids on top of prescribed opioid equivalents. Nonetheless, published case reports documented utilization of modified versions of this strategy in which patients were instructed to either continue or taper their usual illicit opioid while introducing low-dose buprenorphine/naloxone (Brar et al. 2020; Rozylo et al. 2020). In the study by Brar et al. (2020), patients maintained the use of the full-agonist opioid, including illicitly obtained fentanyl, over an 8-day buprenorphine crossover induction, and then abruptly stopped the full agonist on day 8, without a cross-taper. There are also potential ethical considerations with this approach in an outpatient setting, owing to the provider-given instruction for individuals to continue use of illicit opioids, which may further limit the widespread use of this approach.

A 2021 systematic review of 20 studies on crossover dosing of buprenorphine cited wide methodological variations (e.g., inconsistent use of validated withdrawal assessment tools, dosing, and cross-titration opioid used) but a low rate of precipitated withdrawal (all of which involved methadone as the cross-titrated opioid) (Moe et al. 2021). Another review on buprenorphine/naloxone crossover initiations summarized that most initiations began with buprenorphine doses of 0.2–0.5 mg, lasted 4–8 days, and ended when total dosage reached 8–16 mg/day (Ahmed et al. 2021).

Crossover initiations may be helpful for individuals who cannot tolerate even brief periods of withdrawal. They can especially benefit individuals cross-tapering from a prescribed long-acting opioid such as methadone, because low-dose initiation does not require opioids to be held, thus avoiding a withdrawal period that may last for days. Crossover initiations may also be considered when there is increased concern for precipitated withdrawal when a patient has been using illicit opioids. This concern has been heightened owing to increasing nonpharmaceutical fentanyl, fentanyl analogs (including carfentanil), and novel HPSOs in the illicit drug supply in the United States (Armenian et al. 2018).

Although the duration of fentanyl and HPSO activity on the opioid receptor is short, its volume of distribution is large, so it can remain in reserve in the body for at least 3 days (McClain and Hug 1980). Although fentanyl may not produce clinically notable effects hours after administration, when it is displaced by buprenorphine, its presence can become apparent in withdrawal symptoms (De Aquino et al. 2021). Less is known about the pharmacology of fentanyl analogs and novel synthetic opioids, leading to further uncertainty about how long they last in the body and the risk of precipitated withdrawal.

Patient Selection: Alternative Buprenorphine Initiation Strategies
The purpose of exploring alternative strategies for buprenorphine initiations is to minimize the unique risk of buprenorphine-induced precipitated withdrawal in traditional buprenorphine initiation, thereby enhancing treatment engagement and decreasing provider and patient fear. Data on rates of precipitated withdrawal are difficult to obtain, but several studies support the

notion that precipitated withdrawal is a relatively rare event. For example, one study of 36 individuals initiated on buprenorphine prehospital cited zero precipitated withdrawal events (Hern et al. 2022). A retrospective study of office-based initiations cited a "complicated induction" rate of 10%, 90% of which involved individuals taking methadone (Whitley et al. 2010). Another retrospective study in the prefentanyl era of emergency department buprenorphine initiations reported a precipitated withdrawal rate of 0.8% (Herring et al. 2021).

With the advent of increasingly widespread exposure to chronic fentanyl and other HPSO use, clinical experience and case reports have raised the concern that individuals taking these compounds may be at higher risk of precipitated withdrawal (Antoine et al. 2021; Oakley et al. 2021; Silverstein et al. 2019). One self-report study (involving 1,679 individuals from multiple treatment sites) compared the risk of precipitated withdrawal in individuals using fentanyl versus methadone within 48 hours of initiation. The authors reported an odds ratio of 3.3 (fentanyl to methadone) of developing buprenorphine-precipitated withdrawal (Varshneya et al. 2022). In addition to prior chronic use of fentanyl or methadone, other factors associated with higher risk of buprenorphine-precipitated withdrawal include chronic kidney disease, cirrhosis, and concurrent benzodiazepine use (Huhn et al. 2020; Whitley et al. 2010).

Clinical experience and emerging case reports suggest that some individuals may tolerate low-dose or crossover initiations better than high-dose initiations, but appropriate matching of patient to initiation strategy is challenging and not well understood. The working neuropharmacological model proposed by Greenwald et al. (2022) described earlier ("Alternative Buprenorphine Initiation Protocols") provides a framework for understanding the observed challenges in buprenorphine initiation. Building from the earlier description of this model, individuals exposed to chronic high-potency opioids (e.g., fentanyl) with high ALE values may face a more challenging neuroadaptive hurdle (i.e., reversal of tolerance) than those exposed to lower-ALE-value opioids (e.g., heroin). In a low-dose or crossover dose initiation strategy, individuals chronically exposed to high-ALE-value opioids such as fentanyl may therefore benefit from coadministration of a low-ALE-value opioid to "maximize the activation of spare functional MOR so that withdrawal is not experienced while not inhibiting MOR resensitization" (Greenwald et al. 2022, p. 520).

Seen through the lens of this model, high-dose initiations therefore take advantage of the observation that "buprenorphine treats buprenorphine-precipitated withdrawal," since the magnitude of agonist activation and that of tolerance reversal are dose-dependent (Greenwald et al. 2003, 2022; Guo et al. 2021). In other words, larger doses of buprenorphine can accelerate the reversal of tolerance and maximize the agonist effect of buprenorphine by pushing the binding-dissociation equilibrium toward μ activation.

The working neuropharmacological model further suggests that both low-dose and high-dose initiations can therefore be effective in transitioning individuals to buprenorphine who had previously been exposed to both high- and low-ALE-value opioids, with some adjustments to the strategy being made on account of the ALE value of the previously used opioids (i.e., introduction of a concomitant low-ALE-value opioid in individuals previously taking high-ALE-value opioids who are being initiated onto buprenorphine through a low-dose/microdose approach). Nonetheless, the authors of the model highlighted that prospective data on the model are particularly lacking for transitions from high-ALE-value opioids; therefore, until further data accumulate, traditional approaches in line with established guidelines should be considered (Greenwald et al. 2022).

Opioid Antagonists

Originally, behavioral principles were the basis for the use of opioid antagonists to treat OUD. In theory, opioid use that was once operantly reinforced by euphoria would no longer be reinforced if the patients were given a high-enough dosage of an opioid antagonist. In addition, with no regular opioid use, the association between withdrawal symptoms and the environment in which opioids had been used would extinguish (Wikler 1980). Studies of cyclazocine, naloxone, and naltrexone showed them all to be successful in blocking opioid effects, but patients with OUD generally stayed in treatment for only 6–8 weeks on average (Capone et al. 1986; Fram et al. 1989; Resnick et al. 1980).

Naltrexone

Oral naltrexone and LAI naltrexone (Vivitrol) are the only opioid antagonists currently approved for the treatment of OUD. Systematic reviews and meta-analyses have demonstrated the effectiveness of both oral and LAI naltrexone over placebo (Jarvis et al. 2018; Larney et al. 2014; Lim et al. 2022;

Zangiabadian et al. 2022). Additional studies demonstrated that LAI naltrexone retains patients better in treatment and decreases the odds of relapse relative to oral naltrexone and to placebo. Nonetheless, a 2002 systematic review that included 707 individuals in randomized controlled trials showed no statistically significant effect of naltrexone treatment relative to placebo on successful completion of treatment, opioid use during treatment, incarceration during treatment, or mean duration of treatment (Kirchmayer et al. 2002).

Studies comparing the effectiveness of naltrexone relative to methadone and buprenorphine treatment have yielded mixed results. A 2022 systematic review showed that all three medication interventions had higher retention than nonmedication control groups, although methadone treatment showed greater retention in treatment than buprenorphine, and buprenorphine showed greater retention than naltrexone (Lim et al. 2022). In a 2018 head-to-head study, extended-release naltrexone was shown to be less effective than buprenorphine in terms of retention in addiction treatment and abstinence; this finding may be attributable to the need for individuals to undergo withdrawal before extended-release initiation (Lee et al. 2018). The same study found that if individuals were successfully initiated on extended-release naltrexone after withdrawal, the differences in efficacy were no longer present (Lee et al. 2018). Similarly, a 2020 database-review study comparing 40,885 individuals with OUD who received various treatments (nonintensive behavioral health, inpatient detoxification or residential services, buprenorphine, methadone, or naltrexone) reported that treatment with naltrexone was not protective against overdose or serious opioid-related acute care use (Wakeman et al. 2020). Taken together, these data suggest that naltrexone may have clinical utility in the treatment of OUD, but that patient selection and coordination of appropriate initiation (i.e., ensuring safety during the necessary withdrawal period) may be critical for its success.

Patients likely to continue to use naltrexone and to benefit from it are those with established safety-sensitive careers in which opioid agonist and opioid partial agonist treatment is prohibited (e.g., health professionals, pilots) and those with strong social support and high motivation. Up to 70% of such patients are abstinent at 1-year follow-up (Washton et al. 1984). Programs that use additional rehabilitative services have better results than those that provide minimal services. One study compared the effect of naltrexone alone versus naltrexone combined with either contingency management or family counseling (Carroll et al. 2001). Both study conditions improved retention and medication compliance, with the most significant effect seen in the subgroup that attended family counseling.

Oral naltrexone may be given at a dosage of 50 mg/day or, alternatively, 100 mg/day on Mondays and Wednesdays and 150 mg/day on Fridays. It has a long duration of action (24 hours when given in a 50-mg dose, which increases to 72 hours with a dose of 150 mg). Some authors recommend that naltrexone be started slowly and only after a waiting period (e.g., a maximum starting dosage of 50 mg/day only after the patient is opioid free for 7 days or methadone free for 10 days, confirmed by a negative naloxone challenge) (Ginzburg 1984). Unfortunately, patients are at significant risk for relapse during such a waiting period (see next section, "Naltrexone Microinitiation"). Patients who start naltrexone immediately after MSW often complain of insomnia, gastrointestinal distress, hyperalgesia, anergia, anxiety, and dysphoria ("naltrexone flu"). These symptoms usually clear in 2–4 weeks, but the dropout rate is high during this period. Oral naltrexone can be expected to lead to retention of 20%–30% of patients at 6 months (Sullivan et al. 2019).

In 2010, the FDA approved a microsphere injectable depot formulation of naltrexone (Vivitrol) that is given intramuscularly at a dosage of 380 mg/month. Efficacy for OUD was confirmed in a large Russian study (Krupitsky et al. 2011), although questions have been raised regarding the applicability of these findings to the U.S. population, given that agonist and partial agonist therapies are not available in Russia. In clinical practice (as suggested in the Vivitrol package insert [Vivitrol 2022]), individuals who struggle with opioid cravings and relapse in the latter part of the monthly interval may be given an LAI naltrexone injection every 3 weeks, although there are no clinical trials evaluating this frequency. In a study using implantable naltrexone, a naltrexone plasma concentration of 3 ng/mL conferred the lowest risk for heroin use (Hulse et al. 2010). A pharmacokinetic study of LAI naltrexone (Vivitrol) showed that the mean naltrexone plasma concentration dropped below 3 ng/mL after day 21 postinjection (Dunbar et al. 2006). This finding suggests that some individuals may require injections more frequently than every 4 weeks to maintain the most effective naltrexone plasma concentration of 3 ng/mL. Trials using naltrexone for other SUDs, such as methamphetamine use disorder, have used dosing every 3 weeks for all patients in the trial (Trivedi et al. 2021).

Behavioral therapy strategies can improve retention with both oral and depot naltrexone (Rothenberg et al. 2002; Sullivan 2011). Six-month retention rates near 30% have been described for the depot formulation, approaching those of long-term buprenorphine (Sullivan 2011). Although initiation of extended-release naltrexone does not require initiation of oral naltrexone first, many providers and patients may choose to initiate naltrexone orally first for several days before the first injection of extended-release naltrexone to assess for tolerability.

At the dosages of naltrexone used, the effects of as much as 25 mg of injected heroin are blocked. Although toxicity of naltrexone in OUD is low, there have been some reported subtle adverse effects, such as decreased energy (Hollister et al. 1981). Nonaddicted subjects with obesity have been known to develop markedly elevated transaminase levels at a dosage of 300 mg/day PO, indicating that high doses of naltrexone are potentially hepatotoxic (Mitchell et al. 1987; Pfohl et al. 1986). Naltrexone is therefore generally contraindicated in patients with decompensated liver failure or acute hepatitis, and its use in pregnant individuals is also not currently advised because of potential risks of teratogenicity (although the clinical data supporting teratogenicity are lacking, and some research indicates that there may be little to no teratogenicity risk) (Hulse et al. 2001). Other studies, however, suggested that concerns about transaminitis and hepatotoxicity with oral naltrexone may be exaggerated, and extended-release injectable naltrexone may carry even lower risk of this potential complication (Lucey et al. 2008; Mitchell et al. 2012; Vagenas et al. 2014). Nonetheless, baseline and periodic (i.e., every 3–6 months) liver function tests are widely recommended. In addition, baseline pregnancy, HIV, and hepatitis testing are recommended (Substance Abuse and Mental Health Services Administration 2021).

Neither oral nor extended-release naltrexone requires a specialty treatment site (unlike methadone). However, prescribing and administering of extended-release naltrexone does require completion of a REMS program. Logistically, extended-release naltrexone can be challenging to obtain and administer, owing to the need for specialty pharmacy or manufacturer-direct ordering, coordinated delivery, refrigeration, and staff education about proper deep gluteal injection procedures. Extended-release naltrexone comes as a kit with both powdered and liquid components that must be mixed shortly before administration and, once mixed, can become viscous rapidly, requiring prompt administration. These factors may limit extended-release naltrexone's widespread applicability and uptake. Conversely, it may have increased appeal for certain populations because naltrexone is not a DEA-controlled substance, and there is evidence that there may be less stigma associated with naltrexone treatment relative to buprenorphine and methadone (Randall-Kosich et al. 2020).

An additional potential use of naltrexone treatment (either extended-release or oral) is emerging for individuals who elect to discontinue their maintenance opioid (full or partial agonist) OUD treatment. Some patients may want to stop opioid medication, but they may be open to continuing OUD treatment on a nonopioid medication, and they should be offered naltrexone because receiving naltrexone medication for OUD is superior to no medication treatment (Ndegwa et al. 2017).

It is also important to consider the overdose risk in individuals who have been taking naltrexone and then discontinue. Unlike with buprenorphine and methadone, where a certain level of tolerance is maintained throughout treatment, an individual receiving naltrexone maintenance will predictably lose most, if not all, tolerance to opioids over the course of treatment. Therefore, discontinuation of naltrexone treatment followed by resumption of opioid use may carry a heightened risk of overdose, and patients should be clearly advised of this risk.

Naltrexone Microinitiation

Once initiated, naltrexone can be as effective as buprenorphine for preventing relapse in people with OUD. However, induction onto naltrexone has classically required a 1-week opioid-free period, resulting in significantly lower rates of achieving initiation. One report found that 72% of participants had successful induction onto naltrexone versus 94% onto buprenorphine (Lee et al. 2018). The 1-week washout recommendation is because naltrexone is a competitive opioid antagonist with high binding affinity and carries a high risk of precipitated withdrawal. Naltrexone is also relatively long-acting, unlike other opioid antagonists such as naloxone.

To minimize side effects and dropout, novel methods of induction are being developed. These microinitiations start with subtherapeutic doses of naltrexone, then slowly increase to an effective naltrexone dose over multiple days. There is no standardized way to do a naltrexone microinitiation because it is still under study. In one study, participants were given a single 8-mg dose of buprenorphine, followed by a day off opioids, followed by 1 mg naltrexone on day 1, with an increased dose each subsequent day following a protocol of 3 mg, then 12 mg, then 25 mg, then LAI naltrexone (Vivitrol) 380 mg IM by day 5 (Sullivan et al. 2017). Another method started with naltrexone 25–50 µg on day 1 in combination with buprenorphine 4 mg. On day 2, the same dose of naltrexone was given, but buprenorphine was reduced to 2 mg. On day 3, buprenorphine 2 mg was continued, and naltrexone was increased to 50 µg–1 mg. On day 4, buprenorphine was stopped, and naltrexone was increased to 2–6 mg. After that, naltrexone was dosed on the following schedule: day 5, 3–15 mg; day 6, 5–35 mg; and day 7, 13–50 mg (Mannelli et al. 2014).

Considerations Related to Chronic Pain

Current research has shown that although opioids are effective treatment for acute pain, their effectiveness for chronic pain is questionable—they can even worsen the pain in some individuals (Volkow et al. 2018). In a national survey of U.S. adults, only one-third of individuals receiving long-term opioid therapy thought their pain was well controlled (Manhapra 2022). Further complicating long-term opioid therapy, because of tolerance to analgesic effects (which may develop more slowly than tolerance to euphoric effects), a person will predictably require escalating doses of opioids over time just to maintain an effective level of pain control.

Long-term use can also lead to opioid-induced hyperalgesia (OIH) because of neuroadaptations that result in increased sensitivity to pain to compensate for the ongoing presence of opioids that dampen pain. OIH is operationally defined as increased sensitivity to painful stimuli, and it may be mediated by reduction of endogenous opioids and changes in the opioid receptor itself (Hayhurst and Durieux 2016). Tolerance and OIH are often difficult to separate clinically because they both result in reports of increased pain and perceived need for higher opioid doses to control pain. The prevalence of OIH is unclear, but studies show that, as a group, people taking long-term opioids have increased pain sensitivity and that higher doses of opioids are correlated with increased pain sensitivity (Chen et al. 2009). Although a patient may be taking opioids that are legally prescribed for pain, they may still be physically dependent on and may be given increasing doses of a medication that is only worsening their pain in the long term, which puts them at risk for poor outcomes, including withdrawal and overdose.

Some have proposed the term *complex opioid dependence* to describe this phenomenon, which is still in need of intervention despite not always meeting criteria for OUD (Ballantyne et al. 2012). In patients with complex opioid dependence, subclinical withdrawal may be caused by fluctuations in opioid levels that occur each time an opioid is administered and then begins to be metabolized. This subclinical withdrawal can result in hyperalgesia and hyperkatifeia (increased sensitivity to negative emotional states). Pain and emotions may be governed by the level of opioid in the body as the main input, rather than the usual external inputs (Friedman and Nabong 2020). The hyperalgesia and hyperkatifeia are thought to occur as opponent processes to maintain homeostasis in response to the exogenous opioid's effects of reducing pain and aversive emotions. The process may be chronically worsened by increasing doses of opioids, but a patient may perceive the increasing doses to improve the opponent processes because there is an acute temporary boost in the opioid's effects until the body increases the opponent processes once more. This chronic dysregulation of pain and emotions can lead to behavioral changes, so a person with complex opioid dependence will experience suffering, functional impairment, or both. It has been found that even after a chronic opioid for pain has been tapered, this hyperalgesia can persist for years. Manhapra (2022) proposed the new term *opioid-induced chronic pain syndrome* (OICP) for the process just described, to emphasize that it is a medication-induced condition distinct from addiction and distinct from "benign physical dependence." A key part of the proposed OICP definition includes chronic pain that develops while taking chronic opioids for pain and persists whether the opioid dose is stabilized, increased, or reduced and for years after opioid abstinence, indicating that a simple opioid taper by itself is not adequate treatment (Manhapra 2022).

The HHS, the CDC, and the U.S. Department of Veterans Affairs/Department of Defense have all issued guidelines to help clinicians plan treatment if the risks of continuing opioids for chronic pain outweigh the benefits, as in complex opioid dependency. The HHS guidelines, for example, suggest an opioid taper, but if the patient is unable to tolerate the taper because of withdrawal or intolerable pain, then another option may be buprenorphine (U.S. Department of Health and Human Services 2019). Accumulating research and clinical observation show that tapering long-term opioids given for pain is not effective at improving pain or functioning, and that tapering alone may even increase mortality and cause psychiatric destabilization (Manhapra 2022). Evidence suggests that switching from a chronic opioid agonist for pain to buprenorphine or methadone may be more effective and specifically reduces OIH (Axelrod and Reville 2007; Friedman and Nabong 2020). Low-dose naloxone given with an opioid such as buprenorphine may further improve hyperalgesia (La Vincente et al. 2008; Oaks et al. 2018). Research also suggests the optimal treatment includes behavioral interventions to promote improved functioning. CDC guidelines on prescribing opioids for pain were updated in 2022 and emphasize shared decision-making, considering benefit versus risk of opioids on an individual basis rather than recommending mandatory opioid tapers or reductions to set doses (Dowell et al. 2022). In patients already prescribed opioids for pain, the guidelines also emphasize the importance of identifying and treating OUD with appropriate medication, preferably either buprenorphine or methadone, and suggest that any provider who prescribes opioids for pain should get a waiver to prescribe buprenorphine as well for this purpose.

Considerations Related to Pregnancy

Currently, methadone and buprenorphine are both considered first-line treatments of OUD in pregnant individuals. More recent research has shown that the combination product buprenorphine/naloxone appears to be as safe as methadone or buprenorphine for OUD in pregnancy (Link et al. 2020). Naltrexone is also an option; however, the evidence on its safety in pregnancy is limited, so it is not the ideal treatment and would not be an ideal choice for initiation of treatment in pregnancy. Generally, if an individual's symptoms of OUD were stable on a medication before pregnancy, maintaining the same medication while pregnant is logical. Methadone is initiated as in protocols for nonpregnant individuals and will not induce withdrawal or require withdrawal before initiation, so often it is a first choice for initiation of treatment for OUD in pregnancy. Because of physiological changes in pregnancy, methadone has a larger volume of distribution and greater renal clearance, so maintenance dosing is quite different in pregnancy than in other states. Methadone doses that reduce craving and withdrawal during pregnancy are generally higher than those required in nonpregnant people, and many pregnant people do better with split dosing to avoid low serum levels in the second half of the day. Evidence suggests that buprenorphine maintenance dosing may also need to be altered in pregnancy, either with a higher dose or a split dose, but there are no clear guidelines, because buprenorphine in pregnancy is a more recent option than methadone. Clinicians should therefore monitor pregnant patients closely for craving or withdrawal and adjust the dose as necessary (Martin et al. 2020). Buprenorphine initiation needs to be considered carefully because buprenorphine, as a partial opioid agonist, can induce withdrawal from a full-agonist opioid, and there are significant risks of withdrawal in pregnancy, such a miscarriage, preterm labor, fetal distress, and so on. Because of the high risks of withdrawal in pregnancy, and the risk of relapse, MSW alone is not recommended.

Another consideration of OUD treatment in pregnancy is neonatal opioid withdrawal syndrome (NOWS). NOWS occurs when a fetus is exposed to any chronic opioid from the mother's circulation and develops dependence on the opioid. After birth, the neonate is no longer getting opioid exposure and may go through opioid withdrawal. NOWS can be treated with a taper of opioid agonist medication (morphine or methadone) given to the neonate (Weller et al. 2021). Reducing the dose of methadone in the pregnant individual does not seem to reduce NOWS (Rodriguez and Klie 2019). There is research showing that NOWS after buprenorphine is milder than NOWS after methadone exposure in utero (Jones et al. 2010). Although both treatments can produce NOWS at birth, it is important to remember that the risks of untreated OUD during pregnancy are much higher than risks from treated OUD. Pregnant individuals with OUD who are not given a medication treatment for OUD have a much higher risk of overdose death, miscarriage, and other adverse effects than those treated with methadone or buprenorphine, and receiving medication for OUD is associated with increased prenatal care (Rodriguez and Klie 2019).

Individuals receiving methadone and buprenorphine pass a small amount into their breast milk (Ito 2018). If an individual is receiving a stable dose of methadone or buprenorphine with well-controlled OUD, and the infant is monitored and does not show signs of methadone adverse effects such as sedation or respiratory depression, breastfeeding is recommended (Doerzbacher and Chang 2019). Nonetheless, breastfeeding while receiving methadone or buprenorphine should be carefully considered based on individual circumstances. For instance, in the event of dose changes or other potentially interacting medication changes, both mother and infant should be monitored for behavioral and physiological changes that could be indicative of the need for additional supports or changes in treatment.

Considerations Related to Co-occurring Psychiatric Disorders

Psychiatric comorbidities are common in patients with OUD. A 2022 systematic review and meta-analysis found that among those with OUD, the prevalence of depression was about 36%, with a prevalence of 29% for anxiety, 21% for ADHD, 18% for PTSD, and 9% for bipolar disorder (Santo et al. 2022). Comorbid conditions such as PTSD have been associated with increased severity of OUD and increased rates of depression and suicide (Meshberg-Cohen et al. 2021). A prospective cohort study of approximately 900 patients receiving methadone for OUD found that approximately 80% had a psychiatric comorbidity and, more specifically, 42% had at least one other SUD (Rosic et al. 2017). The authors found no association between general psychiatric comorbidity and continued use of the misused opioid, but they did find an association between comorbid tranquilizer and cocaine use disorders and continued opioid misuse. A study of Medicaid enrollees found that 50% of those with OUD had a comorbid SUD (Donohue et al. 2021). Friesen and Kurdyak (2020) found that having a psychiatric comorbidity decreased the odds of a patient voluntarily stopping medication for OUD by 12% but also increased the odds that the treatment center would discharge the patient by 59%.

The research on OUD and comorbid conditions and their effects on treatment is rapidly evolving, but it is clear that it is extremely important to screen for and treat psychiatric comorbidities in patients presenting with OUD and vice versa. It is also specifically important to screen patients with OUD for suicidality, because SUDs are major risk factors for suicide. Care must be taken when diagnosing a non-SUD psychiatric disorder in a patient who has recently been using substances, because the differential includes substance-induced conditions that can mimic symptoms of mood, anxiety, and psychotic disorders. A careful history with timelines of symptoms versus substance use and collateral information—plus monitoring for symptoms after substance use stops—can help differentiate substance-induced conditions from primary psychiatric conditions.

Broadly speaking, medication management of OUD is similar in patients with and without co-occurring psychiatric disorders, in that methadone, buprenorphine, or naltrexone can usually be given. OUD and psychiatric comorbidities should be treated simultaneously, because leaving one condition untreated can worsen outcomes, as shown in a retrospective study of veterans with OUD who were admitted for inpatient MSW of opioids. In the study, there was a very high 4-year all-cause mortality rate of 18%, and veterans with untreated comorbid depression or anxiety had an even higher risk of death, whereas those treated for OUD with a medication had a reduced risk of death (Li et al. 2019).

In certain situations, one OUD medication may be preferred over the other because of the co-occurring disorder or its treatment. For example, a patient may prefer naltrexone if they have co-occurring alcohol use disorder (AUD) because naltrexone can treat both OUD and AUD. There are also many cases in which medication choice for the co-occurring disorder may be guided by the OUD medication that the patient prefers or is already taking. Interactions between medications for OUD and other psychiatric medications are important to consider. Many psychiatric medications can increase or decrease methadone serum levels (discussed earlier in the section "Methadone"); most psychiatric medications do not interact with buprenorphine or naltrexone to change their levels.

The most concerning interactions include increased sedation or respiratory depression, which increases the risk for overdose death. Benzodiazepine use in particular has been associated with an increased rate of overdose death in patients with OUD, owing to the synergistic effects between opioids and benzodiazepines; strikingly, in animal studies, the lethal doses of methadone and buprenorphine were reduced when a benzodiazepine was coadministered (Lintzeris and Nielsen 2010). Benzodiazepines generally do not interact with naltrexone. If a patient with OUD is actively misusing opioids, the mortality risk of prescribing benzodiazepines is extremely high (Park et al. 2020). Even if a patient is receiving a stable dose of methadone with no other opioids in the body, coadministration of diazepam can increase methadone's opioid effects and sedation and worsen memory and attention. Benzodiazepines coadministered with buprenorphine can also increase adverse effects, but the change seems to be milder than with methadone (Lintzeris and Nielsen 2010). Another concern is that benzodiazepines can be misused, and the risks increase if a patient is taking doses higher than prescribed. It is generally safer to avoid prescribing benzodiazepines when a patient is receiving methadone or buprenorphine, but there may be individual cases where the benefits outweigh the risks. These cases would likely be for an individual who is taking moderate doses of benzodiazepines only as prescribed and is not misusing other medications.

In patients with a history of OUD or other SUDs, medications that can cause their own SUDs or that can enhance opioid effects (e.g., benzodiazepines for anxiety disorders or stimulants for ADHD) must be prescribed carefully to avoid iatrogenic SUDs. Nonaddictive medications for anxiety (e.g., selective serotonin reuptake inhibitors) or ADHD (e.g., atomoxetine) would usually be first-line treatments if a patient has co-occurring OUD. If a patient has not received benefit for ADHD or anxiety after adequate trials of nonaddictive medications, and OUD is in remission, there may be individual cases in which the benefits of prescribing the aforementioned medications outweigh the risks; however, there are very limited data on optimal medication choices (Ramey et al. 2023).

Psychotherapy should always be considered when it is indicated for a co-occurring diagnosis, and it may improve OUD outcomes as well, although studies are limited. In patients with comorbid depressive disorders, there is evidence that adding psychotherapy to methadone for OUD can improve outcomes, including reduction in substance use, reduction in OUD severity, and improvement in functioning (Woody et al. 1987). There are very limited data on psychotherapy combined with naltrexone, and data on buprenorphine and psychotherapy are somewhat equivocal; but some studies have shown a benefit to retention and other outcomes (Sofuoglu et al. 2019).

A large number of patients with OUD have a comorbid SUD. SUDs should be treated simultaneously when possible, including tobacco use disorder (TUD). In particular, studies have shown that quitting smoking is associated with lower levels of relapse to other substances (Weinberger et al. 2017). Options for treatment of TUD include the nicotine patch, nicotine gum, bupropion, and varenicline. As stated earlier in this section, AUD can be treated with naltrexone, which is also a medication for OUD, but other FDA-approved options exist, including acamprosate and disulfiram.

Stimulant use, especially methamphetamines, has been increasing in the U.S. population, and a significant proportion of people with OUD have comorbid stimulant use disorder (Chan et al. 2020). Unfortunately, there is no FDA-approved medication for the treatment of stimulant use disorder. Emerging research using psychostimulants shows promise; however, data on treatment of stimulant use disorder specifically comorbid with OUD are limited (Chan et al. 2020). The most effective treatment today for stimulant use disorders is a behavioral therapy called *contingency management*, which involves providing rewards for specific behaviors, such as reduced substance use as measured by drug-free urine samples. Studies have shown that contingency management can reduce not only stimulant use but also risky behaviors, and it increases participation in treatment (Brown and DeFulio 2020). Contingency management can be used adjunctively with medications for treatment of OUD (Sofuoglu et al. 2019). OTPs in particular are well suited to contingency management because they may have built-in rewards (such as the possibility of increased take-home methadone dosing in place of daily dosing at the clinic), and these rewards can be used to reduce stimulant use as well as opioid use (Sofuoglu et al. 2019).

Considerations Related to Opioid Drug Supply Adulterants and Emerging Agents

The illicit opioid drug supply in the United States is increasingly found to contain an ever-expanding array of adulterants. As presented earlier in "Pharmacological Management of Intoxication," the presence of fentanyl and other HPSOs in the supply of illicit opioids (and other drugs) is particularly concerning and is responsible for a majority of the escalating illicit drug use overdose/poisoning deaths in the United States. In addition, other nonopioid adulterants/additives as well as novel synthetic opioids have been increasingly detected and present their own distinctive challenges. Two are briefly reviewed here: xylazine and benzimidazole-opioids (nitazenes).

Xylazine

Xylazine is a potent presynaptic α_2-adrenergic agonist that is approved as a large-animal veterinary sedative. It is structurally similar to clonidine and causes respiratory depression and a sleep-like state. It has never been approved for human indications, owing to concerns related to hypotension and impaired CNS function. Xylazine (also known colloquially as "tranq") emerged in the illicit drug supply around 2009, predominantly in Puerto Rico, and then surfaced along the U.S. Mid-Atlantic (especially Philadelphia). By 2019, xylazine was detected in 31% of fatal opioid overdoses in Philadelphia, and 91% of opioid samples there tested positive for xylazine (Hoffman et al. 2024).

When combined with opioids, such as fentanyl, xylazine may extend the euphoric effect of the opioid but can also increase the likelihood of respiratory depression and death (Friedman et al. 2022; Kariisa et al. 2023). One multicenter cohort study, however, demonstrated that opioid-xylazine overdose was not associated with greater morbidity than opioid overdose alone (Love et al. 2023). One noteworthy potential sequela of xylazine is the development of necrotic skin ulcerations, not necessarily at the site of injection, perhaps resulting from local decreases in tissue perfusion from the systemic effects of xylazine. These lesions typically begin as small round ulcerations, which then coalesce and get deeper with increasing tissue loss; extensor surfaces appear to be affected more commonly (McFadden et al. 2024).

Xylazine-dependent respiratory depression is not reversed by naloxone. Because individuals using substances containing xylazine may also have coexposure to opioids, however, naloxone should still routinely be offered to these individuals and those around them as part of a comprehensive public health community response to substance use. There are no FDA-approved xylazine reversal agents in humans. In animals, tolazoline (a selective α_2-antagonist) is approved for xylazine reversal; human α_2-antagonists, such as yohimbine, have been proposed for xylazine reversal, but this has yet to be meaningfully studied.

It is not yet clear whether there is a distinct xylazine withdrawal syndrome in humans. Such a syndrome is conceivable, given the similarity of xylazine to clonidine, the chronic use of which can lead to a clinically significant withdrawal syndrome on discontinuation, including hypertension, headache, insomnia, and anxiety (Ram and Engelman 1979). Like fentanyl test strips, xylazine test strips (lateral flow immunoassay) are increasingly becoming available as an opportunity for individuals to test their drugs for the presence of xylazine. Xylazine test strips are currently approved in Canada for detection of xylazine in urine samples and have been proposed as effective in detecting xylazine in the unregulated drug supply (Jones and Bailey 2023; Medical Devices Active License Listing 2023), although the evidence base is limited. In the United States, both SAMHSA and the CDC encourage consideration of xylazine test strips as part of a comprehensive community response to illicit drug use (Centers for Disease Control and Prevention 2024b; Substance Abuse and Mental Health Services Administration 2024).

Benzimidazole-Opioids (Nitazenes)

The synthetic benzimidazole-opioids (nitazenes) were first developed in the 1950s but have never been approved for medical use. To date, at least 13 different nitazenes have been identified, the most prevalent of which is isotonitazene (also known colloquially as "iso"). Beginning in 2019, nitazenes emerged in the illicit drug supply and since have become widespread globally (Inter-American Drug Abuse Control Commission 2024). Nitazenes have potency comparable to that of fentanyl, even though they are structurally unrelated (Vandeputte et al. 2021), and they have been increasingly detected in counterfeit prescription medication samples (Ujváry et al. 2021), highlighting the possibility that consumers may not be aware of the presence of nitazenes in the substances that they are using. Nitazenes are comparatively easy and inexpensive to manufacture, and there are no quality or purity manufacturing standards.

In theory, because nitazenes are potent MOR agonists, overdoses and poisonings should be reversible with MOR antagonists such as naloxone or nalmefene. However, there is a dearth of research on the effectiveness of opioid antagonists in relation to nitazene overdose and poisoning (Pergolizzi et al. 2023). Emerging data suggest that nitazene overdose and poisoning may require higher doses of naloxone than fentanyl overdose and poisoning, but further research is needed (Amaducci et al. 2023). Because nitazenes are structurally unrelated to fentanyl, fentanyl test strips are ineffective in detecting their presence in illicit drug supplies, and nitazene-specific test strips are not currently available but are in development (De Vrieze et al. 2024). Almost no literature exists on the effectiveness of standard medications for the treatment of OUD (i.e., buprenorphine, methadone, or naltrexone) in the face of nitazene use. However, given that nitazenes may be both more potent and more effective at stimulating the MOR than fentanyl, it has been proposed that higher doses of buprenorphine may be required to stabilize symptoms in individuals who have been chronically exposed to nitazenes (Chambers et al. 2023).

Key Points

- Opioids can act at a range of neurotransmitter receptor systems, but many of the noteworthy effects of opioids (e.g., analgesia, euphoria, respiratory depression) are mediated primarily through their activation of µ opioid receptors (MORs).
- Development of tolerance and withdrawal in the context of chronic opioid use is physiologically predictable and can contribute to continued use patterns and the development of opioid use disorder (OUD).

Tolerance to analgesic and mood effects of opioids appears to develop more rapidly (in 1–2 weeks) than tolerance to respiratory depression, which can increase the risk of unintentional overdose. Opioid withdrawal can be acute (lasting hours to days) and protracted (less severe but bothersome, lasting for months).
- Pharmacotherapies to facilitate discontinuation of chronic opioid use aim to minimize the experience of the opioid withdrawal syndrome and can be achieved either through controlled introduction of opioid medications that are then gradually tapered (i.e., buprenorphine, methadone) or through the use of medications aimed at ameliorating the symptoms of withdrawal (i.e., clonidine, lofexidine, loperamide, nonsteroidal anti-inflammatory drugs), a process known as medically supervised withdrawal (MSW).
- MSW alone is often insufficient to prevent relapse and mitigate the risk of subsequent opioid overdose (fatal or nonfatal); therefore, long-term pharmacotherapy utilizing buprenorphine, methadone, or naltrexone (the three FDA-approved medications for the treatment of OUD) is imperative, and the duration of maintenance treatment may be indefinite.
- Methadone may be prescribed for pain (by any U.S. Drug Enforcement Administration [DEA]–authorized controlled substance prescriber) or for OUD (can be initiated in acute care hospitals, but is only available in outpatient settings through registered opioid treatment programs [OTPs]). OTPs are highly regulated and structured. Initiation on methadone does not require that the patient first enter opioid withdrawal.
- Buprenorphine is a partial MOR agonist that can be prescribed by any DEA-authorized controlled substance prescriber for either pain or OUD. It has several attractive pharmacological features, such as a ceiling effect on respiratory depression and very high binding affinity. Traditionally, buprenorphine initiation protocols required the individual to first enter opioid withdrawal to prevent precipitated withdrawal, but newer protocols have been proposed that may not require this step.
- Naltrexone may be preferable for patients with safety-sensitive professions. The efficacy of naltrexone is blunted by the need for a period of opioid abstinence before initiation, but once initiated, naltrexone

treatment has similar outcomes to other medications for OUD. Extended-release naltrexone (injectable) may be more efficacious than oral naltrexone because of better treatment adherence.
• Patients with chronic pain, pregnant patients, and patients with co-occurring psychiatric illnesses should all be offered OUD pharmacotherapies, although patient-specific factors may drive which treatment option is optimal.

References

Aghajanian GK, Kogan JH, Moghaddam B: Opiate withdrawal increases glutamate and aspartate efflux in the locus coeruleus: an in vivo microdialysis study. Brain Res 636(1):126–130, 1994 7908850

Ahmed S, Bhivandkar S, Lonergan BB, et al: Microinduction of buprenorphine/naloxone: a review of the literature. Am J Addict 30(4):305–315, 2021 33378137

Amaducci A, Aldy K, Campleman SL, et al: Naloxone use in novel potent opioid and fentanyl overdoses in emergency department patients. JAMA Netw Open 6(8):e2331264, 2023 37642962

American Psychiatric Association: American Psychiatric Association Practice Guidelines for the Treatment of Psychiatric Disorders: Compendium 2006. Washington, DC, American Psychiatric Association, 2006

American Psychiatric Association: Diagnostic and Statistical Manual of Mental Disorders, 5th Edition. Arlington, VA, American Psychiatric Association, 2013

American Psychiatric Association: Diagnostic and Statistical Manual of Mental Disorders, 5th Edition, Text Revision. Washington, DC, American Psychiatric Association, 2022

American Society of Addiction Medicine: Clinical Opiate Withdrawal Scale (COWS). Available at: https://www.asam.org/docs/default-source/education-docs/cows_induction_flow_sheet.pdf?sfvrsn=b577fc2_2. Accessed March 29, 2025.

Anderson IB, Kearney TE: Use of methadone. West J Med 172(1):43–46, 2000 10695444

Antoine D, Huhn AS, Strain EC, et al: Method for successfully inducting individuals who use illicit fentanyl onto buprenorphine/naloxone. Am J Addict 30(1):83–87, 2021 32572978

Armenian P, Vo KT, Barr-Walker J, et al: Fentanyl, fentanyl analogs and novel synthetic opioids: a comprehensive review. Neuropharmacology 134(Pt A):121–32, 2018

Axelrod DJ, Reville B: Using methadone to treat opioid-induced hyperalgesia and refractory pain. J Opioid Manag 3(2):113–114, 2007 17520991

Azar P, Nikoo M, Miles I: Methadone to buprenorphine/naloxone induction without withdrawal utilizing transdermal fentanyl bridge in an inpatient setting: Azar method. Am J Addict 27(8):601–604, 2018 30387894

Azar P, Wong JSH, Mathew N, et al: 48-hour induction of transdermal buprenorphine to sublingual buprenorphine/naloxone: the IPPAS method. J Addict Med 17(2):233–236, 2023 36149002

Bailey GL, Herman DS, Stein MD: Perceived relapse risk and desire for medication assisted treatment among persons seeking inpatient opiate detoxification. J Subst Abuse Treat 45(3):302–305, 2013 23786852

Baldo BA, Rose MA: The anaesthetist, opioid analgesic drugs, and serotonin toxicity: a mechanistic and clinical review. Br J Anaesth 124(1):44–62, 2020 31653394

Ball JC, Ross A: The Effectiveness of Methadone Maintenance Treatment. New York, Springer-Verlag, 1991

Ball J, Corty E, Bond H, et al: The reduction of intravenous heroin use, non-opiate abuse and crime during methadone maintenance treatment: further findings. NIDA Res Monogr 81:224–230, 1988a 3136364

Ball JC, Lange WR, Myers CP, et al: Reducing the risk of AIDS through methadone maintenance treatment. J Health Soc Behav 29(3):214–226, 1988b

Ballantyne JC, Sullivan MD, Kolodny A: Opioid dependence vs addiction: a distinction without a difference? Arch Intern Med 172(17):1342–1343, 2012 22892799

Baxter LE Sr, Campbell A, Deshields M, et al: Safe methadone induction and stabilization: report of an expert panel. J Addict Med 7(6):377–386, 2013 24189172

Bell A, Bennett AS, Jones TS, et al: Amount of naloxone used to reverse opioid overdoses outside of medical practice in a city with increasing illicitly manufactured fentanyl in illicit drug supply. Subst Abus 40(1):52–55, 2019 29558283

Bell J, Seres V, Bowron P, et al: The use of serum methadone levels in patients receiving methadone maintenance. Clin Pharmacol Ther 43(6):623–629, 1988 3378383

Bell J, Bowron P, Lewis J, et al: Serum levels of methadone in maintenance clients who persist in illicit drug use. Br J Addict 85(12):1599–1602, 1990 1981155

Bennett JA, Abrams JT, Van Riper DF, et al: Difficult or impossible ventilation after sufentanil-induced anesthesia is caused primarily by vocal cord closure. Anesthesiology 87(5):1070–1074, 1997 9366458

Bickel WK, Johnson RE, Stitzer ML, et al: A clinical trial of buprenorphine: I. Comparison with methadone in the detoxification of heroin addicts. II. Examination of its opioid blocking properties. NIDA Res Monogr 76:182–188, 1987 2449618

Brar R, Fairbairn N, Sutherland C, et al: Use of a novel prescribing approach for the treatment of opioid use disorder: buprenorphine/naloxone micro-dosing: a case series. Drug Alcohol Rev 39(5):588–594, 2020 32657496

Brown BS, Watters JK, Iglehart AS: Methadone maintenance dosage levels and program retention. Am J Drug Alcohol Abuse 9(2):129–139, 1982 7171077

Brown HD, DeFulio A: Contingency management for the treatment of methamphetamine use disorder: a systematic review. Drug Alcohol Depend 216:108307, 2020 33007699

Bruneau J, Ahamad K, Goyer ME, et al: Management of opioid use disorders: a national clinical practice guideline. CMAJ 190(9):E247–E257, 2018 29507156

Cacciola JS, Alterman AI, Rutherford MJ, et al: The relationship of psychiatric comorbidity to treatment outcomes in methadone maintained patients. Drug Alcohol Depend 61(3):271–280, 2001 11164691

Calsyn DA, Malcy JA, Saxon AJ: Slow tapering from methadone maintenance in a program encouraging indefinite maintenance. J Subst Abuse Treat 30(2):159–163, 2006 16490679

Camí J, Farré M: Drug addiction. N Engl J Med 349(10):975–986, 2003 12954747

Campbell ND, Lovell AM: The history of the development of buprenorphine as an addiction therapeutic. Ann NY Acad Sci 1248:124–139, 2012 22256949

Cao JL, Vialou VF, Lobo MK, et al: Essential role of the cAMP-cAMP response-element binding protein pathway in opiate-induced homeostatic adaptations of locus coeruleus neurons. Proc Natl Acad Sci USA 107(39):17011–17016, 2010 20837544

Cao SS, Dunham SI, Simpson SA: Prescribing buprenorphine for opioid use disorders in the ED: a review of best practices, barriers, and future directions. Open Access Emerg Med 12(12):261–274, 2020 33116962

Capone T, Brahen L, Condren R, et al: Retention and outcome in a narcotic antagonist treatment program. J Clin Psychol 42(5):825–833, 1986 3760220

Carpenter J, Murray BP, Atti S, et al: Naloxone dosing after opioid overdose in the era of illicitly manufactured fentanyl. J Med Toxicol 16(1):41–48, 2020

Carroll KM, Ball SA, Nich C, et al: Targeting behavioral therapies to enhance naltrexone treatment of opioid dependence: efficacy of contingency management and significant other involvement. Arch Gen Psychiatry 58(8):755–761, 2001 11483141

Centers for Disease Control and Prevention: What Can You Do to Test for Fentanyl. Atlanta, GA, Centers for Disease Control and Prevention, April 2, 2024a. Available at: https://www.cdc.gov/stop-overdose/safety/index.html. Accessed November 2, 2024.

Centers for Disease Control and Prevention: What You Should Know About Xylazine. Atlanta, GA, Centers for Disease Control and Prevention, May 16, 2024b. Available at: https://www.cdc.gov/overdose-prevention/about/what-you-should-know-about-xylazine.html. Accessed November 2, 2024.

Chambers LC, Hallowell BD, Zullo AR, et al: Buprenorphine dose and time to discontinuation among patients with opioid use disorder in the era of fentanyl. JAMA Netw Open 6(9):e2334540, 2023 37721749

Chan B, Freeman M, Ayers C, et al: A systematic review and meta-analysis of medications for stimulant use disorders in patients with co-occurring opioid use disorders. Drug Alcohol Depend 216:108193, 2020 32861136

Chang G, Chen L, Mao J: Opioid tolerance and hyperalgesia. Med Clin North Am 91(2):199–211, 2007 17321281

Charney DS, Sternberg DE, Kleber HD, et al: The clinical use of clonidine in abrupt withdrawal from methadone: effects on blood pressure and specific signs and symptoms. Arch Gen Psychiatry 38(11):1273–1277, 1981 7305608

Chen A, Ashburn MA: Cardiac effects of opioid therapy. Pain Med 16(Suppl 1):S27–S31, 2015 26461073

Chen L, Malarick C, Seefeld L, et al: Altered quantitative sensory testing outcome in subjects with opioid therapy. Pain 143(1–2):65–70, 2009 19237249

Cheskin LJ, Fudala PJ, Johnson RE: A controlled comparison of buprenorphine and clonidine for acute detoxification from opioids. Drug Alcohol Depend 36(2):115–121, 1994 7851278

Christie MJ: Cellular neuroadaptations to chronic opioids: tolerance, withdrawal and addiction. Br J Pharmacol 154(2):384–396, 2008 18414400

Ciraulo DA, Ciraulo AN: Substance abuse, in Handbook of Clinical Psychopharmacology. Edited by Tupin JP, Shader RI, Harnett DS. Northvale, NJ, Jason Aronson, 1988, p 143

Ciraulo DA, Hitzemann RJ, Somoza E, et al: Pharmacokinetics and pharmacodynamics of multiple sublingual buprenorphine tablets in dose-escalation trials. J Clin Pharmacol 46(2):179–192, 2006 16432270

Cornish R, Macleod J, Strang J, et al: Risk of death during and after opiate substitution treatment in primary care: prospective observational study in UK General Practice Research Database. BMJ 341:c5475, 2010 20978062

Cushman P, Dole VP: Detoxification of rehabilitated methadone-maintained patients. JAMA 226(7):747–752, 1973 4585339

Dang VC, Christie MJ: Mechanisms of rapid opioid receptor desensitization, resensitization and tolerance in brain neurons. Br J Pharmacol 165(6):1704–1716, 2012 21564086

Darcq E, Kieffer BL: Opioid receptors: drivers to addiction? Nat Rev Neurosci 19(8):499–514, 2018 29934561

De Aquino JP, Parida S, Sofuoglu M: The pharmacology of buprenorphine microinduction for opioid use disorder. Clin Drug Investig 41(5):425–436, 2021 33818748

DePriest AZ, Puet BL, Holt AC, et al: Metabolism and disposition of prescription opioids: a review. Forensic Sci Rev 27(2):115–145, 2015 26227254

Derbel I, Ghorbel A, Akrout FM, et al: Opiate withdrawal syndrome in buprenorphine abusers admitted to a rehabilitation center in Tunisia. Afr Health Sci 16(4):1067–1077, 2016 28479900

de Vries F, Bruin M, Lobatto DJ, et al: Opioids and their endocrine effects: a systematic review and meta-analysis. J Clin Endocrinol Metab 105(3):1020–1029, 2020 31511863

De Vrieze LM, Stove CP, Vandeputte MM: Nitazene test strips: a laboratory evaluation. Harm Reduct J 21(1):159, 2024 39198843

Dhawan A, Rao R, Ambekar A, et al: Methadone Maintenance Treatment in India: A Feasibility and Effectiveness Report. New Delhi, India, United Nations Office on Drugs and Crime, Regional Office for South Asia, 2014

Doerzbacher M, Chang YP: Supporting breastfeeding for women on opioid maintenance therapy: a systematic review. J Perinatol 39(9):1159–1164, 2019 31263203

Dole VP, Joseph H: Long-term outcome of patients treated with methadone maintenance. Ann NY Acad Sci 311:181–189, 1978 283719

Dole VP, Nyswander M: A medical treatment for diacetylmorphine (heroin) addiction: a clinical trial with methadone hydrochloride. JAMA 193:646–650, 1965 14321530

Donohue JM, Jarlenski MP, Kim JY, et al: Use of medications for treatment of opioid use disorder among US Medicaid enrollees in 11 states, 2014–2018. JAMA 326(2):154–164, 2021 34255008

Donroe JH, Tetrault JM: Substance use, intoxication, and withdrawal in the critical care setting. Crit Care Clin 33(3):543–558, 2017 28601134

Dowell D, Ragan KR, Jones CM, et al: CDC Clinical Practice Guideline for Prescribing Opioids for Pain—United States, 2022. MMWR Recomm Rep 71(3):1–95, 2022 36327391

Dunbar JL, Turncliff RZ, Dong Q, et al: Single- and multiple-dose pharmacokinetics of long-acting injectable naltrexone. Alcohol Clin Exp Res 30(3):480–490, 2006 16499489

Dunn KE, Sigmon SC, Strain EC, et al: The association between outpatient buprenorphine detoxification duration and clinical treatment outcomes: a review. Drug Alcohol Depend 119(1–2):1–9, 2011 21741781

Edwards FJ, Wicelinski R, Gallagher N, et al: Treating opioid withdrawal with buprenorphine in a community hospital emergency department: an outreach program. Ann Emerg Med 75(1):49–56, 2020 31732373

Endo Pharmaceuticals: BELBUCA product information: BELBUCA buccal film, buprenorphine buccal film. Malvern, PA, Endo Pharmaceuticals Inc, 2016. Available at: https://www.accessdata.fda.gov/drugsatfda_docs/label/2016/207932s002lbl.pdf. Accessed February 5, 2025.

Fareed A, Stout S, Casarella J, et al: Illicit opioid intoxication: diagnosis and treatment. Subst Abuse 5:17–25, 2011 22879747

Ferrari A, Coccia CP, Bertolini A, et al: Methadone: metabolism, pharmacokinetics and interactions. Pharmacol Res 50(6):551–559, 2004 15501692

Fiellin DA, Pantalon MV, Chawarski MC, et al: Counseling plus buprenorphine-naloxone maintenance therapy for opioid dependence. N Engl J Med 355(4):365–374, 2006 16870915

Fiellin DA, Schottenfeld RS, Cutter CJ, et al: Primary care-based buprenorphine taper vs maintenance therapy for prescription opioid dependence: a randomized clinical trial. JAMA Intern Med 174(12):1947–1954, 2014 25330017

Fram DH, Marmo J, Holden R: Naltrexone treatment: the problem of patient acceptance. J Subst Abuse Treat 6(2):119–122, 1989 2746710

Friedman A, Nabong L: Opioids: pharmacology, physiology, and clinical implications in pain medicine. Phys Med Rehabil Clin N Am 31(2):289–303, 2020 32279731

Friedman J, Montero F, Bourgois P, et al: Xylazine spreads across the US: a growing component of the increasingly synthetic and polysubstance overdose crisis. Drug Alcohol Depend 233:109380, 2022 35247724

Friesen EL, Kurdyak P: The impact of psychiatric comorbidity on treatment discontinuation among individuals receiving medications for opioid use disorder. Drug Alcohol Depend 216:108244, 2020 32861134

Fudala PJ, Jaffe JH, Dax EM, et al: Use of buprenorphine in the treatment of opioid addiction. II. Physiologic and behavioral effects of daily and alternate-day administration and abrupt withdrawal. Clin Pharmacol Ther 47(4):525–534, 1990 2328561

Gerstein DR, Harwood HJ (eds): Treating Drug Problems, Vol 1: A Study of the Evolution, Effectiveness, and Financing of Public and Private Drug Treatment Systems. Washington, DC, National Academy Press, 1990

Ginzburg HM: Naltrexone: Its Clinical Utility (NIDA Treatment Research Report ADM-84-1358). Washington, DC, U.S. Government Printing Office, 1984

Gold MS, Redmond DE Jr, Kleber HD: Clonidine in opiate withdrawal. Lancet 1(8070):929–930, 1978 76860

Gomes T, McCormack D, Bozinoff N, et al: Duration of use and outcomes among people with opioid use disorder initiating methadone and buprenorphine in Ontario: a population-based propensity-score matched cohort study. Addiction 117(7):1972–1981, 2022 35257434

Gordon DB, Stevenson KK, Griffie J, et al: Opioid equianalgesic calculations. J Palliat Med 2(2):209–218, 1999 15859817

Gossop M, Bradley B, Phillips GT: An investigation of withdrawal symptoms shown by opiate addicts during and subsequent to a 21-day in-patient methadone detoxification procedure. Addict Behav 12(1):1–6, 1987 3565107

Greenwald MK, Schuh KJ, Stine SM: Transferring methadone-maintained outpatients to the buprenorphine sublingual tablet: a preliminary study. Am J Addict 12(4):365–374, 2003 14504028

Greenwald MK, Herring AA, Perrone J, et al: A neuropharmacological model to explain buprenorphine induction challenges. Ann Emerg Med 80(6):509–524, 2022 35940992

Grella CE, Wugalter SE, Anglin MD: Predictors of treatment retention in enhanced and standard methadone maintenance treatment for HIV risk reduction. J Drug Issues 27(2):203–224, 1997

Groer CE, Schmid CL, Jaeger AM, et al: Agonist-directed interactions with specific beta-arrestins determine mu-opioid receptor trafficking, ubiquitination, and dephosphorylation. J Biol Chem 286(36):31731–31741, 2011 21757712

Gruber VA, McCance-Katz EF: Methadone, buprenorphine, and street drug interactions with antiretroviral medications. Curr HIV/AIDS Rep 7(3):152–160, 2010 20532839

Gunderson EW, Levin FR, Rombone MM, et al: Improving temporal efficiency of outpatient buprenorphine induction. Am J Addict 20(5):397–404, 2011 21838837

Guo CZ, D'Onofrio G, Fiellin DA, et al: Emergency department-initiated buprenorphine protocols: a national evaluation. J Am Coll Emerg Physicians Open 2(6):e12606, 2021 34877567

Gutstein HB, Akil H: Opioid analgesics, in Goodman and Gilman's The Pharmacological Basis of Therapeutics, 10th Edition. Edited by Hardman JG, Limbird LE, Gilman AG. New York, McGraw Hill, 2001, pp 569–619

Hakansson A, Medvedeo A, Andersson M, et al: Buprenorphine misuse among heroin and amphetamine users in Malmo, Sweden: purpose of misuse and route of administration. Eur Addict Res 13(4):207–215, 2007 17851242

Hämmig R, Kemter A, Strasser J, et al: Use of microdoses for induction of buprenorphine treatment with overlapping full opioid agonist use: the Bernese method. Subst Abuse Rehabil 7:99–105, 2016 27499655

Hawk K, Hoppe J, Ketcham E, et al: Consensus recommendations on the treatment of opioid use disorder in the emergency department. Ann Emerg Med 78(3):434–442, 2021 34172303

Hayhurst CJ, Durieux ME: Differential opioid tolerance and opioid-induced hyperalgesia: a clinical reality. Anesthesiology 124(2):483–488, 2016 26594912

Heishman SJ, Stitzer ML, Bigelow GE, et al: Acute opioid physical dependence in postaddict humans: naloxone dose effects after brief morphine exposure. J Pharmacol Exp Ther 248(1):127–134, 1989 2913267

Hern HG, Lara V, Goldstein D, et al: Prehospital buprenorphine treatment for opioid use disorder by paramedics: first year results of the EMS buprenorphine use pilot. Prehosp Emerg Care 13:1–9, 2022 35420925

Herring AA, Schultz CW, Yang E, et al: Rapid induction onto sublingual buprenorphine after opioid overdose and successful linkage to treatment for opioid use disorder. Am J Emerg Med 37(12):2259–2262, 2019 31239086

Herring AA, Vosooghi AA, Luftig J, et al: High-dose buprenorphine induction in the emergency department for treatment of opioid use disorder. JAMA Netw Open 4(7):e2117128, 2021 34264326

Hill LG, Zagorski CM, Loera LJ: Increasingly powerful opioid antagonists are not necessary. Int J Drug Policy 99:103457, 2022 34560623

Himmelsbach CK: The morphine abstinence syndrome, its nature and treatment. Ann Intern Med 15(5):829–839, 1941

Hoffman GR, Giduturi C, Cordaro NJ, et al: Classics in chemical neuroscience: xylazine. ACS Chem Neurosci 15(11):2091–2098, 2024 38747710

Hollister LE, Johnson K, Boukhabza D, et al: Aversive effects of naltrexone in subjects not dependent on opiates. Drug Alcohol Depend 8(1):37–41, 1981 7297411

Horspool MJ, Seivewright N, Armitage CJ, et al: Post-treatment outcomes of buprenorphine detoxification in community settings: a systematic review. Eur Addict Res 14(4):179–185, 2008 18583914

H.R. 2617–117th Congress (2021–2022): Consolidated Appropriations Act of 2023. December 29, 2022. Available at: https://www.congress.gov/bill/117th-congress/house-bill/2617. Accessed February 5, 2025.

Huhn AS, Hobelmann JG, Oyler GA, et al: Protracted renal clearance of fentanyl in persons with opioid use disorder. Drug Alcohol Depend 214:108147, 2020 32650192

Hulse GK, O'Neill G, Pereira C, et al: Obstetric and neonatal outcomes associated with maternal naltrexone exposure. Aust N Z J Obstet Gynaecol 41(4):424–428, 2001 11787918

Hulse GK, Ngo HT, Tait RJ: Risk factors for craving and relapse in heroin users treated with oral or implant naltrexone. Biol Psychiatry 68(3):296–302, 2010 20537615

Humphreys K, Barreto NB, Alessi SM, et al: Impact of 12 step mutual help groups on drug use disorder patients across six clinical trials. Drug Alcohol Depend 215:108213, 2020 32801112

Hunt DE, Lipton DS, Goldsmith DS, et al: "It takes your heart": the image of methadone maintenance in the addict world and its effect on recruitment into treatment. Int J Addict 20(11–12):1751–1771, 1985 3833809

Indivior: BUPRENEX product information: BUPRENEX intravenous injection, intramuscular injection, buprenorphine HCl intravenous injection, intramuscular injection. North Chesterfield, VA, Indivior Inc, 2023. Available at: https://dailymed.nlm.nih.gov/dailymed/downloadpdffile.cfm?setId=b086772e-d15a-4d13-b1a2-38bfbde1f18c. Accessed February 5, 2025.

Indivior: Indivior Announces FDA Approval of Label Changes for SUBLOCADE® (buprenorphine extended-release) Injection. Indivior, 2025. Available at: https://www.indivior.com/en/media/press-releases/indivior-announces-fda-approval-of-label-changes-for-sublocade-injection. Accessed June 23, 2025.

Inter-American Drug Abuse Control Commission: Information Bulletin: The Emergence of Nitazenes in the Americas. Washington, DC, Inter-American Drug Abuse Commission, Organization of American States, September 2024. Available at: https://www.oas.org/ext/DesktopModules/MVC/OASDnnModules/Views/Item/Download.aspx?type=1&id=1045&lang=1. Accessed November 2, 2024.

Ito S: Opioids in breast milk: pharmacokinetic principles and clinical implications. J Clin Pharmacol 58(Suppl 10):S151–S163, 2018 30248201

Jaffe J, Knapp CM, Ciraulo DA: Opiates: Clinical Aspects, in Substance Abuse: A Comprehensive Textbook. Edited by Lowinson JH, Ruiz P, Millman RB, et al. New York, Lippincott Williams & Wilkins, 2004, pp 158–165

Jarlenski M, Chen Q, Gao A, et al: Association of duration of methadone or buprenorphine use during pregnancy with risk of nonfatal drug overdose among pregnant persons with opioid use disorder in the US. JAMA Netw Open 5(4):e227964, 2022 35438758

Jarvis BP, Holtyn AF, Subramaniam S, et al: Extended-release injectable naltrexone for opioid use disorder: a systematic review. Addiction 113(7):1188–1209, 2018 29396985

Jasinski DR, Pevnick JS, Griffith JD: Human pharmacology and abuse potential of the analgesic buprenorphine: a potential agent for treating narcotic addiction. Arch Gen Psychiatry 35(4):501–516, 1978 215096

Jasinski DR, Johnson RE, Kocher TR: Clonidine in morphine withdrawal. Differential effects on signs and symptoms. Arch Gen Psychiatry 42(11):1063–1066, 1985 2413818

Johnson RE, Chutuape MA, Strain EC, et al: A comparison of levomethadyl acetate, buprenorphine, and methadone for opioid dependence. N Engl J Med 343(18):1290–1297, 2000 11058673

Jones HE, Kaltenbach K, Heil SH, et al: Neonatal abstinence syndrome after methadone or buprenorphine exposure. N Engl J Med 363(24):2320–2331, 2010 21142534

Jones JD, Sullivan MA, Vosburg SK, et al: Abuse potential of intranasal buprenorphine versus buprenorphine/naloxone in buprenorphine-maintained heroin users. Addict Biol 20(4):784–798, 2015 25060839

Jones RT: Dependence in non-addict humans after a single dose of morphine, in Endogenous and Exogenous Opiate Agonists and Antagonists. Edited by Way EL. New York, Pergamon, 1979, pp 557–560

Jones S, Bailey S: Xylazine Test Strips for Drug Checking: CADTH Horizon Scan (July Report No EN0049). Ottawa, ON, Canada, Canadian Agency for Drugs and Technologies in Health, 2023

Joudrey PJ, Adams ZM, Bach P, et al: Methadone access for opioid use disorder during the COVID-19 pandemic within the United States and Canada. JAMA Netw Open 4(7):e2118223, 2021 34297070

Kakko J, Svanborg KD, Kreek MJ, et al: 1-year retention and social function after buprenorphine-assisted relapse prevention treatment for heroin dependence in Sweden: a randomised, placebo-controlled trial. Lancet 361(9358):662–668, 2003 12606177

Kale N: Urine drug tests: ordering and interpreting results. Am Fam Physician 99(1):33–39, 2019 30600984

Kariisa M, O'Donnell J, Kumar S, et al: Illicitly manufactured fentanyl–involved overdose deaths with detected xylazine—United States, January 2019–June 2022. MMWR Morb Mortal Wkly Rep 72(26):721–727, 2023 37384558

King VL, Stoller KB, Hayes M, et al: A multicenter randomized evaluation of methadone medical maintenance. Drug Alcohol Depend 65(2):137–148, 2002 11772475

Kirchmayer U, Davoli M, Verster AD, et al: A systematic review on the efficacy of naltrexone maintenance treatment in opioid dependence. Addiction 97(10):1241–1249, 2002 12359026

Klaire S, Zivanovic R, Barbic SP, et al: Rapid micro-induction of buprenorphine/ naloxone for opioid use disorder in an inpatient setting: a case series. Am J Addict 28(4):262–265, 2019 30901127

Kleber HD: Detoxification from narcotics, in Substance Abuse: Clinical Problems and Perspectives. Edited by Lowinson J, Ruiz P. Baltimore, MD, Williams & Wilkins, 1981, pp 317–338

Kleber HD, Riordan CE, Rounsaville B, et al: Clonidine in outpatient detoxification from methadone maintenance. Arch Gen Psychiatry 42(4):391–394, 1985 3977557

Koob GF: Neurobiology of opioid addiction: opponent process, hyperkatifeia, and negative reinforcement. Biol Psychiatry 87(1):44–53, 2020 31400808

Kornfeld H, Reetz H: Transdermal buprenorphine, opioid rotation to sublingual buprenorphine, and the avoidance of precipitated withdrawal: a review of the literature and demonstration in three chronic pain patients treated with butrans. Am J Ther 22(3):199–205, 2015 23846520

Kornick CA, Kilborn MJ, Santiago-Palma J, et al: QTc interval prolongation associated with intravenous methadone. Pain 105(3):499–506, 2003 14527710

Kosten TR, George TP: The neurobiology of opioid dependence: implications for treatment. Sci Pract Perspect 1(1):13–20, 2002 18567959

Kosten TR, Kleber HD: Buprenorphine detoxification from opioid dependence: a pilot study. Life Sci 42(6):635–641, 1988 3276999

Kosten TR, Rounsaville BJ, Kleber HD: A 2.5 year follow-up of treatment retention and reentry among opioid addicts. J Subst Abuse Treat 3(3):181–189, 1986 3806731

Kosten TR, Rounsaville BJ, Kleber HD: Multidimensionality and prediction of treatment outcome in opioid addicts: 2.5-year follow-up. Compr Psychiatry 28(1):3–13, 1987a 3802797

Kosten TR, Rounsaville BJ, Kleber HD: Predictors of 2.5-year outcome in opioid addicts: pretreatment source of income. Am J Drug Alcohol Abuse 13(1–2):19–32, 1987b 3687883

Krantz MJ, Lewkowiez L, Hays H, et al: Torsade de pointes associated with very-high-dose methadone. Ann Intern Med 137(6):501–504, 2002 12230351

Krantz MJ, Kutinsky IB, Robertson AD, et al: Dose-related effects of methadone on QT prolongation in a series of patients with torsade de pointes. Pharmacotherapy 23(6):802–805, 2003 12820821

Kreek MJ: Methadone in treatment: physiological and pharmacological issues, in Handbook on Drug Abuse. Edited by Dupont RL, Goldstein A, O'Donnell J. Washington, DC, U.S. Government Printing Office, 1979, pp 57–86

Kreek MJ: Health consequences associated with the use of methadone, in Research on the Treatment of Narcotic Addiction: State of the Art (NIDA Res Monograph ADM-83-1281). Edited by Cooper JR, Altman R, Brown BS, et al. Washington, DC, U.S. Government Printing Office, 1983, pp 456–482

Kreek MJ, Levran O, Reed B, et al: Opiate addiction and cocaine addiction: underlying molecular neurobiology and genetics. J Clin Invest 122(10):3387–3393, 2012 23023708

Krotulski AJ, Chapman BP, Marks SJ, et al: Sentanyl: a comparison of blood fentanyl concentrations and naloxone dosing after non-fatal overdose. Clin Toxicol (Phila) 60(2):197–204, 2022 34278904

Krupitsky E, Nunes EV, Ling W, et al: Injectable extended-release naltrexone for opioid dependence: a double-blind, placebo-controlled, multicentre randomised trial. Lancet 377(9776):1506–1513, 2011 21529928

Kuip EJM, Zandvliet ML, Koolen SLW, et al: A review of factors explaining variability in fentanyl pharmacokinetics: focus on implications for cancer patients. Br J Clin Pharmacol 83(2):294–313, 2017 27619152

Kuszmaul AK, Palmer EC, Frederick EK: Lofexidine versus clonidine for mitigation of opioid withdrawal symptoms: a systematic review. J Am Pharm Assoc (2003) 60(1):145–152, 2020

Kutscher E, Barber Grossi M, LaPolla F, et al: Fentanyl test strips for harm reduction: a scoping review. J Addict Med 18(4):373–380, 2024

Lagisetty P, Klasa K, Bush C, et al: Primary care models for treating opioid use disorders: what actually works? A systematic review. PLoS One 12(10):e0186315, 2017 29040331

Lam JKW, Cheung CCK, Chow MYT, et al: Transmucosal drug administration as an alternative route in palliative and end-of-life care during the COVID-19 pandemic. Adv Drug Deliv Rev 160:234–243, 2020 33137363

Larney S, Gowing L, Mattick RP, et al: A systematic review and meta-analysis of naltrexone implants for the treatment of opioid dependence. Drug Alcohol Rev 33(2):115–128, 2014 24299657

La Vincente SF, White JM, Somogyi AA, et al: Enhanced buprenorphine analgesia with the addition of ultra-low-dose naloxone in healthy subjects. Clin Pharmacol Ther 83(1):144–152, 2008 17568402

Leavitt SB: Methadone dosing and safety in the treatment of opioid addiction. Addiction Treatment Forum 12:3, 2003

Lee JD, Nunes EV Jr, Novo P, et al: Comparative effectiveness of extended-release naltrexone versus buprenorphine-naloxone for opioid relapse prevention (X:BOT): a multicentre, open-label, randomised controlled trial. Lancet 391(10118):309–318, 2018 29150198

LeSaint KT, Klapthor B, Wang RC, et al: Buprenorphine for opioid use disorder in the emergency department: a retrospective chart review. West J Emerg Med 21(5):1175–1181, 2020 32970572

Li KJ, Smedberg DL, DeLisi LE: A retrospective 4-year outcome study of veterans admitted to an acute inpatient detoxification unit for opioid use disorder. Am J Addict 28(4):318–323, 2019 31067001

Lim J, Farhat I, Douros A, et al: Relative effectiveness of medications for opioid-related disorders: a systematic review and network meta-analysis of randomized controlled trials. PLoS One 17(3):e0266142, 2022 35358261

Ling W, Charuvastra C, Collins JF, et al: Buprenorphine maintenance treatment of opiate dependence: a multicenter, randomized clinical trial. Addiction 93(4):475–486, 1998 9684386

Ling W, Nadipelli VR, Solem CT, et al: Patient-centered outcomes in participants of a buprenorphine monthly depot (BUP-XR) double-blind, placebo-controlled, multicenter, phase 3 study. J Addict Med 13(6):442–449, 2019 30844878

Ling W, Nadipelli VR, Solem CT, et al: Effects of monthly buprenorphine extended-release injections on patient-centered outcomes: a long-term study. J Subst Abuse Treat 110(Mar):1–8, 2020 31952623

Link HM, Jones H, Miller L, et al: Buprenorphine-naloxone use in pregnancy: a systematic review and metaanalysis. Am J Obstet Gynecol MFM 2(3):100179, 2020 33345863

Lintzeris N, Nielsen S: Benzodiazepines, methadone and buprenorphine: interactions and clinical management. Am J Addict 19(1):59–72, 2010 20132123

Lofwall MR, Walsh SL, Nunes EV, et al: Weekly and monthly subcutaneous buprenorphine depot formulations vs daily sublingual buprenorphine with naloxone for treatment of opioid use disorder: a randomized clinical trial. JAMA Intern Med 178(6):764–773, 2018 29799968

Love JS, Levine M, Aldy K, et al: Opioid overdoses involving xylazine in emergency department patients: a multicenter study. Clin Toxicol (Phila) 61(3):173–180, 2023 37014353

Lucey MR, Silverman BL, Illeperuma A, et al: Hepatic safety of once-monthly injectable extended-release naltrexone administered to actively drinking alcoholics. Alcohol Clin Exp Res 32(3):498–504, 2008 18241321

Magura S, Goldsmith D, Casriel C, et al: The validity of methadone clients' self-reported drug use. Int J Addict 22(8):727–749, 1987 3679632

Mancher M, Leshner AI (eds): Medications for Opioid Use Disorder Save Lives. Washington, DC, National Academies Press, 2019

Manhapra A: Complex persistent opioid dependence—an opioid-induced chronic pain syndrome. Curr Treat Options Oncol 23(7):921–935, 2022 35435616

Mannelli P, Wu L-T, Peindl KS, et al: Extended release naltrexone injection is performed in the majority of opioid dependent patients receiving outpatient induction: a very low dose naltrexone and buprenorphine open label trial. Drug Alcohol Depend 138:83–88, 2014 24602363

Mariani JJ, Mahony AL, Podell SC, et al: Open-label trial of a single-day induction onto buprenorphine extended-release injection for users of heroin and fentanyl. Am J Addict 30(5):470–476, 2021 34223681

Mariolis T, Bosse J, Martin S, et al: A systematic review of the effectiveness of buprenorphine for opioid use disorder compared to other treatments: implications for research and practice. J Addict Res Ther 10(2):379, 2019

Martin CE, Shadowen C, Thakkar B, et al: Buprenorphine dosing for the treatment of opioid use disorder through pregnancy and postpartum. Curr Treat Options Psychiatry 7(3):375–399, 2020 33585165

Martin WR, Jasinski DR, Haertzen CA, et al: Methadone: a reevaluation. Arch Gen Psychiatry 28(2):286–295, 1973 4684295

McCarthy JJ, Graas J, Leamon MH, et al: The use of the methadone/metabolite ratio (MMR) to identify an individual metabolic phenotype and assess risks of poor response and adverse effects: towards scientific methadone dosing. J Addict Med 14(5):431–436, 2020

McCaul ME, Bigelow GE, Stitzer ML, et al: Short-term effects of oral methadone in methadone maintenance subjects. Clin Pharmacol Ther 31(6):753–761, 1982 7075123

McClain DA, Hug CC Jr: Intravenous fentanyl kinetics. Clin Pharmacol Ther 28(1):106–114, 1980 7389247

McFadden R, Wallace-Keeshen S, Petrillo Straub K, et al: Xylazine-associated wounds: clinical experience from a low-barrier wound care clinic in Philadelphia. J Addict Med 18(1):9–12, 2024 38019592

McLellan AT, Childress AR, Ehrman R, et al: Extinguishing conditioned responses during opiate dependence treatment: turning laboratory findings into clinical procedures. J Subst Abuse Treat 3(1):33–40, 1986 2874232

McLellan AT, Lewis DC, O'Brien CP, et al: Drug dependence, a chronic medical illness: implications for treatment, insurance, and outcomes evaluation. JAMA 284(13):1689–1695, 2000 11015800

McNicholas L, Howell EF: Buprenorphine Clinical Practice Guidelines, Field Review Draft, November 17, 2000. Rockville, MD, U.S. Department of Health and Human Services, Substance Abuse and Mental Health Services Administration, Center for Substance Abuse Treatment, Office of Pharmacologic and Alternative Therapies, 2000

Medical Devices Active License Listing: Rapid Response Xylazine Test Strip (Urine): License No 109225. Government of Canada, 2023. Available at: https://health-products.canada.ca/mdall-limh/information?licenceId=109225 &type=active&lang=eng. Accessed November 2, 2024.

Medications for the Treatment of Opioid Use Disorder, 42 CFR Part 8 (2022)
Mello NK, Mendelson JH: Buprenorphine suppresses heroin use by heroin addicts. Science 207(4431):657–659, 1980 7352279
Mendelson J, Jones RT, Welm S, et al: Buprenorphine and naloxone interactions in methadone maintenance patients. Biol Psychiatry 41(11):1095–1101, 1997 9146820
Meshberg-Cohen S, Ross MacLean R, Schnakenberg Martin AM, et al: Treatment outcomes in individuals diagnosed with comorbid opioid use disorder and posttraumatic stress disorder: a review. Addict Behav 122:107026, 2021 34182307
Miller JC, Brooks MA, Wurzel KE, et al: A guide to expanding the use of buprenorphine beyond standard initiations for opioid use disorder. Drugs R D 23(4):339–362, 2023 37938531
Miner NB, Schutzer WE, Zarnegarnia Y, et al: Fentanyl causes naloxone-resistant vocal cord closure: a platform for testing opioid overdose treatments. Drug Alcohol Depend 227:108974, 2021 34492557
Mitchell JE, Morley JE, Levine AS, et al: High-dose naltrexone therapy and dietary counseling for obesity. Biol Psychiatry 22(1):35–42, 1987 3790639
Mitchell MC, Memisoglu A, Silverman BL: Hepatic safety of injectable extended-release naltrexone in patients with chronic hepatitis C and HIV infection. J Stud Alcohol Drugs 73(6):991–997, 2012 23036218
Moe J, Godwin J, Purssell R, et al: Naloxone dosing in the era of ultra-potent opioid overdoses: a systematic review. CJEM 22(2):178–186, 2020 31955714
Moe J, O'Sullivan F, Hohl CM, et al: Short communication: systematic review on effectiveness of micro-induction approaches to buprenorphine initiation. Addict Behav 114:106740, 2021 33352498
Moeller KE, Kissack JC, Atayee RS, et al: Clinical interpretation of urine drug tests: what clinicians need to know about urine drug screens. Mayo Clin Proc 92(5):774–796, 2017 28325505
Moss RB, Carlo DJ: Higher doses of naloxone are needed in the synthetic opioid era. Subst Abuse Treat Prev Policy 14:6, 2019
National Institute on Drug Abuse. Clinical Opiate Withdrawal Scale. Available at: https://nida.nih.gov/sites/default/files/ClinicalOpiateWithdrawalScale.pdf. Accessed March 29, 2025.
Naumann RB, Durrance CP, Ranapurwala SI, et al: Impact of a community-based naloxone distribution program on opioid overdose death rates. Drug Alcohol Depend 204(1):107536, 2019 31494440
Ndegwa S, Pant S, Pohar S, et al: Injectable extended-release naltrexone to treat opioid use disorder, in CADTH Issues in Emerging Health Technologies. Ottawa, ON, Canada, Canadian Agency for Drugs and Technologies in

Health, August 1, 2017. Available at: https://www.ncbi.nlm.nih.gov/books/NBK481477/pdf/Bookshelf_NBK481477.pdf. Accessed February 5, 2025.

Nestler EJ, Hyman SE, Malenka RC: Molecular Neuropharmacology: A Foundation for Clinical Neuroscience. New York, McGraw Hill, 2001

Nielsen S, Dietze P, Lee N, et al: Concurrent buprenorphine and benzodiazepines use and self-reported opioid toxicity in opioid substitution treatment. Addiction 102(4):616–622, 2007 17286641

Nordmann S, Frauger E, Pauly V, et al: Misuse of buprenorphine maintenance treatment since introduction of its generic forms: OPPIDUM survey. Pharmacoepidemiol Drug Saf 21(2):184–190, 2012 22109894

Novick DM, Pascarelli EF, Joseph H, et al: Methadone maintenance patients in general medical practice: a preliminary report. JAMA 259(22):3299–3302, 1988 3373662

Nunes EV, Comer SD, Lofwall MR, et al: Extended-release injection vs sublingual buprenorphine for opioid use disorder with fentanyl use: a post hoc analysis of a randomized clinical trial. JAMA Netw Open 7(6):e2417377, 2024 38916892

Oakley B, Wilson H, Hayes V, et al: Managing opioid withdrawal precipitated by buprenorphine with buprenorphine. Drug Alcohol Rev 40(4):567–571, 2021 33480051

Oaks Z, Stage A, Middleton B, et al: Clinical utility of the cold pressor test: evaluation of pain patients, treatment of opioid-induced hyperalgesia and fibromyalgia with low dose naltrexone. Discov Med 26(144):197–206, 2018 30695679

O'Brien CP, Woody GE, McLellan AT: Enhancing the effectiveness of methadone using psychotherapeutic interventions. NIDA Res Monogr 150:5–18, 1995 8742769

Orexo US: ZUBSOLV product information: ZUBSOLV sublingual tablets, buprenorphine, naloxone sublingual tablets. Morristown, NJ, Orexo US, Inc, 2016. Available at: https://www.accessdata.fda.gov/drugsatfda_docs/label/2016/204242s009lbl.pdf. Accessed February 5, 2025.

O'Rourke TK Jr, Wosnitzer MS: Opioid-induced androgen deficiency (OPIAD): diagnosis, management, and literature review. Curr Urol Rep 17(10):76, 2016 27586511

Park TW, Larochelle MR, Saitz R, et al: Associations between prescribed benzodiazepines, overdose death and buprenorphine discontinuation among people receiving buprenorphine. Addiction 115(5):924–932, 2020 31916306

Pelletier DE, Andrew TA: Common findings and predictive measures of opioid overdoses. Acad Forensic Pathol 7(1):91–98, 2017 31239961

Pergolizzi JV Jr, Raffa RB, Rosenblatt MH: Opioid withdrawal symptoms, a consequence of chronic opioid use and opioid use disorder: current understanding and approaches to management. J Clin Pharm Ther 45(5):892–903, 2020 31986228

Pergolizzi J Jr, Raffa R, LeQuang JAK, et al: Old drugs and new challenges: a narrative review of nitazenes. Cureus 15(6):e40736, 2023 37485167

Pfohl DN, Allen JI, Atkinson RL, et al: Naltrexone hydrochloride (Trexan): a review of serum transaminase elevations at high dosage. NIDA Res Monogr 67:66–72, 1986 3092099

Phillips RH, Salzman M, Haroz R, et al: Elective naloxone-induced opioid withdrawal for rapid initiation of medication-assisted treatment of opioid use disorder. Ann Emerg Med 74(3):430–432, 2019 30773411

Purdue Pharma: BUTRANS product information: BUTRANS transdermal system patch, buprenorphine transdermal system patch. Stamford, CT, Purdue Pharma LP, 2014. Available at: https://www.accessdata.fda.gov/drugsatfda_docs/label/2014/021306s015s019lbl.pdf. Accessed February 5, 2025.

Raheemullah A, Lembke A: Buprenorphine induction without opioid withdrawal: a case series of 15 opioid-dependent inpatients induced on buprenorphine using microdoses of transdermal buprenorphine. Am J Ther 28(4):e504–e508, 2019 31833872

Ram CVS, Engelman K: Abrupt discontinuation of clonidine therapy. JAMA 242(19):2104–2105, 1979 490793

Ramey OL, Bonny AE, Silva Almodóvar A, et al: Gaps in evidence-based treatment of concurrent attention deficit hyperactivity disorder and opioid use disorder: a scoping review. Ann Pharmacother 57(8):978–990, 2023 36510631

Randall-Kosich O, Andraka-Christou B, Totaram R, et al: Comparing reasons for starting and stopping methadone, buprenorphine, and naltrexone treatment among a sample of white individuals with opioid use disorder. J Addict Med 14(4):e44–e52, 2020 31651562

Resnick RB, Schuyten-Resnick E, Washton AM: Assessment of narcotic antagonists in the treatment of opioid dependence. Annu Rev Pharmacol Toxicol 20:463–474, 1980 6992703

Ripamonti C, Groff L, Brunelli C, et al: Switching from morphine to oral methadone in treating cancer pain: what is the equianalgesic dose ratio? J Clin Oncol 16(10):3216–3221, 1998 9779694

Rodriguez CE, Klie KA: Pharmacological treatment of opioid use disorder in pregnancy. Semin Perinatol 43(3):141–148, 2019 30755340

Rosic T, Naji L, Bawor M, et al: The impact of comorbid psychiatric disorders on methadone maintenance treatment in opioid use disorder: a prospective cohort study. Neuropsychiatr Dis Treat 13:1399–1408, 2017 28579787

Rothenberg JL, Sullivan MA, Church SH, et al: Behavioral naltrexone therapy: an integrated treatment for opiate dependence. J Subst Abuse Treat 23(4):351–360, 2002 12495797

Rounsaville BJ, Kosten TR, Kleber HD: The antecedents and benefits of achieving abstinence in opioid addicts: a 2.5-year follow-up study. Am J Drug Alcohol Abuse 13(3):213–229, 1987 3687888

Rozylo J, Mitchell K, Nikoo M, et al: Case report: successful induction of buprenorphine/naloxone using a microdosing schedule and assertive outreach. Addict Sci Clin Pract 15(1):2, 2020 31941547

Ryan Haight Online Pharmacy Consumer Protection Act of 2008. 21 USC 801 note. Public Law 110-425, October 15, 2008. Available at: https://www.congress.gov/110/plaws/publ425/PLAW-110publ425.pdf. Accessed February 5, 2025.

Saiz-Rodríguez M, Ochoa D, Herrador C, et al: Polymorphisms associated with fentanyl pharmacokinetics, pharmacodynamics and adverse effects. Basic Clin Pharmacol Toxicol 124(3):321–329, 2019 30281924

Santo T Jr, Campbell G, Gisev N, et al: Prevalence of mental disorders among people with opioid use disorder: a systematic review and meta-analysis. Drug Alcohol Depend 238:109551, 2022 35797876

Seecof R, Tennant FS Jr: Subjective perceptions to the intravenous "rush" of heroin and cocaine in opioid addicts. Am J Drug Alcohol Abuse 12(1–2):79–87, 1986 3788901

Sees KL, Delucchi KL, Masson C, et al: Methadone maintenance vs 180-day psychosocially enriched detoxification for treatment of opioid dependence: a randomized controlled trial. JAMA 283(10):1303–1310, 2000 10714729

Selley DE, Liu Q, Childers SR: Signal transduction correlates of mu opioid agonist intrinsic efficacy: receptor-stimulated [35S]GTP gamma S binding in mMOR-CHO cells and rat thalamus. J Pharmacol Exp Ther 285(2):496–505, 1998 9580589

Selley DE, Herbert JT, Morgan D, et al: Effect of strain and sex on mu opioid receptor-mediated G-protein activation in rat brain. Brain Res Bull 60(3):201–208, 2003 12754081

Sells SB: Treatment effectiveness, in Handbook on Drug Abuse. Edited by Dupont RE, Goldstein A, O'Donnell J. Washington, DC, U.S. Government Printing Office, 1979, pp 105–118

Senay EC: Methadone maintenance treatment. Int J Addict 20(6–7):803–821, 1985 3908338

Senay EC, Dorus W, Goldberg F, et al: Withdrawal from methadone maintenance: rate of withdrawal and expectation. Arch Gen Psychiatry 34(3):361–367, 1977 843188

Shinderman M, Maxwell S, Brawand-Amey M, et al: Cytochrome P4503A4 metabolic activity, methadone blood concentrations, and methadone doses. Drug Alcohol Depend 69(2):205–211, 2003 12609702

Silverstein SM, Daniulaityte R, Martins SS, et al: "Everything is not right anymore": buprenorphine experiences in an era of illicit fentanyl. Int J Drug Policy 74:76–83, 2019 31563098

Sofuoglu M, DeVito EE, Carroll KM: Pharmacological and behavioral treatment of opioid use disorder. Psychiatr Res Clin Pract 1(1):4–15, 2019

Spahn V, Del Vecchio G, Rodriguez-Gaztelumendi A, et al: Opioid receptor signaling, analgesic and side effects induced by a computationally designed pH-dependent agonist. Sci Rep 8(1):8965, 2018 29895890

Stein M, Herman D, Conti M, et al: Initiating buprenorphine treatment for opioid use disorder during short-term in-patient "detoxification": a randomized clinical trial. Addiction 115(1):82–94, 2020 31430414

Stimmel B, Goldberg J, Rotkopf E, et al: Ability to remain abstinent after methadone detoxification: a six-year study. JAMA 237(12):1216–1220, 1977 576458

Strang J, Bearn J, Gossop M: Lofexidine for opiate detoxification: review of recent randomised and open controlled trials. Am J Addict 8(4):337–348, 1999 10598217

Substance Abuse and Mental Health Services Administration: Federal Guidelines for Opioid Treatment Programs (HHS Publ No SMA-PEP15-FEDGUIDEOTP). Rockville, MD, Substance Abuse and Mental Health Services Administration, January 2015. Available at: https://library.samhsa.gov/sites/default/files/guidelines-opioid-treatment-pep15-fedguideotp.pdf. Accessed February 5, 2025.

Substance Abuse and Mental Health Services Administration: FAQs: Provision of Methadone and Buprenorphine for the Treatment of Opioid Use Disorder in the COVID-19 Emergency. Rockville, MD, Substance Abuse and Mental Health Services Administration, April 2020. Available at: https://www.samhsa.gov/sites/default/files/faqs-for-oud-prescribing-and-dispensing.pdf. Accessed February 5, 2025.

Substance Abuse and Mental Health Services Administration: Medications for Opioid Use Disorder. Treatment Improvement Protocol (TIP) Series 63 (Publ No PEP21-02-01-002). Rockville, MD, Substance Abuse and Mental Health Services Administration, 2021. Available at: https://library.samhsa.gov/product/tip-63-medications-opioid-use-disorder/pep21-02-01-002. Accessed February 5, 2025.

Substance Abuse and Mental Health Services Administration: Fentanyl and Xylazine Test Strips. Rockville, MD, Substance Abuse and Mental Health

Services Administration, January 1, 2024. Available at: https://www.samhsa.gov/medications-substance-use-disorders/medications-counseling-related-conditions/fentanyl-xylazine-test-strips. Accessed November 2, 2024.

Substance Abuse and Mental Health Services Administration: Buprenorphine Telemedicine Prescribing: Questions and Answers. Rockville, MD, Substance Abuse and Mental Health Services Administration, 2025. Available at: https://www.samhsa.gov/substance-use/treatment/statutes-regulations-guidelines/buprenorphine-telemedicine-prescribing. Accessed May 18, 2025.

Sullivan LE, Metzger DS, Fudala PJ, et al: Decreasing international HIV transmission: the role of expanding access to opioid agonist therapies for injection drug users. Addiction 100(2):150–158, 2005 15679744

Sullivan MA: Antagonist maintenance for opioid dependence: the naltrexone story. Presented at the 22nd Annual Meeting of the American Academy of Addiction Psychiatry, Scottsdale, AZ, December 10, 2011

Sullivan M, Bisaga A, Pavlicova M, et al: Long-acting injectable naltrexone induction: a randomized trial of outpatient opioid detoxification with naltrexone vs. buprenorphine. Am J Psychiatry 174(5):459–467, 2017 28068780

Sullivan MA, Bisaga A, Pavlicova M, et al: A randomized trial comparing extended-release injectable suspension and oral naltrexone, both combined with behavioral therapy, for the treatment of opioid use disorder. Am J Psychiatry 176(2):129–137, 2019 30336703

Talton CW: Serotonin syndrome/serotonin toxicity. Fed Pract 37(10):452–459, 2020 33132683

Tennant FS Jr: Inadequate plasma concentrations in some high-dose methadone maintenance patients. Am J Psychiatry 144(10):1349–1350, 1987 3661772

Terasaki D, Smith C, Calcaterra SL: Transitioning hospitalized patients with opioid use disorder from methadone to buprenorphine without a period of opioid abstinence using a microdosing protocol. Pharmacotherapy 39(10):1023–1029, 2019 31348544

Teva Pharmaceuticals USA: CASSIPA product information: CASSIPA sublingual film, buprenorphine naloxone sublingual film. North Wales, PA, Teva Pharmaceuticals USA Inc, 2018. Available at: https://www.accessdata.fda.gov/drugsatfda_docs/label/2018/208042s000lbl.pdf. Accessed February 5, 2025.

Torralva R, Janowsky A: Noradrenergic mechanisms in fentanyl-mediated rapid death explain failure of naloxone in the opioid crisis. J Pharmacol Exp Ther 371(2):453–475, 2019 31492824

Trescot AM, Datta S, Lee M, et al: Opioid pharmacology. Pain Physician 11(2 Suppl):S133–S153, 2008 18443637

Trivedi MH, Walker R, Ling W, et al: Bupropion and naltrexone in methamphetamine use disorder. N Engl J Med 384(2):140–153, 2021 33497547

Ujváry I, Christie R, Evans-Brown M, et al: Dark classics in chemical neuroscience: etonitazene and related benzimidazoles. ACS Chem Neurosci 12(7):1072–1092, 2021 33760580

U.S. Department of Health and Human Services: HHS Guide for Clinicians on the Appropriate Dosage Reduction or Discontinuation of Long-Term Opioid Analgesics. Washington, DC, U.S. Department of Health and Human Services, 2019. Available at: https://www.hhs.gov/system/files/Dosage _Reduction_Discontinuation.pdf. Accessed February 5, 2025.

Vagenas P, Di Paola A, Herme M, et al: An evaluation of hepatic enzyme elevations among HIV-infected released prisoners enrolled in two randomized placebo-controlled trials of extended release naltrexone. J Subst Abuse Treat 47(1):35–40, 2014 24674234

Vandeputte MM, Van Uytfanghe K, Layle NK, et al: Synthesis, chemical characterization, and μ-opioid receptor activity assessment of the emerging group of "nitazene" 2-benzylbenzimidazole synthetic opioids. ACS Chem Neurosci 12(7):1241–1251, 2021 33759494

Varshneya NB, Thakrar AP, Hobelmann JG, et al: Evidence of buprenorphine-precipitated withdrawal in persons who use fentanyl. J Addict Med 16(4):e265–e268, 2022 34816821

Vivitrol [package insert]. Waltham, MA, Alkermes, 2022

Volkow N, Benveniste H, McLellan AT: Use and misuse of opioids in chronic pain. Annu Rev Med 69(1):451–465, 2018 29029586

Wakeman SE, Larochelle MR, Ameli O, et al: Comparative effectiveness of different treatment pathways for opioid use disorder. JAMA Netw Open 3(2):e1920622, 2020 32022884

Walsh SL, Preston KL, Stitzer ML, et al: Clinical pharmacology of buprenorphine: ceiling effects at high doses. Clin Pharmacol Ther 55(5):569–580, 1994 8181201

Washton AM, Pottash AC, Gold MS: Naltrexone in addicted business executives and physicians. J Clin Psychiatry 45(9 Pt 2):39–41, 1984 6088468

Weinberger AH, Platt J, Esan H, et al: Cigarette smoking is associated with increased risk of substance use disorder relapse: a nationally representative, prospective longitudinal investigation. J Clin Psychiatry 78(2):e152–e160, 2017 28234432

Weiss RD, Rao V: The Prescription Opioid Addiction Treatment Study: what have we learned. Drug Alcohol Depend 173(Suppl 1):S48–S54, 2017 28363320

Weiss RD, Potter JS, Fiellin DA, et al: Adjunctive counseling during brief and extended buprenorphine-naloxone treatment for prescription opioid dependence: a 2-phase randomized controlled trial. Arch Gen Psychiatry 68(12):1238–1246, 2011 22065255

Weller AE, Crist RC, Reiner BC, et al: Neonatal opioid withdrawal syndrome (NOWS): a transgenerational echo of the opioid crisis. Cold Spring Harb Perspect Med 11(3):a039669, 2021 32229609

Wesson DR: Revival of medical maintenance in the treatment of heroin dependence. JAMA 259(22):3314–3315, 1988 3373666

Wesson DR, Ling W: The Clinical Opiate Withdrawal Scale (COWS). J Psychoactive Drugs 35(2):253–259, 2003 12924748

Whitley SD, Sohler NL, Kunins HV, et al: Factors associated with complicated buprenorphine inductions. J Subst Abuse Treat 39(1):51–57, 2010 20682186

Wikler A: Opioid Dependence: Mechanisms and Treatment. New York, Plenum, 1980

Williams JT, Christie MJ, Manzoni O: Cellular and synaptic adaptations mediating opioid dependence. Physiol Rev 81(1):299–343, 2001 11152760

Wishik G, Gaeta JM, Racine MW, et al: Substance consumption and intoxication patterns in a medically supervised overdose prevention program for people experiencing homelessness. Subst Abus 42(4):851–857, 2021 33617749

Woody GE, McLellan AT, Luborsky L, et al: Twelve-month follow-up of psychotherapy for opiate dependence. Am J Psychiatry 144(5):590–596, 1987 3578568

Woody GE, McLellan AT, Luborsky L, et al: Psychotherapy in community methadone programs: a validation study. Am J Psychiatry 152(9):1302–1308, 1995 7653685

Zangiabadian M, Golmohammadi S, Nejadghaderi SA, et al: The effects of naltrexone on retention in treatment and being opioid-free in opioid-dependent people: a systematic review and meta-analysis. Front Psychiatry 13:1003257, 2022 36226100

Zhang J, Ferguson SS, Barak LS, et al: Role for G protein-coupled receptor kinase in agonist-specific regulation of mu-opioid receptor responsiveness. Proc Natl Acad Sci U S A 95(12):7157–7162, 1998 9618555

6

Stimulants

Kyle Kampman, M.D.

Cocaine and amphetamines are highly reinforcing drugs that act by increasing monoamine neurotransmission in the CNS. The intoxicating effects of both are similar, although methamphetamines' duration of action is longer. Both cocaine and amphetamines are associated with a withdrawal syndrome; these withdrawal syndromes are not medically significant but may be associated with differences in treatment outcome. Medical consequences of use include cardiovascular, pulmonary, and CNS adverse effects.

There are no medications approved by the FDA for the treatment of either cocaine use disorder or methamphetamine/amphetamine use disorder. Promising pharmacotherapies for cocaine use disorder include topiramate, either alone or in combination with dopamine agonists such as mixed amphetamine salts or phentermine. The use of contingency management, either alone or in combination with pharmacotherapy, has been shown to be beneficial. For methamphetamine use disorder, the combination of bupropion and extended-release injectable naltrexone (XRNT) is promising. In the population of men who have sex with men (MSM), mirtazapine may be beneficial for methamphetamine use disorder.

Neuropharmacology of Cocaine and Amphetamine Use

Both cocaine and amphetamines increase arousal, alertness, and motor activity and are highly reinforcing in humans. The two drugs act by different mechanisms to increase transmission of the monoamine neurotransmitters dopamine, norepinephrine, and serotonin. Although cocaine and amphetamines affect all three neurotransmitters, their activity on dopamine neurotransmission has been most closely associated with their reinforcing effects. Thus, the dopaminergic system has been the main focus of pharmacological strategies to treat cocaine use disorder and methamphetamine/amphetamine use disorder. In addition, chronic cocaine use has been shown to modify other neurotransmitter systems such as those involving GABA and glutamate. These neurotransmitter systems also have been targeted to treat cocaine use disorder and methamphetamine/amphetamine use disorder.

Cocaine increases monoamine transmission by blocking the reuptake of norepinephrine, serotonin, and dopamine into presynaptic neurons (White and Kalivas 1998). By increasing synaptic levels of dopamine in certain brain regions, such as the nucleus accumbens, cocaine induces a strong sense of pleasure. Activation of the nucleus accumbens by natural reinforcers, such as food and sex, ensures that these survival-associated behaviors are maintained. Cocaine artificially elevates dopamine in the nucleus accumbens to levels much higher than those generated by natural stimuli, inducing a tremendous euphoria that far exceeds pleasure resulting from natural reinforcers (Nestler 2005). Laboratory animals given unlimited access to cocaine have been known to use it until they starve (Wise and Bozarth 1985).

Although blockade of norepinephrine reuptake and serotonin reuptake may not be crucial to the euphorigenic and reinforcing properties of cocaine or amphetamines, these neurotransmitter systems may be important in maintaining cocaine and amphetamine use disorders, making them potential targets for pharmacotherapy. For example, norepinephrine may be critically important in stress-induced relapse to cocaine. α_2-Noradrenergic agonists have been shown to decrease stress-induced relapse to cocaine-seeking in rats (Erb et al. 2000). Norepinephrine also appears to be critical for the development of stimulant sensitization, a process in which repeated exposure to stimulants leads to increased psychomotor response and increased dopamine release. Stimulant sensitization is thought to be important for the development of stimulant use disorder. Mice lacking α_1-noradrenergic receptors do not develop this sensitization (Drouin et al. 2002). Likewise, lesioning noradrenergic neurons in the locus coeruleus or depleting central norepinephrine will also block the development of amphetamine sensitization (Archer et al. 1986; Kostowski et al. 1982; for review, see Sofuoglu and Sewell 2009). Serotonin reuptake appears to play an important role in shaping cocaine's euphorigenic and reinforcing properties, although the data are complicated, and no consensus exists for a clear direction for pharmacological intervention (Nonkes et al. 2011).

Non-monoaminergic neurotransmitter effects of cocaine use have been identified and may indicate pharmacological targets in medication development. Chronic cocaine use leads to profound changes in glutamatergic neurotransmission in the limbic system, particularly the nucleus accumbens. These changes appear to be critical in mediating behaviors characteristic of substance use disorder, including drug craving and relapse. Acutely, cocaine administration has little or no effect on extracellular glutamate levels in the nucleus accumbens, but withdrawal from chronic cocaine use reduces basal extracellular glutamate levels (Schmidt and Pierce 2010). Normalization of basal extracellular glutamate levels has been shown to prevent reinstatement of drug-seeking behavior induced by a priming dose of cocaine (Schmidt and Pierce 2010). In rats pretreated with repeated cocaine administrations, cocaine administration increased glutamate release in the nucleus accumbens core. Blockade of the α-amino-3-hydroxy-5-methyl-4-isoxazolepropionic acid (AMPA)-type glutamate receptors blocked the reinstatement of cocaine-primed drug-seeking behavior (Park et al. 2002). Thus, chronic cocaine use appears to alter glutamate activity in the nucleus accumbens, a change that appears to be associated with the relapse process.

Amphetamines and methamphetamines also increase monoaminergic neurotransmission, but their mechanism of action is somewhat different from that of cocaine. Cocaine acts primarily by reuptake blockade, whereas amphetamines both block the reuptake of monoamines and stimulate the release of catecholamines from nerve terminals. Amphetamines and methamphetamines increase cytosolic dopamine and reverse the normal activity of the dopamine transporter, which causes the transporter to release dopamine into the synapse (Brown et al. 2001; Khoshbouei et al. 2003). Amphetamines also appear to stimulate the release of norepinephrine (Azzaro et al. 1974). Amphetamines have much greater activity at the norepinephrine transporter compared with cocaine, and this may have implications for pharmacological treatments. In humans, the subjective effects of amphetamines are closely related to the ability to stimulate the release of norepinephrine (Rothman et al. 2001). Medications that affect noradrenergic neurotransmission may hold more promise for treating methamphetamine/amphetamine use disorder.

Cocaine and amphetamines/methamphetamines also differ in their duration of action. The half-life of amphetamines and methamphetamines (~10 hours) is considerably longer than that of cocaine (1.5 hours). This may lead to different patterns of use for amphetamines and cocaine that could have implications for their associated toxicities and the development of effective medications. Although amphetamines and methamphetamines have the same mechanism of action, methamphetamines are more potent than amphetamines, and methamphetamines are available in a smokeable form (Panenka et al. 2013).

Acute Presentation of Intoxication

Cocaine and amphetamines are CNS stimulants. They produce dose-dependent increases in heart rate and blood pressure along with increased arousal, alertness, and sense of well-being. Both drugs are highly reinforcing and can cause a strong urge to redose. Involuntary motor activity, stereotyped behavior, and psychosis can occur after repeated doses.

Patients with cocaine intoxication often present with agitation, tachycardia, and hypertension. Physical findings may include mydriasis, diaphoresis, hyperthermia, and tachypnea. CNS effects may include paranoia, mania, and delirium. The time course of cocaine intoxication varies with the route of administration and form of cocaine used. Freebase, or crack cocaine, which is smoked, results in rapid onset of effects (within a minute), as does cocaine hydrochloride when injected. Intranasal cocaine use results in a more delayed onset of effects (several minutes). The duration of effects is shortest with smoked cocaine (5–15 minutes) and longest with intranasal cocaine (60–90 minutes) (Zimmerman 2012).

One of the most common drugs used together with cocaine is alcohol. Alcohol use disorder has been shown to occur in about 80% of patients with cocaine use disorder (Stinson et al. 2005). Patients with cocaine use disorder will say that the alcohol reduces the anxiety associated with coming down from cocaine. An important metabolic interaction probably accounts for much of this effect. In the presence of alcohol, some of the cocaine is metabolized to cocaethylene. Cocaethylene is psychoactive, with effects similar to those of cocaine (Pergolizzi et al. 2022). Thus, the presence of cocaethylene prolongs the high and makes coming down more gradual and pleasant.

The acute effects of amphetamines and methamphetamines are similar to those of cocaine. Signs and symptoms include agitation, tachycardia, hypertension, hyperthermia, and psychosis. The time course of methamphetamine intoxication is much longer than that of cocaine. The half-life of methamphetamine is estimated to be 9–25 hours (Schep et al. 2010). Prescription stimulants (amphetamines) can be taken orally, intranasally, or by injection. Methamphetamines are most often smoked (68%) or snorted (31%), and less commonly injected (7%) or orally ingested (3%) (Wood et al. 2008). Like cocaine, smoked and injected methamphetamines have a very rapid onset of effect (within a few minutes), but the duration of action of amphetamines and methamphetamines is much longer than that of cocaine, 10 hours or more (Substance Abuse and Mental Health Services Administration 2021). The opioid fentanyl has been found as a frequent contaminant in amphetamines and methamphetamines purchased on the street. The presence of fentanyl increases the likelihood of overdose and can alter the stimulatory effects of amphetamines and methamphetamines (Kariisa et al. 2019).

Withdrawal Presentation

Cocaine withdrawal symptoms include dysphoric mood, fatigue, sleep disturbance, appetite changes, and irritability (Kampman et al. 1998). Patients entering treatment with severe cocaine withdrawal symptoms often drop out of treatment prematurely and are not likely to attain abstinence from cocaine in outpatient treatment programs (Kampman et al. 1998, 2001, 2002; Mulvaney et al. 1999). Several investigators have noted that patients with cocaine use disorder who experience cocaine withdrawal symptoms report a greater high from experimentally administered cocaine (Newton et al. 2003; Sofuoglu et al. 2003; Uslaner et al. 1999). The increased euphoria that patients with cocaine withdrawal syndrome experience may make the drug more rewarding and therefore more difficult to give up. Because patients with cocaine use disorder who have withdrawal symptoms (cocaine withdrawal syndrome) experience cocaine differently, poor treatment outcomes may result.

Methamphetamine/amphetamine use disorder, like cocaine use disorder, have been linked to a withdrawal syndrome. Amphetamine withdrawal symptoms are similar to cocaine withdrawal symptoms and include increased appetite, increased sleep, and dysphoria. McGregor and colleagues (2005) characterized the nature and time course of amphetamine withdrawal. They reported a two-phase syndrome, with an acute phase lasting 7–10 days, during which patients experienced increased appetite, increased sleep, depression, fatigue, anhedonia, and dysphoria. These symptoms peaked during the first 24 hours after the last use of amphetamines and declined linearly over time. The second, or subacute, phase lasted 2–3 weeks and consisted of similar but more attenuated symptoms. Older patients, patients with more severe dependence, and patients with a longer history of amphetamine use had more severe withdrawal symptoms.

Pharmacological Management of Intoxication and Withdrawal

Mild stimulant intoxication can usually be managed nonpharmacologically by providing a calm, low-stimulation environment, along with supportive care. However, acute agitation is the most common presentation of both cocaine and amphetamine intoxication and may require pharmacological interventions. Physiological and psychological dimensions of agitation in stimulant intoxication can help organize the psychopharmacological approach to mitigating this agitation, including 1) neuromuscular excitation, anxiety, and seizures (managed with GABAergic medications); 2) sympathetic overactivity (managed with sympatholytic medications); and 3) psychosis (managed with neuroleptics). Table 6.1 provides an overview of possible psychopharmacological treatments organized through this framework.

Overall, agitation can be best managed by using sedatives such as benzodiazepines. If indicated, these can be given orally in cases of mild to moderate agitation and intravenously or intramuscularly (e.g., lorazepam 2 mg repeated until agitation is under control, or midazolam 5 mg IM if rapid behavioral control is essential) in cases of severe agitation (Zimmerman 2012). Because benzodiazepines may cause respiratory and

Table 6.1 Examples of psychopharmacological interventions for stimulant intoxication (adults)

Indication and class	Mechanism of action	Dosing	Indications	Other
Neuromuscular excitation, anxiety, seizures				
Benzodiazepines	GABAergic	Lorazepam 1–2 mg PO/IV/IM at frequency guided by clinical judgment of efficacy/need Diazepam 5–10 mg PO/IV at frequency guided by clinical judgment of efficacy/need Midazolam 5 mg IM or 0.01–0.05 mg/kg IV	Excitatory symptoms	IV vs. PO administration based on consideration of access availability or cooperation, availability of medication, and acuity of context (i.e., speed of onset needed)

Table 6.1 Examples of psychopharmacological interventions for stimulant intoxication (adults) *(continued)*

Indication and class	Mechanism of action	Dosing	Indications	Other
Phenobarbital	GABAergic	Incremental 130–260 mg IV/PO Loading (e.g., 5–10 mg/kg)	Excitatory symptoms and benzodiazepines not available or contraindicated, or patient's symptoms not responding to escalating benzodiazepine dosing	PO dosing similar to parenteral dosing Watch for respiratory depression, especially if concurrently administered with (or in proximity to) benzodiazepines
Sympathetic overactivity				
Clonidine	Sympatholytic: α_2-agonism	0.1–0.2 mg every 4 h prn	Anxiety, sympathetic overactivity	Maintain hydration Watch for hypotension
Dexmedetomidine	Sympatholytic: α_2-agonism	0.2–0.4 µg/kg/h and titrate up every 30 min to a maximum of 1.5 µg/kg/h	Critically ill patients in the ICU	Sedation without impairments in ventilation

Stimulants 283

Table 6.1 Examples of psychopharmacological interventions for stimulant intoxication (adults) *(continued)*

Indication and class	Mechanism of action	Dosing	Indications	Other
Nitroprusside	Vasodilation action as a prodrug converted into nitric oxide in blood vessels	IV infusion: 0.5–4 µg/kg/min	Hypertensive crisis	Avoid longer-acting antihypertensives
Psychosis				
Typical neuroleptics	Dopamine antagonism	Haloperidol or droperidol 5 mg IM Haloperidol 0.2–0.67 mg/kg IV	Acute agitation with psychosis, agitation not responding to benzodiazepines	QT prolongation Hyperthermia/neuroleptic malignant syndrome
Atypical neuroleptics	Dopamine antagonism	Olanzapine 2.5–10 mg PO every 2 h Quetiapine 50–100 mg at night Ziprasidone 20 mg	Acute agitation with psychosis, agitation not responding to benzodiazepines, stimulant-induced sleep disruptions	QT prolongation Hyperthermia/neuroleptic malignant syndrome

Table 6.1 Examples of psychopharmacological interventions for stimulant intoxication (adults) *(continued)*

Indication and class	Mechanism of action	Dosing	Indications	Other
Other				
Ketamine	NMDA receptor antagonism	1–5 mg/kg IM depending on severity of agitation	Severe agitation	Rapid onset

Source. Adapted from American Society of Addiction Medicine and American Academy of Addiction Psychiatry (2023).
Note. h = hour; IM = intramuscular; IV = intravenous; min = minute; NMDA = *N*-methyl-D-aspartate; PO = per os.

cardiac depressant effects, the use of antipsychotics, including haloperidol (e.g., 0.2–0.67 mg/kg IV), droperidol (e.g., 5 mg), ziprasidone (e.g., 20 mg), and olanzapine (e.g., 2.5–10 mg every 2 hours prn for behavioral control), has been studied either alone or in combination with benzodiazepines. In several trials, antipsychotic medications have been shown to be safe and effective either alone or in combination with benzodiazepines (Martell et al. 2005; Ruha and Yarema 2006). There are potential risks involved in the use of antipsychotics, however, including lowering of the seizure threshold, worsening of hyperthermia, and prolonging of the QT interval (Martel et al. 2005; Zimmerman 2012). A systematic review suggested that these concerns may not be as significant as previously thought (Connors et al. 2019). Methamphetamine supplies have been contaminated with fentanyl (Amlani et al. 2015). Naloxone may be indicated in cases where concomitant opioid overdose is suspected.

Cocaine and amphetamine withdrawal are generally not medically significant, and there are no FDA-approved pharmacological treatments for either cocaine or methamphetamine withdrawal. The presence of cocaine withdrawal has been shown to be predictive of poor outcome in the outpatient treatment of cocaine use disorder (Kampman et al. 2001, 2002; Mulvaney et al. 1999). In a trial of topiramate for comorbid cocaine and alcohol use disorders, however, patients with more severe cocaine withdrawal symptoms, as measured by high Cocaine Selective Severity Assessment (CSSA) scores, experienced a better symptom response to topiramate ($\leq$300 mg/day). Patients with CSSA scores in the highest tertile (corresponding to patients with CSSA scores >18) on the day of randomization exhibited larger topiramate effects than patients with lower scores. Among subjects with CSSA scores greater than 18 (n = 59), topiramate-treated subjects, on average, submitted significantly more cocaine-negative urine samples during the trial compared with placebo-treated subjects (Kampman et al. 2013). These data suggest that patients with more severe cocaine withdrawal symptoms may benefit from treatment with topiramate at this dose.

Substance Use Disorder Presentation

Repeated use of cocaine and amphetamines can lead to the development of substance use disorder. Characteristics of this disorder include behavioral sensitization, which is a long-lasting increase in behavioral response occurring on repeated presentation of a stimulus (also see the Preface for an overview of the DSM-5-TR [American Psychiatric Association 2022] substance use disorder diagnosis). Behavioral sensitization reliably results in a behavioral response favoring self-administration at subsequent substance presentation (Koob 1996). In this model of drug dependence, intermittent administration of cocaine leads to an increase in the subjective effects of cocaine and cocaine craving, resulting in a loss of control over use and, finally, a substance use disorder. Some preclinical studies and human laboratory studies have shown the development of sensitization to stimulants under controlled conditions (Ahmed and Cador 2006; Schenk and Partridge 1997). However, patients with cocaine use disorder rarely report an increase in the subjective effects of cocaine over time. This observation has led researchers to suggest that the hedonic dysregulation model better explains cocaine addiction. In this model, adaptive processes within the body lead to decreased subjective effects of the drug (tolerance) and a negative affective state when drug use is stopped (withdrawal). Tolerance and withdrawal arise from neurochemical changes in brain reward and stress pathways, inducing a negative motivation state that drives addiction (Koob 1996, 2006).

Other investigators have tried to find a middle ground, proposing that drug craving (the desire to use a drug) and drug liking (the euphoric effects of the drug) are differentially regulated in a model called *incentive sensitization*. They suggest that brain systems that mediate incentive salience (craving) become sensitized to drugs and associated stimuli, while the reward system that regulates euphoric effects becomes tolerant to drugs. The uncoupling of these feelings results in intense craving and drug-seeking behavior without enjoyment of the drugs being sought (Robinson and Berridge 1993, 2001; Small et al. 2009).

Long-Term Management

Although no medications are currently approved to treat cocaine use disorder or methamphetamine/amphetamine use disorder, several medications have shown potential efficacy in controlled clinical trials for cocaine use disorder, and a few have shown efficacy for the treatment of methamphetamine/amphetamine use disorder. Others appear promising based on preliminary trials. Several meta-analyses have not demonstrated clear superiority of any medication for the treatment of cocaine use disorder or methamphetamine/

amphetamine use disorder (Chan et al. 2019; Pani et al. 2011; Ronsley et al. 2020). Medications to treat cocaine use disorder and methamphetamine/amphetamine use disorder are discussed separately. First, I describe medications that have potential efficacy reported in controlled clinical trials, which are grouped according to the neurotransmitter system they are thought to target, followed by promising medications. Finally, I discuss medications found to be efficacious only when used in conjunction with a novel psychosocial treatment called contingency management.

Medications to Treat Cocaine Use Disorder

Dopaminergic Medications

Agonist treatments have been used successfully to treat both opioid and nicotine use disorders. Ideally, in agonist treatment, the medication used should bind to the same receptor as the misused drug, exert similar effects, and demonstrate pharmacological properties that render it less susceptible to misuse than the drug for which it is being substituted. Cocaine has diverse effects in the brain and, unlike nicotine and opiates, does not have a single molecular target. Therefore, finding an effective agonist treatment for cocaine use disorder has been challenging. Table 6.2 presents a summary of medications used to treat cocaine use disorder.

Methylphenidate and Amphetamines

Agonist treatments for cocaine use disorder have thus far focused on the dopaminergic properties of cocaine. Methylphenidate, an amphetamine analog, was ineffective for the treatment of cocaine dependence in one trial (maximum of 45 mg/day) (Grabowski et al. 1997). Levin and colleagues (2007), however, found that among cocaine-dependent patients with comorbid ADHD, methylphenidate therapy was associated with decreased cocaine use (20–40 mg bid). Some success has been achieved with amphetamines and methamphetamines to treat cocaine use disorder. In 2001, Grabowski and colleagues published results of the first pilot trial evaluating dextroamphetamine to treat cocaine dependence (Grabowski et al. 2001). In the 12-week trial, 128 cocaine-dependent patients were randomly assigned to placebo, low-dose dextroamphetamine (30 mg/day), or high-dose dextroamphetamine (60 mg/day). Treatment retention was significantly better in the low-dose amphetamine group. Cocaine use was nonsignificantly lower

Table 6.2 Medications to treat cocaine use disorder (all non-FDA-approved indications)

Class and medication	Dosing	Evidence	Notes
Dopaminergic			
Methylphenidate	45 mg/d maximum	Ineffective (Grabowski et al. 1997)	High dropout rate
	20–40 mg bid	Decreased cocaine use (Levin et al. 2007)	In cocaine-dependent patients with co-occurring ADHD High dropout rate
Amphetamines	Dextroamphetamine 30 and 60 mg/d	Mixed (Grabowski et al. 2004)	Low-dose group had better retention; high-dose cocaine use was nonsignificantly lower High dropout rate
	Methamphetamine IR 30 mg/d and methamphetamine SR 30 mg/d	Mixed (Mooney et al. 2009)	SR formulation had significantly fewer cocaine-positive urine results High dropout rate
Modafinil	200, 400, or 800 mg/d	Positive in human laboratory trials; mixed in clinical trials (Anderson et al. 2009; Dackis et al. 2005; Kampman et al. 2015)	May block effects of cocaine Some evidence of efficacy in cocaine-dependent individuals without alcohol use

Table 6.2 Medications to treat cocaine use disorder (all non-FDA-approved indications) *(continued)*

Class and medication	Dosing	Evidence	Notes
Disulfiram	250 mg/d	Mixed (Oliveto et al. 2011; Perrakis et al. 2000; Pettinati et al. 2008)	Monitor for fulminant hepatic failure; dietary modifications
Bupropion	SR 150–300 mg bid XL 300 mg/d	Individual studies were small with mixed results, but meta-analyses suggested benefit (Castells et al. 2016; Chan et al. 2019)	Especially in individuals with co-occurring tobacco use disorder, opioid use disorder, or depressive disorder
GABAergic and glutamatergic			
Topiramate	200–300 mg/d	Mixed (Johnson et al. 2013; Kampman et al. 2004; Umbricht et al. 2014)	Perhaps more effective in combination with XR mixed amphetamine salts (60 mg/d) (Mariani et al. 2012)
N-acetylcysteine	600–3,600 mg/d	Limited small clinical studies (LaRowe et al. 2006, 2013)	May be effective in helping maintain abstinence

Note. IR = immediate release; SR = sustained release; XL = extended release.

in the high-dose amphetamine group. Dropout rates for all groups were high. In a subsequent trial by the same group involving 120 cocaine- and opioid-dependent patients whose symptoms were stabilized with methadone, significant reductions in cocaine use were seen in patients taking dextroamphetamine 60 mg/day compared with placebo or dextroamphetamine 30 mg/day (Grabowski et al. 2004). Again, treatment retention in this trial was poor, with fewer than 50% of the subjects completing the trial (Grabowski et al. 2004).

In an 8-week trial, immediate-release (IR) methamphetamine 30 mg/day and sustained-release (SR) methamphetamine 30 mg/day were compared with placebo (Mooney et al. 2009). The SR methamphetamine group submitted significantly fewer cocaine-positive urine drug screen samples during the trial (29% SR methamphetamine vs. 66% IR methamphetamine vs. 60% placebo). However, the dropout rate in this trial was high, with only 32% of the patients completing the trial (Mooney et al. 2009). Although the findings, in general, favor amphetamines and methamphetamines, high dropout rates in all the trials make the results difficult to interpret.

Modafinil

Modafinil, a medication approved to treat excessive sleepiness associated with narcolepsy, obstructive sleep apnea, and shift work sleep disorder, is under investigation to treat cocaine dependence. Proposed uses include reduction of cocaine withdrawal symptoms, reduction in cocaine craving, and reduction in cocaine-induced euphoria. As a mild stimulant, modafinil may be able to reduce cocaine withdrawal symptoms (Dackis and O'Brien 2003). Modafinil has been shown to increase dopaminergic neurotransmission by blocking the dopamine transporter, and this may account for its ability to reduce cocaine withdrawal symptoms (Volkow et al. 2009). Modafinil also enhances glutamate neurotransmission (Touret et al. 1994). This medication may therefore be efficacious for cocaine use disorder by ameliorating the glutamate depletion seen in chronic cocaine users (Dackis and O'Brien 2003). Improved baseline glutamatergic tone in the nucleus accumbens prevented reinstatement of cocaine self-administration in an animal model of relapse (Baker et al. 2003).

Modafinil was found to block the euphoric effects of cocaine in three independent human laboratory studies (Dackis et al. 2003; Hart et al. 2008; Malcolm et al. 2002). First, Dackis and colleagues (2003) conducted a double-blind, placebo-controlled cocaine-modafinil interaction trial. Cocaine-dependent patients were given modafinil 200 mg, modafinil 400 mg, or placebo and then challenged with cocaine 30 mg IV. Pretreatment with modafinil significantly blunted cocaine-induced euphoria in one of the subjective measures (Dackis et al. 2003). In a separate, but very similar, human laboratory trial, Malcolm and colleagues (2002) found that modafinil at both 400- and 800-mg doses significantly reduced the response to cocaine, as measured by visual analog scale ratings ("High," "Any drug effect," and "Worth in dollars") compared with cocaine alone. Hart and colleagues (2008) evaluated the effect of modafinil on the self-administration of cocaine in a human laboratory trial. In this trial, the effects of modafinil maintenance (0, 200, and 400 mg/day) on response to smoked cocaine (0, 12, 25, and 50 mg) were examined in non-treatment-seeking cocaine-dependent individuals ($n = 8$). Active doses of cocaine were more likely to be self-administered compared with placebo doses, evoked higher subjective-effect ratings compared with placebo, and elevated cardiovascular measures (i.e., systolic and diastolic blood pressure, heart rate) more than placebo; modafinil at both dosages (200 and 400 mg/day) markedly attenuated the effects of cocaine (Hart et al. 2008).

In several clinical trials of modafinil, the results have been mixed. In a double-blind, placebo-controlled pilot trial of modafinil involving 62 cocaine-dependent patients completed in 2004, patients treated with modafinil 400 mg/day submitted significantly more cocaine metabolite–free urine samples than placebo-treated patients (42% vs. 22%) (Dackis et al. 2005). Modafinil-treated patients were also rated as more improved than placebo-treated patients (Dackis et al. 2005). The results of the pilot trial were partly replicated in a larger multicenter trial involving 210 cocaine-dependent patients (Anderson et al. 2009). In this 16-week trial, cocaine-dependent patients were treated with modafinil 400 mg/day or placebo. In contrast with the pilot trial, in which none of the patients were both cocaine and alcohol dependent, 41% of patients in this trial were both alcohol and cocaine dependent. In the group as a whole, modafinil was not superior to placebo in promoting abstinence from cocaine. Among patients who were not also alcohol dependent, however, both dosages of modafinil were superior to placebo for promoting abstinence from cocaine (Anderson et al. 2009).

Further evidence supports modafinil's potential efficacy in cocaine-dependent patients without alcohol use disorder. In an 8-week trial with

94 cocaine-dependent individuals without comorbid alcohol use disorder, Kampman et al. (2015) found that those treated with modafinil 300 mg/day were significantly more likely to be abstinent from cocaine during the last 3 weeks of the trial than those treated with placebo (23% vs. 9%). Enthusiasm for modafinil is somewhat dampened, however, by the results of a clinical trial by Dackis and colleagues (2012). In this trial, 210 cocaine-dependent patients who were actively using cocaine at baseline were randomly assigned to 8 weeks of modafinil (0, 200, or 400 mg/day) combined with once-weekly cognitive-behavioral therapy (CBT). The investigators found no effect of modafinil at either dosage on cocaine use or cocaine craving.

Disulfiram

The last of the dopaminergic medications to be considered is disulfiram. Disulfiram is an approved treatment for alcohol use disorder and may also be a promising medication for the treatment of cocaine use disorder. Its mechanism of action in the treatment of alcohol dependence is based on its blockade of the enzyme aldehyde dehydrogenase and the subsequent buildup of the toxic metabolite acetaldehyde when alcohol is ingested, which produces a characteristic unpleasant reaction. The effectiveness of disulfiram is hampered by the need for significant vigilance regarding dietary and environmental exposure and low adherence (Enghusen Poulsen et al. 1992; Fuller et al. 1986). Disulfiram is also tied to rare fulminant hepatic failure, requiring close monitoring of liver function (Wright et al. 1988).

Disulfiram blocks the degradation of dopamine by inhibiting the enzyme dopamine β-hydroxylase, which leads to increased levels of dopamine in the brain (Goldstein et al. 1964). This action may affect cocaine use by decreasing the reinforcing properties of cocaine (Hameedi et al. 1995; McCance-Katz et al. 1998). A dopaminergic mechanism of action for disulfiram is supported by a pharmacogenetic trial showing that patients with cocaine use disorder who carried a mutation resulting in higher levels of dopamine transporters, and therefore lower levels of synaptic dopamine, responded better to disulfiram treatment (Kampangkaew et al. 2019).

In several clinical trials conducted from 1998 to 2004, disulfiram 250 mg/day reduced cocaine use in cocaine-dependent patients (Carroll et al. 1998, 2004; George et al. 2000; Petrakis et al. 2000). Petrakis and colleagues (2000) compared disulfiram with placebo in 67 cocaine- and opioid-dependent patients receiving methadone maintenance. They found that disulfiram-treated patients self-reported significantly less cocaine use in a 12-week trial (Petrakis et al. 2000). In a smaller trial with cocaine- and opioid-dependent patients receiving buprenorphine maintenance, disulfiram was significantly better than placebo in reducing cocaine use (George et al. 2000). Carroll and colleagues (2004) at Yale conducted two trials of disulfiram during that time, one in patients with addiction to both alcohol and cocaine and one in patients whose principal drug of dependence was cocaine. In the first trial, disulfiram treatment was associated with significantly better treatment retention as well as a longer duration of abstinence from cocaine and alcohol. In the second trial, disulfiram was associated with less cocaine use as measured by urine drug screens. Patients without a history of alcohol use responded better to disulfiram, confirming disulfiram's specific effect on cocaine use (Carroll et al. 2004).

Disulfiram at a dosage of 250 mg/day was not found to be superior to placebo in reducing cocaine use in a trial involving 161 cocaine- and opioid-dependent patients receiving methadone maintenance. Moreover, lower dosages of disulfiram (62.5 or 125 mg/day) were associated with significantly more cocaine use than placebo (Oliveto et al. 2011). Pettinati and colleagues (2008) found the combination of disulfiram and naltrexone to be better than placebo in promoting sustained abstinence from both cocaine and alcohol in patients with dual cocaine and alcohol dependence.

Bupropion

Bupropion is a dual dopamine and norepinephrine reuptake inhibitor commonly used as a treatment for major depressive disorder and smoking cessation, and it has also been studied as a treatment for cocaine use disorder. Most of the studies of the effects of bupropion on cocaine use have been small and have yielded mixed results. However, a 2016 meta-analysis suggested that bupropion (with dosing of SR bupropion 300 mg bid vs. extended-release [XL] bupropion 300 mg/day) was superior to placebo in achieving sustained abstinence from cocaine, especially in individuals with co-occurring opioid use disorder (Castells et al. 2016). A subsequent systematic review echoed this finding, indicating that despite limited data, bupropion may enhance abstinence in cocaine-dependent individuals (Chan et al. 2019). On account of the findings from these meta-analyses, the American Society of Addiction Medicine (ASAM) and the American Academy of Addiction

Psychiatry (AAAP) included bupropion as a conditional recommendation in their Clinical Practice Guideline on the Management of Stimulant Use Disorder (discussed later in this chapter), especially in individuals who have co-occurring tobacco use disorder or depressive disorders (American Society of Addiction Medicine and American Academy of Addiction Psychiatry 2023).

GABAergic and Glutamatergic Medications (Topiramate)

Mesocortical dopamine neurons receive modulatory inputs from both GABAergic and glutamatergic neurons. GABA is primarily an inhibitory neurotransmitter in the CNS, and activation of GABAergic neurons tends to decrease activation in the dopaminergic reward system. Preclinical trials of medications that foster GABAergic neurotransmission have suggested that these compounds reduce the dopamine response to both cocaine administration and conditioned reminders of prior cocaine use (Dewey et al. 1997; Gerasimov et al. 1999). GABAergic medications also reduce the self-administration of cocaine in animal models (Kushner et al. 1999; Roberts et al. 1996). Therefore, GABAergic medications could prevent relapse either by blocking cocaine-induced euphoria or by reducing craving caused by exposure to conditioned reminders of prior cocaine use. One promising GABAergic medication is topiramate.

On the basis of both its GABA neurotransmission and glutamate neurotransmission effects, topiramate is under investigation for the relapse prevention treatment of cocaine dependence. Topiramate increases cerebral levels of GABA and facilitates GABA neurotransmission (Kuzniecky et al. 1998; Petroff et al. 1999). Topiramate also inhibits glutamate neurotransmission through a blockade of AMPA/kainate receptors (Gibbs et al. 2000). In animal models of cocaine relapse, blockade of AMPA receptors in the nucleus accumbens prevented reinstatement of cocaine self-administration (Cornish and Kalivas 2000).

Kampman and colleagues (2004) conducted two trials of topiramate for cocaine dependence. The first was a 13-week double-blind, placebo-controlled pilot trial of topiramate 200 mg/day involving 40 cocaine-dependent patients with symptoms meeting DSM-IV criteria (American Psychiatric Association 1994). In this trial, topiramate-treated patients were significantly more likely to be abstinent from cocaine during the last 5 weeks of the trial than placebo-treated patients. In addition, among patients who returned for at least one visit after receiving medications, topiramate-treated patients were significantly more likely to achieve at least 3 weeks of continuous abstinence from cocaine than placebo-treated patients (59% vs. 26%), and topiramate-treated patients were significantly more likely than placebo-treated patients to be rated very much improved at their last visit (71% vs. 32%) (Kampman et al. 2004). This initial trial of topiramate was replicated in a second, larger, trial involving 170 cocaine- and alcohol-dependent subjects (Kampman et al. 2013). In this trial, topiramate-treated subjects (300 mg/day) were significantly more likely than placebo-treated subjects to achieve 3 weeks of continuous abstinence from cocaine at the end of the trial. Twenty percent of the topiramate-treated patients were cocaine abstinent, compared with 6% of the placebo-treated patients.

Two other mainly positive trials of topiramate have been conducted. The first of these was conducted by Johnson and colleagues (2013). In this trial, 142 cocaine-dependent patients were treated for 12 weeks with either topiramate (300 mg/day) or identical placebo. Topiramate-treated patients had significantly more cocaine nonuse days than placebo-treated patients during weeks 6–12 of the trial. Cocaine nonuse days were determined by self-reporting and verified by urine drug screens. The other positive trial involved 60 men who used freebase (crack) cocaine (Baldaçara et al. 2016). In this trial, topiramate was found to reduce cocaine use early in treatment. Subjects were randomly assigned to either topiramate (≥200 mg/day, titrated over several weeks) or a placebo. During the first 4 weeks of the trial, topiramate-treated patients used significantly less cocaine, as measured by the quantity used and frequency of use, and they spent significantly less money on cocaine. At the conclusion of the 12-week trial, however, there were no significant differences between topiramate- and placebo-treated subjects in any outcome variable (Baldaçara et al. 2016).

There have been three negative trials of topiramate. Two involved patients with comorbid cocaine and opioid dependence. Umbricht and colleagues (2014) evaluated the efficacy of topiramate with and without contingency management in 171 cocaine- and opioid-dependent patients receiving methadone maintenance whose symptoms met DSM-IV criteria. The patients were randomly assigned to one of four groups that received either topiramate (titrated to 300 mg/day) or placebo and monetary voucher incentives that were either contingent (contingency management [CM] group) or noncontingent (non-CM group) on drug abstinence. The primary outcome measures were cocaine abstinence and treatment retention. Neither topiramate nor CM was effective in reducing cocaine use. There was no significant difference in cocaine abstinence between the topiramate and placebo-treated groups or between the CM-treated and the non-CM-treated groups. There was also no significant topiramate/CM interaction (Umbricht et al. 2014).

The second negative trial involved 50 cocaine- and opioid-dependent individuals receiving methadone maintenance who were randomly assigned to receive topiramate up to 300 mg/day or identical placebo. Topiramate was not superior to placebo in reducing cocaine use (Pirnia et al. 2018). Third, Nuijten et al. (2014) conducted a trial of topiramate involving 74 patients with freebase (crack) cocaine dependence. The patients were randomly assigned to receive either 12 weeks of topiramate (titrated to 300 mg/day) plus CBT or 12 weeks of CBT only. The primary outcome measure was treatment retention. Secondary outcomes included cocaine and other substance use. Adherence to topiramate treatment was low. Topiramate did not improve treatment retention, nor did it reduce cocaine and other substance use.

Combination of Dopaminergic and GABA/Glutamate Medications

On the basis of the positive trials of long-acting dopamine agonists and topiramate for cocaine use disorder, Mariani and colleagues (2012) evaluated the combination of topiramate and extended-release mixed amphetamine salts (MAS-ER) for the treatment of cocaine use disorder. Eighty-one cocaine-dependent patients were randomly assigned to receive either a combination of MAS-ER plus topiramate or all placebo for 12 weeks. MAS-ER doses were titrated over 2 weeks to a maximum dosage of 60 mg/day, and topiramate doses were titrated over 6 weeks to a maximum dosage of 300 mg/day. Significantly more patients in the topiramate plus MAS-ER group achieved 3 consecutive weeks of abstinence during the trial (33.3%) compared with the placebo group (16.7%). The combination treatment was most effective for participants with a high baseline frequency of cocaine use.

This promising pilot trial was replicated in a larger multicenter trial involving 127 adults with cocaine use disorder who used cocaine at least 9 days in the month before entering the trial. MAS-ER was titrated to a maximum dosage of 60 mg/day and topiramate to a maximum dosage of 100 mg bid. The proportion of participants achieving 3 abstinent weeks at the end of the trial was significantly greater in the group treated with topiramate and MAS-ER (14.1%) compared with the placebo group (0.0%) (Levin et al. 2020).

Most recently, Rush and colleagues (2021) evaluated the combination of the dopamine agonist phentermine with topiramate in a human laboratory trial. In this trial, patients received maintainence with combinations of topiramate (0, 50, or 100 mg/day) and phentermine (0, 15, or 30 mg/day). After 7 days of medication administration, patients participated in a human trial during which they were able to self-administer various doses of cocaine. Maintenance on topiramate or phentermine alone significantly decreased cocaine self-administration. However, combining topiramate and phentermine decreased cocaine self-administration much more than either topiramate or phentermine alone (Rush et al. 2021).

Other Medications

A few other medications have shown promise in preclinical and early clinical trials. These include dopamine D_3 receptor medications and N-acetylcysteine (NAC).

Dopamine Antagonists

Dopamine is central to the reinforcing effects of all drugs of abuse, including alcohol and cocaine. Therefore, dopamine antagonists were among the first medications considered for the treatment of cocaine dependence. The two main groups of dopamine receptors are the D_1–D_5 family and the D_2–D_3 family. Several representatives of antagonists to both groups of dopamine receptors have been evaluated for cocaine dependence treatment and have not been found to be efficacious. D_1 receptor antagonists such as ecopipam were simply ineffective (McCance-Katz et al. 2001). D_2 antagonists, although sometimes effective at reducing either cocaine or cue-induced craving in human laboratory studies, either had intolerable side effects or proved ineffective in clinical trials (Amato et al. 2007; Grabowski et al. 2000; Kampman et al. 2003; Loebl et al. 2008; Sayers et al. 2005).

D_3 receptor antagonists may be more effective than D_2 receptor antagonists. The high concentration of D_3 receptors in limbic structures suggests that these receptors may be most important in drug reward and addiction (Heidbreder et al. 2005). D_3 receptors have the highest affinity of all dopamine receptors for exogenous dopamine, again suggesting a predominant role for these receptors in reward and addiction (Levant 1997; Sokoloff et al. 2006). The net effect of D_3 receptor antagonism is a slight increase in dopaminergic tone, which may be useful in chronic cocaine users, who generally have decreased dopaminergic tone (Heidbreder et al. 2005). Thus, D_3 receptor antagonism may be a better strategy than D_1 or D_2 receptor blockade to treat cocaine dependence. D_3 antagonist medications, therefore, may reduce cocaine-induced euphoria, craving for cocaine, or relapse to cocaine caused by stress.

The preclinical trials with D_3 receptor antagonists predict clinical usefulness, because in almost every animal model of addiction, D_3 receptor antagonists appear to be useful to treat cocaine dependence. The D_3 receptor antagonist SB-277011 blocked both the acquisition and the expression of cocaine-induced conditioned place preference (Vorel et al. 2002). D_3 receptor antagonists also reduced cocaine-induced reinstatement of self-administration as well as conditioned cue-induced reinstatement of cocaine self-administration (Di Ciano et al. 2003; Vorel et al. 2002), and they lowered the breakpoint in progressive ratio self-administration models (Xi et al. 2006). D_3 receptor antagonists also reduced stress-induced reinstatement of cocaine self-administration (Xi et al. 2004). As a result of these data, clinical trials with D_3 receptor antagonists are currently underway.

N-Acetylcysteine

The last of the promising medications is NAC, an amino acid and a cysteine prodrug. In preclinical and some early pilot clinical trials, NAC has shown potential utility in the treatment of addictive disorders. Through stimulation of the cysteine-glutamate antiporters, NAC may increase extracellular glutamate. This modulates the release of glutamate in response to drug-taking via stimulation of metabotropic glutamate autoreceptors. Preclinical studies have suggested that levels of glutamate in the nucleus accumbens mediate reward-seeking behavior (Kalivas and Volkow 2005; McFarland et al. 2003). Low levels of extracellular glutamate in the nucleus accumbens are associated with chronic cocaine exposure. This reduction in glutamate release may block drug-seeking behaviors and drug craving. In rats, NAC pretreatment blocked the reinstatement of drug-seeking behavior induced by cocaine or conditioned cues of cocaine (Baker et al. 2003). In a human laboratory trial, NAC 600 mg/day reduced cocaine craving in non-treatment-seeking cocaine-dependent men and women (LaRowe et al. 2007). In an open-label trial, NAC was safe and well tolerated in cocaine-dependent patients at dosages of 1,200, 2,400, or 3,600 mg/day (LaRowe et al. 2006). In one double-blind, placebo-controlled trial of NAC for cocaine use disorder, 11 patients with cocaine use disorder were randomly assigned to receive NAC 1,200 mg/day, NAC 2,400 mg/day, or placebo and were treated for 8 weeks. In the groups as a whole, there was no effect of NAC. Among patients who were cocaine abstinent at the start of the trial, however, patients receiving NAC 2,400 mg/day had a longer time to relapse and lower craving ratings (LaRowe et al. 2013). NAC may therefore be effective in helping maintain abstinence from cocaine.

Medications to Treat Methamphetamine and Amphetamine Use Disorders

The effort to find medications to treat methamphetamine/amphetamine use disorder started much more recently than the search for a medication to treat cocaine use disorder. Consequently, fewer medications have been tested. Similarities between the mechanisms of action of amphetamines and methamphetamines and those of cocaine have suggested that medications effective for cocaine dependence also may be effective for methamphetamine/amphetamine use disorder, and several medications tested for treatment of cocaine use disorder are currently undergoing or are about to undergo testing for treatment of methamphetamine/amphetamine use disorder. Thus far, bupropion and the combination of bupropion and XRNT have shown evidence of potential efficacy in controlled clinical trials. In addition, mirtazapine has shown evidence of efficacy in special populations of patients with methamphetamine use disorder (see the later section "Special Populations").

Bupropion, an antidepressant medication, acts primarily as a reuptake inhibitor of dopamine and norepinephrine. It has also been shown to be effective in treating nicotine dependence. Bupropion's mechanism of action in the treatment of nicotine and methamphetamine dependence may be related to its effects on dopamine reuptake. It is thought to potentially alleviate stimulant withdrawal symptoms by facilitating dopamine neurotransmission. As noted earlier in this chapter, bupropion has been tested for treatment of cocaine dependence in the past and in some studies was found to be ineffective (Margolin et al. 1995), whereas in other meta-analyses it has shown some promise (Castells et al. 2016; Chan et al. 2019). For methamphetamine use disorder, bupropion is more promising.

Although several systematic reviews and meta-analyses have demonstrated that bupropion alone may not be effective for all who use amphetamines or methamphetamines, closer analysis of the individual studies reveals the possible utility of bupropion in certain subgroups (Chan et al. 2019; Lee et al. 2018; Siefried et al. 2020). For instance, bupropion SR (150 mg bid) was tested for the treatment of methamphetamine dependence in 151 methamphetamine-dependent patients (Elkashef et al. 2008). In the group as a whole, bupropion treatment resulted in a nonsignificant trend toward more weeks of abstinence compared with placebo. In a subgroup of patients in the trial with less methamphetamine use at baseline, bupropion treatment was associated with significantly more weeks of abstinence for methamphetamine compared with placebo treatment (Elkashef et al. 2008). This finding was replicated in a subsequent trial involving 73 methamphetamine-dependent outpatients (Shoptaw et al. 2008). Among light methamphetamine users (defined as zero, one, or two amphetamine-positive urine samples out of six during a 2-week baseline), patients treated with bupropion SR (150 mg bid) had significantly more methamphetamine-free weeks measured by negative urine drug screen results than placebo-treated patients (Shoptaw et al. 2008). This finding suggests that bupropion may be efficacious for individuals with less severe methamphetamine use (typically considered <18 days of use per month). Finally, Heinzerling and colleagues (2014) found that bupropion SR (150 mg bid) was not more efficacious than placebo for the treatment of methamphetamine/amphetamine use disorder overall, but in a small subgroup of highly adherent patients, bupropion was associated with significantly higher rates of abstinence than in the nonadherent patients.

Naltrexone has also been found in some (but not all) trials to be associated with improvement in symptoms of methamphetamine/amphetamine use disorder. Jayaram-Lindström and colleagues (2008) evaluated naltrexone (50 mg/day) as a treatment for methamphetamine/amphetamine use disorder in a 12-week, double-blind, placebo-controlled trial involving 55 patients with the disorder. Patients treated with naltrexone had significantly fewer amphetamine-positive urine results during the trial compared with placebo-treated patients (Jayaram-Lindström et al. 2008). Coffin and colleagues (2018) randomly assigned 100 patients with methamphetamine/amphetamine use disorder to XRNT 380 mg every 4 weeks or identical placebo in a 12-week trial. They found that naltrexone was not superior to placebo in promoting amphetamine abstinence as measured by urine drug screens. XRNT was well tolerated in the trial (Coffin et al. 2018).

Based on the positive findings with bupropion and naltrexone, Trivedi and colleagues (2021) conducted a multicenter two-stage, double-blind, placebo-controlled trial with the use of a sequential parallel comparison design to evaluate the efficacy and safety of XRNT (380 mg every 3 weeks) plus oral bupropion XL (450 mg/day) in adults with moderate or severe methamphetamine use disorder. In the first stage of the trial, patients with methamphetamine use disorder were randomly assigned to receive XRNT-bupropion or matching injectable and oral placebo for 6 weeks. Those in the placebo group who did not have a response in the first stage underwent rerandomization in stage 2 and were assigned in a 1:1 ratio to receive XRNT-bupropion or placebo for an additional 6 weeks. Urine samples were obtained from patients twice a week. The primary outcome was a response defined as at least three methamphetamine-negative urine samples out of four obtained at the end of the first or second stage. In this trial, the combination of bupropion and XRNT was significantly better than placebo. The weighted average response across the two stages was a 13.6% response with XRNT-bupropion and a 2.5% response to placebo (Trivedi et al. 2021). Although it was not explicitly studied, the introduction of naltrexone pharmacotherapy, alone or in combination with bupropion, could provide some protection against inadvertent overdose resulting from opioid-adulterated (e.g., high-potency synthetic opioid) stimulants.

Topiramate influences GABA and glutamate neurotransmission (as described in the section "GABAergic and Glutamatergic Medications") and is a potential pharmacotherapy for several different substance use disorders, including methamphetamine/amphetamine use disorder, although the studies are limited. Two randomized controlled trials demonstrated decreased methamphetamine use via urine toxicology screening in those prescribed topiramate 200 mg/day (Chan et al. 2019; Elkashef et al. 2012; Lee et al. 2018; Rezaei et al. 2016).

Psychostimulants (e.g., dextroamphetamine, methylphenidate) have also been studied in the treatment of methamphetamine/amphetamine use disorder, although the studies have been small and evidence is limited. Similar to the discussion of bupropion earlier in this section, a meta-analysis (38 studies included) of the use of methylphenidate did not demonstrate overall benefit in methamphetamine use or treatment retention, but subgroup analysis suggested that methylphenidate may, in fact, have been beneficial in achieving short-term abstinence in the subset of individuals who received higher doses of methylphenidate (Tardelli et al. 2020). Two additional systematic reviews also support the possibility that methylphenidate may be beneficial in reducing methamphetamine use and cravings, and that individuals with a moderate to high frequency of use (>10 days per month) may be more likely to experience a response (Lee et al. 2018; Siefried et al. 2020), as drawn from the studies that have examined this treatment (Konstenius et al. 2010, 2014; Ling et al. 2014; Miles et al. 2013). Table 6.3 describes medications used to treat methamphetamine/amphetamine use disorder.

Psychostimulant replacement therapy is currently not approved by the FDA, carries significant potential risk, and has been studied in limited, highly controlled research study contexts only. Nonetheless, the recently published ASAM/AAAP Clinical Practice Guideline on the Management of Stimulant Use Disorder (American Society of Addiction Medicine and American Academy of Addiction Psychiatry 2023) provides limited endorsement of consideration of this treatment based on the current evidence in conjunction with expert clinical experience, as discussed later in this chapter.

Combining Contingency Management With Medications

Voucher-based reinforcement therapy (VBRT) is a form of reinforcement program (known more broadly as CM) that capitalizes on the motivational processes that underpin substance use and addiction. VBRT is a behavioral treatment intervention for substance use disorders, in which patients receive vouchers redeemable for goods and services in the community contingent on achieving a predetermined therapeutic goal. VBRT has been shown to be highly effective in promoting initial abstinence from cocaine among cocaine-dependent patients (Higgins et al. 1994). Researchers have begun to combine VBRT with medications to augment medication response in cocaine-dependent patients. In several trials, patients receiving the combination of VBRT and medications have responded better than patients receiving medications alone or VBRT alone. For example, Kosten and colleagues (2003) tested the efficacy of desipramine and VBRT in cocaine- and opiate-dependent patients receiving buprenorphine maintenance. Previously, desipramine had not been found to be consistently efficacious for the treatment of cocaine dependence when combined with standard psychosocial treatment. In the trial, patients received desipramine or placebo with VBRT or a noncontingent voucher control. Cocaine-free and combined cocaine- and opiate-free urine samples increased more rapidly over time in subjects receiving desipramine or VBRT. Those receiving both VBRT and desipramine had significantly more drug-free urine samples than did the other three groups (Kosten et al. 2003).

In a double-blind, placebo-controlled trial of bupropion and VBRT, the combination of bupropion and VBRT was superior to bupropion alone, placebo, and VBRT alone in promoting abstinence from cocaine in cocaine-dependent patients (Poling et al. 2006). Similar results were found for the combination of the selective serotonin reuptake inhibitor (SSRI) citalopram and VBRT (Moeller et al. 2007). Several SSRIs have been tested to treat cocaine dependence, but like desipramine, SSRIs have not been found to be consistently efficacious for the treatment of cocaine dependence when used in association with standard psychosocial treatment. The use of VBRT as a psychosocial treatment platform appears to be highly effective in increasing the efficacy of certain medications to treat cocaine dependence.

Significant Medical and Psychiatric Considerations

Cocaine and amphetamines have similar mechanisms of action and consequently have similar medical complications associated with their use. Both agents increase monoamine activity and potentiate acute sympathetic effects on the cardiovascular system, resulting in increased heart rate, blood pressure, and peripheral vasoconstriction (Kevil et al. 2019; Vongpatanasin et al. 1999). Therefore, the most serious medical complications of stimulants involve the cardiovascular system, the pulmonary system, and the CNS.

Both cocaine and amphetamines increase the rate of cardiovascular disease. The mechanism behind cocaine-induced myocardial ischemia includes increased myocardial oxygen demand, which is accompanied by

Table 6.3 Medications to treat methamphetamine/amphetamine use disorder (all non-FDA-approved indications)

Class	Medication	Dosing	Evidence	Notes
Dopaminergic	Bupropion	Bupropion SR 150 mg bid	Perhaps more effective for those who use less at baseline (Elkashef et al. 2008; Heinzerling et al. 2014; Shoptaw et al. 2008)	Less use at baseline typically defined as <18 d/mo Use caution in individuals with seizure disorders or eating disorders May be considered in those with co-occurring tobacco use disorder and/or depressive disorder
Dopaminergic	Methylphenidate	Methylphenidate XR 18–180 mg/d Methylphenidate SR 54 mg/d	Perhaps more effective for those who use more frequently (>10 d/mo) and those who receive higher doses, although evidence is mixed (Konstenius et al. 2010, 2014; Ling et al. 2014; Miles et al. 2013)	May be considered in those with co-occurring ADHD

Table 6.3 Medications to treat methamphetamine/amphetamine use disorder (all non-FDA-approved indications) *(continued)*

Class	Medication	Dosing	Evidence	Notes
GABAergic and glutamatergic	Topiramate	200 mg/d	May be helpful in reducing the amount taken and prevent relapse in those already abstinent (Elkashef et al. 2012) Small study shows potential benefit in reducing use, improving addiction severity index scores (Rezaei et al. 2016)	May be considered in those with co-occurring alcohol use disorder May suppress appetite/weight, so may be problematic for those already underweight courtesy of stimulant use
μ Opioid receptor antagonist	Naltrexone (monotreatment)	50 mg/d PO 380 mg/mo XR IM	Mixed: the PO study showed benefit (Jayaram-Lindström et al. 2008), whereas the injectable study showed no benefit (Coffin et al. 2018)	May be considered in those with co-occurring alcohol use disorder, or those with co-occurring opioid use disorder already taking naltrexone, or possibly to prevent opioid overdose from fentanyl-adulterated stimulants

Table 6.3 Medications to treat methamphetamine/amphetamine use disorder (all non-FDA-approved indications) *(continued)*

Class	Medication	Dosing	Evidence	Notes
Combination	Naltrexone and bupropion	Bupropion 450 mg/d ER naltrexone 380 mg/mo	Significantly fewer urine toxicology results positive for amphetamines (Trivedi et al. 2021)	May be considered in those with co-occurring alcohol use disorder and/or tobacco use disorder, those with co-occurring opioid use disorder already taking naltrexone, or possibly to prevent opioid overdose from fentanyl-adulterated stimulants
Other	Mirtazapine	30 mg/d	A small study (Colfax et al. 2011) replicated in a larger study (Coffin et al. 2020) showed fewer methamphetamine-positive urine test results and a decrease in risky sexual behaviors	Studies have been in population of men who have sex with men May help restore normal sleep architecture following stimulant-induced disruption

Note. d = day; mo = month; PO = per os; SR = sustained release; XR = extended release.

coronary vasoconstriction and a prothrombotic state (Havakuk et al. 2017). Individuals using cocaine often present to the emergency department with chest pain (Substance Abuse and Mental Health Services Administration 2011). Mittleman and colleagues (1999) found that among cocaine consumers, the risk of myocardial infarction onset was elevated 24 times over baseline in the 60 minutes after cocaine use. Likewise, methamphetamine use has been associated with cardiovascular disease, which represents the second leading cause of death among users, following accidental overdose (Darke et al. 2017). Postmortem studies of individuals using methamphetamine have found unexpectedly high rates of coronary artery disease among this group (Karch et al. 1999; Kaye et al. 2008). In addition, methamphetamine and cocaine can both cause cardiac arrythmias (Darke et al. 2017; Havakuk et al. 2017). Methamphetamine use has been shown to be associated with a 27% increased risk of sudden cardiac death (Parekh et al. 2018).

Inhalation of smoked cocaine is associated with lung disease. An acute pulmonary syndrome, referred to colloquially as "crack lung," results from smoking crack or freebase cocaine and is characterized by fever, shortness of breath, hemoptysis, hypoxemia, and respiratory failure (Mégarbane and Chevillard 2013). It occurs up to 48 hours after cocaine inhalation and is characterized by radiological evidence of alveolitis (Forrester et al. 1990). Methamphetamine use has been associated with pulmonary hypertension, and this syndrome presents frequently with fatigue, chest pain, dyspnea, and syncope (Chin et al. 2006; Schaiberger et al. 1993).

Both cocaine use and methamphetamine use have been associated with cerebral vascular accidents (stroke). Cocaine use has been specifically associated with both ischemic and hemorrhagic stroke. Insufflated cocaine has been more associated with hemorrhagic stroke relative to ischemic stroke, whereas smoked cocaine is equally associated with both ischemic and hemorrhagic stroke (Treadwell and Robinson 2007). Among methamphetamine users, hemorrhagic stroke is more common. In case reports and series, 80% of methamphetamine-related strokes reported were hemorrhagic (Lappin et al. 2017).

Both cocaine use and methamphetamine/amphetamine use are associated with the development of psychotic symptoms, with amphetamine use more likely to cause more prolonged episodes of psychosis. Amphetamine-induced psychotic symptoms occur in approximately 40% of users (Fiorentini et al. 2021). Prominent symptoms include auditory, visual, and tactile hallucinations as well as ideas of reference and paranoid delusions (Glasner-Edwards and Mooney 2014). Although, in most cases, the psychotic symptoms are brief and recede after intoxication, about 25% of patients who experience psychotic symptoms have a persistent psychosis that can last for more than a month after they become abstinent. Risk factors for the development of psychotic symptoms include amount and duration of use and earlier age at onset (Fiorentini et al. 2021). Antipsychotics can be used for acute treatment of psychosis, and sedatives can be used to control agitation. Long-term treatment should focus on abstinence from amphetamines/methamphetamines (Glasner-Edwards and Mooney 2014).

Cocaine-induced psychosis is relatively common among cocaine users, occurring in 29%–86% (Fiorentini et al. 2021). It is generally brief, lasting only a few days in most cases. Symptoms include paranoid delusion and auditory/visual hallucinations. Risk factors include quantity of cocaine used, using cocaine from a young age, and the presence of psychiatric comorbidity. Route of cocaine use is also a risk factor, with intravenous use being associated with a greater risk of psychosis (Roncero et al. 2014). Cocaine-induced psychosis is generally treated with behavioral measures aimed at keeping the patient calm. Benzodiazepines or sedating antipsychotics may be used to manage acute agitation. Antipsychotics rarely need to be continued for more than a few days, because the psychosis is usually brief (Tang et al. 2014).

Depression and anxiety can often occur in both methamphetamine/amphetamine use disorder and cocaine use disorder. These symptoms can be associated with cocaine or amphetamine withdrawal, as discussed earlier, but are also seen in individuals using stimulants after withdrawal is over. In one trial, 60% of those using methamphetamine experienced moderate to severe anxiety or depression after the resolution of acute withdrawal (Duncan et al. 2022). Similarly, depressive disorders have been seen in 11%–50% of cocaine users (López and Becoña 2007). For both cocaine use disorder and methamphetamine/amphetamine use disorder, the presence of comorbid anxiety or depression is associated with poorer drug use and mood/anxiety outcomes.

Special Populations

MSM represent a population at risk for stimulant use disorder. Gay and bisexual men are three times more likely to use illicit substances than their heterosexual counterparts (Maxwell et al. 2019). Methamphetamine use among MSM is prevalent and associated with medical and social risks, including HIV transmission (Colfax et al. 2010).

Mirtazapine is an antidepressant medication with multiple mechanisms of action. It facilitates norepinephrine, serotonin, and dopamine release in mesocorticolimbic areas involved in drug reward, craving, and drug-seeking (Devoto et al. 2004; Haddjeri et al. 1998; Nakayama et al. 2004). In addition, mirtazapine is highly sedating without the significant sleep architecture disruption seen with other sedative-hypnotic medications. Given this mechanism of action, mirtazapine has been proposed to reduce methamphetamine craving and withdrawal symptoms (Colfax et al. 2011).

Investigators have evaluated mirtazapine for the treatment of methamphetamine use disorder in an MSM population in two trials, and they found it to be effective in reducing methamphetamine use and associated risky sexual behaviors. In the first trial, 60 sexually active MSM with methamphetamine use disorder were randomly assigned to receive either mirtazapine 30 mg/day or placebo for 12 weeks (Colfax et al. 2011). Participants assigned to the mirtazapine group had fewer methamphetamine-positive urine test results compared with participants assigned to the placebo group. In addition, risky sexual behaviors decreased significantly more among patients taking mirtazapine compared with those taking placebo (Colfax et al. 2011). This pilot trail was replicated in a larger trial involving 120 community-recruited adult cisgender men, transgender men, and transgender women with methamphetamine use disorder who had sex with men, who were sexually active, and who were actively using methamphetamines (Coffin et al. 2020). Patients were randomly assigned to receive either mirtazapine 30 mg/day or placebo for 24 weeks, with a follow-up 12 weeks after stopping medications. Patients receiving mirtazapine had fewer methamphetamine-positive urine test results at 12, 24, and 36 weeks. Mirtazapine-treated patients compared with placebo-treated patients had fewer episodes of condomless anal sex with partners who were serodiscordant for HIV, and they had fewer episodes of condomless receptive anal sex with partners who were serodiscordant at week 24 (Coffin et al. 2020). Mirtazapine appears to be a promising treatment in this population of patients with methamphetamine use disorder, and further study will be needed to determine whether mirtazapine may also be beneficial in a broader population of individuals who use methamphetamines.

American Society of Addiction Medicine and American Academy of Addiction Psychiatry Clinical Guideline on the Management of Stimulant Use Disorder

In 2023, the ASAM and the AAAP published a comprehensive clinical guideline on the treatment of stimulant use disorders, a portion of which is dedicated to providing practical guidance regarding pharmacotherapies for these disorders. The guideline was compiled by a 13-member committee tasked with developing recommendations based on a review of existing research literature and evaluation of its quality in combination with expert clinical judgment (American Society of Addiction Medicine and American Academy of Addiction Psychiatry 2023). As such, the guideline can be viewed as an effort to evaluate, organize, and translate the extant scientific literature to inform and encourage clinical practice. The guideline is, therefore, a practical attempt to resolve potentially conflicting research findings by combining the literature with expert clinical judgment.

It is beyond the scope of this chapter to review all the recommendations provided in the ASAM/AAAP guideline, but in brief, the pharmacotherapeutic recommendations made in the guideline largely line up with those described in this chapter. The guideline authors do encourage the consideration of off-label pharmacotherapies for the treatment of stimulant use disorders, including consideration of the use of psychostimulant medications to treat stimulant use disorders (both cocaine use disorder and amphetamine use disorder), despite the relative lack of consistent, robust research supporting their use in this manner. The guideline authors encourage careful risk-benefit calculations when considering use of stimulant pharmacotherapy, and they recommend that this approach be undertaken by only those clinicians who are board certified in addiction medicine or addiction psychiatry and by those with commensurate training, competencies, and capacity for close patient monitoring. Long-acting formulations of methylphenidate and amphetamine pharmacotherapies are preferred, and the guideline authors describe this recommendation as a low-certainty, conditional recommendation, which acknowledges that the evidence base is lacking and is based on individual clinical situations (e.g., patient values, resource availability, setting).

Vaccines for Cocaine and Methamphetamine Use Disorders

Vaccination against infectious disease has become a mainstay of modern medicine. As the science of immunology advanced, it became clear that vaccines could be developed against other molecules in addition to infectious pathogens. This finding led to the study of vaccines for a number of diseases, including addiction. Because there were no effective medications for the treatment of cocaine use disorder and methamphetamine/amphetamine use disorder, vaccines for these two illnesses became the focus of intense study. Cocaine and methamphetamines are too small to invoke an immune response on their own, but if bonded to a larger molecule such as a protein, the cocaine (methamphetamine) protein complex could trigger the production of antibodies that would subsequently bind to cocaine or methamphetamines. The resulting cocaine or methamphetamine antibody complex would be too large to pass through the blood–brain barrier (Ozgen and Blume 2019); thus, the vaccine could prevent the drug from entering the brain and triggering a response, or at least slow the rapid buildup of drug in the brain that is associated with drug euphoria. Vaccines for the treatment of both cocaine use disorder and methamphetamine/amphetamine use disorder have been studied. However, clinical trials thus far have only been conducted for cocaine use disorder (Bloom and Bushell 2022).

Cocaine vaccine development started in the mid- to late 1990s, when a number of possible vaccines were tested in rodents. These vaccines were shown to significantly reduce cocaine levels in the brains of immunized rats (Ozgen and Blume 2019). Human vaccine trials with a vaccine made from succinyl norcocaine conjugated to a cholera toxin were conducted. This vaccine, named TACD, was evaluated in two clinical trials. In the first phase II trial, 18 subjects with cocaine use disorder were given either a low or high dose of the vaccine. The high-dose group was significantly more likely to maintain cocaine-free urine results compared with the low-dose group (Martell et al. 2005). A second, larger trial involving 300 patients with cocaine use disorder was conducted. Patients were randomly assigned to placebo or active vaccine. Patients who achieved high vaccine levels were more likely to complete the trial. However, there was no difference between the placebo and active vaccine groups in cocaine-free urine results, even among patients who achieved high antibody levels (Kosten et al. 2014). Although the results of the two trials were not completely negative, the development of a truly effective vaccine for cocaine use disorder has not been achieved.

Key Points

- Stimulants such as cocaine and amphetamine are highly reinforcing and increase alertness, arousal, sympathetic tone, and motor activity via increases in monoamine neurotransmission, especially dopamine, norepinephrine, and serotonin, although to different extents and through different mechanisms.
- Both cocaine and amphetamine/methamphetamine have similar intoxication and withdrawal syndrome symptom profiles, although the extent and duration of each can vary by substance; methamphetamine, for example, is typically more pronounced and longer lasting. Management of stimulant intoxication is largely symptomatic, targeting agitation with sedative-hypnotics, and in some cases neuroleptics (although caution is necessary with the latter). Stimulant withdrawal is generally not medically significant, although withdrawal may drive relapse. Some evidence suggests that topiramate may be beneficial to those who experience severe cocaine withdrawal.
- Cocaine use disorder and methamphetamine/amphetamine use disorder are significant clinical problems, and there are currently no medications approved by the FDA for their treatment.
- Off-label stimulant agonist treatment trials aimed at stabilizing dopamine transmission (methylphenidate/amphetamine, modafinil) have been conducted to treat stimulant use disorders, but the results are mixed and difficult to interpret or generalize. Similarly, trials of disulfiram were initially promising but have not sustained their promise.
- Of trials examining the effect of GABAergic and glutamatergic medications, topiramate has been most studied and has had mixed outcomes. Nonetheless, topiramate, especially when combined with long-acting mixed amphetamine salts, seems promising for treatment of cocaine use disorder.
- Bupropion and naltrexone trials have had mixed results for the treatment of methamphetamine/amphetamine use disorder. A trial of combined bupropion and extended-release (injectable) naltrexone showed promise.

- Contingency management is the most effective treatment for cocaine use disorder.
- Stimulant use is associated with significant cardiovascular, pulmonary, and CNS complications, and providers should be aware of, and monitor for, these risks.
- Mirtazapine may be effective for methamphetamine/amphetamine use disorder in the population of men who have sex with men.

References

Ahmed SH, Cador M: Dissociation of psychomotor sensitization from compulsive cocaine consumption. Neuropsychopharmacology 31(3):563–571, 2006 16034440

Amato L, Minozzi S, Pani PP, et al: Antipsychotic medications for cocaine dependence. Cochrane Database Syst Rev (3):CD006306, 2007 17636840

American Psychiatric Association: Diagnostic and Statistical Manual of Mental Disorders, 4th Edition. Washington, DC, American Psychiatric Association, 1994

American Psychiatric Association: Diagnostic and Statistical Manual of Mental Disorders, 5th Edition, Text Revision. Washington, DC, American Psychiatric Association, 2022

American Society of Addiction Medicine, American Academy of Addiction Psychiatry: Clinical Practice Guideline on the Management of Stimulant Use Disorder, Appendix N. New York, American Society of Addiction Medicine/American Academy of Addiction Psychiatry, 2023. Available at: https://downloads.asam.org/sitefinity-production-blobs/docs/default-source/quality-science/stud_guideline_document_final.pdf. Accessed February 6, 2025.

Amlani A, McKee G, Khamis N, et al: Why the FUSS (Fentanyl Urine Screen Study)? A cross-sectional survey to characterize an emerging threat to people who use drugs in British Columbia, Canada. Harm Reduct J 12:54, 2015 26577516

Anderson AL, Reid MS, Li SH, et al: Modafinil for the treatment of cocaine dependence. Drug Alcohol Depend 104(1–2):133–139, 2009 19560290

Archer T, Fredriksson A, Jonsson G, et al: Central noradrenaline depletion antagonizes aspects of d-amphetamine-induced hyperactivity in the rat. Psychopharmacology (Berl) 88(2):141–146, 1986 3081924

Azzaro AJ, Ziance RJ, Rutledge CO: The importance of neuronal uptake of amines for amphetamine-induced release of 3H-norepinephrine from isolated brain tissue. J Pharmacol Exp Ther 189(1):110–118, 1974 4823286

Baker DA, McFarland K, Lake RW, et al: N-acetyl cysteine-induced blockade of cocaine-induced reinstatement. Ann NY Acad Sci 1003:349–351, 2003 14684458

Baldaçara L, Cogo-Moreira H, Parreira BL, et al: Efficacy of topiramate in the treatment of crack cocaine dependence: a double-blind, randomized, placebo-controlled trial. J Clin Psychiatry 77(3):398–406, 2016 27046312

Bloom BT, Bushell MJ: Vaccines against drug abuse: are we there yet? Vaccines (Basel) 10(6):860, 2022 35746468

Brown JM, Hanson GR, Fleckenstein AE: Regulation of the vesicular monoamine transporter-2: a novel mechanism for cocaine and other psychostimulants. J Pharmacol Exp Ther 296(3):762–767, 2001 11181904

Carroll KM, Nich C, Ball SA, et al: Treatment of cocaine and alcohol dependence with psychotherapy and disulfiram. Addiction 93(5):713–727, 1998 9692270

Carroll KM, Fenton LR, Ball SA, et al: Efficacy of disulfiram and cognitive behavior therapy in cocaine-dependent outpatients: a randomized placebo-controlled trial. Arch Gen Psychiatry 61(3):264–272, 2004 14993114

Castells X, Cunill R, Pérez-Mañá C, et al: Psychostimulant drugs for cocaine dependence. Cochrane Database Syst Rev 9(9):CD007380, 2016 27670244

Chan B, Kondo K, Freeman M, et al: Pharmacotherapy for cocaine use disorder: a systematic review and meta-analysis. J Gen Intern Med 34(12):2858–2873, 2019 31183685

Chin KM, Channick RN, Rubin LJ: Is methamphetamine use associated with idiopathic pulmonary arterial hypertension? Chest 130(6):1657–1663, 2006 17166979

Coffin PO, Santos GM, Hern J, et al: Extended-release naltrexone for methamphetamine dependence among men who have sex with men: a randomized placebo-controlled trial. Addiction 113(2):268–278, 2018 28734107

Coffin PO, Santos GM, Hern J, et al: Effects of mirtazapine for methamphetamine use disorder among cisgender men and transgender women who have sex with men: a placebo-controlled randomized clinical trial. JAMA Psychiatry 77(3):246–255, 2020 31825466

Colfax G, Santos G-M, Chu P, et al: Amphetamine-group substances and HIV. Lancet 376(9739):458–474, 2010 20650520

Colfax GN, Santos GM, Das M, et al: Mirtazapine to reduce methamphetamine use: a randomized controlled trial. Arch Gen Psychiatry 68(11):1168–1175, 2011 22065532

Connors NJ, Alsakha A, Larocque A, et al: Antipsychotics for the treatment of sympathomimetic toxicity: a systematic review. Am J Emerg Med 37(10):1880–1890, 2019 30639129

Cornish JL, Kalivas PW: Glutamate transmission in the nucleus accumbens mediates relapse in cocaine addiction. J Neurosci 20(15):RC89, 2000 10899176

Dackis C, O'Brien C: Glutamatergic agents for cocaine dependence. Ann NY Acad Sci 1003:328–345, 2003 14684456

Dackis CA, Lynch KG, Yu E, et al: Modafinil and cocaine: a double-blind, placebo-controlled drug interaction study. Drug Alcohol Depend 70(1):29–37, 2003 12681523

Dackis CA, Kampman KM, Lynch KG, et al: A double-blind, placebo-controlled trial of modafinil for cocaine dependence. Neuropsychopharmacology 30(1):205–211, 2005 15525998

Dackis CA, Kampman KM, Lynch KG, et al: A double-blind, placebo-controlled trial of modafinil for cocaine dependence. J Subst Abuse Treat 43(3):303–312, 2012 22377391

Darke S, Kaye S, Duflou J: Rates, characteristics and circumstances of methamphetamine-related death in Australia: a national 7-year study. Addiction 112(12):2191–2201, 2017 28603836

Devoto P, Flore G, Pira L, et al: Mirtazapine-induced corelease of dopamine and noradrenaline from noradrenergic neurons in the medial prefrontal and occipital cortex. Eur J Pharmacol 487(1–3):105–111, 2004 15033381

Dewey SL, Chaurasia CS, Chen CE, et al: GABAergic attenuation of cocaine-induced dopamine release and locomotor activity. Synapse 25(4):393–398, 1997 9097399

Di Ciano P, Underwood RJ, Hagan JJ, et al: Attenuation of cue-controlled cocaine-seeking by a selective D3 dopamine receptor antagonist SB-277011-A. Neuropsychopharmacology 28(2):329–338, 2003 12589386

Drouin C, Darracq L, Trovero F, et al: Alpha1b-adrenergic receptors control locomotor and rewarding effects of psychostimulants and opiates. J Neurosci 22(7):2873–2884, 2002 11923452

Duncan Z, Kippen R, Sutton K, et al: Correlates of anxiety and depression in a community cohort of people who smoke methamphetamine. Aust NZ J Psychiatry 56(8):964–973, 2022 34558302

Elkashef AM, Rawson RA, Anderson AL, et al: Bupropion for the treatment of methamphetamine dependence. Neuropsychopharmacology 33(5):1162–1170, 2008 17581531

Elkashef A, Kahn R, Yu E, et al: Topiramate for the treatment of methamphetamine addiction: a multi-center placebo-controlled trial. Addiction 107(7):1297–1306, 2012 22221594

Enghusen Poulsen H, Loft S, Andersen JR, et al: Disulfiram therapy: adverse drug reactions and interactions. Acta Psychiatr Scand Suppl 86(S369):59–65, discussion 65–66, 1992 1471554

Erb S, Hitchcott PK, Rajabi H, et al: Alpha-2 adrenergic receptor agonists block stress-induced reinstatement of cocaine seeking. Neuropsychopharmacology 23(2):138–150, 2000 10882840

Fiorentini A, Cantù F, Crisanti C, et al: Substance-induced psychoses: an updated literature review. Front Psychiatry 12:694863, 2021 35002789

Forrester JM, Steele AW, Waldron JA, et al: Crack lung: an acute pulmonary syndrome with a spectrum of clinical and histopathologic findings. Am Rev Respir Dis 142(2):462–467, 1990 2382909

Fuller RK, Branchey L, Brightwell DR, et al: Disulfiram treatment of alcoholism: a Veterans Administration cooperative study. JAMA 256(11):1449–1455, 1986 3528541

George TP, Chawarski MC, Pakes J, et al: Disulfiram versus placebo for cocaine dependence in buprenorphine-maintained subjects: a preliminary trial. Biol Psychiatry 47(12):1080–1086, 2000 10862808

Gerasimov MR, Ashby CR Jr, Gardner EL, et al: Gamma-vinyl GABA inhibits methamphetamine, heroin, or ethanol-induced increases in nucleus accumbens dopamine. Synapse 34(1):11–19, 1999 10459167

Gibbs JW III, Sombati S, DeLorenzo RJ, et al: Cellular actions of topiramate: blockade of kainate-evoked inward currents in cultured hippocampal neurons. Epilepsia 41(Suppl 1):10–16, 2000 10768293

Glasner-Edwards S, Mooney LJ: Methamphetamine psychosis: epidemiology and management. CNS Drugs 28(12):1115–1126, 2014 25373627

Goldstein M, Anagnoste B, Lauber E, et al: Inhibition of dopamine-beta-hydroxylase by disulfiram. Life Sci (1962) 3:763–767, 1964 14203977

Grabowski J, Roache JD, Schmitz JM, et al: Replacement medication for cocaine dependence: methylphenidate. J Clin Psychopharmacol 17(6):485–488, 1997 9408812

Grabowski J, Rhoades H, Silverman P, et al: Risperidone for the treatment of cocaine dependence: randomized, double-blind trial. J Clin Psychopharmacol 20(3):305–310, 2000 10831016

Grabowski J, Rhoades H, Schmitz J, et al: Dextroamphetamine for cocaine-dependence treatment: a double-blind randomized clinical trial. J Clin Psychopharmacol 21(5):522–526, 2001 11593078

Grabowski J, Rhoades H, Stotts A, et al: Agonist-like or antagonist-like treatment for cocaine dependence with methadone for heroin dependence: two double-blind randomized clinical trials. Neuropsychopharmacology 29(5):969–981, 2004 15039761

Haddjeri N, Blier P, de Montigny C: Acute and long-term actions of the antidepressant drug mirtazapine on central 5-HT neurotransmission. J Affect Disord 51(3):255–266, 1998 10333981

Hameedi FA, Rosen MI, McCance-Katz EF, et al: Behavioral, physiological, and pharmacological interaction of cocaine and disulfiram in humans. Biol Psychiatry 37(8):560–563, 1995 7619981

Hart CL, Haney M, Vosburg SK, et al: Smoked cocaine self-administration is decreased by modafinil. Neuropsychopharmacology 33(4):761–768, 2008 17568397

Havakuk O, Rezkalla SH, Kloner RA: The cardiovascular effects of cocaine. J Am Coll Cardiol 70(1):101–113, 2017 28662796

Heidbreder CA, Gardner EL, Xi ZX, et al: The role of central dopamine D3 receptors in drug addiction: a review of pharmacological evidence. Brain Res Brain Res Rev 49(1):77–105, 2005 15960988

Heinzerling KG, Swanson AN, Hall TM, et al: Randomized, placebo-controlled trial of bupropion in methamphetamine-dependent participants with less than daily methamphetamine use. Addiction 109(11):1878–1886, 2014 24894963

Higgins ST, Budney AJ, Bickel WK, et al: Incentives improve outcome in outpatient behavioral treatment of cocaine dependence. Arch Gen Psychiatry 51(7):568–576, 1994 8031230

Jayaram-Lindström N, Hammarberg A, Beck O, et al: Naltrexone for the treatment of amphetamine dependence: a randomized, placebo-controlled trial. Am J Psychiatry 165(11):1442–1448, 2008 18765480

Johnson BA, Ait-Daoud N, Wang XQ, et al: Topiramate for the treatment of cocaine addiction: a randomized clinical trial. JAMA Psychiatry 70(12):1338–1346, 2013 24132249

Kalivas PW, Volkow ND: The neural basis of addiction: a pathology of motivation and choice. Am J Psychiatry 162(8):1403–1413, 2005 16055761

Kampangkaew JP, Spellicy CJ, Nielsen EM, et al: Pharmacogenetic role of dopamine transporter (SLC6A3) variation on response to disulfiram treatment for cocaine addiction. Am J Addict 28(4):311–317, 2019 31087723

Kampman KM, Volpicelli JR, McGinnis DE, et al: Reliability and validity of the Cocaine Selective Severity Assessment. Addict Behav 23(4):449–461, 1998 9698974

Kampman KM, Alterman AI, Volpicelli JR, et al: Cocaine withdrawal symptoms and initial urine toxicology results predict treatment attrition in outpatient cocaine dependence treatment. Psychol Addict Behav 15(1):52–59, 2001 11255939

Kampman KM, Volpicelli JR, Mulvaney F, et al: Cocaine withdrawal severity and urine toxicology results from treatment entry predict outcome in medication trials for cocaine dependence. Addict Behav 27(2):251–260, 2002 11817766

Kampman KM, Pettinati H, Lynch KG, et al: A pilot trial of olanzapine for the treatment of cocaine dependence. Drug Alcohol Depend 70(3):265–273, 2003 12757964

Kampman KM, Pettinati H, Lynch KG, et al: A pilot trial of topiramate for the treatment of cocaine dependence. Drug Alcohol Depend 75(3):233–240, 2004 15283944

Kampman KM, Pettinati HM, Lynch KG, et al: A double-blind, placebo-controlled trial of topiramate for the treatment of comorbid cocaine and alcohol dependence. Drug Alcohol Depend 133(1):94–99, 2013 23810644

Kampman KM, Lynch KG, Pettinati HM, et al: A double blind, placebo controlled trial of modafinil for the treatment of cocaine dependence without co-morbid alcohol dependence. Drug Alcohol Depend 155:105–110, 2015 26320827

Karch SB, Stephens BG, Ho CH: Methamphetamine-related deaths in San Francisco: demographic, pathologic, and toxicologic profiles. J Forensic Sci 44(2):359–368, 1999 10097363

Kariisa M, Scholl L, Wilson N, et al: Drug overdose deaths involving cocaine and psychostimulants with abuse potential—United States, 2003–2017. MMWR Morb Mortal Wkly Rep 68(17):388–395, 2019 31048676

Kaye S, Darke S, Duflou J, et al: Methamphetamine-related fatalities in Australia: demographics, circumstances, toxicology and major organ pathology. Addiction 103(8):1353–1360, 2008 18855825

Kevil CG, Goeders NE, Woolard MD, et al: Methamphetamine use and cardiovascular disease. Arterioscler Thromb Vasc Biol 39(9):1739–1746, 2019 31433698

Khoshbouei H, Wang H, Lechleiter JD, et al: Amphetamine-induced dopamine efflux: a voltage-sensitive and intracellular Na+-dependent mechanism. J Biol Chem 278(14):12070–12077, 2003 12556446

Konstenius M, Jayaram-Lindström N, Beck O, et al: Sustained release methylphenidate for the treatment of ADHD in amphetamine abusers: a pilot study. Drug Alcohol Depend 108(1–2):130–133, 2010 20015599

Konstenius M, Jayaram-Lindström N, Guterstam J, et al: Methylphenidate for attention deficit hyperactivity disorder and drug relapse in criminal offenders with substance dependence: a 24-week randomized placebo-controlled trial. Addiction 109(3):440–449, 2014 24118269

Koob GF: Drug addiction: the yin and yang of hedonic homeostasis. Neuron 16(5):893–896, 1996 8630244

Koob GF: The neurobiology of addiction: a neuroadaptational view relevant for diagnosis. Addiction 101(Suppl 1):23–30, 2006 16930158

Kosten T, Oliveto A, Feingold A, et al: Desipramine and contingency management for cocaine and opiate dependence in buprenorphine maintained patients. Drug Alcohol Depend 70(3):315–325, 2003 12757969

Kosten TR, Domingo CB, Shorter D, et al: Vaccine for cocaine dependence: a randomized double-blind placebo-controlled efficacy trial. Drug Alcohol Depend 140:42–47, 2014 24793366

Kostowski W, Płaźnik A, Puciłowski O, et al: Effect of lesions of the brain noradrenergic systems on amphetamine-induced hyperthermia and locomotor stimulation. Acta Physiol Pol 33(4):383–387, 1982 7184321

Kushner SA, Dewey SL, Kornetsky C: The irreversible gamma-aminobutyric acid (GABA) transaminase inhibitor gamma-vinyl-GABA blocks cocaine self-administration in rats. J Pharmacol Exp Ther 290(2):797–802, 1999 10411594

Kuzniecky R, Hetherington H, Ho S, et al: Topiramate increases cerebral GABA in healthy humans. Neurology 51(2):627–629, 1998 9710056

Lappin JM, Darke S, Farrell M: Stroke and methamphetamine use in young adults: a review. J Neurol Neurosurg Psychiatry 88(12):1079–1091, 2017 28835475

LaRowe SD, Mardikian P, Malcolm R, et al: Safety and tolerability of N-acetylcysteine in cocaine-dependent individuals. Am J Addict 15(1):105–110, 2006 16449100

LaRowe SD, Myrick H, Hedden S, et al: Is cocaine desire reduced by N-acetylcysteine? Am J Psychiatry 164(7):1115–1117, 2007 17606664

LaRowe SD, Kalivas PW, Nicholas JS, et al: A double-blind placebo-controlled trial of N-acetylcysteine in the treatment of cocaine dependence. Am J Addict 22(5):443–452, 2013 23952889

Lee NK, Jenner L, Harney A, et al: Pharmacotherapy for amphetamine dependence: a systematic review. Drug Alcohol Depend 191:309–337, 2018 30173086

Levant B: The D3 dopamine receptor: neurobiology and potential clinical relevance. Pharmacol Rev 49(3):231–252, 1997 9311022

Levin FR, Evans SM, Brooks DJ, et al: Treatment of cocaine dependent treatment seekers with adult ADHD: double-blind comparison of methylphenidate and placebo. Drug Alcohol Depend 87(1):20–29, 2007 16930863

Levin FR, Mariani JJ, Pavlicova M, et al: Extended release mixed amphetamine salts and topiramate for cocaine dependence: a randomized clinical replication trial with frequent users. Drug Alcohol Depend 206:107700, 2020 31753736

Ling W, Chang L, Hillhouse M, et al: Sustained-release methylphenidate in a randomized trial of treatment of methamphetamine use disorder. Addiction 109(9):1489–1500, 2014 24825486

Loebl T, Angarita GA, Pachas GN, et al: A randomized, double-blind, placebo-controlled trial of long-acting risperidone in cocaine-dependent men. J Clin Psychiatry 69(3):480–486, 2008 18294021

López A, Becoña E: Depression and cocaine dependence. Psychol Rep 100(2):520–524, 2007 17564228

Malcolm RJ, Donovan CL, Devane A, et al: Influence of modafinil, 400 or 800 mg/day on subjective effects of intravenous cocaine in non-treatment seeking volunteers. Drug Alcohol Depend 66(Suppl 1):S110, 2002

Margolin A, Kosten TR, Avants SK, et al: A multicenter trial of bupropion for cocaine dependence in methadone-maintained patients. Drug Alcohol Depend 40(2):125–131, 1995 8745134

Mariani JJ, Pavlicova M, Bisaga A, et al: Extended-release mixed amphetamine salts and topiramate for cocaine dependence: a randomized controlled trial. Biol Psychiatry 72(11):950–956, 2012 22795453

Martel M, Sterzinger A, Miner J, et al: Management of acute undifferentiated agitation in the emergency department: a randomized double-blind trial of droperidol, ziprasidone, and midazolam. Acad Emerg Med 12(12):1167–1172, 2005 16282517

Martell BA, Mitchell E, Poling J, et al: Vaccine pharmacotherapy for the treatment of cocaine dependence. Biol Psychiatry 58(2):158–164, 2005 16038686

Maxwell S, Shahmanesh M, Gafos M: Chemsex behaviours among men who have sex with men: a systematic review of the literature. Int J Drug Policy 63:74–89, 2019 30513473

McCance-Katz EF, Kosten TR, Jatlow P: Disulfiram effects on acute cocaine administration. Drug Alcohol Depend 52(1):27–39, 1998 9788003

McCance-Katz EF, Kosten TA, Kosten TR: Going from the bedside back to the bench with ecopipam: a new strategy for cocaine pharmacotherapy development. Psychopharmacology (Berl) 155(4):327–329, 2001 11441421

McFarland K, Lapish CC, Kalivas PW: Prefrontal glutamate release into the core of the nucleus accumbens mediates cocaine-induced reinstatement of drug-seeking behavior. J Neurosci 23(8):3531–3537, 2003 12716962

McGregor C, Srisurapanont M, Jittiwutikarn J, et al: The nature, time course and severity of methamphetamine withdrawal. Addiction 100(9):1320–1329, 2005 16128721

Mégarbane B, Chevillard L: The large spectrum of pulmonary complications following illicit drug use: features and mechanisms. Chem Biol Interact 206(3):444–451, 2013 24144776

Miles SW, Sheridan J, Russell B, et al: Extended-release methylphenidate for treatment of amphetamine/methamphetamine dependence: a randomized, double-blind, placebo-controlled trial. Addiction 108(7):1279–1286, 2013 23297867

Mittleman MA, Mintzer D, Maclure M, et al: Triggering of myocardial infarction by cocaine. Circulation 99(21):2737–2741, 1999 10351966

Moeller FG, Schmitz JM, Steinberg JL, et al: Citalopram combined with behavioral therapy reduces cocaine use: a double-blind, placebo-controlled trial. Am J Drug Alcohol Abuse 33(3):367–378, 2007 17613964

Mooney ME, Herin DV, Schmitz JM, et al: Effects of oral methamphetamine on cocaine use: a randomized, double-blind, placebo-controlled trial. Drug Alcohol Depend 101(1–2):34–41, 2009 19058926

Mulvaney FD, Alterman AI, Boardman CR, et al: Cocaine abstinence symptomatology and treatment attrition. J Subst Abuse Treat 16(2):129–135, 1999 10023610

Nakayama K, Sakurai T, Katsu H: Mirtazapine increases dopamine release in prefrontal cortex by 5-HT1A receptor activation. Brain Res Bull 63(3):237–241, 2004 15145142

Nestler EJ: The neurobiology of cocaine addiction. Sci Pract Perspect 3(1):4–10, 2005 18552739

Newton TF, Kalechstein AD, Tervo KE, et al: Irritability following abstinence from cocaine predicts euphoric effects of cocaine administration. Addict Behav 28(4):817–821, 2003 12726795

Nonkes LJ, van Bussel IP, Verheij MM, et al: The interplay between brain 5-hydroxytryptamine levels and cocaine addiction. Behav Pharmacol 22(8):723–738, 2011 22015806

Nuijten M, Blanken P, van den Brink W, et al: Treatment of crack-cocaine dependence with topiramate: a randomized controlled feasibility trial in The Netherlands. Drug Alcohol Depend 138:177–184, 2014 24629631

Oliveto A, Poling J, Mancino MJ, et al: Randomized, double blind, placebo-controlled trial of disulfiram for the treatment of cocaine dependence in methadone-stabilized patients. Drug Alcohol Depend 113(2–3):184–191, 2011 20828943

Ozgen MH, Blume S: The continuing search for an addiction vaccine. Vaccine 37(36):5485–5490, 2019 31266675

Panenka WJ, Procyshyn RM, Lecomte T, et al: Methamphetamine use: a comprehensive review of molecular, preclinical and clinical findings. Drug Alcohol Depend 129(3):167–179, 2013 23273775

Pani PP, Trogu E, Vecchi S, et al: Antidepressants for cocaine dependence and problematic cocaine use. Cochrane Database Syst Rev (12):CD002950, 2011 22161371

Parekh JD, Jani V, Patel U, et al: Methamphetamine use is associated with increased risk of stroke and sudden cardiac death: analysis of the nationwide inpatient sample database. JACC Cardiovasc Interv 11:S29, 2018

Park WK, Bari AA, Jey AR, et al: Cocaine administered into the medial prefrontal cortex reinstates cocaine-seeking behavior by increasing AMPA receptor-mediated glutamate transmission in the nucleus accumbens. J Neurosci 22(7):2916–2925, 2002 11923456

Pergolizzi J, Breve F, Magnusson P, et al: Cocaethylene: when cocaine and alcohol are taken together. Cureus 14(2):e22498, 2022 35345678

Petrakis IL, Carroll KM, Nich C, et al: Disulfiram treatment for cocaine dependence in methadone-maintained opioid addicts. Addiction 95(2):219–228, 2000 10723850

Petroff OA, Hyder F, Mattson RH, et al: Topiramate increases brain GABA, homocarnosine, and pyrrolidinone in patients with epilepsy. Neurology 52(3):473–478, 1999 10025774

Pettinati HM, Kampman KM, Lynch KG, et al: A double blind, placebo-controlled trial that combines disulfiram and naltrexone for treating co-occurring cocaine and alcohol dependence. Addict Behav 33(5):651–667, 2008 18079068

Pirnia B, Soleimani AA, Malekanmehr P, et al: Topiramate for the treatment of dually dependent on opiates and cocaine: a single-center placebo-controlled trial. Iran J Public Health 47(9):1345–1353, 2018 30320009

Poling J, Oliveto A, Petry N, et al: Six-month trial of bupropion with contingency management for cocaine dependence in a methadone-maintained population. Arch Gen Psychiatry 63(2):219–228, 2006 16461866

Rezaei F, Ghaderi E, Mardani R, et al: Topiramate for the management of methamphetamine dependence: a pilot randomized, double-blind, placebo-controlled trial. Fundam Clin Pharmacol 30(3):282–289, 2016 26751259

Roberts DC, Andrews MM, Vickers GJ: Baclofen attenuates the reinforcing effects of cocaine in rats. Neuropsychopharmacology 15(4):417–423, 1996 8887996

Robinson TE, Berridge KC: The neural basis of drug craving: an incentive-sensitization theory of addiction. Brain Res Brain Res Rev 18(3):247–291, 1993 8401595

Robinson TE, Berridge KC: Incentive-sensitization and addiction. Addiction 96(1):103–114, 2001 11177523

Roncero C, Daigre C, Grau-López L, et al: An international perspective and review of cocaine-induced psychosis: a call to action. Subst Abus 35(3):321–327, 2014 24927026

Ronsley C, Nolan S, Knight R, et al: Treatment of stimulant use disorder: a systematic review of reviews. PLoS One 15(6):e0234809, 2020 32555667

Rothman RB, Baumann MH, Dersch CM, et al: Amphetamine-type central nervous system stimulants release norepinephrine more potently than they release dopamine and serotonin. Synapse 39(1):32–41, 2001 11071707

Ruha AM, Yarema MC: Pharmacologic treatment of acute pediatric methamphetamine toxicity. Pediatr Emerg Care 22(12):782–785, 2006 17198209

Rush CR, Stoops WW, Lile JA, et al: Topiramate-phentermine combinations reduce cocaine self-administration in humans. Drug Alcohol Depend 218:108413, 2021 33290875

Sayers SL, Campbell EC, Kondrich J, et al: Cocaine abuse in schizophrenic patients treated with olanzapine versus haloperidol. J Nerv Ment Dis 193(6):379–386, 2005 15920378

Schaiberger PH, Kennedy TC, Miller FC, et al: Pulmonary hypertension associated with long-term inhalation of "crank" methamphetamine. Chest 104(2):614–616, 1993 8101799

Schenk S, Partridge B: Sensitization and tolerance in psychostimulant self-administration. Pharmacol Biochem Behav 57(3):543–550, 1997 9218279

Schep LJ, Slaughter RJ, Beasley DMG: The clinical toxicology of metamfetamine. Clin Toxicol (Phila) 48(7):675–694, 2010 20849327

Schmidt HD, Pierce RC: Cocaine-induced neuroadaptations in glutamate transmission: potential therapeutic targets for craving and addiction. Ann N Y Acad Sci 1187:35–75, 2010 20201846

Shoptaw S, Heinzerling KG, Rotheram-Fuller E, et al: Randomized, placebo-controlled trial of bupropion for the treatment of methamphetamine dependence. Drug Alcohol Depend 96(3):222–232, 2008 18468815

Siefried KJ, Acheson LS, Lintzeris N, et al: Pharmacological treatment of methamphetamine/amphetamine dependence: a systematic review. CNS Drugs 34(4):337–365, 2020 32185696

Small AC, Kampman KM, Plebani J, et al: Tolerance and sensitization to the effects of cocaine use in humans: a retrospective study of long-term cocaine users in Philadelphia. Subst Use Misuse 44(13):1888–1898, 2009 20001286

Sofuoglu M, Sewell RA: Norepinephrine and stimulant addiction. Addict Biol 14(2):119–129, 2009 18811678

Sofuoglu M, Dudish-Poulsen S, Brown SB, et al: Association of cocaine withdrawal symptoms with more severe dependence and enhanced subjective response to cocaine. Drug Alcohol Depend 69(3):273–282, 2003 12633913

Sokoloff P, Diaz J, Le Foll B, et al: The dopamine D3 receptor: a therapeutic target for the treatment of neuropsychiatric disorders. CNS Neurol Disord Drug Targets 5(1):25–43, 2006 16613552

Stinson FS, Grant BF, Dawson DA, et al: Comorbidity between DSM-IV alcohol and specific drug use disorders in the United States: results from the National Epidemiologic Survey on Alcohol and Related Conditions. Drug Alcohol Depend 80(1):105–116, 2005 16157233

Substance Abuse and Mental Health Services Administration: Drug Abuse Warning Network, 2009: National Estimates of Drug-Related Emergency Department Visits (HHS Publ No SMA-11-4659). Rockville, MD, Substance

Abuse and Mental Health Services Administration, 2011. Available at: https://www.samhsa.gov/data/sites/default/files/DAWN2k11ED/DAWN2k11ED/DAWN2k11ED.pdf. Accessed November 26, 2012.

Substance Abuse and Mental Health Services Administration: Treatment for Stimulant Use Disorders. Treatment Improvement Protocol (TIP) Series 33 (Publ No PEP21-02-01-004). Rockville, MD, Substance Abuse and Mental Health Services Administration, 2021. Available at: https://library.samhsa.gov/sites/default/files/pep21-02-01-004.pdf. Accessed February 6, 2025.

Tang Y, Martin NL, Cotes RO: Cocaine-induced psychotic disorders: presentation, mechanism, and management. J Dual Diagn 10(2):98–105, 2014 25392252

Tardelli VS, Bisaga A, Arcadepani FB, et al: Prescription psychostimulants for the treatment of stimulant use disorder: a systematic review and meta-analysis. Psychopharmacology (Berl) 237(8):2233–2255, 2020 32601988

Touret M, Sallanon-Moulin M, Fages C, et al: Effects of modafinil-induced wakefulness on glutamine synthetase regulation in the rat brain. Brain Res Mol Brain Res 26(1–2):123–128, 1994 7854038

Treadwell SD, Robinson TG: Cocaine use and stroke. Postgrad Med 83(980):389–394, 2007 17551070

Trivedi MH, Walker R, Ling W, et al: Bupropion and naltrexone in methamphetamine use disorder. N Engl J Med 384(2):140–153, 2021 33497547

Umbricht A, DeFulio A, Winstanley EL, et al: Topiramate for cocaine dependence during methadone maintenance treatment: a randomized controlled trial. Drug Alcohol Depend 140:92–100, 2014 24814607

Uslaner J, Kalechstein A, Richter T, et al: Association of depressive symptoms during abstinence with the subjective high produced by cocaine. Am J Psychiatry 156(9):1444–1446, 1999 10484960

Volkow ND, Fowler JS, Logan J, et al: Effects of modafinil on dopamine and dopamine transporters in the male human brain: clinical implications. JAMA 301(11):1148–1154, 2009 19293415

Vongpatanasin W, Mansour Y, Chavoshan B, et al: Cocaine stimulates the human cardiovascular system via a central mechanism of action. Circulation 100(5):497–502, 1999 10430763

Vorel SR, Ashby CR Jr, Paul M, et al: Dopamine D3 receptor antagonism inhibits cocaine-seeking and cocaine-enhanced brain reward in rats. J Neurosci 22(21):9595–9603, 2002 12417684

White FJ, Kalivas PW: Neuroadaptations involved in amphetamine and cocaine addiction. Drug Alcohol Depend 51(1–2):141–153, 1998 9716936

Wise RA, Bozarth MA: Brain mechanisms of drug reward and euphoria. Psychiatr Med 3(4):445–460, 1985 2893431

Wood E, Stoltz JA, Zhang R, et al: Circumstances of first crystal methamphetamine use and initiation of injection drug use among high-risk youth. Drug Alcohol Rev 27(3):270–276, 2008 18368608

Wright C IV, Vafier JA, Lake CR: Disulfiram-induced fulminating hepatitis: guidelines for liver-panel monitoring. J Clin Psychiatry 49(11):430–434, 1988 3053669

Xi Z-X, Gilbert J, Campos AC, et al: Blockade of mesolimbic dopamine D3 receptors inhibits stress-induced reinstatement of cocaine-seeking in rats. Psychopharmacology (Berl) 176(1):57–65, 2004 15083257

Xi Z-X, Newman AH, Gilbert JG, et al: The novel dopamine D3 receptor antagonist NGB 2904 inhibits cocaine's rewarding effects and cocaine-induced reinstatement of drug-seeking behavior in rats. Neuropsychopharmacology 31(7):1393–1405, 2006 16205781

Zimmerman JL: Cocaine intoxication. Crit Care Clin 28(4):517–526, 2012 22998988

7

Sedatives, Hypnotics, or Anxiolytics

Christopher Blazes, M.D.
Stephen Leung, M.D.

Sedative medications (also known as *anxiolytics* or *tranquilizers*) are defined as any group of the CNS depressants that have been developed for the therapeutic purpose of their calming effect. Hypnotic medications induce sleep. Medications such as barbiturates and chloral hydrate are sedative-hypnotics, which were used widely in the past but have fallen out of favor because of their narrow therapeutic window. Benzodiazepine receptor agonists (BzRAs), which include benzodiazepines and the nonbenzodiazepine hypnotic medications also known as *Z drugs* (zolpidem [Ambien], eszopiclone [Lunesta], and zaleplon [Sonata]), are now the most commonly used medications in this class.

Benzodiazepines are useful and effective medications in the right circumstances and are among the most effective treatments for acute mania, agitation, and seizures (Dubovsky and Marshall 2022). They also are effective muscle relaxants. However, BzRAs are most commonly prescribed for anxiety and insomnia, for which there is limited evidence supporting their long-term efficacy (Buysse 2013; Rickels and Moeller 2019; Riemann and Perlis 2009). BzRAs are among the most commonly prescribed psychiatric medications (Moore and Mattison 2017), with one study reporting their use by more than 12% of the U.S. population between 2015 and 2016 (Maust et al. 2019).

Benzodiazepines have been prescribed predominantly by psychiatrists (16%) and primary care physicians, nurse practitioners, and physician assistants (70%) (the IQVIA National Prescription Audit, with data extracted in 2021). Of note, these data can be somewhat misleading because there are roughly 10 times as many primary care prescribers as there are psychiatrists.

Despite the dangers, benzodiazepines have been prescribed for many years, with little awareness of their negative consequences and potential for misuse. Little attention has been paid to the emerging crisis of benzodiazepine misuse, despite the fact that it has become a growing public health problem (Lembke et al. 2018).

National data suggest that the nonbenzodiazepine hypnotic Z drugs are less frequently misused than their benzodiazepine counterparts (0.5% vs. 2% reporting past-year misuse in the general population, respectively). Those who misuse Z drugs tend to be older, have less severe psychiatric symptoms, report fewer co-occurring substance use issues, and report use more specifically tied to sleep difficulties relative to those who misuse benzodiazepines (McHugh et al. 2023).

Historical Perspective

In 1955, Leo Sternbach (Hoffman-La Roche Pharmaceuticals) serendipitously synthesized the first benzodiazepine, chlordiazepoxide. Following on the heels of that discovery, Hoffmann-La Roche subsequently introduced diazepam in 1960 (Lader 1991; Wick 2013). This compound was found to be very effective as an anxiolytic, as an agent to induce sleep (hypnotic), and as a muscle relaxant. Hoffmann-La Roche continued to experiment on similar compounds and subsequently developed diazepam under the brand name Valium in 1963. Contemporaneously, the deaths of Judy Garland and Marilyn Monroe were attributed to barbiturate overdoses in the 1960s, with widespread media coverage (Wick 2013). Benzodiazepines were heavily marketed as being less toxic and less likely to cause dependence than other medications that were available at that time, most specifically barbiturates.

These medications emerged at a time when direct-to-prescriber marketing strategies were used heavily by pharmaceutical companies to enhance the sales of their products. Benzodiazepines were marketed to physicians as being safe and effective for treating the everyday stressors of life (Wick 2013), which may have contributed to pathologizing normal conditions. They were also heavily marketed to the psychoanalytic community as an effective way to deepen the therapeutic alliance. These factors contributed to perceived low risk associated with benzodiazepine use. Furthermore, benzodiazepines were classified by the U.S. Drug Enforcement Administration as Schedule IV controlled substances (low potential for abuse, low potential for dependence), which further supported the industry claims of relatively low risk for misuse. These standards of scheduling and regulation are consistent even outside of the United States. To this day, benzodiazepines remain Schedule IV agents.

In 2020, however, the FDA released a Drug Safety Communication mandating that all benzodiazepine package inserts include a boxed warning acknowledging "serious risks of abuse, addiction, physical dependence, and withdrawal reactions" (U.S. Food and Drug Administration 2020). Those with a history of other substance use disorders (SUDs) are at a particularly high risk for misuse of benzodiazepines (Licata and Rowlett 2008).

Pharmacology and Neurobiology

Nonbenzodiazepine Hypnotic Medications

BzRAs bind to the GABA type A receptor ($GABA_A$) and act as positive allosteric modulators increasing receptor affinity for GABA. Although benzodiazepines and Z drugs share this fundamental mechanism of action, they are chemically distinct; in addition, although Z drugs are noted to perhaps have lower risk of physiological dependence and addiction (Chiaro et al. 2018; Ebbens and Verster 2010; Schifano et al. 2019), withdrawal effects (including seizures) and cases of addiction have nonetheless been reported (Barbosa Eyler and Utria Castro. 2021; Cubała and Landowski 2007; Victorri-Vigneau et al. 2014), but typically in patients who have been taking high dosages (e.g., zolpidem 450–600 mg/day). Perhaps related to their unique chemical structure and consequent interactions at the benzodiazepine receptor binding sites, Z drugs can potentially cause rare side effects such as fugue states (especially zolpidem), hallucinations, and amnesia (Stone et al. 2008; Toner et al. 2000; Yang et al. 2005). Furthermore, limited data suggest that in high doses, zolpidem may have a paradoxical euphoric stimulatory effect in some individuals (Lyu et al. 2022; Sabe et al. 2019).

The literature on Z drug misuse is comparatively scant relative to that of benzodiazepines. Recent data suggested a potential uptick in Z drug use, especially zolpidem, during the COVID-19 pandemic (both in the United States and internationally), possibly due to consequent increases in anxiety and insomnia during that period (de Lima et al. 2024). Nonetheless, in clinical practice, the treatment approach for Z drug misuse or use disorder is similar to that for benzodiazepines. Therefore, the majority of this chapter focuses more specifically on benzodiazepine misuse and treatment approaches.

Benzodiazepines

The term *benzodiazepine* refers to agents with a structural core consisting of a benzene ring fused to a diazepine ring. Variations on the benzodiazepine ring structure have produced the triazolo (e.g., alprazolam, triazolam, estazolam), 2-keto (e.g., diazepam), 3-hydroxy (e.g., lorazepam, oxazepam), and imidazo (e.g., midazolam) agents that produce similar clinical actions: sedative, hypnotic, anxiolytic, muscle relaxant, and anticonvulsant effects.

Benzodiazepines change the receptor conformation to allow increased frequency of chloride ion channel opening, thereby enhancing the inhibitory effect of GABA. Barbiturates, by comparison, increase the duration of chloride ion channel opening when GABA is bound (Miller and Aricescu 2014). Activation of $GABA_A$ receptors, which are ligand-gated ion channels, leads to hyperpolarization and inhibition of neurotransmission (Sigel and Ernst 2018).

The $GABA_A$ receptor is a heteropentameric protein composed of different subunit families (α_{1-6}, β_{1-3}, γ_{1-3}, δ, ε, θ, π, and ρ_{1-3}; Olsen 2018) (Figure 7.1). The benzodiazepine-specific $GABA_A$ receptor is typically composed of two α subunits, two β subunits, and a γ subunit. GABA binds at the interface between α and β subunits. Benzodiazepines and Z drugs have specific binding sites at the interface between α and γ subunits. The sedative effects of benzodiazepines are associated with the presence of α_1 subunits in the

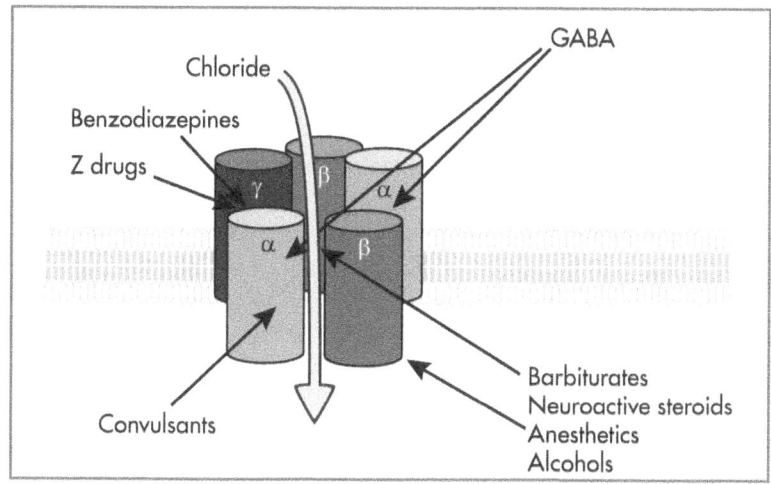

Figure 7.1 Model GABA$_A$ receptor showing drug binding sites.

GABA$_A$ receptor structure (the GABA$_{A1}$ receptor subtype) (McKernan et al. 2000), and the presence of α_2 units in this receptor may be required for the antianxiety effect (Löw et al. 2000). The Z drugs (Pritchett and Seeburg 1990; Sanna et al. 2002) bind to GABA$_{A1}$ receptors more selectively, permitting them to act as hypnotic agents that, compared with benzodiazepines, are less likely to produce antianxiety and anticonvulsant effects.

Chronic BzRA exposure results in complex neuronal adaptations that include the downregulation of the number and function of GABA$_A$ receptors, as well as opponent processes such as compensatory glutamatergic potentiation (Allison and Pratt 2003; Barnes 1996). The end result is decreased endogenous GABA activity and increased excitability of the glutamate system. These neuroadaptations represent a new homeostasis as the body tries to overcome the CNS-depressant effects of the drug and are the root cause of tolerance, dependence, and withdrawal (Allison and Pratt 2003; Bateson 2002; Wafford 2005).

It is important to differentiate physiological dependence from SUD (detailed later in "Substance Use Disorder Presentation"). Physiological dependence is a condition caused by chronic use of a tolerance-forming drug, in which abrupt or gradual drug withdrawal causes unpleasant physical symptoms. Physiological dependence on benzodiazepines has been known to occur rapidly with regular use (Pétursson 1994) and can happen with low-dose benzodiazepine use as well as in high therapeutic dose ranges (Rickels et al. 1986). Factors that may be predictive of withdrawal severity include shorter elimination half-life and higher potency (Wolf and Griffiths 1991), as in the specific case of alprazolam, which has been shown to produce dependence in 7 days (Ait-Daoud et al. 2018). Specific dose ranges at which different benzodiazepines will produce tolerance and withdrawal have not been elucidated in humans, because of the heterogeneity of existing data (Vinkers and Olivier 2012) and significant variations in how individuals respond to benzodiazepines (Busto and Sellers 1991).

Tolerance has been shown to develop within days to weeks of initiation of use (Committee on the Review of Medicines 1980). In 1991, the American Psychiatric Association Benzodiazepine Dependence, Toxicity, and Abuse Task Force concluded that tolerance was probably more pronounced for the anticonvulsant and sedative-hypnotic effects than for the anxiolytic effects, and the report described that it would be unusual for patients with anxiety disorders to incrementally increase their daily dose (Salzman 1991). In clinical practice, whether tolerance is truly dissociable between the anticonvulsant, sedative-hypnotic, and anxiolytic effects of benzodiazepines is unclear. Many patients, for instance, may be prescribed benzodiazepines for anxiety but, in fact, are more likely seeking the hypnotic effect to relieve restlessness, irritability, or agitation.

Because physiological dependence can develop so quickly, it has been recommended that benzodiazepines (even at a low dosage) be prescribed for a maximum of 7–14 days to minimize the risk (Meier et al. 1988; National Institute for Health and Care Excellence 2022). Despite this knowledge, long-term use of benzodiazepines increased from 1999 to 2014, with approximately 80% of BzRA prescription recipients reporting medium (6–24 months) or long-term (>24 months) use (Kaufmann et al. 2018).

The onset of action for oral benzodiazepines is first determined by the rate of absorption from the gastrointestinal tract, and the duration of action is determined by lipid solubility and rate of clearance (Greenblatt et al. 1990). Benzodiazepines are, as a class, lipophilic, and the rapidity of onset of clinical effects is determined by how quickly they cross the blood–brain barrier. Diazepam, for example, is more lipophilic than other benzodiazepines and therefore has a quicker onset of action than alprazolam, although the latter is notorious for a more severe withdrawal syndrome, partially because of its shorter half-life and consequently a more aggressive rebound syndrome (Ait-Daoud et al. 2018). Once equilibration is achieved between the brain concentration and systemic circulation, the brain concentration remains proportional to the protein-unbound plasma concentration until the agent is metabolized and cleared. Withdrawal symptoms are more likely to occur on discontinuation of short-half-life benzodiazepines (Greenblatt et al. 1990).

Most benzodiazepines first undergo oxidative metabolism through the hepatic microsomal system, followed by glucuronide conjugation, although some noteworthy metabolic differences between benzodiazepines exist. Oxidative metabolism involves N-dealkylation or aliphatic hydroxylation. Cytochrome P450 (CYP) 3A4 mediates the metabolism of several benzodiazepines, including triazolam, alprazolam, and midazolam. Of clinical significance, however, oxazepam, temazepam, and lorazepam are solely metabolized through glucuronidation and are thus less affected by impairments in oxidative metabolism due to age, disease (e.g., cirrhosis), or drug–drug interactions resulting from competition for hepatic oxidative resources.

Commonly used benzodiazepines and Z drugs are outlined in Table 7.1. It is difficult to rank the addictive potential of the various benzodiazepines and Z drugs, although diazepam, lorazepam, and alprazolam have been associated with higher rates of misuse (Griffiths and Wolf 1990; Votaw et al. 2019).

Intoxication Presentation

Benzodiazepine intoxication is marked by sedation and CNS depression. Some patients may exhibit a paradoxical reaction to benzodiazepines, which manifests as behavioral disinhibition, hyperactivity, or outright agitation. There are few pathognomonic signs of benzodiazepine intoxication beyond the hallmark features of CNS depression, but patients can also present with diplopia, dysarthria, and ataxia (Gaudreault et al. 1991). The severity of impaired consciousness can vary widely based on the amount and type of benzodiazepine ingested as well as the presence of additional CNS depressants (e.g., alcohol, Z drugs, and opioids). The clinical features of an isolated benzodiazepine overdose are usually mild, and supportive therapy is sufficient in most cases (Busto et al. 1980). Therefore, the severely obtunded, comatose, or medically unstable patient warrants a thorough evaluation

Table 7.1 Approximate oral benzodiazepine receptor agonist dose equivalency

Generic name	Trade name	Dose (mg), equal to phenobarbital 30 mg	Therapeutic dose range (mg/d)	Half-life (active metabolite) (h)
Alprazolam	Xanax	1	0.75–6	12–15 (1)
Chlordiazepoxide	Librium	25–50	15–100	5–30 (36–200)
Clonazepam	Klonopin	0.5–1	0.5–4	19–60
Clorazepate	Tranxene	7.5–15	15–60	2–2.5 (≤200)
Diazepam	Valium	10	4–40	20–100 (36–200)
Flurazepam	Dalmane	15	15–30	2–3 (25–100)
Lorazepam	Ativan	2	1–6	10–20
Oxazepam	Serax	10–30	10–120	7–20
Temazepam	Restoril	15–20	15–30	7–14 (4–15)
Triazolam	Halcion	0.25	0.125–0.5	2–4
Eszopiclone	Lunesta	2[a]	1–3	4–8
Zolpidem	Ambien	20[a]	5–10	2–4
Zaleplon	Sonata	20[a]	5–20	1–2

Source. Adapted from Ashton (2005); Baldwin (2021); Lader (2011); Sadock et al. (2015); Smith and Wesson (2004); Soyka (2017).
[a]Phenobarbital equivalence has not been demonstrated for the Z drugs; the listed doses are approximately equivalent to diazepam 10 mg.

for additional toxidromes beyond isolated benzodiazepine intoxication. Stabilization of the patient's airway, breathing, and circulation should not be delayed. Endotracheal intubation and supplemental oxygen may be necessary.

In most situations, information gathered from the patient or through collateral sources will implicate benzodiazepines as the culprit for intoxication. The index of suspicion should be raised if the patient has a history of anxiety or if a prescription drug monitoring program query reveals concerning benzodiazepine prescriptions. A urine drug screen should be ordered, but results may be falsely negative depending on the type of benzodiazepine ingested. Routine benzodiazepine immunoassays often do not detect alprazolam, lorazepam, and clonazepam (Owen et al. 2012). Z drugs are detected in urine only by mass spectroscopy (Gunja 2013).

Flumazenil is a competitive antagonist at the $GABA_A$ benzodiazepine receptor that can reverse benzodiazepine-induced sedation (An and Godwin 2016). Experts discourage the use of flumazenil in the so-called "coma cocktail," given the risk of precipitating benzodiazepine withdrawal and seizures (Sivilotti 2016). Flumazenil-induced seizures may be difficult to treat, because the flumazenil itself would render subsequently administered benzodiazepines ineffective as anticonvulsants. Flumazenil is typically reserved for the reversal of iatrogenic oversedation from benzodiazepines during medical procedures and in cases of accidental pediatric ingestion. In addition, optimal dosing of flumazenil is unclear, with some suggesting that the manufacturer-recommended dosing of 0.2 mg given over 15 seconds might be overly aggressive. An alternative dosing regimen has been proposed of flumazenil 0.01 mg/kg over 1 minute in sequential dosing to a maximum of 1 mg or until the desired effects have been achieved or toxicity has emerged (An and Godwin 2016). A patient who requires resuscitation is likely to have used other substances, and the pharmacological reversal of other potential overdoses (i.e., opioids) should take precedence.

Withdrawal Presentation

Acute Withdrawal

Abrupt discontinuation of benzodiazepines produces a state of hyperexcitability in the CNS, which can manifest as an acute withdrawal syndrome akin to alcohol withdrawal (MacKinnon and Parker 1982). Withdrawal symptoms can also emerge when benzodiazepine doses are rapidly reduced after long-term treatment. Severe withdrawal syndromes can occur from discontinuation or gradual reduction from even low doses of benzodiazepines (Lader 1987). Mild benzodiazepine withdrawal symptoms include depression, anxiety, insomnia, dizziness, headache, anorexia, hyperacusis, and photophobia (MacKinnon and Parker 1982; Marriott and Tyrer 1993). Severe symptoms include nausea, vomiting, vertigo, sweating, tremor, tachycardia, muscle twitches and spasms, seizures, confusion, psychosis, and hallucinations (Pétursson 1994). Some withdrawal symptoms, such as anxiety and insomnia, are often more severe than pretreatment and are likely related to a rebound phenomenon, thus complicating the picture. This increased severity has also been shown to happen as a result of tolerance during the course of treatment.

The onset of benzodiazepine withdrawal is highly variable. Symptoms have been shown to occur within 24 hours on discontinuation of short-acting benzodiazepines, with longer-acting benzodiazepines demonstrating a lag period of up to 7 days before onset of withdrawal symptoms. A review of alprazolam (a short-acting benzodiazepine) demonstrated that the withdrawal syndrome associated with alprazolam discontinuation tends to be more severe than other benzodiazepine withdrawal syndromes, even when alprazolam is carefully tapered (Ait-Daoud et al. 2018). Various studies reviewed by Ait-Daoud et al. suggest a more complicated rebound anxiety (at times, more severe than pretreatment anxiety), dissociation, delirium, and suicidal and homicidal ideation. The severity of alprazolam withdrawal may require ICU-level care because of hyperadrenergic states, with some case reports of symptoms refractory to treatment with other benzodiazepines owing to incomplete cross-tolerance (Sachdev et al. 2014).

It is also important that clinicians are aware of the kindling effect, which is postulated to happen with repeated episodes of withdrawal from benzodiazepines. *Kindling* describes a physiological sensitization that happens with repeated episodes of withdrawal. With each cessation attempt, individuals have increased neuroexcitability and are at higher risk for experiencing more severe withdrawal symptoms (Allison and Pratt 2003). The mechanism of the kindling effect is currently not well understood. The glutamate system has been implicated, with 2-amino-3-hydroxy-5-methyl-4-isoxazolepropionic acid receptors, a subtype of glutamate receptors, being altered by repeated withdrawals from benzodiazepines (Allison and Pratt 2003). Although the kindling effect is widely accepted to exist within alcohol withdrawal, this effect may in fact be even more prominent with benzodiazepines, in our experience. Patients who misuse benzodiazepines or take more than prescribed may be frequently experiencing mild withdrawal phenomena, thus increasing the risk of more severe withdrawal over time.

Pseudowithdrawal

Pseudowithdrawal symptoms from benzodiazepines are defined as symptoms occurring when patients begin to exhibit minor withdrawal symptoms without any changes to their overall dose (Ashton 1991). This phenomenon was initially described in double-blind studies in which study participants believed they were randomly assigned to receive a dose reduction when, in reality, their dose was maintained (Winokur and Rickels 1981). The etiology for pseudowithdrawal is likely multifactorial, with anticipatory anxiety playing a role. Patients taking short-acting benzodiazepines may also be prone to experiencing "miniwithdrawal" between doses characterized by increasing anxiety, panic, and cravings (Ashton 1984). Highly anxious or neurotic patients may be hyperaware of their internal bodily sensations and misinterpret these as withdrawal symptoms, when somatic preoccupation may be a more accurate description.

Postacute Withdrawal Syndrome

After resolution of acute benzodiazepine withdrawal, many patients will go on to develop a *postacute withdrawal syndrome* that can last for weeks to months. This syndrome is also referred to as *postwithdrawal syndrome, prolonged withdrawal syndrome,* or *protracted withdrawal syndrome*. A follow-up study of patients successfully treated for benzodiazepine dependence showed that symptoms may persist after 1–5 years (Golombok et al. 1987), consistent with historical observations (Ashton 1991; Smith and Wesson 1983). Benzodiazepine postacute withdrawal syndrome has not been well documented in the literature, perhaps because of the heterogeneity of its presentation and lack of incentives guiding research in this area. It has long been established that benzodiazepines can produce a protracted withdrawal syndrome characterized by persistent anxiety, depression, tinnitus, paresthesia, nonspecific motor symptoms, and irritable bowel symptoms (Ashton 1991). Subtle diminishment of cognitive function (referred to colloquially as "benzo brain"), poor frustration tolerance, insomnia, and irritability are also commonly reported. The symptoms are also known to wax and wane in severity, and they can also completely resolve and reoccur during periods of stress, thus sometimes leading to new potential misdiagnoses. The severity of this protracted withdrawal syndrome seems to be associated with a prolonged duration of treatment with benzodiazepines, as well as with shorter-acting and higher-potency benzodiazepines (Cosci and Chouinard 2020). In our experience, benzodiazepine postacute withdrawal syndrome is the rule rather than the exception, and treatment with anticonvulsants may have benefit. We recommend educating patients about the protracted withdrawal course and providing reassurance that "this too shall pass" with extended abstinence.

Pharmacological Management of Intoxication and Withdrawal

Outpatient Management

Outpatient management of benzodiazepine withdrawal is focused on gradual tapering of long-standing benzodiazepines. Benzodiazepine tapers can be an arduous process for both patient and clinician. It is important to set expectations early regarding the estimated length of the taper as well as the high likelihood of rebound phenomenon and withdrawal symptoms. Even with careful tapering and treatment with ancillary medications, a certain level of distress is to be expected, and patients should be encouraged to contact their providers in between appointments with questions and concerns. Throughout the duration of outpatient treatment, the clinician should evaluate the patient's clinical progress and be vigilant for signs and symptoms that may warrant a higher level of care. Medical and psychiatric emergencies should be triaged and referred to the appropriate levels of care. Warning signs include ongoing benzodiazepine use, new illicit substance use, worsening depression, and emergence of suicidal thinking.

Taper

For patients who have been chronically using long-acting benzodiazepines (e.g., clonazepam, diazepam, chlordiazepoxide), we recommend directly tapering the benzodiazepine that they are taking. This is the most intuitive approach, and patients may be more comfortable sticking to the benzodiazepine they are familiar with.

A slow and gradual taper may mitigate the emergence of withdrawal symptoms. There is no consensus regarding the optimal pace of a benzodiazepine taper (Soyka 2017). A 10%–25% daily dose reduction every 1–2 weeks is reasonable and allows for flexibility. Whenever possible, consider tapering daytime doses before nighttime doses to mitigate rebound insomnia. Clinical experience shows that patients are able to tolerate more aggressive dose reductions at the beginning of the taper; a taper deceleration may be needed toward the second half as withdrawal symptoms emerge. Flexibility is key, and sometimes a short pause in the taper is warranted if the patient becomes severely symptomatic or if there are new stressors in the patient's life (e.g., unexpected loss, unemployment, relationship turmoil, medical illness).

Switch and Taper

For patients who have been chronically using short-acting benzodiazepines (e.g., alprazolam, lorazepam) or multiple benzodiazepines, it may be advantageous to first switch and consolidate to a long-acting benzodiazepine in divided doses. Although there are no high-quality studies that evaluate this approach, long-acting benzodiazepines have more predictable effects after achieving steady state and are more conducive to tapering in our experience.

Once a thorough quantification of the patient's daily benzodiazepine intake has been completed, the patient's approximate daily benzodiazepine requirement can be determined using Table 7.1. Note that dose equivalence will vary individually, and some patients may require more or less than the approximated dose from Table 7.1, especially if consolidating across multiple benzodiazepines or illicit benzodiazepines with impurities. Once the patient's symptoms have been stabilized on a standing dosage of a single long-acting benzodiazepine (e.g., clonazepam, diazepam, chlordiazepoxide) taken in divided doses, a fixed-dose taper can be started with the same principles outlined earlier in this section.

Some patients may benefit from initiating antiepileptics or α_2-agonists at points during the taper to mitigate withdrawal symptoms that emerge. The use of these agents is discussed in the following sections.

Inpatient Management

In cases of severe sedative-hypnotic use disorders, failed outpatient tapers, high medical complexity, high risk of complex withdrawal, or co-occurring

SUDs, inpatient treatment with closer monitoring may be appropriate. Clinicians should be aware of previous episodes of sedative-hypnotic withdrawal before initiating a taper or detoxification protocol, because the kindling effect can predispose the patient to a more complicated course. Prescribers should also be very mindful of prescribing benzodiazepines to patients who have had a previous history of tolerance or withdrawal, because subsequent withdrawals might be more complicated.

More rapid tapers (i.e., 20%–25% reduction every 4 days; see Harada et al. 2024) and the use of adjunct antiepileptics can be conducted in residential or hospitalized settings. Inpatient withdrawal management protocols for benzodiazepine detoxification administered at either hospital-based or inpatient detoxification facilities vary significantly, depending on the facility and the comfort of the practitioners. Lorazepam is commonly used in ICUs and when treating patients with significant active medical comorbidities, because it is shorter-acting, is available in intravenous form, and has no active metabolites, making it more easily titratable. Long-acting benzodiazepines such as chlordiazepoxide and diazepam are commonly used in the residential setting; they have the benefit of requiring less frequent dosing and may be self-tapering because of their long half-lives and active metabolites.

In the inpatient setting, we recommend implementing Clinical Institute Withdrawal Assessment for Alcohol—Revised (CIWA-Ar) or Clinical Institute Withdrawal Assessment for Benzodiazepines (CIWA-B) protocols for more frequent monitoring of vital signs and clinical status. The CIWA-B has been studied as a variation of the CIWA-Ar for the specific monitoring of benzodiazepine withdrawal (Busto et al. 1989), although its usefulness may be limited because of lack of staff familiarity with the protocol. Although symptom-triggered approaches are generally superior to fixed-dose approaches to the treatment of alcohol withdrawal (Saitz et al. 1994), either approach is reasonable for the treatment of benzodiazepine withdrawal. A randomized trial of 44 patients comparing symptom-triggered diazepam tapering with fixed-dose diazepam tapering in an inpatient setting revealed similar outcomes in withdrawal severity, duration of inpatient treatment, amount of diazepam administered, attrition from treatment, and benzodiazepine use 1 month postdischarge (McGregor et al. 2003).

Phenobarbital is a long-acting barbiturate that was studied for the treatment of barbiturate dependence (Smith and Wesson 1971) and subsequently used in the treatment of benzodiazepine withdrawal, especially in the setting of benzodiazepine polydrug combinations and high-dose benzodiazepine dependence (Landry et al. 1992; Smith and Wesson 1983). Researchers proposed converting the patient's estimated daily use of all sedative-hypnotics to phenobarbital equivalents, up to a maximum of phenobarbital 500 mg/day, and stabilization with phenobarbital divided doses three to four times per day, followed by a taper of 30 mg/day. They recommended checking for three features of intoxication: sustained horizontal nystagmus, slurred speech, and ataxia. Scheduled doses of phenobarbital were withheld in the presence of nystagmus. If all three features of intoxication were present, two doses of phenobarbital were withheld and the total daily dose of phenobarbital was reduced by 50% the following day.

There have been data suggesting that phenobarbital improves certain outcomes in severe alcohol withdrawal, including decreased number of ICU days, hospital length of stay, ventilator use, and antipsychotic use (Nelson et al. 2019; Tidwell et al. 2018). Given the pathophysiological similarities between alcohol and benzodiazepine withdrawal states, phenobarbital would appear to be an attractive candidate for the treatment of severe benzodiazepine withdrawal. Anecdotally, we have observed that more and more residential facilities are developing comfort with and having success using phenobarbital.

There have been no high-quality trials that examined phenobarbital in this capacity, and therefore, no optimal phenobarbital protocol exists for benzodiazepine withdrawal. A retrospective medical record review of 310 patients treated with a 3-day fixed-dose phenobarbital taper for benzodiazepine dependence at Johns Hopkins Bayview Medical Center demonstrated safety and efficacy (Kawasaki et al. 2012). The 3-day phenobarbital taper begins with an initial dose of 200 mg, followed by 100 mg every 4 hours for five doses, 60 mg every 4 hours for four doses, and 60 mg every 8 hours for three doses. The standardized protocol does not require conversion of sedative-hypnotic doses to phenobarbital equivalents. Instead, trained nurses from the dedicated detoxification unit hold doses for sedation—at least one dose of phenobarbital was held in 25.8% of admissions, which was more common among those receiving methadone or buprenorphine for opioid detoxification. Notably, delirium occurred in only 1% of patients, and no seizures occurred during treatment despite 13.9% of patients having a history of seizures. One of the main advantages of this protocol is that phenobarbital did not have to be dose adjusted for those receiving buprenorphine or methadone; in addition, despite phenobarbital's induction of CYP, no increases in methadone maintenance doses were required.

Adjunctive Medication Strategies

No medications have been approved by the FDA for benzodiazepine dependence or withdrawal symptom management, and use of the medications described in this section is considered off-label. Many belong to the anticonvulsant class, which has been more extensively studied for the treatment of alcohol withdrawal (Hammond et al. 2015) and may have some analogous benefit as adjunctive treatment for benzodiazepine withdrawal. To minimize polypharmacy, we recommend gradually tapering off all off-label medications on symptom resolution or finding the lowest effective dose that prevents symptom recurrence.

Carbamazepine

Carbamazepine causes inhibition of action potentials and decreased synaptic transmission through modulation of voltage-gated sodium channels (Maan et al. 2021). Potential downstream mechanisms of carbamazepine pertinent to benzodiazepine withdrawal include GABAergic activity and blockade of *N*-methyl-D-aspartate receptors (Barrons and Roberts 2010). In an open-label study of nine patients with benzodiazepine dependence, carbamazepine was started at 200 mg bid and titrated up to 600–800 mg/day in an inpatient setting either before or during abrupt discontinuation of long-standing benzodiazepines (Ries et al. 1989). Before treatment, five patients were using alprazolam 1.5–15 mg/day, whereas the remaining four patients were using long-acting benzodiazepines ranging from diazepam 20 mg/day to chlordiazepoxide 2,000 mg/day. Although the study was small and nonblinded, all patients were successfully detoxified off benzodiazepines, with no significant withdrawal symptoms or rescue doses of benzodiazepines required.

In a double-blind, randomized, placebo-controlled trial of 40 patients, carbamazepine started at 200 mg bid and titrated up to 800 mg/day during an outpatient benzodiazepine taper (25% per week) was associated with significantly more patients free of benzodiazepines 5 weeks posttaper (Schweizer et al. 1991). Only patients taking lorazepam, diazepam, or alprazolam totaling up to 40 mg/day diazepam equivalents were included.

Patients randomly assigned to carbamazepine reported less-severe withdrawal symptoms, although the difference was not statistically significant. Carbamazepine was abruptly discontinued 2–4 weeks after the completion of the benzodiazepine taper, although we generally recommend that anticonvulsants be gradually tapered to discontinuation. Attention should be paid to carbamazepine's autoinduction of CYP, drug–drug interactions (including oral contraceptives and warfarin), black box warnings on agranulocytosis, and Category D teratogenic effects.

Valproate

The antiepileptic action of valproate is attributable to blockage of voltage-dependent sodium currents (Löscher 2002). There is evidence that valproate potentiates GABAergic functions, and it also has effects on neuronal excitation mediated by the N-methyl-D-aspartate subtype of glutamate receptors (Löscher 2002). A small double-blind, placebo-controlled trial showed that treatment with valproate (divalproex sodium 500–2,500 mg/day) before an outpatient benzodiazepine taper (25% per week) significantly improved rates of taper completion and benzodiazepine abstinence at 5 weeks (Rickels et al. 1999). There was no significant improvement in benzodiazepine withdrawal severity. Potential adverse reactions included hepatitis, pancreatitis, and myelosuppression. Because of the risk of neural tube defects, valproate should not be used in pregnancy, and alternatives should be considered in people who may become pregnant.

Gabapentin and Pregabalin

Gabapentin and pregabalin are structurally related to GABA and exhibit inhibitory effects on voltage-gated calcium channels at the $\alpha_2\delta_1$ subunit, resulting in decreased neurotransmitter release and attenuation of postsynaptic excitability (Sills 2006). Neither gabapentin nor pregabalin binds directly to GABA receptors, although gabapentin has been shown to have GABAergic effects. Gabapentin and pregabalin are not hepatically metabolized and can be used for patients with renal impairment as long as they are renally dosed.

There has been growing evidence supporting the use of gabapentin in the treatment of alcohol withdrawal and alcohol use disorder (Leung et al. 2018; Mason et al. 2014; Myrick et al. 2009). Although the use of gabapentin for benzodiazepine withdrawal has been limited to case reports (Crockford et al. 2001), the similarity between alcohol and benzodiazepine withdrawal pathophysiology, combined with gabapentin's relatively safe profile, makes it a useful adjunct medication. We recommend starting gabapentin 600–900 mg/day in two to three divided doses. For more severe withdrawal, the total daily dosage can be increased by 300 mg every 1–2 days, up to 1,800 mg/day. Larger doses at bedtime may help with sleep.

Pregabalin is an effective first-line treatment for generalized anxiety disorder (Slee et al. 2019) in Europe, but it is limited to off-label use in this capacity within the United States, where it is a Schedule V controlled substance (U.S. Drug Enforcement Administration 2005). A small case series and a small open-label study found that pregabalin dosages of 225–900 mg/day were effective in the treatment of benzodiazepine withdrawal and dependence (Oulis and Konstantakopoulos 2010). In a double-blind, placebo-controlled trial, a nonsignificantly higher proportion of patients treated with pregabalin remained benzodiazepine free (Hadley et al. 2012). However, that study was underpowered because of the high attrition rate, and study participants were switched from their long-term benzodiazepines to alprazolam (contrary to conventional tapering strategies outlined earlier in this section).

Both gabapentin and pregabalin have been shown to enhance the euphoria of opioids including buprenorphine (Baird et al. 2014) and to increase the risk of opioid overdose and other opioid-related adverse events (Gomes et al. 2017). Therefore, these medications should be used with caution in patients who are taking opioids, including buprenorphine. Their abuse potential appears to be very limited outside concomitant use of opioids (Bonnet and Scherbaum 2017), but case reports have described both gabapentinoid-related SUDs and withdrawal syndromes (Mersfelder and Nichols 2016).

Oxcarbazepine

As a structural analog to carbamazepine, oxcarbazepine also blocks sodium channels, but it modulates calcium channels differently, is not a potent inducer of CYP, and overall has a more favorable side-effect profile (Beydoun et al. 2020). Oxcarbazepine has been hypothesized to reduce glutamatergic transmission (Koethe et al. 2007). In a small case series of 10 patients undergoing rapid inpatient benzodiazepine detoxification, oxcarbazepine was started at 150 mg and titrated up to 1,200 mg/day over 12 days while diazepam was simultaneously tapered (Croissant et al. 2008). Before treatment, participants reported using an average of 91 mg/day of diazepam equivalents (SD = 100.5 mg/day). For patients with low-dose diazepam dependence (≤30 mg/day), diazepam was tapered by 5 mg/day every 2 days. For patients with high-dose diazepam dependence (>30 mg/day), diazepam was tapered by 25% every 2 days until reaching 30 mg/day, at which point they were switched to the low-dose taper. All patients were successfully detoxified without withdrawal symptoms.

Propranolol

A small double-blind, placebo-controlled study of 40 patients evaluating propranolol (20–40 mg tid) for benzodiazepine withdrawal did not demonstrate any significant benefit (Tyrer et al. 1981). Another small double-blind, placebo-controlled study of 31 patients found that abrupt benzodiazepine discontinuation with propranolol treatment (40 mg tid) was significantly worse than a gradual benzodiazepine taper (Cantopher et al. 1990). It is unsurprising that propranolol failed to demonstrate any benefit in both of these studies when benzodiazepines were abruptly discontinued and substituted with propranolol, because they share no similarities in their mechanism of action. Propranolol should not be used as monotherapy for benzodiazepine withdrawal, and there are no high-quality studies that have evaluated propranolol as an adjunct to a gradual benzodiazepine taper or another taper strategy.

Clonidine

Clonidine, an α_2-agonist, is well suited to be used as an adjunctive treatment for benzodiazepine or alcohol withdrawal. Clonidine directly addresses the hyperadrenergic pathophysiological state of withdrawal by decreasing norepinephrine release and noradrenergic tone (Muzyk et al. 2011). It has had mixed results in the treatment of benzodiazepine withdrawal. Initial case reports demonstrated success (Ashton 1984; Keshavan and Crammer 1985; Vinogradov et al. 1986), but the benefits were not replicated in subsequent studies (Fyer et al. 1988; Joyce et al. 1990). Although withdrawal or panic symptoms were still prominent despite clonidine treatment, Fyer et al. (1988) noted that alprazolam was successfully tapered off for 9 of 12 patients—a higher success rate than that in a previous study by the same group without adjunctive clonidine (Fyer et al. 1987). Joyce et al. (1990) postulated that clonidine may be useful in withdrawal states marked by significant anxiety, which has been our experience as well.

Despite inconclusive evidence of clonidine's efficacy for benzodiazepine withdrawal, no serious adverse events were reported in the aforementioned studies. Thus, clonidine remains a relatively safe medication, provided blood pressure can be carefully monitored for hypotension. In our experience, clonidine can be effective as adjunctive treatment, especially when there are additional indications for clonidine (e.g., hypertension, opioid withdrawal, ADHD). We prefer transdermal clonidine over oral clonidine because the former achieves more steady plasma concentrations with less variability (Burris and Mroczek 1986). Clonidine patches (0.1 mg/24 hours) can be applied every 7 days and increased to 0.2-mg patches if well tolerated. Alternatively, oral clonidine can be started at 0.1 mg tid and gradually increased up to 0.3 mg tid or qid. On resolution of withdrawal symptoms, clonidine should be gradually tapered to minimize the risk of rebound hypertension. Table 7.2 presents a summary of pharmacotherapies for benzodiazepine withdrawal.

Substance Use Disorder Presentation

BzRAs have been shown to activate the reward pathway by increasing the firing of dopamine neurons in the ventral tegmental area through effects of α_1-containing $GABA_A$ receptors in nearby interneurons (Tan et al. 2010), thus causing dopamine release in the nucleus accumbens (a common characteristic of all drugs of abuse). A sedative, hypnotic, or anxiolytic use disorder is diagnosed when there is a problematic pattern of use leading to clinically significant impairment or distress, as manifested by DSM-5 criteria (American Psychiatric Association 2022), which are reviewed elsewhere. The population most likely to misuse benzodiazepines are young adults ages 18–25 (Maust et al. 2019), and misuse in this population has been shown to be correlated with greater risk of developing a sedative-hypnotic use disorder (Chen et al. 2009). Misuse includes taking without a prescription, taking more than prescribed, taking in a route different than intended (e.g., intravenous or intranasal; Sheehan et al. 1991), or taking for a purpose not as prescribed.

It is worth noting that, as with the opioid epidemic, the pendulum has swung from overprescribing to deprescribing of benzodiazepines, so middle-aged and older adults who have taken prescription benzodiazepines long-term may have experienced inappropriate discontinuations or rapid dose reductions (Oldenhof et al. 2019). Although they may exhibit tolerance and withdrawal due to physiological dependence, their symptoms may not meet DSM-5 criteria for an SUD that could warrant such decreases or discontinuations. Patient education has been shown to be effective at helping older adults discontinue benzodiazepines (Tannenbaum et al. 2014), yet a substantial number of patients will struggle to discontinue or reduce their benzodiazepine use without specialized treatment—a testament to the addictive potential of benzodiazepines and the strong attachment that some patients have to these substances.

Long-Term Management Approaches to the Disorder

There are no evidence-based long-term management approaches after successful discontinuation of benzodiazepines. As with other SUDs, it is important to focus on relapse prevention. In addition to preventing relapse to benzodiazepines, it is prudent to routinely assess for problematic alcohol use, because patients may turn to alcohol as another sedative with similar effects.

The symptoms that initially drove the patient to use benzodiazepines should be evaluated and treated. Selective serotonin reuptake inhibitors should be considered if there is a primary anxiety disorder. Patients with anxiety may also benefit from cognitive-behavioral therapy (CBT), alone or in combination with pharmacotherapy. There is moderate-quality evidence that CBT plus taper is more likely to result in successful discontinuation of benzodiazepines compared with taper alone, although CBT alone without a taper was not found to have benefit in two small trials (Darker et al. 2015).

Patients who chronically used benzodiazepines for insomnia are at significant risk of relapse after benzodiazepine discontinuation (Morin et al. 2005). Proper sleep hygiene techniques and CBT for insomnia should be tried before pharmacotherapy. Melatonin, trazodone, and mirtazapine are commonly used for sleep and are safe at low doses. Compared with trazodone, mirtazapine has more potential for weight gain but may be a better treatment for anxiety (Slee et al. 2019). Doxepin is approved by the FDA for insomnia at doses of 3 and 6 mg, at which it acts primarily at histamine receptors without significant anticholinergic effects (Schroeck et al. 2016). Consultation with a sleep medicine specialist may be helpful for more complex sleep disorders.

Table 7.2 Summary of inpatient and outpatient pharmacotherapies for benzodiazepine withdrawal[a]

Medication	Dose	Notes
Outpatient		
Taper medication that the patient is currently taking	Set based on current dose patient is taking	Taper rate depends on how the patient tolerates the rate of decrease; 10%–25% decreases every 1–2 wk are usually a reasonable starting rate Consider adjunctive antiepileptics and/or α_2-agonists for breakthrough symptoms
Switch to longer-acting benzodiazepine and taper	Quantify total daily dose of short-acting medication and convert to equivalent dose of longer-acting benzodiazepine (i.e., clonazepam, chlordiazepoxide, diazepam; see Table 7.1)	Taper rate depends on how the patient tolerates the rate of decrease; 10%–25% decreases every 1–2 wk are usually a reasonable starting rate If breakthrough symptoms occur and are not managed by adjusting longer-acting benzodiazepine taper, then consider discontinuing long-acting medication and restarting and tapering original short-acting medication Consider adjunctive antiepileptics and/or α_2-agonists for breakthrough symptoms
Inpatient[b]		
Taper strategies as above for outpatient settings	Varies Symptom-triggered and fixed dosing strategies can be considered	May consider faster tapers (i.e., 20%–25% reductions every 4 d) if close monitoring is possible (CIWA-A or CIWA-B)

Table 7.2 Summary of inpatient and outpatient pharmacotherapies for benzodiazepine withdrawal[a] *(continued)*

Medication	Dose	Notes
Phenobarbital	Convert estimated total daily dose of benzodiazepine to phenobarbital equivalent (phenobarbital ≤500 mg/d), divided into 3–4 doses/d, followed by taper of phenobarbital 30 mg/d	Watch for signs of phenobarbital intoxication (sustained horizontal nystagmus, slurred speech, ataxia). If nystagmus is present, withhold 1 dose. If all 3 signs are present, withhold 2 doses and decrease total daily dose by 50% the following day (Smith and Wesson 1983). No high-quality studies to date on this pharmacotherapy for this indication
	Johns Hopkins Bayview Medical Center approach (Kawasaki et al. 2012): Initial dose of phenobarbital 200 mg; then 100 mg every 4 h × 5 doses; then 60 mg every 4 h × 4 doses; then 60 mg every 8 h × 3 doses	Doses held for sedation (conducted on unit with trained nurses)
Carbamazepine	Start 200 mg bid, titrate up to 600–800 mg total daily dose (Ries et al. 1989; Schweizer et al. 1991)	Although studies abruptly discontinued medication, tapers are prudent. Not in pregnancy

Table 7.2 Summary of inpatient and outpatient pharmacotherapies for benzodiazepine withdrawal[a] (continued)

Medication	Dose	Notes
Valproate	500–2,500 mg/d starting 5 d before benzodiazepine taper (Rickels et al. 1999)	Not in pregnancy
Gabapentin/pregabalin	Gabapentin: 600–900 mg/d in 2–3 divided doses, titrate up by 300 mg/d if needed to maximum of 1,800 mg/d	Data limited to case reports. Can also load larger proportion of total daily dose in evening, to facilitate sleep
	Pregabalin: 225–900 mg/d (Oulis and Konstantakopoulos 2010)	Use with caution in individuals who also have opioid use
Oxcarbazepine	Start 150 mg/d and titrate up to 1,200 mg/d over 12 d (while benzodiazepine is concurrently tapered) (Croissant et al. 2008)	Data limited to case reports
Propranolol	20–40 mg tid (Cantopher et al. 1990; Tyrer et al. 1981)	Data limited to case reports. Not to be used as monotherapy

Sedative, Hypnotics, or Anxiolytics 351

Table 7.2 Summary of inpatient and outpatient pharmacotherapies for benzodiazepine withdrawal[a] *(continued)*

Medication	Dose	Notes
Clonidine	Oral: start 0.1 mg tid, and increase to 0.3 mg tid to qid prn	Inconclusive results, but also no adverse events noted in studies
	Transdermal: 0.1 mg/24 h patch, increase to 0.2 mg/24 h patch prn	Watch for hypotension
		Taper to discontinue and watch for rebound hypertension when discontinued

Note. CIWA-A = Clinical Institute Withdrawal Assessment for Alcohol; CIWA-B = Clinical Institute Withdrawal Assessment for Benzodiazepines; d = day; h = hour; wk = week.

[a]Data are further limited when considering pharmacotherapies for discontinuation of Z drugs, but case reports suggest that strategies employed for benzodiazepine withdrawal pharmacotherapy may be effective for Z drugs as well (Awasthi and Vohra 2023; Barbosa Eyler and Utria Castro 2021).

[b]Consider if sedative-hypnotic use disorder is severe, outpatient tapers have failed, high medical or psychiatric complexity is present, withdrawal risk is high, or severe co-occurring other substance use disorders are present.

Some patients appear to have a wide range of enduring neurological symptoms after chronic exposure to benzodiazepines. More research is needed to further explore these two heuristics—benzodiazepine induced neurological dysfunction (BIND) and complex persistent benzodiazepine dependence (CPBD)—but they do seem to bring light to the complexity and refractory nature of a subgroup of patients with chronic exposure to benzodiazepines (Peng et al. 2022a; Ritvo et al. 2023).

Significant Medical or Physiological Considerations

Older Adults

The American Geriatrics Society advises against using benzodiazepines or nonbenzodiazepine hypnotics in older adults. Despite these recommendations, benzodiazepines continue to be increasingly prescribed in large doses for prolonged periods of time to this group with the highest risk of serious adverse effects from these medications (Markota et al. 2016). Older adults are relatively more sensitive to the effects of benzodiazepines, which can increase the risk of cognitive impairment, delirium, falls, hip fractures, and motor vehicle accidents (Bakken et al. 2014; Fick et al. 2019). The Z drugs have similar adverse effects and have contributed to increased emergency department visits and hospitalizations (Fick et al. 2019).

Retrospective cohort studies suggest that benzodiazepines and Z drugs increase the risk of all-cause mortality (Weich et al. 2014; Xu et al. 2020). Benzodiazepines have also been associated with increased suicide risk, potentially mediated by increased aggression and behavioral disinhibition (Dodds 2017).

As described earlier, most benzodiazepines are hepatically metabolized by microsomal oxidation or demethylation, followed by glucuronide conjugation (Griffin et al. 2013). The exceptions are lorazepam, oxazepam, and temazepam, which require only glucuronide conjugation. These three benzodiazepines may be safer in individuals with hepatic dysfunction or those taking other medications that are hepatically metabolized. Older adults are particularly vulnerable to adverse effects because of age-related physiological changes in drug metabolism and elimination (Griffin et al. 2013). Aging is associated with higher body fat (Kuerbis et al. 2014), resulting in increased volume of distribution and accumulation of lipophilic benzodiazepines and their active metabolites. Active benzodiazepine metabolites can accumulate with repeated dosing, making estimation of half-lives challenging, especially in the setting of kidney disease, because benzodiazepines are excreted almost entirely in the urine.

Strategies to successfully reach long-term abstinence from benzodiazepines in older adults are not well described in the literature. We recommend taking a patient-centered approach that includes risk-benefit analysis, involving the patient's family in treatment planning, and maximizing the patient's daily functioning and quality of life. In some instances, continuing benzodiazepines, albeit at the lowest effective dose, may be indicated, especially if prior discontinuation attempts resulted in medical or psychiatric decompensation.

Pregnant Individuals

Benzodiazepines cross the placenta and have been associated with preterm delivery and low birth weight (Shyken et al. 2019), although there is no increased risk of major congenital malformations (Grigoriadis et al. 2019). In a cohort study of 201,275 pregnancies with neonates exposed to opioids, in utero coexposure to benzodiazepines was associated with increased relative risk (1.49) of neonatal abstinence syndrome (Huybrechts et al. 2017). Surprisingly, coexposure to gabapentin with nonsteroidal anti-inflammatory drugs was associated with an even higher relative risk (1.61), whereas no significant association was found for Z drugs and antipsychotics.

Benzodiazepines have been associated with a neonatal withdrawal syndrome (referred to colloquially as "floppy infant syndrome") that is characterized by low Apgar scores, apneic spells, hypotonia, and difficulty feeding (McElhatton 1994). There is no consensus on whether long-term benzodiazepines should be tapered off during pregnancy, especially because maternal anxiety may have negative outcomes on pregnancy (Shyken et al. 2019). Shyken et al. proposed switching from short-acting to long-acting benzodiazepines, followed by a protracted taper over weeks to months.

Special Populations

Co-occurring Opioid Use Disorder

According to the National Institute on Drug Abuse, 16% of opioid-related overdose deaths in 2019 also involved benzodiazepines. Concomitant prescribing of benzodiazepines and opioids increases the risk of overdose (Sun et al. 2017); still, concomitant prescriptions have been on the rise (Hwang et al. 2016). It is commonly known that the combination of benzodiazepines and opioids significantly increases the risk of respiratory suppression and accidental overdose. Benzodiazepines should generally be avoided in patients taking buprenorphine or methadone (but their coprescription is not absolutely contraindicated), yet many report concurrent use with methadone, which carries greater risks of opioid toxicity compared with buprenorphine (Nielsen et al. 2007). There may be a decreased risk of respiratory depression when benzodiazepines are combined with buprenorphine compared with methadone, yet benzodiazepine-related deaths have been reported with buprenorphine (Lintzeris and Nielsen 2010). Buprenorphine and methadone can be lifesaving for opioid use disorder and should not be withheld from patients taking benzodiazepines if the benefits outweigh the risks (U.S. Food and Drug Administration 2017). Nonetheless, the FDA has issued a black box warning for both opioids and benzodiazepines, cautioning prescribers about the risks associated with coprescribing these medications.

Benzodiazepine tapering among patients receiving buprenorphine or methadone has not been extensively studied. A review by Lintzeris and Nielsen (2010) suggested that patients have difficulty tolerating tapers and may return to illicit benzodiazepines, and that some cases may warrant benzodiazepine maintenance treatment as a form of harm reduction. In most cases, a trial of benzodiazepine taper is warranted, and the dose of methadone or buprenorphine should be kept stable for the duration of the taper (Baldwin 2021).

Women

Studies in the United States have not demonstrated consistent gender differences, with some data indicating similar rates of benzodiazepine misuse between men and women (Votaw et al. 2019) and others showing higher rates of misuse among men despite women reporting higher rates of any benzodiazepine use (Maust et al. 2019). Outside of the United States, rates of benzodiazepine use and misuse are higher among women.

Young Adults

Benzodiazepine misuse among young adults is especially concerning because younger age of misuse is associated with greater risk of developing a sedative-hypnotic use disorder (Chen et al. 2009). Benzodiazepines are also the third most commonly misused illicit or prescription substance among adults and adolescents in the United States (Johnston et al. 2018).

A new threat to young adults has been the rise of designer benzodiazepines. A category of novel psychoactive substances, designer benzodiazepines are synthetic compounds commonly sold online as research chemicals to evade regulatory bodies. Their exact pharmacodynamic or receptor binding profiles have not been systematically studied (Greenblatt and Greenblatt 2019), but like traditional benzodiazepines, they exert their effect at $GABA_A$ receptors. They may be more potent and more addictive than traditional benzodiazepines (Peng et al. 2022a). Some designer benzodiazepines were developed decades ago by pharmaceutical companies but never approved for medical use, whereas others are novel substances that have been identified only in the illicit market. The European Monitoring Centre for Drugs and Drug Addiction (2018; now the European Union Drugs Agency) actively monitors 23 designer benzodiazepines, more than half of which were only detected since 2015 (Zawilska and Wojcieszak 2019). In the United States, the designer benzodiazepine etizolam is not listed under the Controlled Substances Act but has been declared a controlled substance in Alabama, Arkansas, Arizona, Florida, Georgia, Indiana, Mississippi, and Virginia.

Data from the U.S. National Poison Data System for 2014–2017 indicated that the two most common designer benzodiazepines were etizolam and clonazolam, and they tended to be most commonly used by males (median age 25 years) (Carpenter et al. 2019). It has been suspected that use of designer benzodiazepines increased during the COVID-19 pandemic (Zaami et al. 2020), because they can be purchased online. Purchasing designer benzodiazepines online may require a certain technological proficiency with the dark web and cryptocurrency as form of payment (Shapiro et al. 2019). Some users willingly seek out designer benzodiazepines, whereas other users unknowingly purchase these compounds sold as counterfeit alprazolam (Blumenberg et al. 2020).

The rise of designer benzodiazepines presents multiple challenges. Standard urine drug screens may fail to detect these substances, and confirmatory liquid chromatography and mass spectrometry is often needed (Peng et al. 2022b). Case reports indicate that diazepam, phenobarbital, valproate, and gabapentin have been used in treatment of withdrawal and cravings (Hauck et al. 2022; Peng et al. 2022; Shapiro et al. 2019), although more research is needed.

Key Points

- Benzodiazepine receptor agonists (BzRAs) are used most commonly as anxiolytics and hypnotics and can be used safely by many individuals, but they are often prescribed over a longer period than initially intended, and some vulnerable individuals can experience unintended side effects.
- Despite being previously marketed as being non-habit-forming, evidence and clinical experience suggest that BzRAs do have misuse potential related to their ability to activate brain reward circuitry.
- BzRAs can have significant adverse effects and complications, which are especially dangerous when used in combination with other CNS depressants.
- Discontinuing long-term BzRAs can be achieved by an outpatient benzodiazepine taper or with inpatient withdrawal management in the hospital or residential treatment facility. Benzodiazepine-sparing protocols include the adjunctive use of antiepileptic medications, phenobarbital, and antihypertensive agents.
- BzRA withdrawal is highly variable and in complex cases can be prolonged, uncomfortable, and even dangerous because of the kindling effect.
- In many patients who have used BzRAs long term, a postacute withdrawal syndrome can last months to years and contributes to frequent relapses after successful tapers.
- Elevated glutamatergic tone present in the BzRA withdrawal state leads to many of the sequelae of the withdrawal syndrome and can be treated through the combination of GABAergic medications and α_2-agonists (e.g., clonidine) that decrease noradrenergic tone.
- Novel psychoactive substances, including designer benzodiazepines, are becoming increasingly available on the recreational and online drug market.
- Decision-making around discontinuation of long-standing benzodiazepines should include risk-benefit analysis, because the process of

deprescribing can lead to clinical destabilization in certain populations. In some cases, continuation of benzodiazepines is warranted.

References

Ait-Daoud N, Hamby AS, Sharma S, et al: A review of alprazolam use, misuse, and withdrawal. J Addict Med 12(1):4–10, 2018 28777203

Allison C, Pratt JA: Neuroadaptive processes in GABAergic and glutamatergic systems in benzodiazepine dependence. Pharmacol Ther 98(2):171–195, 2003 12725868

American Psychiatric Association: Diagnostic and Statistical Manual of Mental Disorders, 5th Edition, Text Revision. Washington, DC, American Psychiatric Association, 2022

An H, Godwin J: Flumazenil in benzodiazepine overdose. CMAJ 188(17–18):E537, 2016 27920113

Ashton H: Benzodiazepine withdrawal: an unfinished story. Br Med J (Clin Res Ed) 288(6424):1135–1140, 1984 6143582

Ashton H: Protracted withdrawal syndromes from benzodiazepines. J Subst Abuse Treat 8(1–2):19–28, 1991 1675688

Ashton H: The diagnosis and management of benzodiazepine dependence. Curr Opin Psychiatry 18(3):249–255, 2005 16639148

Awasthi H, Vohra A: Abrupt withdrawal from chronic high-dose zolpidem use: a case report of resulting delirium. Cureus 15(11):e49025, 2023 38024021

Baird CRW, Fox P, Colvin LA: Gabapentinoid abuse in order to potentiate the effect of methadone: a survey among substance misusers. Eur Addict Res 20(3):115–118, 2014 24192603

Bakken MS, Engeland A, Engesæter LB, et al: Risk of hip fracture among older people using anxiolytic and hypnotic drugs: a nationwide prospective cohort study. Eur J Clin Pharmacol 70(7):873–880, 2014 24810612

Baldwin DS: Clinical management of withdrawal from benzodiazepine anxiolytic and hypnotic medications. Addiction 117(5):1472–1482, 2021 34542216

Barbosa Eyler GE, Utria Castro JV: Zolpidem dependence and withdrawal: a case report of generalized seizures. Rev Colomb Psiquiatr (Engl Ed). S0034-7450(21)00131-1, 2021 34446256

Barnes EM Jr: Use-dependent regulation of GABAA receptors. Int Rev Neurobiol 39(39):53–76, 1996 8894844

Barrons R, Roberts N: The role of carbamazepine and oxcarbazepine in alcohol withdrawal syndrome. J Clin Pharm Ther 35(2):153–167, 2010 20456734

Bateson AN: Basic pharmacologic mechanisms involved in benzodiazepine tolerance and withdrawal. Curr Pharm Des 8(1):5–21, 2002 11812247

Beydoun A, DuPont S, Zhou D, et al: Current role of carbamazepine and oxcarbazepine in the management of epilepsy. Seizure 83:251–263, 2020 33334546

Blumenberg A, Hughes A, Reckers A, et al: Flualprazolam: report of an outbreak of a new psychoactive substance in adolescents. Pediatrics 146(1):e20192953, 2020 32581001

Bonnet U, Scherbaum N: How addictive are gabapentin and pregabalin? A systematic review. Eur Neuropsychopharmacol 27(12):1185–1215, 2017 28988943

Burris JF, Mroczek WJ: Transdermal administration of clonidine: a new approach to antihypertensive therapy. Pharmacotherapy 6(1):30–34, 1986 3952004

Busto U, Sellers EM: Pharmacologic aspects of benzodiazepine tolerance and dependence. J Subst Abuse Treat 8(1–2):29–33, 1991 1675689

Busto U, Kaplan HL, Sellers EM: Benzodiazepine-associated emergencies in Toronto. Am J Psychiatry 137(2):224–227, 1980 6101526

Busto UE, Sykora K, Sellers EM: A clinical scale to assess benzodiazepine withdrawal. J Clin Psychopharmacol 9(6):412–416, 1989 2574193

Buysse DJ: Insomnia. JAMA 309(7):706–716, 2013 23423416

Cantopher T, Olivieri S, Cleave N, et al: Chronic benzodiazepine dependence: a comparative study of abrupt withdrawal under propranolol cover versus gradual withdrawal. Br J Psychiatry 156:406–411, 1990 1971767

Carpenter JE, Murray BP, Dunkley C, et al: Designer benzodiazepines: a report of exposures recorded in the National Poison Data System, 2014–2017. Clin Toxicol (Phila) 57(4):282–286, 2019 30430874

Chen C-Y, Storr CL, Anthony JC: Early-onset drug use and risk for drug dependence problems. Addict Behav 34(3):319–322, 2009 19022584

Chiaro G, Castelnovo A, Bianco G, et al: Severe chronic abuse of zolpidem in refractory insomnia. J Clin Sleep Med 14(7):1257–1259, 2018 29991431

Committee on the Review of Medicines: Systematic review of the benzodiazepines: guidelines for data sheets on diazepam, chlordiazepoxide, medazepam, clorazepate, lorazepam, oxazepam, temazepam, triazolam, nitrazepam, and flurazepam: Committee on the Review of Medicines. Br Med J 280(6218):910–912, 1980 7388368

Cosci F, Chouinard G: Acute and persistent withdrawal syndromes following discontinuation of psychotropic medications. Psychother Psychosom 89(5):283–306, 2020 32259826

Crockford D, White WD, Campbell B: Gabapentin use in benzodiazepine dependence and detoxification. Can J Psychiatry 46(3):287, 2001 11320686

Croissant B, Grosshans M, Diehl A, et al: Oxcarbazepine in rapid benzodiazepine detoxification. Am J Drug Alcohol Abuse 34(5):534–540, 2008 18821451

Cubała WJ, Landowski J: Seizure following sudden zolpidem withdrawal. Prog Neuropsychopharmacol Biol Psychiatry 31(2):539–540, 2007 16950552

Darker CD, Sweeney BP, Barry JM, et al: Psychosocial interventions for benzodiazepine harmful use, abuse or dependence. Cochrane Database Syst Rev 2015(5):CD009652, 2015 26106751

de Lima WD, da Silva MD, de Souza Costa E, et al: Abusive use of zolpidem as a result of COVID-19 and perspectives of continuity of the problem in the post-pandemic period. Curr Neuropharmacol 22(10):1578–1582, 2024 37811654

Dodds TJ: Prescribed benzodiazepines and suicide risk: a review of the literature. Prim Care Companion CNS Disord 19(2):16r02037, 2017 28257172

Dubovsky SL, Marshall D: Benzodiazepines remain important therapeutic options in psychiatric practice. Psychother Psychosom 91(5):307–334, 2022 35504267

Ebbens MM, Verster JC: Clinical evaluation of zaleplon in the treatment of insomnia. Nat Sci Sleep 2:115–126, 2010 23616704

European Monitoring Centre for Drugs and Drug Addiction: Perspectives on Drugs: The Misuse of Benzodiazepines Among High-Risk Opioid Users in Europe. 2018. Available at: http://www.emcdda.europa.eu/system/files/publications/2733/Misuse of benzos_POD2015.pdf. Accessed February 7, 2025.

Fick DM, Semla TP, Steinman M, et al: American Geriatrics Society 2019 updated AGS Beers Criteria® for potentially inappropriate medication use in older adults. J Am Geriatr Soc 67(4):674–694, 2019 30693946

Fyer AJ, Liebowitz MR, Gorman JM, et al: Discontinuation of alprazolam treatment in panic patients. Am J Psychiatry 144(3):303–308, 1987 3826428

Fyer AJ, Liebowitz MR, Gorman JM, et al: Effects of clonidine on alprazolam discontinuation in panic patients: a pilot study. J Clin Psychopharmacol 8(4):270–274, 1988 3209718

Gaudreault P, Guay J, Thivierge RL, et al: Benzodiazepine poisoning: clinical and pharmacological considerations and treatment. Drug Saf 6(4):247–265, 1991 1888441

Golombok S, Higgitt A, Fonagy P, et al: A follow-up study of patients treated for benzodiazepine dependence. Br J Med Psychol 60(Pt 2):141–149, 1987 2887197

Gomes T, Juurlink DN, Antoniou T, et al: Gabapentin, opioids, and the risk of opioid-related death: a population-based nested case-control study. PLoS Med 14(10):e1002396, 2017 28972983

Greenblatt DJ, Miller LG, Shader RI: Neurochemical and pharmacokinetic correlates of the clinical action of benzodiazepine hypnotic drugs. Am J Med 88(3 Suppl 1):S18–S24, 1990 1968714

Greenblatt HK, Greenblatt DJ: Designer benzodiazepines: a review of published data and public health significance. Clin Pharmacol Drug Dev 8(3):266–269, 2019 30730611

Griffin CE III, Kaye AM, Bueno FR, et al: Benzodiazepine pharmacology and central nervous system-mediated effects. Ochsner J 13(2):214–223, 2013 23789008

Griffiths RR, Wolf B: Relative abuse liability of different benzodiazepines in drug abusers. J Clin Psychopharmacol 10(4):237–243, 1990 1981067

Grigoriadis S, Graves L, Peer M, et al: Benzodiazepine use during pregnancy alone or in combination with an antidepressant and congenital malformations: systematic review and meta-analysis. J Clin Psychiatry 80(4):18r12412, 2019 31294935

Gunja N: The clinical and forensic toxicology of Z-drugs. J Med Toxicol 9(2):155–162, 2013 23404347

Hadley SJ, Mandel FS, Schweizer E: Switching from long-term benzodiazepine therapy to pregabalin in patients with generalized anxiety disorder: a double-blind, placebo-controlled trial. J Psychopharmacol 26(4):461–470, 2012 21693549

Hammond CJ, Niciu MJ, Drew S, et al: Anticonvulsants for the treatment of alcohol withdrawal syndrome and alcohol use disorders. CNS Drugs 29(4):293–311, 2015 25895020

Harada T, Tatebayashi K, Nakai M: Successful rapid benzodiazepine detoxification in an acute care hospital: a case report. J Community Hosp Intern Med Perspect 14(4):93–96, 2024 39391115

Hauck TS, Rochon S, Bahra P, et al: Outpatient treatment of chronic designer benzodiazepine use: a case report. J Addict Med 16(2):e137–e139, 2022 33900229

Huybrechts KF, Bateman BT, Desai RJ, et al: Risk of neonatal drug withdrawal after intrauterine co-exposure to opioids and psychotropic medications: cohort study. BMJ 358:j3326, 2017 28768628

Hwang CS, Kang EM, Kornegay CJ, et al: Trends in the concomitant prescribing of opioids and benzodiazepines, 2002–2014. Am J Prev Med 51(2):151–160, 2016 27079639

Johnston LD, Miech RA, O'Malley PM, et al: Monitoring the Future: National Survey Results on Drug Use 1975–2017: Overview, Key Findings on Adolescent Drug Use. Ann Arbor, MI, Institute for Social Research, The University of Michigan, 2018. Available at: https://monitoringthefuture.org/wp-content/uploads/2022/08/mtf-overview2017.pdf. Accessed February 8, 2025.

Joyce EM, Moodley P, Keshavan MS, et al: Failure of clonidine treatment in benzodiazepine withdrawal. J Psychopharmacol 4(1):42–45, 1990 22282926

Kaufmann CN, Spira AP, Depp CA, et al: Long-term use of benzodiazepines and nonbenzodiazepine hypnotics, 1999–2014. Psychiatr Serv 69(2):235–238, 2018 29089011

Kawasaki SS, Jacapraro JS, Rastegar DA: Safety and effectiveness of a fixed-dose phenobarbital protocol for inpatient benzodiazepine detoxification. J Subst Abuse Treat 43(3):331–334, 2012 22285834

Keshavan MS, Crammer JL: Clonidine in benzodiazepine withdrawal. Lancet 1(8441):1325–1326, 1985 2860507

Koethe D, Juelicher A, Nolden BM, et al: Oxcarbazepine: efficacy and tolerability during treatment of alcohol withdrawal: a double-blind, randomized, placebo-controlled multicenter pilot study. Alcohol Clin Exp Res 31(7):1188–1194, 2007 17511748

Kuerbis A, Sacco P, Blazer DG, et al: Substance abuse among older adults. Clin Geriatr Med 30(3):629–654, 2014 25037298

Lader M: Long-term anxiolytic therapy: the issue of drug withdrawal. J Clin Psychiatry 48(Suppl):12–16, 1987 2891684

Lader M: History of benzodiazepine dependence. J Subst Abuse Treat 8(1–2):53–59, 1991 1675692

Lader M: Benzodiazepines revisited: will we ever learn? Addiction 106(12):2086–2109, 2011 21714826

Landry MJ, Smith DE, McDuff DR, et al: Benzodiazepine dependence and withdrawal: identification and medical management. J Am Board Fam Pract 5(2):167–175, 1992 1575069

Lembke A, Papac J, Humphreys K: Our other prescription drug problem. N Engl J Med 378(8):693–695, 2018 29466163

Leung JG, Rakocevic DB, Allen ND, et al: Use of a gabapentin protocol for the management of alcohol withdrawal: a preliminary experience expanding from the consultation-liaison psychiatry service. Psychosomatics 59(5):496–505, 2018 29735241

Licata SC, Rowlett JK: Abuse and dependence liability of benzodiazepine-type drugs: GABA(A) receptor modulation and beyond. Pharmacol Biochem Behav 90(1):74–89, 2008 18295321

Lintzeris N, Nielsen S: Benzodiazepines, methadone and buprenorphine: interactions and clinical management. Am J Addict 19(1):59–72, 2010 20132123

Löscher W: Basic pharmacology of valproate: a review after 35 years of clinical use for the treatment of epilepsy. CNS Drugs 16(10):669–694, 2002 12269861

Löw K, Crestani F, Keist R, et al: Molecular and neuronal substrate for the selective attenuation of anxiety. Science 290(5489):131–134, 2000 11021797

Lyu X, Hu Y, Zhao Y, et al: Euphoric effect induced by zolpidem: a case study of magnetoencephalography. Gen Psychiatr 35(1):e100729, 2022 35243205

Maan JS, Duong T, Saadabadi A: Carbamazepine. Treasure Island, FL, StatPearls, 2021. Available at: http://www.ncbi.nlm.nih.gov/pubmed/29494062. Accessed February 7, 2025.

MacKinnon GL, Parker WA: Benzodiazepine withdrawal syndrome: a literature review and evaluation. Am J Drug Alcohol Abuse 9(1):19–33, 1982 6133446

Markota M, Rummans TA, Bostwick JM, et al: Benzodiazepine use in older adults: dangers, management, and alternative therapies. Mayo Clin Proc 91(11):1632–1639, 2016 27814838

Marriott S, Tyrer P: Benzodiazepine dependence: avoidance and withdrawal. Drug Saf 9(2):93–103, 1993 8104417

Mason BJ, Quello S, Goodell V, et al: Gabapentin treatment for alcohol dependence: a randomized clinical trial. JAMA Intern Med 174(1):70–77, 2014 24190578

Maust DT, Lin LA, Blow FC: Benzodiazepine use and misuse among adults in the United States. Psychiatr Serv 70(2):97–106, 2019 30554562

McElhatton PR: The effects of benzodiazepine use during pregnancy and lactation. Reprod Toxicol 8(6):461–475, 1994 7881198

McGregor C, Machin A, White JM: In-patient benzodiazepine withdrawal: comparison of fixed and symptom-triggered taper methods. Drug Alcohol Rev 22(2):175–180, 2003 12850904

McHugh RK, Votaw VR, Trapani EW, et al: Prevalence and correlates of the misuse of z-drugs and benzodiazepines in the National Survey on Drug Use and Health. Front Psychiatry 14:1129447, 2023 36970272

McKernan RM, Rosahl TW, Reynolds DS, et al: Sedative but not anxiolytic properties of benzodiazepines are mediated by the GABA(A) receptor α1 subtype. Nat Neurosci 3(6):587–592, 2000 10816315

Meier PJ, Ziegler WH, Neftel K: Benzodiazepine: practice and problems of its use [in German]. Schweiz Med Wochenschr 118(11):381–392, 1988 3287602

Mersfelder TL, Nichols WH: Gabapentin: abuse, dependence, and withdrawal. Ann Pharmacother 50(3):229–233, 2016 26721643

Miller PS, Aricescu AR: Crystal structure of a human GABAA receptor. Nature 512(7514):270–275, 2014 24909990

Moore TJ, Mattison DR: Adult utilization of psychiatric drugs and differences by sex, age, and race. JAMA Intern Med 177(2):274–275, 2017 27942726

Morin CM, Bélanger L, Bastien C, et al: Long-term outcome after discontinuation of benzodiazepines for insomnia: a survival analysis of relapse. Behav Res Ther 43(1):1–14, 2005 15531349

Muzyk AJ, Fowler JA, Norwood DK, et al: Role of α2-agonists in the treatment of acute alcohol withdrawal. Ann Pharmacother 45(5):649–657, 2011 21521867

Myrick H, Malcolm R, Randall PK, et al: A double-blind trial of gabapentin versus lorazepam in the treatment of alcohol withdrawal. Alcohol Clin Exp Res 33(9):1582–1588, 2009 19485969

National Institute for Health and Care Excellence: Medicines Associated With Dependence or Withdrawal Symptoms: Safe Prescribing and Withdrawal Management for Adults. London, National Institute for Health and Care Excellence, April 20, 2022. Available at: https://www.nice.org.uk/guidance/ng215/resources/medicines-associated-with-dependence-or-withdrawal-symptoms-safe-prescribing-and-withdrawal-management-for-adults-pdf-66143776880581. Accessed February 7, 2025.

Nelson AC, Kehoe J, Sankoff J, et al: Benzodiazepines vs barbiturates for alcohol withdrawal: analysis of 3 different treatment protocols. Am J Emerg Med 37(4):733–736, 2019 30685075

Nielsen S, Dietze P, Lee N, et al: Concurrent buprenorphine and benzodiazepines use and self-reported opioid toxicity in opioid substitution treatment. Addiction 102(4):616–622, 2007 17286641

Oldenhof E, Anderson-Wurf J, Hall K, et al: Beyond prescriptions monitoring programs: the importance of having the conversation about benzodiazepine use. J Clin Med 8(12):2143, 2019 31817181

Olsen RW: GABAA receptor: positive and negative allosteric modulators. Neuropharmacology 136(Pt A):10–22, 2018 29407219

Oulis P, Konstantakopoulos G: Pregabalin in the treatment of alcohol and benzodiazepines dependence. CNS Neurosci Ther 16(1):45–50, 2010 20070788

Owen GT, Burton AW, Schade CM, et al: Urine drug testing: current recommendations and best practices. Pain Physician 15(3 Suppl):ES119–ES133, 2012 22786451

Peng L, Lawrence D, Levander XA: Challenges of diagnosing and managing designer benzodiazepine dependence and withdrawal. J Addict Med 16(2):249–251, 2022a 34001772

Peng L, Meeks T, Blazes C: Complex persistent benzodiazepine dependence—when benzodiazepine deprescribing goes awry. JAMA Psychiatry 79(7):639-640, 2022b 35583897

Pétursson H: The benzodiazepine withdrawal syndrome. Addiction 89(11):1455–1459, 1994 7841856

Pritchett DB, Seeburg PH: γ-aminobutyric acidA receptor α5-subunit creates novel type II benzodiazepine receptor pharmacology. J Neurochem 54(5):1802–1804, 1990 2157817

Rickels K, Moeller HJ: Benzodiazepines in anxiety disorders: reassessment of usefulness and safety. World J Biol Psychiatry 20(7):514–518, 2019 30252578

Rickels K, Case WG, Schweizer EE, et al: Low-dose dependence in chronic benzodiazepine users: a preliminary report on 119 patients. Psychopharmacol Bull 22(2):407–415, 1986 2877472

Rickels K, Schweizer E, Garcia España F, et al: Trazodone and valproate in patients discontinuing long-term benzodiazepine therapy: effects on withdrawal symptoms and taper outcome. Psychopharmacology (Berl) 141(1):1–5, 1999 9952057

Riemann D, Perlis ML: The treatments of chronic insomnia: a review of benzodiazepine receptor agonists and psychological and behavioral therapies. Sleep Med Rev 13(3):205–214, 2009 19201632

Ries RK, Roy-Byrne PP, Ward NG, et al: Carbamazepine treatment for benzodiazepine withdrawal. Am J Psychiatry 146(4):536–537, 1989 2929759

Ritvo AD, Foster DE, Huff C, et al: Long-term consequences of benzodiazepine-induced neurologic dysfunction: a survey. PLoS One 18(6):e0285584, 2023 37384788

Sabe M, Kashef H, Gironi C, et al: Zolpidem stimulant effect: Induced mania case report and systematic review of cases. Prog Neuropsychopharmacol Biol Psychiatry 94:109643, 2019 31071363

Sachdev G, Gesin G, Christmas AB, et al: Failure of lorazepam to treat alprazolam withdrawal in a critically ill patient. World J Crit Care Med 3(1):42–44, 2014 24834401

Sadock B, Sadock V, Ruiz P: Preparations and doses of medications acting on the benzodiazepine receptor available in the United States, in Kaplan and Sadock's Synopsis of Psychiatry, 11th Edition. Philadelphia, PA, Wolters Kluwer Health, 2015, p 949

Saitz R, Mayo-Smith MF, Roberts MS, et al: Individualized treatment for alcohol withdrawal: a randomized double-blind controlled trail. JAMA 272(7):519–523, 1994 8046805

Salzman C: The APA Task Force report on benzodiazepine dependence, toxicity, and abuse. Am J Psychiatry 148(2):151–152, 1991 1987812

Sanna E, Busonero F, Talani G, et al: Comparison of the effects of zaleplon, zolpidem, and triazolam at various GABA(A) receptor subtypes. Eur J Pharmacol 451(2):103–110, 2002 12231378

Schifano F, Chiappini S, Corkery JM, et al: An insight into Z-drug abuse and dependence: an examination of reports to the European Medicines Agency database of suspected adverse drug reactions. Int J Neuropsychopharmacol 22(4):270–277, 2019 30722037

Schroeck JL, Ford J, Conway EL, et al: Review of safety and efficacy of sleep medicines in older adults. Clin Ther 38(11):2340–2372, 2016 27751669

Schweizer E, Rickels K, Case WG, et al: Carbamazepine treatment in patients discontinuing long-term benzodiazepine therapy: effects on withdrawal severity and outcome. Arch Gen Psychiatry 48(5):448–452, 1991 2021297

Shapiro AP, Krew TS, Vazirian M, et al: Novel ways to acquire designer benzodiazepines: a case report and discussion of the changing role of the internet. Psychosomatics 60(6):625–629, 2019 31072627

Sheehan MF, Sheehan DV, Torres A, et al: Snorting benzodiazepines. Am J Drug Alcohol Abuse 17(4):457–468, 1991 1684083

Shyken JM, Babbar S, Babbar S, et al: Benzodiazepines in pregnancy. Clin Obstet Gynecol 62(1):156–167, 2019 30628916

Sigel E, Ernst M: The benzodiazepine binding sites of GABAA receptors. Trends Pharmacol Sci 39(7):659–671, 2018 29716746

Sills GJ: The mechanisms of action of gabapentin and pregabalin. Curr Opin Pharmacol 6(1):108–113, 2006 16376147

Sivilotti MLA: Flumazenil, naloxone and the "coma cocktail." Br J Clin Pharmacol 81(3):428–436, 2016 26469689

Slee A, Nazareth I, Bondaronek P, et al: Pharmacological treatments for generalised anxiety disorder: a systematic review and network meta-analysis. Lancet 393(10173):768–777, 2019 30712879

Smith DE, Wesson DR: Phenobarbital technique for treatment of barbiturate dependence. Arch Gen Psychiatry 24(1):56–60, 1971 5538852

Smith DE, Wesson DR: Benzodiazepine dependency syndromes. J Psychoactive Drugs 15(1–2):85–95, 1983 6136575

Smith DE, Wesson DR: Benzodiazepines and their phenobarbital withdrawal equivalents, in The American Psychiatric Publishing Textbook of Substance Abuse Treatment, 3rd Edition. Edited by Galanter M, Kleber HD. Washington, DC, American Psychiatric Publishing, 2004, p 243

Soyka M: Treatment of benzodiazepine dependence. N Engl J Med 376(12):1147–1157, 2017 28328330

Stone JR, Zorick TS, Tsuang J: Dose-related illusions and hallucinations with zaleplon. Clin Toxicol (Phila) 46(4):344–345, 2008 17852167

Sun EC, Dixit A, Humphreys K, et al: Association between concurrent use of prescription opioids and benzodiazepines and overdose: retrospective analysis. BMJ 356:j760, 2017 28292769

Tan KR, Brown M, Labouèbe G, et al: Neural bases for addictive properties of benzodiazepines. Nature 463(7282):769–774, 2010 20148031

Tannenbaum C, Martin P, Tamblyn R, et al: Reduction of inappropriate benzodiazepine prescriptions among older adults through direct patient education: the EMPOWER cluster randomized trial. JAMA Intern Med 174(6):890–898, 2014 24733354

Tidwell WP, Thomas TL, Pouliot JD, et al: Treatment of alcohol withdrawal syndrome: phenobarbital vs CIWA-Ar protocol. Am J Crit Care 27(6):454–460, 2018 30385536

Toner LC, Tsambiras BM, Catalano G, et al: Central nervous system side effects associated with zolpidem treatment. Clin Neuropharmacol 23(1):54–58, 2000 10682233

Tyrer P, Rutherford D, Huggett T: Benzodiazepine withdrawal symptoms and propranolol. Lancet 1(8219):520–522, 1981 6111632

U.S. Drug Enforcement Administration: Schedules of controlled substances: placement of pregabalin into Schedule V: final rule. Fed Regist 70(144):43633–43635, 2005 16050051

U.S. Food and Drug Administration: FDA urges caution about withholding opioid addiction medications from patients taking benzodiazepines or CNS depressants: careful medication management can reduce risks. Rockville, MD, Drug Safety Communications, 2017. Available at: https://www.fda.gov/media/127688/download. Accessed February 8, 2025.

U.S. Food and Drug Administration: FDA requiring Boxed Warning updated to improve safe use of benzodiazepine drug class. FDA Drug Safety Communication, 2020

Victorri-Vigneau C, Gérardin M, Rousselet M, et al: An update on zolpidem abuse and dependence. J Addict Dis 33(1):15–23, 2014 24467433

Vinkers CH, Olivier B: Mechanisms underlying tolerance after long-term benzodiazepine use: a future for subtype-selective GABAA receptor modulators? Adv Pharmacol Sci 2012:416864, 2012 22536226

Vinogradov S, Reiss AL, Csernansky JG: Clonidine therapy in withdrawal from high-dose alprazolam treatment. Am J Psychiatry 143(9):1188, 1986 2875667

Votaw VR, Geyer R, Rieselbach MM, et al: The epidemiology of benzodiazepine misuse: a systematic review. Drug Alcohol Depend 200(1):95–114, 2019 31121495

Wafford KA: GABAA receptor subtypes: any clues to the mechanism of benzodiazepine dependence? Curr Opin Pharmacol 5(1):47–52, 2005 15661625

Weich S, Pearce HL, Croft P, et al: Effect of anxiolytic and hypnotic drug prescriptions on mortality hazards: retrospective cohort study. BMJ 348:g1996, 2014 24647164

Wick JY: The history of benzodiazepines. Consult Pharm 28(9):538–548, 2013 24007886

Winokur A, Rickels K: Withdrawal and pseudowithdrawal from diazepam therapy. J Clin Psychiatry 42(11):442–444, 1981 7298586

Wolf B, Griffiths RR: Physical dependence on benzodiazepines: differences within the class. Drug Alcohol Depend 29(2):153–156, 1991 1686752

Xu KY, Hartz SM, Borodovsky JT, et al: Association between benzodiazepine use with or without opioid use and all-cause mortality in the United States, 1999–2015. JAMA Netw Open 3(12):e2028557, 2020 33295972

Yang W, Dollear M, Muthukrishnan SR: One rare side effect of zolpidem: sleepwalking: a case report. Arch Phys Med Rehabil 86(6):1265–1266, 2005 15954071

Zaami S, Marinelli E, Varì MR: New trends of substance abuse during COVID-19 pandemic: an international perspective. Front Psychiatry 11:700, 2020 32765328

Zawilska JB, Wojcieszak J: An expanding world of new psychoactive substances—designer benzodiazepines. Neurotoxicology 73:8–16, 2019 30802466

8

Hallucinogens and Phencyclidine

Jeffrey DeVido, M.D., M.T.S.
Martin Epson, M.D., J.D., M.T.S.

Hallucinogens are a heterogeneous group of substances, with use patterns in humans ranging from the pathological to potentially therapeutic. Few categories of substances can claim as rich and varied a relationship with humanity as hallucinogens, the breadth of different chemicals included under its category, or the diversity of use patterns and contexts in which they are consumed. Arguably, no other class of substances currently generates the same degree of medical, social, and political intrigue as hallucinogens.

This well-studied class of substances can have significant effects on the perception of reality, an effect that has been proposed to have both potential therapeutic value and cultural and spiritual importance, while at the same time (like all other psychoactive substances) the potential for deleterious consequences, including use disorders and addiction. Therefore, a full understanding of hallucinogens is simultaneously timely and uniquely complex, because understanding the impact of these substances requires synthesis of their known neuropharmacology alongside an appreciation of the broader cultural history and contextual use of these substances.

The use of hallucinogens in human society dates back millennia (Bogenschutz and Johnson 2016; Meyerhoefer 2011; Samorini 2019). An imprecise name, because they do not generally generate true hallucinations (sensory experiences in the absence of an actual referent), the term *hallucinogen* has become the preferred term for these substances in scientific and medical circles. They are often referred to by other monikers based on the experiences they trigger: *psychedelics* (originating from the combination of the Greek terms *psukhē*, meaning "mind," and *dēloun*, meaning "reveal" or "make visible"), *entheogens* (for spiritual experiences), or *oneirogens* (inducing a dream-like state with intact consciousness) (Davis et al. 2017; Meyerhoefer 2011; Nichols 2016; Schenberg et al. 2014). In traditional settings, they are often used for their potential to alter the processing of the cognitive, perceptual, and emotional experience of reality.

The use of hallucinogens can be further categorized based on the setting in which they are used: traditional, clinical, or artistic and recreational (Hartogsohn 2017). In traditional settings, hallucinogens can play sacred and symbolic roles in rites, rituals, and religious or spiritual faith activities (Schultes and Hofmann 1979). Use of ayahuasca, psilocybin, mescaline, and ibogaine, for example, originated in religious-spiritual settings embedded in cultural-community frames (Fotiou 2016; Williams et al. 2022).

Interest in these compounds led to multidisciplinary space within clinical settings and in clinical research, spawning a new field unto itself, now referred to as *psychedelic medicine*. Stemming from this, subjective (Carhart-Harris and Nutt 2010, 2013; van Amsterdam et al. 2015), naturalistic/observational (Bouso et al. 2012), and population-based (Hendricks et al. 2015) data suggest a possible positive association between hallucinogen use and mental health (Carhart-Harris and Goodwin 2017). Simultaneously, clinical experience also demonstrates that recreational use of these substances can have both subjectively positive effects (e.g., on artistic endeavors, religious-spiritual development) and negative impacts on behavior and function (e.g., use disorders/addiction, agitated psychotic-like experiences).

Although many of the hallucinogens used today can trace their origins to traditional cultural settings, a noteworthy exception to this pathway was the accidental discovery of lysergic acid diethylamide (LSD) in 1943 by Albert Hoffman that produced the "prototypical classic hallucinogen" (Bogenschutz and Johnson 2016). The result of this serendipitous discovery was nearly 20 years of steady investigation of hallucinogens used as treatment for a variety of human maladies, including alcohol use disorder (AUD), other substance use disorders (SUDs), pain disorders, and various mental illnesses, and as a psychotherapeutic enhancement tool (Mangini 1998).

Nearly 10,000 scientific articles on LSD were authored during that period alone (Passie et al. 2008). By the early 1970s, most controlled human research with LSD ended due to a combination of tighter drug control policies, decreased government funding, and widespread recreational use that was perceived to be connected to social turmoil (Lee and Shlain 1985). Although the initial research on LSD failed to convincingly demonstrate medical utility, interest in the medical value of hallucinogens nonetheless persisted, and a more recent research renaissance has continued these investigations of hallucinogens in an increasingly wider array of areas such as for the treatment of depression, eating disorders, PTSD, anxiety, OCD, and addictive disorders, as well as to support improvement in general mental well-being (Bogenschutz and Johnson 2016; Bogenschutz et al. 2015; Carhart-Harris et al. 2021; George et al. 2022; Krebs and Johansen 2012; Mans et al. 2021; Mash et al. 2018; Pollan 2019; Reiff et al. 2020; Spriggs et al. 2021; Teixeira et al. 2022; Vargas et al. 2021). Furthermore, hallucinogens have experienced a sociopolitical revival resulting in political movements in some states (e.g., California, Colorado, Oregon), with aims to deregulate or, in some cases, legalize hallucinogen use (Basen 2021; Blistein 2019; Hayes 2021; Miles and Townsend 2021).

Misuse of hallucinogens can result in a range of deleterious consequences, including behavioral patterns of use consistent with addiction (hallucinogen use disorder). Most hallucinogens, however, are generally less euphorigenic than other typically misused substances, and many produce rapid tolerance to acute effects that generally precludes daily intoxication, resulting in a decreased likelihood of the habitual use patterns seen with other, more euphorigenic substances. Altogether, these factors make hallucinogens somewhat more complex to risk-stratify and categorize than other psychoactive substances.

In this chapter, we review the various substances that are categorized as hallucinogens or hallucinogen-like. We examine the psychopharmacology and neurobiology of hallucinogens as a general class of substances and describe the common features of intoxication that these substances share. General principles of pharmacological management of intoxication and withdrawal as well as maintenance pharmacological approaches are reviewed. Given the heterogeneity of chemicals that are categorized as hallucinogens, we also separately review attributes of several common hallucinogenic substances. In addition, given the burgeoning interest in hallucinogens as a treatment for addiction, we briefly review the current evidence base examining this potential therapeutic application (Vollenweider and Preller 2020).

Although it is not a typical hallucinogen (and not one whose use originated in a traditional cultural context), phencyclidine (PCP), a dissociative anesthetic, is reviewed in this chapter, given that it shares some key clinical features with hallucinogens, including a potentially common final pathway in prefrontal glutamatergic modulation (Vollenweider and Kometer 2010).

In this book, ketamine and 3,4-methylenedioxymethamphetamine (MDMA), which are often also considered alongside hallucinogens, are reviewed in Chapter 9 ("Club Drugs and Inhalants").

Hallucinogens

Represented Substances

A number of substances have been categorized as hallucinogens; usually they are differentiated by neurobiological action, psychoactive effect, or chemical structure. So-called *classic hallucinogens* are commonly believed to wield their psychoactive properties through agonism of serotonin (5-hydroxytryptamine [5-HT]) type 2A (5-HT$_{2A}$) receptors. LSD, psilocybin, mescaline, and *N,N*-dimethyltryptamine (DMT) are examples of classic hallucinogens. *Nonclassic hallucinogens* have neurobiological action through nonspecific serotonin mechanisms (e.g., MDMA, covered separately in Chapter 9), *N*-methyl-D-aspartate (NMDA) receptor or glutamatergic modulation (e.g., phencyclidine), κ opioid receptor (KOR) agonism (e.g., salvinorin A/*Salvia divinorum*, ibogaine), or other miscellaneous or combinations of different neurotransmitter systems.

By chemical structure, hallucinogens are commonly separated into two broad categories: the phenethylamines (e.g., mescaline, MDMA) and the indoleamines (e.g., LSD, psilocybin, DMT, harmaline, ibogaine). Table 8.1 organizes a partial list of these compounds based on these criteria.

Common Psychoactive and Physiological Effects of Hallucinogens

The psychoactive and physiological effects of hallucinogens can vary widely by substance, dose, and route of administration. Psychologically, hallucinogens have the potential to impact processing of the cognitive, perceptual, and emotional understanding of self and reality; in other words, they have the potential to alter consciousness. They can change the sentient awareness of internal and external existence, which can challenge an individual's understanding of consciousness at large (Presti 2021). Categorization based on experience organizes the various alterations of consciousness that hallucinogens engender (which may exist simultaneously during intoxication) and includes the following: perceptual changes, experiential changes, and mystical-type or transpersonal experiences (Presti 2017). Table 8.2 summarizes the physiological and psychological effects of hallucinogens.

Physiologically, the effects of hallucinogen ingestion are variable and depend on magnitude of exposure (dose) and route of administration. LSD, for example, can result in mild sympathetic system stimulation (e.g., pupillary dilation, mild increases in heart rate and blood pressure) and hyperreflexia. DMT, PCP, and psilocybin also have mild sympathomimetic effects, whereas salvinorin A/*S. divinorum* does not. In some instances, reports of marked sympathetic activation may actually be tied to psychological activation (e.g., anxiety, panic) driven by setting and context of use.

The physiological and psychological manifestations of hallucinogen intoxication are mediated by the interactions of the various hallucinogenic chemicals with the array of different neurotransmitter systems they impact. How these interactions result in the intoxication experience unique to hallucinogens remains a topic of much research, especially as the experience is increasingly investigated as a potential therapeutic clinical tool. Neuroimaging studies have implicated several brain regions and their associated neural networks as being particularly involved in the experience of hallucinogen intoxication (Carhart-Harris et al. 2012, 2014, 2016; Vollenweider et al. 1997).

Specifically, temporary decreases in resting state functional connectivity in major resting state networks (i.e., the default-mode network [DMN]) and novel patterns of neural network communication have been demonstrated in response to hallucinogen ingestion. The term *default-mode network* refers to

Table 8.1 Hallucinogens and distinguishing features

Class and chemical name	Common or street name	Source	Dosage and route (duration of action)	Major neurobiological target	Notes
Indole-alkylamines					
Lysergic acid diethylamide (LSD)	acid, blotter	Synthetic	50–200 μg PO (8–14 h)	5-HT$_{2A}$ partial agonist	Distributed on small squares of blotting paper, drops of liquid, gel-caps, small pills
Psilocybin	magic mushrooms, shrooms	*Psilocybe cubensis*, *Psilocybe azurescens*, many other subspecies; synthesis	10–50 mg, 1–5 g dried mushroom, quite variable/PO (4–8 h)	5-HT$_{2A}$ partial agonist	Psilocybin is converted in the body to psilocin, the actual active hallucinogen Continued shamanic use in Mexico Bruising of mushroom turns blue

Table 8.1 Hallucinogens and distinguishing features (continued)

Class and chemical name	Common or street name	Source	Dosage and route (duration of action)	Major neurobiological target	Notes
Dimethyltryptamine (DMT)	yopo, cohoba, businessman's trip	*Psychotria viridis*, *Anadenanthera peregrina*, *Mimosa hostilis*, many other natural sources; synthetic	5–40 mg smoked, inhaled snuff (30–60 min)	5-HT$_{2A}$ partial agonist	Continued shamanic use in Amazon region
Dimethyltryptamine + monoamine oxidase inhibitors; harmala β-carbolines (ayahuasca)	daime, yaje, hoasca, vine of the soul	*P. viridis* (DMT) + *Banisteriopsis caapi* (monoamine oxidase inhibitor)	Variable/PO (2–4 h)	5-HT$_{2A}$ partial agonist	Brewed as a tea; religious sacrament

Table 8.1 Hallucinogens and distinguishing features *(continued)*

Class and chemical name	Common or street name	Source	Dosage and route (duration of action)	Major neurobiological target	Notes
Ibogaine		*Tabernanthe iboga*	200–300 mg PO (≥12 h)	Likely 5-HT$_{2A}$ partial agonist	Religious sacrament; long-acting metabolites may contribute to purported anti-opioid withdrawal benefits
Phenyl-alkylamines					
3,4,5-Trimethoxyphenylethylamine	mescaline, peyote, san pedro	*Lophophora williamsii*, *Echinopsis pachanoi*, other cacti; synthetic	200–500 mg, 10–20 g or 5–10 dried peyote buttons, 1 kg fresh *E. pachanoi* PO (6–12 h)	5-HT$_{2A}$ partial agonist	Religious sacrament

Table 8.1 Hallucinogens and distinguishing features *(continued)*

Class and chemical name	Common or street name	Source	Dosage and route (duration of action)	Major neurobiological target	Notes
Entactogenic phenyl-alkylamines					
3,4-Methylenedioxymethamphetamine (MDMA)	ecstasy, X, XTC, rolls, molly	Synthetic	80–150 mg PO (4–6 h)	5-HT release and depletion	Mildly hallucinogenic at high doses
3,4-Methylenedioxyamphetamine (MDA)	love drug, adam	Synthetic	75–160 mg PO (4–8 h)	5-HT release and depletion	—
4-Bromo-2,5-dimethoxyphenethylamine	2C-B, nexus	Synthetic	5–30 mg PO (4–8 h)	Unknown	—
4-Chloro-2,5-dimethoxyamphetamine (DOC)		Synthetic	1–5 mg PO (4–8 h)	Unknown	Has been found on blotting paper
4-Methyl-2,5-dimethoxyamphetamine	DOM, STP	Synthetic	1–10 mg PO (14–20 h)	Unknown	Higher doses used in the 1960s resulted in many emergency department visits

Table 8.1 Hallucinogens and distinguishing features *(continued)*

Class and chemical name	Common or street name	Source	Dosage and route (duration of action)	Major neurobiological target	Notes
Dissociative					
Ketamine	special K, vitamin K, K-hole	Synthetic	25–50 mg IM, 50–100 mg PO or snorted/insufflated (IM 1–2 h; PO 1–4 h)	NMDA antagonist	Subanesthetic dose: lost sense of time, space, verbal skills, balance, and drooling
Dextromethorphan	DXM, robo, DM	Synthetic	100–600 mg PO (4–8 h)	NMDA antagonist	—
Phencyclidine (PCP)	angel dust	Synthetic	3–10 mg PO (8–24 h)	NMDA antagonist	—

Table 8.1 Hallucinogens and distinguishing features *(continued)*

Class and chemical name	Common or street name	Source	Dosage and route (duration of action)	Major neurobiological target	Notes
Other					
Salvinorin A	salvia, sally D, diviner's sage	*Salvia divinorum*	250–750 mg (smoked), 2–10 g dried leaves PO smoked (smoked 30–60 minutes; PO 1–3 h)	κ-Opioid selective agonist	Atypical hallucinogen; no longer found in the wild
Scopolamine and atropine/datura, Jimson weed, loco weed, Thorn apple, angel's trumpet, belladonna, deadly nightshade		*Datura stramonium*, *Atropa belladonna*, many related species	Highly variable/PO (12–48 h)	Competitive muscarinic acetylcholine antagonist	Plants of the Solanaceae family contain various ratios of scopolamine to atropine; blurred vision

Table 8.1 Hallucinogens and distinguishing features *(continued)*

Class and chemical name	Common or street name	Source	Dosage and route (duration of action)	Major neurobiological target	Notes
Muscimol (5-[aminomethyl]-3-isoxazolol)/fly agaric, amanita		*Amanita muscaria, A. pantherina*	1–30 g dried mushrooms PO (5–10 h)	GABA$_A$ agonist Glutamate receptors	Shamanic use in eastern Siberia; more than 600 species of agarics, easy to misidentify; some are extremely poisonous such as "death cap" *A. phalloides*; mushrooms also contain ibotenic acid; as it dries/ages, decarboxylation of ibotenic acid creates muscimol

5-HT = 5-hydroxytryptamine (serotonin); NMDA = *N*-methyl-D-aspartate; PO = per os.

Table 8.2 Hallucinogen physiological and psychological effects

Physical effects[a]	Psychological effects
Slight to moderate	**Usual**
Diaphoresis	Acute cognitive alterations with loosening of association, inability for goal-directed thinking, and memory disturbance
Hyperreflexia	
Hypertension or hypotension	
Hyperthermia	Altered experience of time and space
Motor incoordination	Altered body image
Neuroendocrine alteration	Dream-like state
Palpitation	Increased suggestibility
Tachycardia	Intensification and lability of affect with euphoria, anxiety, depression, and/or cathartic expressions
Tremor	Lassitude, indifference, and/or detachment
	Sensory activation with illusion, pseudo-hallucination, hallucination, and/or synesthesia
Moderate to strong	**Positive**
Arousal	Delight in novelty
Insomnia	Mystical experience
Mydriasis	Sense of perceiving deeper layers of the world, oneself, and others ("consciousness expansion")
	Sense of profound discovery/healing
Occasional	**Negative**
Blurred vision	Depersonalization
Diarrhea	Derealization
Nausea/vomiting	Hysteria
Nystagmus	Impaired judgment
Piloerection	Impulsivity
Salivation	Megalomania
	Odd behavior
	Panic
	Paranoid ideation
	Psychosomatic complaint
	Suicidal ideation

[a]Some effects are reactions to psychological content (e.g., increased heart rate and nausea due to anxiety), and complaints can depend on factors such as mindset, setting, dose, and supervision. Intoxicated individuals may also deny physical impairment or claim increased energy, sharpened mental acuity, and improved sensory perception.

the resting (or default) state of the brain, which is most active during spontaneous, undirected thought (mind-wandering) and significantly involves the posterior cingulate cortex (PCC) and medial prefrontal cortex (mPFC). The PCC and the mPFC are brain hubs involved in introspective thought and emotion processing, respectively, and together are responsible for generating a sense of self as distinct from others and our surroundings. The disintegration of the DMN seen in response to hallucinogen ingestion therefore results in diverse, unusual communication patterns between brain regions that are hypothesized to account for the novel experiences of self, thought, and environment associated with hallucinogen consumption. The creation of novel thought patterns through temporary DMN disintegration not only accounts for the phenomenology seen in hallucinogen intoxication but also provides the foundation for the potential therapeutic benefits documented and proposed in the literature, because DMN hyperactivity is implicated in the genesis and maintenance of several mental illnesses (e.g., anxiety, depression, and SUDs) (Millière et al. 2018).

General Principles of Hallucinogen Intoxication Management

The physiological and psychological effects of most hallucinogen intoxications alone are rarely life-threatening even in overdose, with some notable exceptions (e.g., ibogaine). For individuals with significant underlying medical vulnerabilities, the mild sympathetic activation produced by several hallucinogens may pose a hypothetical risk that should be monitored and managed appropriately. Importantly, however, the altered states of consciousness resulting from hallucinogen use can drive behaviors that may be immediately life-threatening.

The primary objective of hallucinogen intoxication management, therefore, is ensuring the safety of the individual and those around them until the altered state of consciousness has subsided. Containment of the individual in a low-stimulus environment (e.g., dimly lit, quiet environment with minimal distractions) remains the first-line management strategy. No hallucinogen antidote medications are supported by the literature or clinical experience. Targeted symptomatic medications are commonly used, though, in situations in which agitation or other behaviors pose an immediate threat to the individual or those around them. Typically, benzodiazepine sedative-hypnotic medications are sufficient to mitigate immediate threats to safety (e.g., diazepam 5–10 mg PO or IV; lorazepam 1–2 mg PO, IV, or IM). Although elements of hallucinogen intoxication can appear frankly psychotic, there is little evidence to support the efficacy of neuroleptic medications in the management of acute intoxication. Nonetheless, in circumstances in which safety is significantly compromised, clinicians may opt to administer neuroleptics alongside benzodiazepines or other sedative-hypnotics (e.g., risperidone, olanzapine 5–10 mg PO). More recent commentary cautions the use of haloperidol, in particular, because it was found to exacerbate the subjective effects of healthy volunteers when studying psilocybin (Malcolm and Thomas 2022).

General Principles of Hallucinogen Withdrawal Management

Despite many hallucinogens producing rapid, clinically significant tolerance, no hallucinogen-specific withdrawal syndrome is recognized. In some instances, chronic heavy use of certain hallucinogens may result in alterations in mood or anxiety that can be treated symptomatically. These consequences of chronic use of hallucinogens are not a traditional withdrawal syndrome, though, and may be the result of other factors such as co-consumed substances or psychological processing of behaviors and experiences that occurred during intoxication.

A Note About Flashback Phenomena and Hallucinogen Persisting Perception Disorder

Background

Flashback phenomena and hallucinogen persisting perception disorder (HPPD) are not strictly considered withdrawal phenomena. They are considered here because they are necessarily temporally situated after the use of the hallucinogen has been discontinued, sometimes long after.

Hallucinogen *aftereffects*, also known as *flashbacks*, are late drug effects that can emerge after the acute effects have worn off, and they have been a topic of much uncertainty and debate. These aftereffects were first described as "a repetition of the acute phase of the experience days or even weeks after the initial doses" (Sandison and Whitelaw 1957, p. 337). Because flashbacks appear suddenly and unexpectedly, often at inappropriate times, they are usually associated with foreboding or dread and a loss of control or "going mad." In other instances, the response to a flashback may be one of enjoyment and pleasure, perceived as a welcoming "free trip."

In a 2021 systematic review of the literature, Vis et al. (2021) found a total of 66 relevant publications encompassing 97 unique individuals reporting HPPD symptoms, the majority of which (37.1%) were triggered by LSD use. Of those reporting HPPD, 76% described symptoms consistent with what is known as *Alice in Wonderland syndrome* (AIWS). In AIWS, symptoms fall into three different categories: 1) visual distortions, such as macropsia and micropsia; 2) time distortions, such as quick- or slow-motion phenomena; and 3) body distortions, such as macrosomatognosia and microsomatognosia (Vis et al. 2021). Although the majority of those experiencing HPPD reported perceptions consistent with the prior intoxication state, 38% described perceptual symptoms not clearly linked to prior intoxication states, leading the authors to surmise that HPPD is "characterized by changes in the *content* of consciousness and an attentional shift from exogenous to endogenous phenomena" rather than the alteration in state of consciousness often experienced in acute hallucinogen intoxication (Vis et al. 2021, p. 1).

There are some triggers known for the induction of flashback phenomena. Examples include being in the same environmental circumstances (i.e., being in the same place as prior ingestion, listening to the same music) or being in states where the level of CNS excitation is similar or control over the experience is diminished (e.g., being tired, hypnagogic states, cannabis or alcohol intoxication) (Holland and Passie 2011).

These aftereffects very rarely occur under medically controlled conditions, as shown by different surveys about complications in therapeutic and experimental use (Malleson 1971; Studerus et al. 2011). However, they may happen more often in uncontrolled circumstances (Baggott et al. 2011).

Management Strategies for Hallucinogen Persisting Perception Disorder

For patients complaining of HPPD, reassurance that the persisting phenomena are not reflective of cognitive damage is important. Atypical antipsychotics have been reported to aggravate the condition (for review, see Halpern and Pope 2003), although some case reports have reported benefit (Subramanian and Doran 2014). Management with a sedative-hypnotic, such as diazepam or lorazepam, may be effective, especially for those with chronic complaints associated with anxiety. This off-label pharmacotherapy cautiously targeting specific symptoms (e.g., anxiety, depression, persisting psychotic symptoms) demonstrates a high degree of success, with one systematic review finding that 63% of patients who received some pharmacotherapy reported a positive outcome (Vis et al. 2021).

Hallucinogenic Substance–Specific Review

Lysergic Acid Diethylamide

Background

LSD is the most widely used hallucinogenic drug. In both its somatic and psychological effects, LSD is representative of most of the other classic hallucinogenic drugs and remains the most rigorously researched hallucinogen. LSD is a semisynthetic substance derived from lysergic acid as found in the parasitic rye fungus *Claviceps purpurea*. LSD is listed as a Schedule I controlled substance by the U.S. Drug Enforcement Administration (DEA).

Pharmacodynamics

The pharmacology and mechanisms of action of LSD and the interaction of LSD with neurotransmitter receptors is complex, and its mechanisms of action are incompletely understood (Carhart-Harris et al. 2016; Hintzen and Passie 2010; Nichols 1986). LSD acts as a 5-HT autoreceptor agonist on 5-HT$_{1A}$ receptors in the locus coeruleus, the raphe nuclei, and the cortex. It inhibits firing and 5-HT release by these cells. It also acts as a partial agonist on the postsynaptic 5-HT$_{1A}$ site. The hallucinogenic effect of LSD has been primarily linked to its agonism of the 5-HT$_2$ receptor. Therefore, LSD is probably best called a mixed 5-HT$_2$/5-HT$_1$ receptor agonist/partial agonist (Pierce and Peroutka 1989; Sanders-Bush et al. 1988).

Pharmacokinetics

LSD is completely absorbed in the digestive tract (Rothlin 1957; Rothlin and Cerletti 1956). The threshold oral dose for measurable sympathomimetic effects in humans is 0.5–1.0 µg/kg (Greiner et al. 1958). After LSD 100–250 µg, psychological and sympathomimetic effects persist, reaching their peak after 1.5–2.5 hours (Hoch 1956). The distribution of LSD across tissue and organ systems is yet to be quantified for humans. The presence of considerable amounts in the brain and cerebrospinal fluid of rats and cats indicates that LSD may easily pass the blood–brain barrier (Axelrod et al. 1957). The half-life of LSD in humans is 175 minutes (Aghajanian and Bing 1964; Upshall and Wailling 1972).

Tolerance to the effects of LSD occurs rapidly in humans and animals. Tolerance to autonomic and psychological effects of LSD occurs in humans after a few moderate daily doses (Abramson et al. 1956; Belleville et al. 1956; Cholden et al. 1955). Reduction in receptor density is a possible mechanism for the development of tolerance to LSD.

There have been no documented human deaths from an LSD overdose attributable to toxicity (Hendricks et al. 2015; Hintzen and Passie 2010; Nichols 2018); rather, the deaths associated with LSD use are tied to the potentially profound effects on judgment and perception and the resultant behaviors. Empirical studies showed no evidence of teratogenic or mutagenic effects from use of LSD in humans (Leuner 1981; Robinson et al. 1974; Smart and Bateman 1968).

Acute and Chronic Effects

Physiological effects
LSD-induced sympathetic stimulation is evidenced by pupillary dilation, mild increases in heart rate and blood pressure (Dimascio et al. 1957; Forrer and Goldner 1951), and slight blood glucose elevation (Hollister and Sjoberg 1964; Liddell and Weil-Malherbe 1953). Typically there is no change in respiration rate, and increases in body temperature are seen only rarely. Initial nausea, decreased appetite, temporary mild headache, dizziness, and inner trembling may occur in some subjects. The most consistent neurological effect is an exaggeration of the patellar (and other deep tendon) reflexes (Belleville et al. 1956). More unusual signs include slight unsteadiness of gait to full ataxia.

Psychological effects
A moderate oral dose (75–150 µg) of LSD will significantly alter the state of consciousness, including stimulation of various affective states, enhanced capacity for introspection, and altered psychological functioning in the direction of hypnagogia and dreams (Farthing 1992). The acute psychological effects of LSD last 6–10 hours, depending on the dose applied. Typical perceptual changes include illusions, pseudo-hallucinations, and synesthesias, as well as alterations of thinking and time experience (see Table 8.3). Changes in body image and ego function also often occur (Katz et al. 1968; Savage 1955). Occasionally, religious, spiritual, and mystical experiences may occur.

Major surveys indicate that LSD is safe when administered in medically supervised settings (Cohen 1960; Malleson 1971). Traumatic experiences ("bad trips") can have long-lasting effects, including mood swings and (rarely) flashback phenomena (Strassman 1984). These reports of bad trips are primarily confined to LSD recreational and social ingestion experiences—in other words, outside the research or controlled clinical settings. The most common unpleasant reaction is an episode of anxiety or panic, characterized by severe, terrifying thoughts and feelings, fear of losing control, fear of insanity or death, or despair (Strassman 1984). In these cases, dangerous behavior is a possibility. Other complications include temporary paranoid ideation, temporary depressive mood swings, and increase in psychic lability in the days after the LSD experience (Grof 1975; Leuner 1981).

Conversely, it has been shown that under controlled and supportive conditions, LSD experiences may have lasting positive effects on attitude and personality in healthy humans (Griffiths et al. 2006, 2008; Haden and Woods 2020; Hendricks et al. 2015; McGlothlin et al. 1967).

As in treatment for intoxication with other substances, treatment of LSD intoxication includes providing a comfortable and quiet environment in which empathic communication is used to talk down the patient. In some cases, administration of a benzodiazepine may be indicated. Neuroleptics do not have an immediate effect and are therefore indicated only in the rare instance of severe, long-lasting LSD reactions with significant psychotic features that are endangering safety.

Psilocybin

Background

Approximately half of the more than 200 mushrooms in the genus *Psilocybe* produce psilocybin, and they have a widespread, near-global distribution, including in the United States (Stamets 1996). Historically, psilocybin-containing mushrooms have been used sacramentally by Indigenous cultures—a use that persists in some regions to this day (e.g., Mexico) (Wasson and Heim 1958). Psychoactive mushroom consumer availability was not significant until the mid-1970s, when drug aficionados produced guides for collecting wild mushrooms (Pollock 1975) and pamphlets on methods of cultivation (Oss and Oeric 1976).

The prodrug psilocybin (4-phosphoryloxy-N,N-dimethyltryptamine) and its active metabolite psilocin (4-hydroxy-N,N-dimethyltryptamine) are

Table 8.3 Typical sensory and psychological effects under the influence of a medium dose of LSD (100–200 mg PO), mescaline (300–500 mg PO), or psilocybin (15–25 mg PO)

Type	Effect
Sensory alterations (visual, auditory, taste, olfactory, kinesthetic)	Illusion
	Pseudo-hallucination
	Intensification of color perception
	Metamorphosis-like change in objects and faces
	Intense (kaleidoscopic or scenic) visual imagery with transforming content
Alterations of affectivity	Intensification of emotional experience: euphoria, dysphoria, anxiety, mood swings
	Mystical-type experiences
Alterations of thinking	Less abstract and more imaginative thought
	Broader and unusual associations
	Shortened attention span
	Delusions
Alterations of body perceptions	Change in body image
	Unusual inner perception of bodily processes
	Metamorphic alteration of body contours
Memory changes	Re-experiencing of significant biographical memories
	Hypermnesia
	Age regression

substituted hallucinogenic indolealkylamines. Total content of psilocybin varies with mushroom, subspecies, and preparation, but the most commonly used mushroom, *P. cubensis*, contains 5–11 mg psilocybin/g dried mushroom.

Synthetic psilocybin is very complicated to manufacture but has been used in research contexts. Consequently, most of the illegal drug market trade in psilocybin has occurred with naturally derived fungal sources. Psilocybin was used clinically in the 1960s in psychotherapy (Passie 2004) and has been evaluated in a range of experimental studies. Examples of its use include induction of mystical-type experiences (Griffiths et al. 2006) and treatment of advanced-stage cancer anxiety (Grob et al. 2011), various psychiatric disorders such as depression (Balon 2022), anxiety in patients with terminal cancer (Griffiths et al. 2016), OCD (Moreno et al. 2006), and addictive disorders (see later section "Psilocybin in Substance Use Disorder Treatment"). Psilocybin remains a DEA Schedule I controlled substance in the United States.

Pharmacodynamics

Psilocybin interacts mainly with serotonergic neurotransmission (5-HT_{1A}, 5-HT_{1D}, 5-HT_{2A}, and 5-HT_{2C} receptor subtypes). It binds with high affinity at 5-HT_{2A} and to a lesser extent at 5-HT_{1A} receptors (McKenna et al. 1990). It should be noted that unlike LSD, psilocybin and its active metabolite psilocin have no affinity for dopamine D_2 receptors (Creese et al. 1975). A double-blind, placebo-controlled study with ketanserin (a reference standard 5-HT_{2A} receptor antagonist) showed complete blocking of effects of psilocybin (Vollenweider et al. 1998). Despite significant tolerance that occurs with repeated use of psilocybin, neither physical dependence nor a withdrawal syndrome develops.

Pharmacokinetics

Psilocybin is readily absorbed following oral administration and is widely distributed throughout the body (Hopf and Eckert 1974; Passie et al. 2002). There are four main metabolites of psilocybin, including the active metabolite psilocin. Psychological effects occur with plasma levels of 4–6 µg/mL (Hasler et al. 1997), usually within 70–90 minutes after doses of 8–25 mg PO. The half-life of psilocybin is 163.3 ± 63.5 minutes (Hasler et al. 1997), and the mean elimination half-life of psilocin is 50 minutes. The plasma concentration can vary widely between individuals, with the maximum plasma concentration at approximately 80 minutes (Hasler et al. 1997). The elimination of the glucuronidated metabolites as well as unaltered psilocybin (3%–10%) occurs through the kidneys. Approximately two-thirds of the renal excretion of psilocin is completed after 3 hours (Hasler et al. 1997).

Acute and Chronic Effects

Ingestion of *Psilocybe* mushrooms can, in some cases, cause nausea and vomiting, but serious toxicity in humans is rare. There are only three documented cases of human fatalities attributed to psilocybin toxicity, and in each, the direct cause-effect relationship between consumption and death is challenging to prove (Gerault and Picart 1996; Lim et al. 2012). Although there are some data to suggest a dose-dependent correlation between psilocybin and QTc prolongation, the clinical significance of this relationship is believed to be minimal (Dahmane et al. 2021). Peak intoxication occurs approximately within the first 2 hours, diminishing over the subsequent 3–4 hours.

Physiological effects within the usual dose range (10–25 mg PO) include mydriasis, slight changes in heart and breathing rate, and discrete hyperglycemic and hypertonic effects (Passie et al. 2002). Electrolyte levels, liver enzyme activity, and blood glucose levels are unaffected (Delay et al. 1958; Hollister 1961), as are measures of endocrine function (e.g., cortisol, prolactin, and growth hormone levels) (Gouzoulis-Mayfrank et al. 1999). There is no evidence of mutagenic or teratogenic effects (Passie et al. 2002).

The psychopathological phenomena induced by psilocybin are virtually identical to those of LSD (described in the previous subsection). At a moderate dose (12–20 mg PO), psilocybin was found to produce an altered state of consciousness marked by stimulation of affective states, enhanced ability for introspection, and altering of psychological functioning (Studerus et al. 2011). Especially noteworthy are perceptual changes such as illusions, synesthesias, and alterations of thought, time sense, and body experience (Bogenschutz and Johnson 2016).

Most individuals who ingest psilocybin display an erratic pattern of use. The intense and consciousness-altering/expanding effects of psilocybin appear to limit frequency of its use. Daily consumption of psilocybin results in acute tolerance, and such users are virtually absent in the scientific literature (Riley and Blackman 2008).

Complications arising from use and misuse of psilocybin (e.g., emergency department visits) occur with less frequency than with most other hallucinogens (Barbee et al. 2009). This may be partially dependent on its short duration of action—that is, troubled individuals may find the intoxication resolving before being evaluated in crisis. Complications may consist of overarousal with severe panic reactions (bad trips), which can be treated by transferring the person to a quiet environment and offering empathic supportive reassurances. In some clinical situations, the use of a benzodiazepine may be indicated. Although somatic effects of psilocybin rarely present danger, one must be attentive for the potential co-ingestion (or ingestion in error) of other, more toxic mushrooms.

Dimethyltryptamine and Related Chemicals
Background

DMT is a major hallucinogen with unusual psychological effects (Strassman et al. 1994). It is derived from different plant sources and animal venoms and is also produced endogenously by humans (Barker et al. 2012). Despite much conjecture (Callaway 1988; Strassman 2001), endogenous DMT's physiological functions are still unknown, although it has been found to be an endogenous σ_1 receptor regulator agonist (Fontanilla et al. 2009). In the United States, illicit DMT usually appears as a synthetic or extracted powder. DMT is found in and can be extracted from common plants growing in much of the United States, including the root bark of the prairie bundleflower (*Desmanthus illinoensis*) (Halpern 2004).

Many Indigenous peoples of Latin America (especially in Brazil, Colombia, and Peru) have used DMT for spiritual purposes for hundreds of years to the present. It is prepared as a powdered snuff from the seeds of *Anadenanthera peregrina* or the bark of *Virola* sp. trees. Ayahuasca (the Quechua translation is "vine of the soul") is a DMT concoction, but it is orally active because it also contains natural, reversible monoamine oxidase inhibitors from the vine *Banisteriopsis caapi* (Schultes and Hofmann 1979), which prevent degradation of DMT by gut-lined monoamine oxidase enzymes (Naranjo 1979). Ayahuasca in the form of a tea is a sacrament of syncretic religions (Tupper 2008). The U.S. Supreme Court has deemed ayahuasca religious use to be constitutionally protected under the Religious Freedom Restoration Act of 1993 (Anderson et al. 2012; *Gonzales v. O Centro Espírita Beneficente União do Vegetal* 2006). A survey of American members of the Santo Daime religion appear to not have psychiatric sequelae from the use of ayahuasca in a religious setting (Halpern et al. 2008). The traditional use of ayahuasca embedded in a cultural context tends to deploy many of the exclusionary criteria found in clinical trials and unregulated hallucinogen treatment centers (i.e., psychotic disorders, cardiovascular disease, current or recent substance use, metabolic abnormalities). Ayahuasca use in these settings typically involves experienced guides during sessions.

The hallucinogenic methoxylated derivative of DMT, 5-methoxy-*N*,*N*-dimethyltryptamine (5-MeO-DMT), is found naturally in a wide variety of plant species as well as in the glandular secretions of the Sonoran Desert toad (*Incilius alvarius*), also known as the Colorado River toad (Barsuglia et al.

2018). In addition to 5-MeO-DMT, the Sonoran Desert toad's secretions contain another chemically related natural hallucinogen, 5-hydroxy-N,N-dimethyltryptamine (5-HO-DMT, or bufotenine). Together, 5-MeO-DMT and 5-HO-DMT serve a venomous protective role for the toad, but they are potently hallucinogenic if consumed by humans. 5-MeO-DMT and 5-HO-DMT are most typically consumed orally, or the toad secretions are dried and added to other organic matter (e.g., parsley) and smoked. Several U.S. celebrities have publicly shared accounts of their transformative experiences related to 5-MeO-DMT and 5-HO-DMT consumption, bringing these chemicals into more mainstream awareness (Chung 2021; Gastelum 2021). DMT, 5-MeO-DMT, and 5-HO-DMT are all Schedule I controlled substances in the United States.

Pharmacodynamics

DMT, 5-MeO-DMT, and 5-HO-DMT are all believed to exert their hallucinogenic effects via high-affinity agonism of $5-HT_2$ and $5-HT_{1A}$ receptors, much like other classic indoleamine hallucinogens. 5-MeO-DMT is 4–10 times more potent than DMT at the $5-HT_{1A}$ receptor (McKenna and Towers 1984; Ott 1999), and 5-HO-DMT has a much greater affinity for the $5-HT_{2A}$ receptor than 5-MeO-DMT (Spencer et al. 1987).

Pharmacokinetics

When a small amount of DMT (10–20 mg) or 5-MeO-DMT (6–20 mg) is smoked alone or on a substrate of tobacco, parsley, or marijuana, intoxication occurs within seconds, achieves peak effects within 2–3 minutes, and then clears over the next 15 minutes for DMT and 40 minutes for 5-MeO-DMT (Cakic et al. 2010; Shen et al. 2010). The ayahuasca preparation of DMT intoxicates for 3–4 hours, peaking within the first hour, and is typically associated with a considerable amount of nausea and vomiting (Riba et al. 2001). DMT and 5-MeO-DMT are metabolized through demethylation via cytochrome P450 (CYP) 2D6 and deamination via monoamine oxidase A. 5-MeO-DMT is metabolized in the human body to 5-HO-DMT, which can help account for 5-MeO-DMT's longer duration of action relative to DMT.

Acute and Chronic Effects

The psychological effects of DMT, 5-MeO-DMT, and 5-HO-DMT, especially when they appear very rapidly as with smoking or intranasal insufflation, can be very frightening and can lead to severe nonintentional injuries because of disorientation, motor incoordination, and unrealistic thoughts and behaviors. Supervision and a secure environment help to ameliorate these risks. Severe complications appear to be very rare, especially when the oral route is used, and also may not show up in clinical settings because of the very short duration of action of DMT (15–90 minutes).

The somatic effects of DMT consist of a dose-dependent rise in blood pressure and pulse rate and a sympathomimetic excitation syndrome with hallucinations and overarousal. In some cases, high doses or overdoses may lead to epileptic seizures. With orally ingested ayahuasca, the psychological effects of DMT are milder and are very similar to those of LSD and psilocybin. Most people in religious ayahuasca prayer services report significant "spiritual," "cleansing," and "mystical" experiences. In the higher dose range, some very unusual experiences (e.g., contact with "alien creatures," elves, and gnomes; experiences of tunnels or lights; and even "encounters with god-like entities") were reported (Strassman 2001). Those who have consumed toad venom report an experience of anxiolysis, enhanced libido, and "ego death" along with auditory and visual hallucinations at higher doses (Chung 2021; Sandroni 2001).

No deaths have been reported from ayahuasca or other DMT/monoamine oxidase inhibitor combinations. If panic reactions and bad trips are seen in emergency department settings, they may be treated with diazepam 5–10 mg IV or equivalent doses of other benzodiazepines. However, deaths have been reported following consumption of toad venom, which may result from the presence of additional venoms, such as digoxin-like cardiac glycosides (Brubacher et al. 1996; Hitt and Ettinger 1986), as well as the particular toxicity of 5-HO-DMT (Kostakis and Byard 2009).

Mescaline

Background

The principal hallucinogenic compound of the peyote cactus, *Lophophora williamsii*, is mescaline (3,4,5-trimethoxyphenethylamine), although more than 60 other alkaloids are found as well (Anderson 1996). Mescaline has never been commonly synthesized and distributed for illicit purposes in the United States on a significant scale. Peyote use is protected by the American Indian Religious Freedom Act Amendments of 1994 and is almost solely consumed in religious ceremonies of the Native American Church. Peyote contains at most 1.5% mescaline sulfate. A potent mescaline intoxication is achieved with approximately 5 mg/kg or more. Mescaline is primarily consumed orally (as tablets, or more commonly as cactus buds that are chewed or dried and steeped into a tea); it can also be smoked or insufflated. A typical oral dose is 20–500 mg, with a concoction containing mescaline 200–400 mg representing three to six cactus buds or 10–20 g of dried peyote (Dinis-Oliveira et al. 2019; Kapadia and Fayez 1970; Nichols 2004). Mescaline is a Schedule I controlled substance in the United States.

Pharmacodynamics

Like other classic hallucinogens, mescaline's hallucinogenic activity is due to its agonism at the 5-HT$_2$ family of receptors, especially 5-HT$_{2A}$ and 5-HT$_{2B}$ (Aghajanian and Marek 1999; Dinis-Oliveira et al. 2019). Because of side-chain structural similarities to amphetamines, mescaline has been shown to induce mild dopaminergic activity (Trulson et al. 1983), but the clinical significance of this effect is uncertain. Mescaline has been shown to have some cross-tolerance with other classic hallucinogens (LSD, psilocybin); like other hallucinogens, tolerance develops rapidly (over 3–4 days) and is restored after 4 days of abstinence (Freedman 1969; Kapadia and Fayez 1970).

Pharmacokinetics

Mescaline is rapidly absorbed from the gastrointestinal tract and binds with hepatic proteins, distributes rapidly to the kidneys and liver, and has low lipophilicity, accounting for its relatively low blood–brain barrier permeability. Relative to other hallucinogens, mescaline is much less potent and demonstrates a prolonged time to peak intoxication (2–4 hours) and a much longer duration of action (10–12 hours) (Nichols 2004). Unlike many other hallucinogens, metabolism of mescaline does not appear to pass through CYP isoforms to a significant extent, but rather through a combination of amine oxidases (liver, lung) and *N*-acetylation (brain) (Dinis-Oliveira et al. 2019; Wu et al. 1997).

Acute and Chronic Effects

Peyote has a bitter, acrid taste, which itself often induces nausea and vomiting (rather than being a result of the chemical mescaline) (Carstairs and Cantrell 2010). Although mescaline intoxication shares many psychological effects with other classic hallucinogens, it nonetheless has some unique characteristics. Typically, sensory intensifications occur, such as sound, smell, and touch hypersensitivity and pitch distortions, as well as light and color being experienced as more brilliant. Geometrization of three-dimensional objects is unique to mescaline intoxication and is described as a distorted perception of dimensionality akin to Cubist paintings. Time can be experienced as passing more slowly, and there can be a sense of altogether transcendence of regular time, space, and earthly limits, culminating in a sense of communing with God or other deities (Bressloff et al. 2002; Dinis-Oliveira et al. 2019; Foster Olive 2007).

Mescaline poisoning has been documented and is characterized by any combination of hyperreflexia, tachycardia, agitation, seizures, and hyperthermia (Carstairs and Cantrell 2010). Despite one documented case of prolonged psychosis similar to schizophrenia (Kapadia and Fayez 1970), longitudinal studies of Native Americans exposed to mescaline in religious ceremonies have demonstrated no long-term psychological or cognitive sequela (Halpern et al. 2005). As extrapolated from animal experiments, the median lethal dose of mescaline in humans is projected to be an amount beyond what could be reasonably consumed. Although mescaline has been shown in monkeys to cross the placental barrier, peyote use in pregnancy has not demonstrated adverse fetal outcomes (Gilmore 2001).

Salvia Divinorum and Salvinorin A

Background

Salvinorin A is found in the perennial mint *S. divinorum*, a plant initially cultivated in Oaxaca, Mexico, where it has been used for spiritual, medicinal, and divinatory purposes. Early studies isolated salvinorin A as the principal psychoactive constituent responsible for the plant's hallucinogenic effects.

Leaves of the *S. divinorum* plant are commonly chewed, brewed into teas, and dried and smoked. Other routes of administration include inhalation via volatilization or the use of tinctures for buccal absorption (Babu et al. 2008). Salvinorin A/*S. divinorum* is not controlled by the Controlled Substances Act; nonetheless, at least 15 U.S. states have taken steps to criminalize possession or use of salvinorin A/*S. divinorum*, and more than 13 nations have made salvinorin A/*S. divinorum* illegal. It has an image of being relatively safe and cannot be detected by established drug tests, contributing to its attractiveness to some individuals for recreational use.

Pharmacodynamics

Salvinorin A is a neoclerodane diterpene alkaloid, structurally unrelated to any other hallucinogen, and a potent and selective agonist at the KOR (Roth et al. 2002). Its effects are not mediated by the 5-HT$_{2A}$ receptor, the classic target of other hallucinogens (Listos et al. 2011). Nonetheless, its mechanism of action is not fully understood (Cunningham et al. 2011), and preclinical data suggest that KOR agonists are less reinforcing than other opioid receptor agonists (Shippenberg et al. 2001). Doses as small as 200 µg can produce biological effects in humans, highlighting the high potency of salvinorin A.

Pharmacokinetics

Salvinorin A is only minimally absorbed through the mouth, while most is degraded in the gastrointestinal tract. After oral consumption, onset of effect is within 10–15 minutes, peaking at 20–40 minutes and typically resolving within 1 hour (Dalgarno 2007; Siebert 1994). Following inhalation of the dried leaves or vaporized extract, onset of effect is within 30 seconds, with peak effect at 2–5 minutes and resolution after 30 minutes (Johnson et al. 2011; Siebert 1994). Salvinorin A's high lipophilicity accounts for its rapid biodistribution, high plasma protein binding, and swift movement across the blood–brain barrier. Salvinorin A is rapidly metabolized by blood esterases as well as CYP2D6, CYP2C18, CYP1A1, and CYP2E1 isoforms (Teksin et al. 2009) and is renally excreted. After inhalation, the half-life is approximately 50 minutes (Maqueda et al. 2016).

Acute and Chronic Effects

If taken orally, leaves or extracts containing salvinorin A have a mild effect, often compared to cannabis. When inhaled, vaporized, or smoked, its effects can be much more pronounced. The psychological effects of salvinorin A consist of mood changes and hallucination-like experiences depending on dose (and extract concentration) (González et al. 2006). Intense hallucinatory-like effects typically last between 10 and 15 minutes (González et al. 2006). In previous studies, hallucinogenic effects appeared similar to those produced by intravenous DMT (Strassman et al. 1994) and higher oral doses of psilocybin (Griffiths et al. 2006). Salvinorin A does not significantly increase heart rate or blood pressure (Johnson et al. 2011).

There are no reports of acute or chronic toxicity or deaths from overdose on *S. divinorum*. Fatigue, confusion, tachycardia, and dizziness are commonly reported side effects (Baggott et al. 2010). More serious are reports of intense fear, panic, paranoia, and irritability (Brito-da-Costa et al. 2021; Nyi et al. 2010). Loss of consciousness and dangerously unrealistic and potentially self-destructive behaviors have regularly been reported, perhaps related to a sense of "near-death" experience similar to those described in intense ketamine experiences (Doss et al. 2020). Unpleasant aftereffects include reports of tiredness, heaviness of the head, dizziness, physical exhaustion, and slowed mental function (Doss et al. 2020). In laboratory studies, no evidence was found for persisting psychotic-like symptoms or depression and anxiety following *S. divinorum* consumption (Addy 2012; Brito-da-Costa et al. 2021), despite conflicting reports that *S. divinorum* may precipitate depressive illness (Wu et al. 2011).

There are no substances known to antagonize the effects of salvinorin A. No serious physiological symptoms seem to occur with moderate to high doses of this drug, although users become less aware of their surroundings as the dose increases. Should an intoxicated individual present to an emergency department, treatment is to protect the individual from serious injury and potentially self-destructive behavior because of disorientation. Diazepam (5–10 mg IV) or other benzodiazepines for treatment of panic and excitation may be indicated in more severe cases. Typically, the intoxication state lasts no longer than 2 hours, even with higher doses.

The abuse potential of *S. divinorum* appears to be lower than that of other substances of misuse, because it is primarily used in a sporadic or intermittent pattern, and many of those who have used *S. divinorum* report a dislike for the intoxication experience (Baker et al. 2009; Khey et al. 2008). There are no reports of a withdrawal syndrome from acute use of salvinorin A.

Other Plant Alkaloids

Importantly, care should be taken to ensure that other botanicals have not been inadvertently co-consumed or consumed through botanical misidentification. In particular, the alkaloids atropine, hyoscyamine, and scopolamine are found in jimson weed (*Datura stramonium*), nightshade (*Atropa belladonna*), mandrake (*Mandragora officinarum*), and henbane (*Hyoscyamus niger*) (Emboden 1980; Fodor 1971; Gyermek 1997). In overdose, these plants induce a toxic anticholinergic delirium that lasts hours to days and may be life-threatening. These tropane alkaloids are absorbed rapidly from the gastrointestinal tract (Grynkiewicz and Gadzikowska 2008), and initial effects may be perceived 1.5–4 hours after ingestion. Effects in the medium and higher dose range may persist for 24–48 hours. Significant intoxications show the following vegetative effects: dilation of pupils with inability to accommodate, dryness of mouth, difficulty swallowing, urinary retention, hyperreflexia, and muscle weakness (Inch and Brimblecombe 1974). With higher doses, seizures and coma may occur (Diker et al. 2007). Typical psychological effects of these related tropane alkaloids are as follows: clouding of consciousness, euphoria, dysphoria, excitation, confusion, depersonalization, sensory illusions and hallucinations (mainly visual), somnolence, memory disorders and amnesia, sudden outbursts of anger, anxiety, paranoid ideation, delusions, bizarre and disorganized speech, and talking to imaginary people (Ketchum et al. 1973; Longo 1966). Treatment of acute intoxication is mainly aimed at removing plant material from the gastrointestinal tract, keeping the patient safe, and reversing severe anticholinergic sequelae. As an antidote to antagonize the major physiological effects, intravenous physostigmine (0.02 mg/kg) is indicated and may be repeated, if necessary. Neostigmine is not indicated because it does not pass the blood–brain barrier.

Ibogaine

Background

Ibogaine (12-methoxyibogamine) was first isolated in 1901 and is one of a dozen naturally occurring monoterpenoid indole alkaloids identified and extracted from the African shrub *Tabernanthe iboga* root bark (Davis et al. 2017; Heink et al. 2017; Iyer et al. 2021; Schenberg et al. 2014). Iboga alkaloids have been found in a wide range of Apocynaceae family plants globally (Iyer et al. 2021). Traditional ibogaine has been used orally for shamanic ceremonies (Bwiti religion) in cohesive social networks that include initiates overseen by supervisors organized by seniority (Ravalec et al. 2007). Most often linked to Gabon and Cameroon, iboga is also used in other parts of West Africa for its purported antipyretic, analgesic, and antihypertensive effects. Ibogaine has particular notoriety for its professed antiaddictive effects through a reported reduction in craving for cocaine, amphetamine, and heroin. The antiaddictive effects of ibogaine on heroin use in particular were popularized by the chronicles of Howard Lotsoff, who used heroin and noted the relief of opioid withdrawal symptoms and facilitation of long-term recovery from heroin use disorder (Ona et al. 2021).

Ibogaine hydrochloride can be produced through semisynthesis from voacangine, which itself comes the African *Voacanga africana* tree (Davis et al. 2017; Iyer et al. 2021). Ibogaine (combined with its active metabolite noribogaine [12-hydroxyibogamine]) induces a variety of psychotropic effects, ranging from dissociative to psychedelic to oneirophrenic (inducing a dream-like state with intact consciousness) (Davis et al. 2017; Heink et al. 2017; Schenberg et al. 2014).

In low doses, ibogaine has been shown to have mild psychostimulatory effects; at higher doses, it can have hallucinogenic and tremorigenic effects (Cappendijk and Dzoljic 1993; Glick et al. 1993). Ibogaine is a Schedule I illegal substance in the United States, thereby restricting its availability for clinical research and treatment. However, ibogaine is either uncontrolled or legal in other parts of the world, notably Mexico, contributing to the establishment of ibogaine-based SUD treatment destinations in that country (Becker 2018).

Pharmacodynamics

Ibogaine and noribogaine have activity through a broad array of neurotransmitter systems, including NMDA (weak antagonism), KORs and μ opioid receptors (weak agonism), σ_2 receptors (high-affinity agonism), serotonin and dopamine transporter modulation, and noncompetitive inhibition of nicotinic acetylcholine receptors ($\alpha_1\beta_1$ and $\alpha_3\beta_4$ subtypes) (Wasko et al. 2018). Unlike classic hallucinogens, ibogaine's hallucinogenic properties cannot be attributed to 5-HT_{2A} receptor agonism; rather, they are believed to be related to its weak agonism/partial agonism at KORs (similar to, but to a much lesser degree than, salvinorin A) (Maillet et al. 2015). Dissociative properties are postulated to be mediated through ibogaine's weak NMDA receptor antagonism (similar to, but to a much lesser degree than, phencyclidine and ketamine) (Mash et al. 1995). Ibogaine and noribogaine have minimal effect on dopamine and norepinephrine transmission and may actually prevent monoamine efflux. Ibogaine's and noribogaine's noncompetitive dopamine transporter inhibition may result in clinically insignificant dopamine reuptake inhibition that nonetheless could blunt the effects of cocaine and other stimulant self-administration (Bulling et al. 2012). Notably, unlike ibogaine, noribogaine does not bind to the σ_2 receptor, and noribogaine has a higher binding affinity for opioid receptors than ibogaine.

Pharmacokinetics

Ibogaine demonstrates dose-dependent nonlinear oral bioavailability, with larger oral doses corresponding to higher bioavailability (Jeffcoat et al. 1994). Typical doses vary depending on the desired effect, with 10–30 mg used for neuromuscular stimulation (8-mg tablets were marketed in France for this purpose as Lambarene between 1939 and 1970) and 19.3 ± 6.9 mg/

kg used for addiction treatment (Maciulaitis et al. 2008). Doses in excess of 100 mg/kg have demonstrated a range of negative sequalae, including nausea, ataxia, seizures, QTc prolongation, cardiotoxicity, intense hallucinatory experiences, and death (Alper et al. 2012; Breuer et al. 2015; Mash et al. 2000). Ibogaine undergoes first-pass CYP2D6 demethylation to produce its principal metabolite, noribogaine, which, like its parent molecule, has psychoactive activity (Baumann et al. 2001) and is excreted primarily through the renal and gastrointestinal pathways (Jeffcoat et al. 1994). The time to peak drug concentration of ibogaine is 2 hours, and its half-life is 4–7 hours. The time to peak drug concentration of noribogaine is approximately 5 hours (Maciulaitis et al. 2008). Ibogaine's lipophilicity likely accounts for its wide distribution throughout the body, including in the CNS, after oral dosing (Hough et al. 2000). The median lethal dose observed in animal models (mice) is projected as 260 mg/kg (Schenberg et al. 2014).

Acute and Chronic Effects

As described earlier in this section, ibogaine demonstrates dose-dependent variability in physiological effects. At low doses, administration of ibogaine has neuromuscular and psychostimulatory effects. At increasing doses, the antiaddictive and hallucinatory effects become manifest, with toxic effects (i.e., cardiotoxicity, neurotoxicity, and death) at progressively higher doses (Meisner et al. 2016; O'Hearn et al. 1993).

The boundaries between doses that produce toxic and desirable effects can be variable and perhaps overlapping, resulting in a relatively narrow therapeutic window. This narrow window, combined with a more extensive set of medical exclusionary criteria, limits the use of ibogaine in both research and real-world applications.

After oral consumption of ibogaine-containing preparations at doses intended to target the hallucinogenic or antiaddictive effects, the intoxication experience has been characterized as having three phases (Alper 2001). Phase 1 (acute phase) begins within 1–3 hours after administration and can last upwards of 4–8 hours. This phase is characterized by delivery of (usually visual) long-term memory–inspired "vision" or "waking dream" states (oneirogenic), in which individuals describe contact with transcendent beings or passage along lengthy pathways. Phase 2 (evaluative phase) begins 4–8 hours after administration and can last 8–20 hours. This phase is characterized by a gradual decrease in the intensity of the acute-phase dream states, replaced by an introspective evaluative state wherein focus shifts to reflecting on the internal subjective experiences produced by the acute-phase dream states. The third phase (residual stimulation phase) begins 12–24 hours after ingestion, can last upwards of 24–72 hours, and is marked by a gradual return in attention from the intensely internally focused states of the acute and evaluative phases to normal attentiveness to the external environment, with only residual subjective alertness or arousal, including decreased need for sleep (Maciulaitis et al. 2008). Long-term consequences of ibogaine use (either positive or negative) are not well studied.

Given its narrow therapeutic window, acute clinical management of ibogaine intoxication involves close monitoring and potential treatment of cardiovascular and neurological status (Hoelen et al. 2009). Management of hallucinatory or dissociative symptoms involves general reassurance and placement in a minimally stimulating environment, along with administration of sedative-hypnotic medications in situations in which safety is a concern despite taking the measures described in this subsection.

Phencyclidine Review

Background

PCP (1-[1-phenylcyclohexyl] piperidine) was first tested on humans in 1957. Given in doses of 0.25 mg/kg IV, PCP produced anesthesia and was consequently manufactured as an analgesic (Sernyl). Anesthesia can be achieved without the patient being unconscious or losing autonomic reflexes, leading to the proposition that PCP's analgesia is coupled with a dissociative state in which the CNS is disconnected from sensory input from interoception (i.e., the body state, or a "dissociative anesthesia").

After a short period of use, it became clear that PCP induces alienating trance and dream-like states, which can be invasive and frightening and ultimately led to a halt in anesthetic use. A few years later, the PCP derivative ketamine was tested, and it was found to have more benign side effects and therefore marketed as a surrogate for PCP. Currently, PCP may be diverted from veterinary sources or manufactured illegally. In the United States, PCP is a Schedule II controlled substance.

PCP has appeared on the illicit market as a powder, a tablet, a liquid, or crystals in capsules, and it is smoked, intranasally insufflated, or consumed orally. PCP may be sprayed on parsley, mint, oregano, or other leaves that can be smoked. The oral dose of PCP (tablet) is estimated to be 1–6 mg, and laced cigarettes may contain 1–10 mg PCP (Beech et al. 1961; Garey 1979; Petersen and Stillman 1978).

Dextromethorphan

The PCP-like substance and readily available agent dextromethorphan has become more commonly misused. It is an easily accessible over-the-counter antitussive in the United States. When used in large quantities (>2 mg/kg), dextromethorphan has been associated with a dissociative effect similar to that of PCP and ketamine. Symptoms of intoxication and treatment are essentially the same as with PCP and ketamine, but the effects are more numbing than the other two (Romanelli and Smith 2009; Silva and Dinis-Oliveira 2020).

Furthermore, since the 1990s, illicit synthesis of additional related dissociative agents similar to PCP and dextromethorphan has been reported, many of which are poorly recognized and their effects incompletely characterized (Wallach and Brandt 2018).

Pharmacokinetics

PCP is water and lipid soluble, allowing it to be administered conveniently via various routes, and is extensively distributed in the body. Intoxication occurs within 1–5 minutes when smoked or within 15 minutes to 1 hour when ingested orally, and it lasts for 4–7 hours (although it can last ≥48 hours). Intoxication generally resolves after 20 hours, with users reporting a "come-down" period (characterized by hypersomnia, depressed mood, social isolation, and a schizophrenia-like psychotic state) lasting 6–24 hours after intoxication. A delirious or mental disorganization syndrome lasting up to 4–6 weeks may follow acute intoxication. Following a 2- to 3-day binge, it can take users 2–4 days to return to their baseline.

Because of its lipophilicity, PCP is stored in fatty tissue, from which it slowly diffuses. Its half-life varies widely, ranging from 10 hours to more than 72 hours (after extensive daily use). PCP is eliminated by hepatic hydroxylation mediated by hepatic microsomal enzymes and subsequent renal excretion (Laurenzana and Owens 1997; Petersen and Stillman 1978). Interestingly, PCP also demonstrates enterohepatic recirculation whereby it recirculates through the gut, which (when combined with slow release from fat stores) contributes to its prolonged intoxication state. Approximately

10% of total PCP is excreted in the urine and can be detected by suitable screening methods (Jushchyshyn et al. 2006; Shebley et al. 2006).

Evidence of hematological, hepatic, or renal toxicity was not found in chronic use of PCP, even for periods greater than 6 months. Lethal doses for PCP are 200 mg PO or greater (Gable 2004).

Pharmacodynamics

PCP demonstrates complex pharmacodynamics, but it acts primarily as a noncompetitive NMDA receptor antagonist through the so-called PCP receptor site (Chen and Weston 1960; Lodge and Johnson 1990). It also exerts dose-dependent effects to a lesser degree at opioid, muscarinic, GABA/benzodiazepine, and various other voltage-gated receptors (Petersen and Stillman 1978; Roth et al. 2013; Rothman et al. 1989). At substantially higher doses (i.e., those that cause blockade of the NMDA receptor), PCP (but not ketamine) blocks monoamine reuptake, increasing synaptic levels of dopamine and norepinephrine. This action may underpin the stimulatory effects during high-dose PCP intoxication, which can include agitation and violence.

PCP targets many of the reward systems in the brain via dopamine-reuptake inhibition, NMDA antagonism, and μ opioid receptor affinity (Vignon et al. 1989). PCP increases firing of dopamine neurons (Freeman and Bunney 1984) and may reduce cortical GABAergic function (Grunze et al. 1996) while disinhibiting glutamatergic transmission in the prefrontal cortex (Moghaddam et al. 1997; Vollenweider and Kometer 2010) and the ventral tegmental area (Mathé et al. 1998). This increase in glutamatergic transmission stimulates mesocorticolimbic dopaminergic transmission (Jentsch et al. 1998). Long-term abuse of PCP leads to reduced frontal lobe blood flow and glucose utilization (Hertzmann et al. 1990; Wu et al. 1991).

Acute and Chronic Effects

In volunteers, PCP effects were shown to be dose related and sometimes produced profound mental effects, including changes in body image, loss of ego boundaries, and depersonalization associated with feelings of estrangement, isolation, and dependency. Affectively charged experiences, characterized by negativism, hostility, or apathy, can be evoked in some subjects. Thinking is slowed, with disruption of attention span, inability to sustain organized directed thought, and impairment of learning. Subjects tend to present as distractible and perseverative. Time sense is disturbed, with underestimation of time intervals (Pradhan 1984).

The typical PCP experience is characterized by a feeling of numbness, as if the user no longer possesses a body. This effect is caused by interruption of sensory and proprioceptive input to the brain, from which the brain generates the body image in the usual state of consciousness. These sensations are relatively stable (i.e., not particularly sensitive to internal or environmental context and setting, unlike most other hallucinogens). Paranoid ideation is common, contributing to omnipotent or magical thinking and fueling unrealistic behavior or panic. In contrast with most other psychedelics, users of PCP are not always aware that they are experiencing drug effects ("pseudo-hallucinations") and therefore may experience real hallucinations that may promote irrational behaviors (Bertron et al. 2018).

Dramatic nystagmus (often vertical beating) may be used to identify intoxication, because no other recreational drugs induce this sign. In general, grave impairment of motor and sensory functions makes normal physical activities dangerous during the acute effects of the drug. PCP acts on the CNS and the peripheral nervous system and causes bronchodilation and moderate stimulation of the sympathetic and cardiovascular systems. Consequently, at higher doses, PCP can produce sympathomimetic signs such as hypertension, tachycardia, and diaphoresis and cholinergic signs including bronchospasm, xerostomia, urinary retention, flushing, and miosis. Overdoses of more than 100 mg PCP may result in convulsions, coma, and death from respiratory arrest. There is also a risk of hypertensive crisis and in rare cases intracerebral hemorrhage, and PCP has been shown to be a direct cardiac irritant, thereby inducing arrhythmias and vasospasm (Bertron et al. 2018).

In acute PCP intoxication with coma, creatine phosphokinase (CPK) levels greater than 500 U/L are frequently found. CPK levels higher than 20,000 U/L and rhabdomyolysis can occur and may precede myoglobinuria and renal failure (Hoogwerf et al. 1979). In addition, muscle tone becomes exaggerated, and patients may exhibit hyperreflexia and myoclonic, dystonic, or choreoathetoid movements such as opisthotonos and torticollis (Bey and Patel 2007).

The typical user of PCP tries it, but a few times or only occasionally; chronic usage is much less common. If a pattern of chronic use develops, the dangers of persisting dissociation become more evident. Effects of chronic PCP use are listed in Table 8.4.

Those who do use PCP chronically may complain of anxiety or nervousness, personality changes, or social isolation during and after periods of regular PCP use and may seek psychiatric care. Severe depression and even repeated suicide attempts are possible (Brodrick and Mitchell 2016; Poklis et al. 1990). In some cases, chronic PCP use can produce a long-lasting schizophrenia-like presentation including both positive and negative symptoms of schizophrenia (Javitt 2012; Javitt and Zukin 1991).

Tolerance develops with chronic use of PCP, resulting in consumption of higher doses to achieve the desired subjective effects (Rocha et al. 2017). Psychological dependence marked by craving for the drug after discontinuation can precipitate reuse, but a physiological withdrawal syndrome does not appear with the use of PCP in humans (although withdrawal symptoms have been reported in animals) (Knox et al. 2017; Nabeshima et al. 1986).

Phencyclidine Intoxication Management

The acute toxicity of PCP is often misdiagnosed because of its similarity to schizophrenic episodes. When recognized, clinical management includes attention to and stabilization of the patient's airway, breathing, circulation, thermoregulation, and neurological status as well as supportive measures to prevent injury and help patients cope with disorientation. Sensory stimulation should be minimized, because it increases agitation and may exacerbate hallucinatory effects. If safety is a concern owing to behavioral dysregulation, the use of a benzodiazepine, such as diazepam (5–10 mg IV) or lorazepam (1–4 mg IV or IM), appears most appropriate to manage agitation. Some patients require repeated doses of diazepam 10–15 mg or lorazepam 1–4 mg to control restlessness and agitation during prolonged recovery periods.

For severe PCP intoxication, it may be necessary to add a neuroleptic antipsychotic (e.g., haloperidol 5 mg IV or IM) to ensure the patient's safety. However, neuroleptics should be used with caution for two reasons. First, there is no proof that neuroleptics reduce or shorten psychotic symptoms in PCP intoxication (Bowers et al. 1990); in some cases, they have produced prolonged, severe hypotension and hyperthermia (Bey and Patel 2007). Second, phenothiazines, like haloperidol, may in their own right induce dystonic and anticholinergic reactions, result in poikilothermia, and lower the seizure threshold.

There is no known antidote for the toxic effects of PCP. If restraint is needed for safety purposes, chemical restraints are preferred over physical restraints because the latter may exacerbate rhabdomyolysis, the most common cause of morbidity and mortality in these patients (Olmedo 2002). Continuous cardiac monitoring should be considered because of the frequency and severity of cardiac symptoms with PCP overdoses. Treatment also includes efforts to decrease gastrointestinal absorption of the drug (activated charcoal).

In the past, urinary acidification was used to enhance PCP elimination, but this is no longer recommended because acidic urine increases the risk of acute tubular necrosis secondary to myoglobinuria in rhabdomyolysis. Furthermore, only approximately 10% of PCP is excreted in the urine (Bey and Patel 2007).

Intravenous diazepam in doses of 10–15 mg followed by intravenous phenytoin has been effective in the control of seizures. Diazoxide and hydralazine have both been used to reduce blood pressure. Diphenhydramine 50 mg or 1 mg/kg IV can be used to treat PCP-induced dystonic symptoms.

Because PCP-induced seizures, myoclonic activity, and trauma may result in rhabdomyolysis, serum potassium, blood urea nitrogen, creatinine, and CPK should be measured.

Substance Use Disorder Treatment With Hallucinogens: Psychedelic Medicine

Background

Interest in therapeutic utility of hallucinogens for SUD has reemerged in recent decades. A systematic review found 70 studies on ClinicalTrials.gov investigating the utility of hallucinogens in treating psychiatric disorders alone (with PTSD, major depressive disorder, anxiety, and SUDs being most represented). Only 21 of those 70 had published results, indicating that much more will soon be added to our scientific understanding of the therapeutic value of these chemicals (Siegel et al. 2021).

It is beyond the scope of this chapter to review the full array of research into the potential therapeutic value of hallucinogens across all medical and psychiatric domains. (For a recent comprehensive review of the topic, see Gomez-Escolar et al. 2024.) Because hallucinogens are unique among psychoactive substances in their potential both for misuse and to treat non-hallucinogen-related substance misuse, comment on this field is warranted, with samples from clinical, traditional, and social settings.

Hallucinogens and Phencyclidine 407

Table 8.4 Effects of phencyclidine

Type	Effect
Regular somatic effects	Increased blood pressure
	Tachycardia
	Nystagmus
	Miosis
	Blurred vision
Rarely observed somatic effects	Nausea, vomiting
	Hypersalivation
	Hyperpyrexia
	Rhabdomyolysis
	Flushing
	Bronchospasm
Acute psychiatric effects	Euphoria/dysphoria
	Agitation
	Hallucinations
	Dissociation from the environment
	Dissociation from the body
	Sensation of floating
	Delusional and omnipotent thinking
	Aggression
	Bizarre behavior
Effects of chronic use	Psychological dependence
	Confusion
	Depression
	Memory disturbances
	Psychosis
	Personality changes
	Flashbacks (rare)

Finally, the research posited in this section is to be taken within the context of appreciating the generally limited and often methodologically inconsistent nature of the studies from which the data have been culled. This area of research demands greater rigorous study before widespread applicability is achievable. Nonetheless, from these early and often small studies, an intriguing signal emerges that warrants consideration.

Lysergic Acid Diethylamide in Substance Use Disorder Treatment

LSD reliably produces the psychedelic experience that has been correlated with positive clinical outcomes (Bogenschutz and Johnson 2016; Yaden et al. 2021). It appears that the level of this mystical psychedelic experience is linked to the greater positive outcomes cited by research into classic hallucinogens in the treatment of SUDs (Bogenschutz and Johnson 2016; Majić et al. 2015; Yaden et al. 2021).

Early research into the use of LSD in the treatment of SUDs is fraught with methodological challenges (i.e., underpowered, inconsistent controlling) (Mangini 1998). Nonetheless, a meta-analysis of pooled data from six randomized controlled trials (1966–1970) with 536 subjects administered median doses of 500 μg LSD demonstrated decreases in problematic alcohol use (59% in the LSD treatment group vs. 38% in the control group) (Krebs and Johansen 2012). Two studies from the 1960s and 1970s involved using LSD for treatment of opioid use disorder: one enrolled 70 subjects using a single session of 140 μg LSD, and the other included 78 subjects using a single 300- to 500-μg dose with preparation and follow-up sessions with formerly incarcerated individuals (Ludwig and Levine 1965; Savage and McCabe 1973). The later study demonstrated a 25% versus 5% abstinence rate at 12-month follow-up (see also Bogenschutz and Johnson 2016). In both studies, LSD was administered in a controlled setting in conjunction with extensive preparatory and concurrent psychotherapy.

Psilocybin in Substance Use Disorder Treatment

Psilocybin is a leading candidate for demonstrating consistent clinical effectiveness in treatment of a host of mental health conditions, including SUDs. As described earlier in the subsection on psilocybin, its relatively positive safety profile potentially contributes to its utility as a treatment agent. A two-center double-blind randomized controlled trial for psilocybin in the treatment of individuals with a DSM-IV-based (American Psychiatric Association 1994) diagnosis of alcohol dependence (25 mg/70 kg at 4 weeks and 25–40 mg/70 kg at 8 weeks vs. diphenhydramine 50–100 mg) demonstrated significant decreases in the percentage of heavy drinking days in the psilocybin versus diphenhydramine group (9.7% vs. 23.6%), and decreases in number of standard drinks consumed per day were also reported. No adverse events were reported. The 95 participants in this study were also offered a concurrent 12-week manualized psychotherapy course that included motivational enhancement and cognitive-behavioral therapy, and the pharmacotherapy was administered in two day-long monitored sessions (Bogenschutz et al. 2022).

Psilocybin has also been studied in the treatment of tobacco use disorder, with a 2014 open-label pilot study demonstrating 80% abstinence (n = 12 of 15 subjects) at 6-month follow-up after receiving two to three sessions of psilocybin 20–30 mg/70 kg in conjunction with 15 weeks of manualized psychotherapy (Johnson et al. 2014). The intensity of the psychedelic/mystical experience appeared to correlate directly with the observed positive outcome (Garcia-Romeu et al. 2014).

Of the 79 studies utilizing psilocybin, as identified in a search of ClinicalTrials.gov (conducted on October 22, 2022), 5 were investigating its use in the treatment of AUD and 4 were investigating its use for tobacco use disorder, opioid use disorder, methamphetamine use disorder, and cocaine use disorder (1 study each). A central research question that will need to be further explored is whether the intense spiritual or mystical experiences are requisite for the potential beneficial effects of agents such as psilocybin (Bogenschutz and Johnson 2016; Bogenschutz et al. 2015, 2022).

Ayahuasca in Traditional Use Systems and Impact on Substance Use Disorders

There are no current clinical trials examining ayahuasca in its traditional setting. However, its potential use as a therapeutic agent is embedded in these cultural-spiritual-religious contexts where communal ritual spaces (*salãos*) and use of trained guides (*ayahuasceros*) can transcend simple biochemical effects (Talin and Sanabria 2017; Tupper 2008). Long-term studies of members of ayahuasca-consuming religious groups suggest lower incidence of AUD compared with control groups (Talin and Sanabria 2017). Furthermore, accounts from naturalistic use indicate that ayahuasca can play a role in controlling AUD symptoms and SUD symptoms generally (Yaden et al. 2021). An observational study conducted as follow-up from a Canadian ayahuasca retreat for nicotine, cocaine, and AUD also found positive and lasting changes in substance use patterns (Yaden et al. 2021).

Mescaline in Traditional Healing Settings and Impact on Substance Use Disorders

Several reports assert that peyote consumption, as part of the rituals of the Native American Church and in specialized residential treatment programs offering culturally sensitive treatment for AUD and other addictions, may have efficacy. These reports, however, have yet to be validated in double-blind clinical studies (Agin-Liebes et al. 2021; Bogenschutz and Johnson 2016; Calabrese 1997; Halpern 1996; Uthaug et al. 2022). A survey of users of various forms of mescaline reported less-intense mystical or transcendent experiences compared with individuals who used ayahuasca or psilocybin, yet those who used mescaline and had intense positive and memorable experiences also described improvements in their problematic relationships to alcohol or other drugs (Agin-Liebes et al. 2021; Uthaug et al. 2022).

Ibogaine in Treatment Settings

Ibogaine has gained notoriety for its potential as an antiaddictive agent through a reported reduction in craving for cocaine, amphetamine, and heroin (Davis et al. 2017; Schenberg et al. 2014). Animal studies demonstrate reductions in signs of opioid withdrawal as well as in the self-administration of alcohol, cocaine, and amphetamine (Iyer et al. 2021; Schenberg et al. 2014). The requisite exclusionary criteria, given the cardiotoxic and other side effects, long duration of sessions, potential severe side effects, and resource intensities, make deployment of ibogaine in common therapeutic settings challenging (Schenberg et al. 2014).

Despite these challenges, ibogaine has been used for a variety of SUDs (particularly alcohol, stimulants, and opioids), and case reports document improvements in cravings associated with opioid use disorder (Davis et al. 2017; Iyer et al. 2021; Schenberg et al. 2014). In the limited small studies that have examined the antiaddictive effects of ibogaine on opioid use, acute reduction in craving and the intensity of the withdrawal experience is reported to occur within 1–2 hours of single-dose 6–29 mg/kg administration, with resolution of withdrawal within 1 week. In studies examining the antiaddictive effects of ibogaine on those undergoing cocaine detoxification, significant decreases in craving were reported at 36 hours (Baumann et al. 2001; Maciulaitis et al. 2008).

Possible Mechanism of Action of Hallucinogens in the Treatment of Substance Use Disorders

Clear mechanisms of action for such a diverse groups of substances on conditions such as SUDs have yet to be defined. However, hallucinogen-induced promotion of neuroplasticity continues to gain traction (Brouwer and Carhart-Harris 2021; de Vos et al. 2021; Ly et al. 2018; Talin and Sanabria 2017). Brouwer and Carhart-Harris (2021) described the "pivotal" mental state that is "hyper-plastic" and more ready for positive psychological change, and hallucinogens may promote such hyperplastic states. More specifically, hallucinogens may contribute to a temporary dissolution of ego (experience or sense of self as distinct from others and the environment, as opposed to the traditional Freudian conceptualization of ego) that is intertwined with the often-maladaptive patterns of thinking and behavior that can reinforce and perpetuate SUDs. The ego is sustained by the DMN (described in the section "Common Psychoactive and Physiological Effects of Hallucinogens"), and temporary dissolution of this network by hallucinogens may allow for greater openness and behavioral/cognitive flexibility, alongside positive shifts in attitude, mood, and social connections, which altogether can support fundamental personal changes in cognition and outlook that favor recovery.

Key Points

- Hallucinogens are a chemically diverse group of substances that are both naturally occurring and synthetically manufactured and have a long, rich history with human culture. Originally, their use was confined to culturally specific ritual-ceremonial contexts. Currently, hallucinogens continue to have a role in traditional cultural contexts, while they also have proposed therapeutic potential as well as the potential for misuse and deleterious consequences through intoxication syndromes (common) and the development of hallucinogen use disorder (less common).
- All hallucinogens have the potential to change processing of the cognitive, perceptual, and emotional understanding of the self and reality—in other words, to alter consciousness.

- Intoxication syndromes are common with hallucinogens, whereas withdrawal syndromes are rare.
- Most hallucinogens have a relatively benign side-effect profile, with some notable exceptions (phencyclidine, ibogaine); recreational use outside of controlled research or culturally specific contexts appears to increase the likelihood of negative consequences of use.
- Hallucinogens can be categorized by their chemical structure, their purported main neurobiological mechanism of action, and the context in which they are used or the effects that result from their use.
- Classic hallucinogens (LSD, psilocybin, dimethyltryptamine, mescaline) are believed to primarily work through agonism of 5-HT_{2A} receptors.
- Generally, intoxication syndromes can be managed conservatively by placing the individual in a low-stimulus environment and providing supportive reassurances. When intoxication is severe, sedative-hypnotic medications can be used and are preferred over neuroleptic medications, which have little evidence of efficacy in many hallucinogen intoxications but may have a role for extremely agitated patients for whom safety concerns are present.

References

Abramson H, Jarvik M, Gorin M, et al: Lysergic acid diethylamine (LSD 25): XVII. Tolerance development and its relationship to a theory of psychosis. J Psychol 41:81–86, 1956

Addy PH: Acute and post-acute behavioral and psychological effects of salvinorin A in humans. Psychopharmacology (Berl) 220(1):195–204, 2012 21901316

Aghajanian GK, Bing OH: Persistence of lysergic acid diethylamide in the plasma of human subjects. Clin Pharmacol Ther 5:611–614, 1964 14209776

Aghajanian GK, Marek GJ: Serotonin and hallucinogens. Neuropsychopharmacology 21(2 Suppl):16S–23S, 1999 10432484

Agin-Liebes G, Haas TF, Lancelotta R, et al: Naturalistic use of mescaline is associated with self-reported psychiatric improvements and enduring positive life changes. ACS Pharmacol Transl Sci 4(2):543–552, 2021 33860184

Alper KR: Ibogaine: a review. Alkaloids Chem Biol 56:1–38, 2001 11705103

Alper KR, Stajić M, Gill JR: Fatalities temporally associated with the ingestion of ibogaine. J Forensic Sci 57(2):398–412, 2012 22268458

American Psychiatric Association: Diagnostic and Statistical Manual of Mental Disorders, 4th Edition. Washington, DC, American Psychiatric Association, 1994

Anderson BT, Labate BC, Meyer M, et al: Statement on ayahuasca. Int J Drug Policy 23(3):173–175, 2012 22459485

Anderson EF: Peyote: The Divine Cactus. Tucson, AZ, University of Arizona Press, 1996

Axelrod J, Brady RO, Witkop B, et al: The distribution and metabolism of lysergic acid diethylamide. Ann NY Acad Sci 66(3):435–444, 1957 13425233

Babu KM, McCurdy CR, Boyer EW: Opioid receptors and legal highs: Salvia divinorum and Kratom. Clin Toxicol (Phila) 46(2):146–152, 2008 18259963

Baggott MJ, Erowid E, Erowid F, et al: Use patterns and self-reported effects of salvia divinorum: an internet-based survey. Drug Alcohol Depend 111(3):250–256, 2010 20627425

Baggott MJ, Coyle JR, Erowid E, et al: Abnormal visual experiences in individuals with histories of hallucinogen use: a Web-based questionnaire. Drug Alcohol Depend 114(1):61–67, 2011 21035275

Baker LE, Panos JJ, Killinger BA, et al: Comparison of the discriminative stimulus effects of salvinorin A and its derivatives to U69,593 and U50,488 in rats. Psychopharmacology (Berl) 203(2):203–211, 2009 19153716

Balon R: Are magic mushrooms really magic? Psilocybin in the treatment of depression. J Clin Psychopharmacol 42(6):515–516, 2022 36251379

Barbee G, Berry-Cabán C, Barry J, et al: Analysis of mushroom exposures in Texas requiring hospitalization, 2005–2006. J Med Toxicol 5(2):59–62, 2009 19415588

Barker SA, McIlhenny EH, Strassman R: A critical review of reports of endogenous psychedelic N, N-dimethyltryptamines in humans: 1955–2010. Drug Test Anal 4(7–8):617–635, 2012 22371425

Barsuglia J, Davis AK, Palmer R, et al: Intensity of mystical experiences occasioned by 5-MeO-DMT and comparison with a prior psilocybin study. Front Psychol 9:2459, 2018 30574112

Basen R: Academic centers start to take psychedelics seriously: "You're not sticking your neck out as much as you would 10 years ago," one director says. MedPage Today, November 24, 2021. Available at: https://www.medpagetoday.com/special-reports/exclusives/95865. Accessed November 29, 2021.

Baumann MH, Rothman RB, Pablo JP, et al: In vivo neurobiological effects of ibogaine and its O-desmethyl metabolite, 12-hydroxyibogamine (noribogaine), in rats. J Pharmacol Exp Ther 297(2):531–539, 2001 11303040

Becker D: Ibogaine: One Man's Journey to Mexico for Psychedelic Addiction Treatment. WBUR News, September 10, 2018. Available at: https://www.wbur.org/news/2018/09/10/ibogaine-psychedelic-opioid-misuse-therapy. Accessed November 14, 2018.

Beech HR, Davies BM, Morgenstern FS: Preliminary investigations of the effects of Sernyl upon cognitive and sensory processes. J Ment Sci 107:509–513, 1961 13688613

Belleville RE, Fraser HF, Isbell H, et al: Studies on lysergic acid diethylamide (LSD-25): 1. Effects in former morphine addicts and development of tolerance during chronic intoxication. AMA Arch Neurol Psychiatry 76(5):468–478, 1956 13371962

Bertron JL, Seto M, Lindsley CW: DARK classics in chemical neuroscience: phencyclidine (PCP). ACS Chem Neurosci 9(10):2459–2474, 2018 29953199

Bey T, Patel A: Phencyclidine intoxication and adverse effects: a clinical and pharmacological review of an illicit drug. Cal J Emerg Med 8(1):9–14, 2007 20440387

Blistein J: Oakland decriminalizes magic mushrooms, other natural psychedelics: city council unanimously passes new resolution weeks after Denver voters approved similar measure. Rolling Stone, June 5, 2019. Available at: https://www.rollingstone.com/culture/culture-news/oakland-decriminalize-magic-mushrooms-natural-psychedelics-844879/. Accessed November 29, 2021.

Bogenschutz MP, Johnson MW: Classic hallucinogens in the treatment of addictions. Prog Neuropsychopharmacol Biol Psychiatry 64:250–258, 2016 25784600

Bogenschutz MP, Forcehimes AA, Pommy JA, et al: Psilocybin-assisted treatment for alcohol dependence: a proof-of-concept study. J Psychopharmacol 29(3):289–299, 2015 25586396

Bogenschutz MP, Ross S, Bhatt S, et al: Percentage of heavy drinking days following psilocybin-assisted psychotherapy vs placebo in the treatment of adult patients with alcohol use disorder: a randomized clinical trial. JAMA Psychiatry 79(10):953–962, 2022 36001306

Bouso JC, González D, Fondevila S, et al: Personality, psychopathology, life attitudes and neuropsychological performance among ritual users of Ayahuasca: a longitudinal study. PLoS One 7(8):e42421, 2012 22905130

Bowers MB Jr, Mazure CM, Nelson JC, et al: Psychotogenic drug use and neuroleptic response. Schizophr Bull 16(1):81–85, 1990 1970670

Bressloff PC, Cowan JD, Golubitsky M, et al: What geometric visual hallucinations tell us about the visual cortex. Neural Comput 14(3):473–491, 2002 11860679

Breuer L, Kasper BS, Schwarze B, et al: "Herbal seizures": atypical symptoms after ibogaine intoxication: a case report. J Med Case Rep 9:243, 2015 26518760

Brito-da-Costa AM, Dias-da-Silva D, Gomes NGM, et al: Pharmacokinetics and pharmacodynamics of salvinorin A and Salvia divinorum: clinical and forensic aspects. Pharmaceuticals (Basel) 14(2):116, 2021 33546518

Brodrick J, Mitchell BG: Hallucinogen persisting perception disorder and risk of suicide. J Pharm Pract 29(4):431–434, 2016 25631475

Brouwer A, Carhart-Harris RL: Pivotal mental states. J Psychopharmacol 35(4):319–352, 2021 33174492

Brubacher JR, Ravikumar PR, Bania T, et al: Treatment of toad venom poisoning with digoxin-specific Fab fragments. Chest 110(5):1282–1288, 1996 8915235

Bulling S, Schicker K, Zhang YW, et al: The mechanistic basis for noncompetitive ibogaine inhibition of serotonin and dopamine transporters. J Biol Chem 287(22):18524–18534, 2012 22451652

Cakic V, Potkonyak J, Marshall A: Dimethyltryptamine (DMT): subjective effects and patterns of use among Australian recreational users. Drug Alcohol Depend 111(1–2):30–37, 2010 20570058

Calabrese JD: Spiritual healing and human development in the Native American Church: toward a cultural psychiatry of peyote. Psychoanal Rev 84(2):237–255, 1997 9211587

Callaway JC: A proposed mechanism for the visions of dream sleep. Med Hypotheses 26(2):119–124, 1988 3412201

Cappendijk SL, Dzoljic MR: Inhibitory effects of ibogaine on cocaine self-administration in rats. Eur J Pharmacol 241(2–3):261–265, 1993 8243561

Carhart-Harris RL, Goodwin GM: The therapeutic potential of psychedelic drugs: past, present, and future. Neuropsychopharmacology 42(11):2105–2113, 2017 28443617

Carhart-Harris RL, Nutt D: User perceptions of the benefits and harms of hallucinogenic drug use: a web-based questionnaire study. J Subst Use 15(4):283–300, 2010

Carhart-Harris RL, Nutt DJ: Experienced drug users assess the relative harms and benefits of drugs: a web-based survey. J Psychoactive Drugs 45(4):322–328, 2013 24377171

Carhart-Harris RL, Erritzoe D, Williams T, et al: Neural correlates of the psychedelic state as determined by fMRI studies with psilocybin. Proc Natl Acad Sci USA 109(6):2138–2143, 2012 22308440

Carhart-Harris RL, Leech R, Hellyer PJ, et al: The entropic brain: a theory of conscious states informed by neuroimaging research with psychedelic drugs. Front Hum Neurosci 8:20, 2014 24550805

Carhart-Harris RL, Muthukumaraswamy S, Roseman L, et al: Neural correlates of the LSD experience revealed by multimodal neuroimaging. Proc Natl Acad Sci USA 113(17):4853–4858, 2016 27071089

Carhart-Harris R, Giribaldi B, Watts R, et al: Trial of psilocybin versus escitalopram for depression. N Engl J Med 384(15):1402–1411, 2021 33852780

Carstairs SD, Cantrell FL: Peyote and mescaline exposures: a 12-year review of a statewide poison center database. Clin Toxicol (Phila) 48(4):350–353, 2010 20170392

Chen GM, Weston JK: The analgesic and anesthetic effect of 1-(1-phenylcyclohexyl) piperidine HCl on the monkey. Anesth Analg 39:132–137, 1960 13809588

Cholden LS, Kurland A, Savage C: Clinical reactions and tolerance to LSD in chronic schizophrenia. J Nerv Ment Dis 122(3):211–221, 1955 13295823

Chung G: Christina Haack reveals she smoked psychedelic toad venom and says it "reset my brain." People, July 8, 2021. Available at: https://people.com/home/christina-haack-reveals-she-smoked-psychedelic-toad-venom-and-says-it-reset-my-brain/. Retrieved November 17, 2021.

Cohen S: Lysergic acid diethylamide: side effects and complications. J Nerv Ment Dis 130:30–40, 1960 13811003

Creese I, Burt DR, Synder SH: The dopamine receptor: differential binding of d-LSD and related agents to agonist and antagonist states. Life Sci 17(11):1715–1719, 1975 1207384

Cunningham CW, Rothman RB, Prisinzano TE: Neuropharmacology of the naturally occurring kappa-opioid hallucinogen salvinorin A. Pharmacol Rev 63(2):316–347, 2011 21444610

Dahmane E, Hutson PR, Gobburu JVS: Exposure-response analysis to assess the concentration-QTc relationship of psilocybin/psilocin. Clin Pharmacol Drug Dev 10(1):78–85, 2021 32250059

Dalgarno P: Subjective effects of Salvia divinorum. J Psychoactive Drugs 39(2):143–149, 2007 17703708

Davis AK, Barsuglia JP, Windham-Herman AM, et al: Subjective effectiveness of ibogaine treatment for problematic opioid consumption: short- and long-term outcomes and current psychological functioning. J Psychedelic Stud 1(2):65–73, 2017 30272050

Delay J, Pichot P, Lemperiere T, et al: The psychophysiological effects of psilocybine [in French]. C R Hebd Seances Acad Sci 247(16):1235–1238, 1958 13608992

de Vos CMH, Mason NL, Kuypers KPC: Psychedelics and neuroplasticity: a systematic review unraveling the biological underpinnings of psychedelics. Front Psychiatry 12:724606, 2021 34566723

Diker D, Markovitz D, Rothman M, et al: Coma as a presenting sign of Datura stramonium seed tea poisoning. Eur J Intern Med 18(4):336–338, 2007 17574113

Dimascio A, Greenblatt M, Hyde RW: A study of the effects of L.S.D.: physiologic and psychological changes and their interrelations. Am J Psychiatry 114(4):309–317, 1957 13458494

Dinis-Oliveira RJ, Pereira CL, da Silva DD: Pharmacokinetic and pharmacodynamic aspects of peyote and mescaline: clinical and forensic repercussions. Curr Mol Pharmacol 12(3):184–194, 2019 30318013

Doss MK, May DG, Johnson MW, et al: The acute effects of the atypical dissociative hallucinogen salvinorin A on functional connectivity in the human brain. Sci Rep 10(1):16392, 2020 33009457

Emboden W: Narcotic Plants, 2nd Edition. New York, MacMillan, 1980

Farthing G: The Psychology of Consciousness. Englewood Cliffs, NJ, Prentice Hall, 1992

Fodor G: The tropane alkaloids, in The Alkaloids: Chemistry and Physiology, Vol XIII. Edited by Manske R. New York, Academic Press, 1971, pp 351–396

Fontanilla D, Johannessen M, Hajipour AR, et al: The hallucinogen N,N-dimethyltryptamine (DMT) is an endogenous sigma-1 receptor regulator. Science 323(5916):934–937, 2009 19213917

Forrer GR, Goldner RD: Experimental physiological studies with lysergic acid diethylamide (LSD-25). AMA Arch Neurol Psychiatry 65(5):581–588, 1951 14818479

Foster Olive M: Drugs: The Straight Facts: Peyote and Mescaline. New York, Chelsea House Publishers, 2007

Fotiou E: The globalization of ayahuasca shamanism and the erasure of indigenous shamanism. Anthropology of Consciousness 27(2):151–179, 2016

Freedman DX: The psychopharmacology of hallucinogenic agents. Annu Rev Med 20:409–418, 1969 4894506

Freeman AS, Bunney BS: The effects of phencyclidine and N-allylnormetazocine on midbrain dopamine neuronal activity. Eur J Pharmacol 104(3–4):287–293, 1984 6094217

Gable RS: Comparison of acute lethal toxicity of commonly abused psychoactive substances. Addiction 99(6):686–696, 2004 15139867

Garcia-Romeu A, Griffiths RR, Johnson MW: Psilocybin-occasioned mystical experiences in the treatment of tobacco addiction. Curr Drug Abuse Rev 7(3):157–164, 2014 25563443

Garey RE: PCP (phencyclidine): an update. J Psychedelic Drugs 11(4):265–275, 1979 42808

Gastelum A: Mike Tyson says he "died" after smoking psychedelic toad venom. Sports Illustrated, 2021. Available at: https://web.archive.org/web/20211117173356/https://www.si.com/boxing/2021/11/17/mike-tyson-says-he-died-smoking-psychedelic-toad-venom. Accessed November 17, 2021.

George DR, Hanson R, Wilkinson D, et al: Ancient roots of today's emerging renaissance in psychedelic medicine. Cult Med Psychiatry 46(4):890–903, 2022 34476719

Gerault A, Picart D: Intoxication mortelle à la suite de la consommation volontaire et en groupe de champignons hallucinogènes. Bulletin Trimestriel Société Mycologique de France 112(1):1–14, 1996

Gilmore HT: Peyote use during pregnancy. S D J Med 54(1):27–29, 2001 11211421

Glick SD, Rossman K, Wang S, et al: Local effects of ibogaine on extracellular levels of dopamine and its metabolites in nucleus accumbens and striatum: interactions with D-amphetamine. Brain Res 628(1–2):201–208, 1993 8313148

Gomez-Escolar A, Folch-Sanchez D, Stefaniuk J, et al: Current perspectives on the clinical research and medicalization of psychedelic drugs for addiction treatments: safety, efficacy, limitations and challenges. CNS Drugs 38(10):771–789, 2024 39033264

Gonzales v O Centro Espírita Beneficente União do Vegetal, 546 U.S. 418 (2006)

González D, Riba J, Bouso JC, et al: Pattern of use and subjective effects of Salvia divinorum among recreational users. Drug Alcohol Depend 85(2):157–162, 2006 16720081

Gouzoulis-Mayfrank E, Schreckenberger M, Sabri O, et al: Neurometabolic effects of psilocybin, 3,4-methylenedioxyethylamphetamine (MDE) and d-methamphetamine in healthy volunteers: a double-blind, placebo-controlled PET study with [18F]FDG. Neuropsychopharmacology 20(6):565–581, 1999 10327426

Greiner T, Burch NR, Edelberg R: Psychopathology and psychophysiology of minimal LSD-25 dosage; a preliminary dosage-response spectrum. AMA Arch Neurol Psychiatry 79(2):208–210, 1958 13497365

Griffiths RR, Richards WA, McCann U, et al: Psilocybin can occasion mystical-type experiences having substantial and sustained personal meaning and spiritual significance. Psychopharmacology (Berl) 187(3):268–283, discussion 284–292, 2006 16826400

Griffiths RR, Richards WA, Johnson MW, et al: Mystical-type experiences occasioned by psilocybin mediate the attribution of personal meaning and spiritual significance 14 months later. J Psychopharmacol 22(6):621–632, 2008 18593735

Griffiths RR, Johnson MW, Carducci MA, et al: Psilocybin produces substantial and sustained decreases in depression and anxiety in patients with life-threatening cancer: a randomized double-blind trial. J Psychopharmacol 30(12):1181–1197, 2016 27909165

Grob CS, Danforth AL, Chopra GS, et al: Pilot study of psilocybin treatment for anxiety in patients with advanced-stage cancer. Arch Gen Psychiatry 68(1):71–78, 2011 20819978

Grof S: Realms of the Unconscious: Observations From LSD research. New York, Viking, 1975

Grunze HC, Rainnie DG, Hasselmo ME, et al: NMDA-dependent modulation of CA1 local circuit inhibition. J Neurosci 16(6):2034–2043, 1996 8604048

Grynkiewicz G, Gadzikowska M: Tropane alkaloids as medicinally useful natural products and their synthetic derivatives as new drugs. Pharmacol Rep 60(4):439–463, 2008 18799813

Gyermek L: Tropane alkaloids, in Pharmacology of Antimuscarinic Agents. Edited by Gyermek L. Boca Raton, FL, CRC Press, 1997, pp 47–160

Haden M, Woods B: LSD overdoses: three case reports. J Stud Alcohol Drugs 81(1):115–118, 2020 32048609

Halpern JH: The use of hallucinogens in the treatment of addiction. Addict Res 4(2):177–189, 1996

Halpern JH: Hallucinogens and dissociative agents naturally growing in the United States. Pharmacol Ther 102(2):131–138, 2004 15163594

Halpern JH, Pope HG Jr: Hallucinogen persisting perception disorder: what do we know after 50 years? Drug Alcohol Depend 69(2):109–119, 2003 12609692

Halpern JH, Sherwood AR, Hudson JI, et al: Psychological and cognitive effects of long-term peyote use among Native Americans. Biol Psychiatry 58(8):624–631, 2005 16271313

Halpern JH, Sherwood AR, Passie T, et al: Evidence of health and safety in American members of a religion who use a hallucinogenic sacrament. Med Sci Monit 14(8):SR15–SR22, 2008 18668010

Hartogsohn I: Constructing drug effects: a history of set and setting. Drug Sci Policy Law 3(1):2050324516683325, 2017

Hasler F, Bourquin D, Brenneisen R, et al: Determination of psilocin and 4-hydroxyindole-3-acetic acid in plasma by HPLC-ECD and pharmacokinetic profiles of oral and intravenous psilocybin in man. Pharm Acta Helv 72(3):175–184, 1997 9204776

Hayes E: Oregon's medicinal psychedelic mushrooms program moves forward. Portland Business Journal, November 15, 2021. Available at: https://www

.bizjournals.com/portland/news/2021/11/08/oregons-psilocybin-program
-moves-forward.html. Accessed November 29, 2021.

Heink A, Katsikas S, Lange-Altman T: Examination of the phenomenology of the ibogaine treatment experience: role of altered states of consciousness and psychedelic experiences. J Psychoactive Drugs 49(3):201–208, 2017 28266890

Hendricks PS, Thorne CB, Clark CB, et al: Classic psychedelic use is associated with reduced psychological distress and suicidality in the United States adult population. J Psychopharmacol 29(3):280–288, 2015 25586402

Hertzmann M, Reba RC, Kotlyarov EV: Single photon emission computed tomography in phencyclidine and related drug abuse. Am J Psychiatry 147(2):255–256, 1990 2301671

Hintzen A, Passie T: The Pharmacology of LSD: A Critical Review. New York, Oxford University Press, 2010

Hitt M, Ettinger DD: Toad toxicity. N Engl J Med 314(23):1517–1518, 1986 3702971

Hoch P: Studies in routes of administration and counteracting drugs, in Lysergic Acid Diethylamide and Mescaline in Experimental Psychiatry. Edited by Cholden L. New York, Grune & Stratton, 1956, pp 8–12

Hoelen DW, Spiering W, Valk GD: Long-QT syndrome induced by the antiaddiction drug ibogaine. N Engl J Med 360(3):308–309, 2009 19144953

Holland D, Passie T: Flashback-Phänomene als Nachwirkung von Halluzinogeneinnahme. Berlin, Germany, VWB Publishers, 2011

Hollister LE: Clinical, biochemical and psychologic effects of psilocybin. Arch Int Pharmacodyn Ther 130:42–52, 1961 13715376

Hollister LE, Sjoberg BM: Clinical syndromes and biochemical alterations following mescaline, lysergic acid diethylamide, psilocybin and a combination of the three psychotomimetic drugs. Compr Psychiatry 5:170–178, 1964 14156873

Hoogwerf B, Kern J, Bullock M, et al: Phencyclidine-induced rhabdomyolysis and acute renal failure. Clin Toxicol 14(1):47–53, 1979 436384

Hopf A, Eckert H: Distribution patterns of 14-C-psilocin in the brains of various animals. Act Nerv Super (Praha) 16(1):64–66, 1974 4454947

Hough LB, Bagal AA, Glick SD: Pharmacokinetic characterization of the indole alkaloid ibogaine in rats. Methods Find Exp Clin Pharmacol 22(2):77–81, 2000 10849889

Inch TD, Brimblecombe RW: Antiacetylcholine drugs: chemistry, stereochemistry, and pharmacology. Int Rev Neurobiol 16:67–144, 1974 4606226

Iyer RN, Favela D, Zhang G, et al: The iboga enigma: the chemistry and neuropharmacology of iboga alkaloids and related analogs. Nat Prod Rep 38(2):307–329, 2021 32794540

Javitt DC: Twenty-five years of glutamate in schizophrenia: are we there yet? Schizophr Bull 38(5):911–913, 2012 22987849

Javitt DC, Zukin SR: Recent advances in the phencyclidine model of schizophrenia. Am J Psychiatry 148(10):1301–1308, 1991 1654746

Jeffcoat A, Cook C, Hill J, et al: Disposition of [^{3}H] in the rat, in Problems of Drug Dependence, 1993: Proceedings of the 55th Annual Scientific Meeting, the College on Problems of Drug Dependence, Inc., Vol II (NIDA Publ No 94-3749). Rockville, MD, National Institutes of Health, 1994. Available at: https://archives.nida.nih.gov/sites/default/files/monograph141.pdf. Accessed February 9, 2025.

Jentsch JD, Tran A, Taylor JR, et al: Prefrontal cortical involvement in phencyclidine-induced activation of the mesolimbic dopamine system: behavioral and neurochemical evidence. Psychopharmacology (Berl) 138(1):89–95, 1998 96944531

Johnson MW, MacLean KA, Reissig CJ, et al: Human psychopharmacology and dose-effects of salvinorin A, a kappa opioid agonist hallucinogen present in the plant Salvia divinorum. Drug Alcohol Depend 115(1–2):150–155, 2011 21131142

Johnson MW, Garcia-Romeu A, Cosimano MP, et al: Pilot study of the 5-HT2AR agonist psilocybin in the treatment of tobacco addiction. J Psychopharmacol 28(11):983–992, 2014 25213996

Jushchyshyn MI, Wahlstrom JL, Hollenberg PF, et al: Mechanism of inactivation of human cytochrome P450 2B6 by phencyclidine. Drug Metab Dispos 34(9):1523–1529, 2006 16782764

Kapadia GJ, Fayez MB: Peyote constituents: chemistry, biogenesis, and biological effects. J Pharm Sci 59(12):1699–1727, 1970 5499699

Katz MM, Waskow IE, Olsson J: Characterizing the psychological state produced by LSD. J Abnorm Psychol 73(1):1–14, 1968 5639999

Ketchum JS, Sidell FR, Crowell EB Jr, et al: Atropine, scopolamine, and Ditran: comparative pharmacology and antagonists in man. Psychopharmacology (Berl) 28(2):121–145, 1973 4694622

Khey DN, Miller BL, Griffin OH: Salvia divinorum use among a college student sample. J Drug Educ 38(3):297–306, 2008 19157046

Knox LT, Jing Y, Bawazier-Edgecombe J, et al: Effects of withdrawal from repeated phencyclidine administration on behavioural function and brain arginine metabolism in rats. Pharmacol Biochem Behav 153:45–59, 2017 27986516

Kostakis C, Byard RW: Sudden death associated with intravenous injection of toad extract. Forensic Sci Int 188(1–3):e1–e5, 2009 19303230

Krebs TS, Johansen PØ: Lysergic acid diethylamide (LSD) for alcoholism: meta-analysis of randomized controlled trials. J Psychopharmacol 26(7):994–1002, 2012 22406913

Laurenzana EM, Owens SM: Metabolism of phencyclidine by human liver microsomes. Drug Metab Dispos 25(5):557–563, 1997 9152594

Lee MA, Shlain B: Acid Dreams: The Complete Social History of LSD: The CIA, the Sixties, and Beyond. New York, Grove Press, 1985

Leuner H: Halluzinogene: Psychische Grenzzustände in Forschung und Psychotherapie. Berlin, Huber, 1981

Liddell DW, Weil-Malherbe H: The effects of methedrine and of lysergic acid diethylamide on mental processes and on the blood adrenaline level. J Neurol Neurosurg Psychiatry 16(1):7–13, 1953 13023434

Lim TH, Wasywich CA, Ruygrok PN: A fatal case of "magic mushroom" ingestion in a heart transplant recipient. Intern Med J 42(11):1268–1269, 2012 23157524

Listos J, Merska A, Fidecka S: Pharmacological activity of salvinorin A, the major component of Salvia divinorum. Pharmacol Rep 63(6):1305–1309, 2011 22358078

Lodge D, Johnson KM: Noncompetitive excitatory amino acid receptor antagonists. Trends Pharmacol Sci 11(2):81–86, 1990 2156365

Longo VG: Behavioral and electroencephalographic effects of atropine and related compounds. Pharmacol Rev 18(2):965–996, 1966 5328390

Ludwig AM, Levine J: A controlled comparison of five brief treatment techniques employing LSD, hypnosis, and psychotherapy. Am J Psychother 19:417–435, 1965 14339608

Ly C, Greb AC, Cameron LP, et al: Psychedelics promote structural and functional neural plasticity. Cell Rep 23(11):3170–3182, 2018 29898390

Maciulaitis R, Kontrimaviciute V, Bressolle FM, et al: Ibogaine, an anti-addictive drug: pharmacology and time to go further in development: a narrative review. Hum Exp Toxicol 27(3):181–194, 2008 18650249

Maillet EL, Milon N, Heghinian MD, et al: Noribogaine is a G-protein biased κ-opioid receptor agonist. Neuropharmacology 99:675–688, 2015 26302653

Majić T, Schmidt TT, Gallinat J: Peak experiences and the afterglow phenomenon: when and how do therapeutic effects of hallucinogens depend on psychedelic experiences? J Psychopharmacol 29(3):241–253, 2015 25670401

Malcolm B, Thomas K: Serotonin toxicity of serotonergic psychedelics. Psychopharmacology (Berl) 239(6):1881–1891, 2022 34251464

Malleson N: Acute adverse reactions to LSD in clinical and experimental use in the United Kingdom. Br J Psychiatry 118(543):229–230, 1971 4995932

Mangini M: Treatment of alcoholism using psychedelic drugs: a review of the program of research. J Psychoactive Drugs 30(4):381–418, 1998 9924844

Mans K, Kettner H, Erritzoe D, et al: Sustained, multifaceted improvements in mental well-being following psychedelic experiences in a prospective opportunity sample. Front Psychiatry 12:647909, 2021 34267683

Maqueda AE, Valle M, Addy PH, et al: Naltrexone but not ketanserin antagonizes the subjective, cardiovascular, and neuroendocrine effects of salvinorin-A in humans. Int J Neuropsychopharmacol 19(7):pyw016, 2016 26874330

Mash DC, Staley JK, Pablo JP, et al: Properties of ibogaine and its principal metabolite (12-hydroxyibogamine) at the MK-801 binding site of the NMDA receptor complex. Neurosci Lett 192(1):53–56, 1995 7675310

Mash DC, Kovera CA, Pablo J, et al: Ibogaine: complex pharmacokinetics, concerns for safety, and preliminary efficacy measures. Ann NY Acad Sci 914:394–401, 2000 11085338

Mash DC, Duque L, Page B, et al: Ibogaine detoxification transitions opioid and cocaine abusers between dependence and abstinence: clinical observations and treatment outcomes. Front Pharmacol 9:529, 2018 29922156

Mathé JM, Nomikos GG, Schilström B, et al: Non-NMDA excitatory amino acid receptors in the ventral tegmental area mediate systemic dizocilpine (MK-801) induced hyperlocomotion and dopamine release in the nucleus accumbens. J Neurosci Res 51(5):583–592, 1998 9512002

McGlothlin W, Cohen S, McGlothlin MS: Long lasting effects of LSD on normals. Arch Gen Psychiatry 17(5):521–532, 1967 6054248

McKenna DJ, Towers GH: Biochemistry and pharmacology of tryptamines and beta-carbolines: a minireview. J Psychoactive Drugs 16(4):347–358, 1984 6394730

McKenna DJ, Repke DB, Lo L, et al: Differential interactions of indolealkylamines with 5-hydroxytryptamine receptor subtypes. Neuropharmacology 29(3):193–198, 1990 2139186

Meisner JA, Wilcox SR, Richards JB: Ibogaine-associated cardiac arrest and death: case report and review of the literature. Ther Adv Psychopharmacol 6(2):95–98, 2016 27141291

Meyerhoefer M: Serotonergic hallucinogens, in Addiction Medicine. Edited by Johnson B. New York, Springer, 2011, pp 585–602

Miles A, Townsend M: California Senate passes bill to decriminalize psychedelic drugs. Fox40 News, June 2, 2021. Available at: https://fox40.com/news/local-news/california-senate-passes-bill-to-decriminalize-psychedelic-drugs/. Accessed November 29, 2021.

Millière R, Carhart-Harris RL, Roseman L, et al: Psychedelics, meditation, and self-consciousness. Front Psychol 9:1475, 2018 30245648

Moghaddam B, Adams B, Verma A, et al: Activation of glutamatergic neurotransmission by ketamine: a novel step in the pathway from NMDA receptor blockade to dopaminergic and cognitive disruptions associated with the prefrontal cortex. J Neurosci 17(8):2921–2927, 1997 9092613

Moreno FA, Wiegand CB, Taitano EK, et al: Safety, tolerability, and efficacy of psilocybin in 9 patients with obsessive-compulsive disorder. J Clin Psychiatry 67(11):1735–1740, 2006 17196053

Nabeshima T, Ishikawa K, Yamaguchi K, et al: Methysergide-induced precipitated withdrawal syndrome in phencyclidine-dependent rats. Neurosci Lett 69(3):275–278, 1986 3763058

Naranjo P: Hallucinogenic plant use and related indigenous belief systems in the Ecuadorian Amazon. J Ethnopharmacol 1(2):121–145, 1979 542010

Nichols DE: Differences between the mechanism of action of MDMA, MBDB, and the classic hallucinogens: identification of a new therapeutic class: entactogens. J Psychoactive Drugs 18(4):305–313, 1986 2880944

Nichols DE: Hallucinogens. Pharmacol Ther 101(2):131–181, 2004 14761703

Nichols DE: Psychedelics. Pharmacol Rev 68(2):264–355, 2016 26841800

Nichols DE: Dark classics in chemical neuroscience: lysergic acid diethylamide (LSD). ACS Chem Neurosci 9(10):2331–2343, 2018 29461039

Nyi PP, Lai EP, Lee DY, et al: Influence of age on Salvia divinorum use: results of an Internet survey. J Psychoactive Drugs 42(3):385–392, 2010 21053761

O'Hearn E, Long DB, Molliver ME: Ibogaine induces glial activation in parasagittal zones of the cerebellum. Neuroreport 4(3):299–302, 1993 8477052

Olmedo R: Phencyclidine and Ketamine, in Goldfrank's Toxicologic Emergencies. Edited by Goldfrank LR. New York, McGraw Hill, 2002, pp 1034–1045

Ona G, Rocha JM, Bouso JC, et al: The adverse events of ibogaine in humans: an updated systematic review of the literature (2015–2020). Psychopharmacology (Berl) 239(6):1977–1987, 2021 34406452

Oss O, Oeric O: Magic Mushroom Growers Guide. Berkeley, CA, And/Or Press, 1976

Ott J: Pharmahuasca: human pharmacology of oral DMT plus harmine. J Psychoactive Drugs 31(2):171–177, 1999 10438001

Passie T: A History of the use of psilocybin in psychotherapy, in Teonancatl: Sacred Mushroom of Visions. Edited by Metzner R. Rochester, VT, Park Street Press, 2004, pp 109–134

Passie T, Seifert J, Schneider U, et al: The pharmacology of psilocybin. Addict Biol 7(4):357–364, 2002 14578010

Passie T, Halpern JH, Stichtenoth DO, et al: The pharmacology of lysergic acid diethylamide: a review. CNS Neurosci Ther 14(4):295–314, 2008 19040555

Petersen RC, Stillman RC: Phencyclidine: an overview. NIDA Res Monogr (21):1–17, 1978 101864

Pierce PA, Peroutka SJ: Hallucinogenic drug interactions with neurotransmitter receptor binding sites in human cortex. Psychopharmacology (Berl) 97(1):118–122, 1989 2540505

Poklis A, Graham M, Maginn D, et al: Phencyclidine and violent deaths in St. Louis, Missouri: a survey of medical examiners' cases from 1977 through 1986. Am J Drug Alcohol Abuse 16(3–4):265–274, 1990 2288325

Pollan M: How to Change Your Mind: The New Science of Psychedelics. New York, Penguin Books, 2019

Pollock S: The psilocybin mushroom pandemic. J Psychedelic Drugs 7:73–84, 1975

Pradhan SN: Phencyclidine (PCP): some human studies. Neurosci Biobehav Rev 8(4):493–501, 1984 6514253

Presti DE: Altered states of consciousness: drug-induced states, in The Blackwell Companion to Consciousness, 2nd Edition. Edited by Schneider S, Velmans M. New York, Wiley, 2017, pp 171–186

Presti DE: Expanding a science of consciousness, in Consciousness Unbound: Liberating Mind From the Tyranny of Materialism. Edited by Kelly EF, Marshall P. Lanham, MD, Rowman & Littlefield, 2021, pp 323–358

Ravalec V, Mallendi, Paicheler A: Iboga: The Visionary Root of African Shamanism. Rochester, NY, Park Street Press, 2007

Reiff CM, Richman EE, Nemeroff CB, et al: Psychedelics and psychedelic-assisted psychotherapy. Am J Psychiatry 177(5):391–410, 2020 32098487

Riba J, Rodríguez-Fornells A, Urbano G, et al: Subjective effects and tolerability of the South American psychoactive beverage ayahuasca in healthy volunteers. Psychopharmacology (Berl) 154(1):85–95, 2001 11292011

Riley SC, Blackman G: Between prohibitions: patterns and meanings of magic mushroom use in the UK. Subst Use Misuse 43(1):55–71, 2008 18189205

Robinson JT, Chitham RG, Greenwood RM, et al: Chromosome aberrations and LSD: a controlled study in 50 psychiatric patients. Br J Psychiatry 125(0):238–244, 1974 4422173

Rocha A, Hart N, Trujillo KA: Differences between adolescents and adults in the acute effects of PCP and ketamine and in sensitization following intermittent administration. Pharmacol Biochem Behav 157:24–34, 2017 28442368

Romanelli F, Smith KM: Dextromethorphan abuse: clinical effects and management. J Am Pharm Assoc (2003) 49(2):e20–25; quiz e26–e27, 2009 19289333

Roth BL, Baner K, Westkaemper R, et al: Salvinorin A: a potent naturally occurring nonnitrogenous kappa opioid selective agonist. Proc Natl Acad Sci USA 99(18):11934–11939, 2002 12192085

Roth BL, Gibbons S, Arunotayanun W, et al: The ketamine analogue methoxetamine and 3- and 4-methoxy analogues of phencyclidine are high affinity and selective ligands for the glutamate NMDA receptor. PLoS One 8(3):e59334, 2013 23527166

Rothlin E: Lysergic acid diethylamide and related substances. Ann NY Acad Sci 66(3):668–676, 1957 13425249

Rothlin E, Cerletti A: Pharmacology of LSD-25, in Lysergic Acid Diethylamide and Mescaline in Experimental Psychiatry. Edited by Cholden L. New York, Grune & Stratton, 1956, pp 1–7

Rothman RB, Reid AA, Monn JA, et al: The psychotomimetic drug phencyclidine labels two high affinity binding sites in guinea pig brain: evidence for N-methyl-D-aspartate-coupled and dopamine reuptake carrier-associated phencyclidine binding sites. Mol Pharmacol 36(6):887–896, 1989 2557536

Samorini G: The oldest archeological data evidencing the relationship of Homo sapiens with psychoactive plants: a worldwide overview. J Psychedelic Stud 3(2):63–80, 2019

Sanders-Bush E, Burris KD, Knoth K: Lysergic acid diethylamide and 2,5-dimethoxy-4-methylamphetamine are partial agonists at serotonin receptors linked to phosphoinositide hydrolysis. J Pharmacol Exp Ther 246(3):924–928, 1988 2843634

Sandison RA, Whitelaw JD: Further studies in the therapeutic value of lysergic acid diethylamide in mental illness. J Ment Sci 103(431):332–343, 1957 13429304

Sandroni P: Aphrodisiacs past and present: a historical review. Clin Auton Res 11(5):303–307, 2001 11758796

Savage C: Variations in ego feeling induced by D-lysergic acid diethylamide (LSD-25). Psychoanal Rev 42(1):1–16, 1955 14371878

Savage C, McCabe OL: Residential psychedelic (LSD) therapy for the narcotic addict: a controlled study. Arch Gen Psychiatry 28(6):808–814, 1973 4575166

Schenberg EE, de Castro Comis MA, Chaves BR, et al: Treating drug dependence with the aid of ibogaine: a retrospective study. J Psychopharmacol 28(11):993–1000, 2014 25271214

Schultes RE, Hofmann A: Plants of the Gods: Origins of Hallucinogenic Use. New York, McGraw Hill, 1979

Shebley M, Jushchyshyn MI, Hollenberg PF: Selective pathways for the metabolism of phencyclidine by cytochrome P450 2B enzymes: identification of electrophilic metabolites, glutathione, and N-acetyl cysteine adducts. Drug Metab Dispos 34(3):375–383, 2006 16326815

Shen HW, Jiang XL, Winter JC, et al: Psychedelic 5-methoxy-N,N-dimethyltryptamine: metabolism, pharmacokinetics, drug interactions, and pharmacological actions. Curr Drug Metab 11(8):659–666, 2010 20942780

Shippenberg TS, Chefer VI, Zapata A, et al: Modulation of the behavioral and neurochemical effects of psychostimulants by kappa-opioid receptor systems. Ann NY Acad Sci 937:50–73, 2001 11458540

Siebert DJ: Salvia divinorum and salvinorin A: new pharmacologic findings. J Ethnopharmacol 43(1):53–56, 1994 7526076

Siegel AN, Meshkat S, Benitah K, et al: Registered clinical studies investigating psychedelic drugs for psychiatric disorders. J Psychiatr Res 139:71–81, 2021 34048997

Silva AR, Dinis-Oliveira RJ: Pharmacokinetics and pharmacodynamics of dextromethorphan: clinical and forensic aspects. Drug Metab Rev 52(2):258–282, 2020 32393072

Smart RG, Bateman K: The chromosomal and teratogenic effects of lysergic acid diethylamide: a review of the current literature. Can Med Assoc J 99(16):805–810, 1968 4878647

Spencer DG Jr, Glaser T, Traber J: Serotonin receptor subtype mediation of the interoceptive discriminative stimuli induced by 5-methoxy-N,N-dimethyltryptamine. Psychopharmacology (Berl) 93(2):158–166, 1987 3122248

Spriggs MJ, Douglass HM, Park RJ, et al: Study protocol for "Psilocybin as a treatment for anorexia nervosa: a pilot study." Front Psychiatry 12:735523, 2021 34744825

Stamets P: Psilocybin Mushrooms of the World. Berkeley, CA, Ten Speed Press, 1996

Strassman RJ: Adverse reactions to psychedelic drugs: a review of the literature. J Nerv Ment Dis 172(10):577–595, 1984 6384428

Strassman RJ: DMT: the Spirit Molecule. Rochester, VT, Park Street Press, 2001

Strassman RJ, Qualls CR, Uhlenhuth EH, et al: Dose-response study of N,N-dimethyltryptamine in humans: II. Subjective effects and preliminary results of a new rating scale. Arch Gen Psychiatry 51(2):98–108, 1994 8297217

Studerus E, Kometer M, Hasler F, et al: Acute, subacute and long-term subjective effects of psilocybin in healthy humans: a pooled analysis of experimental studies. J Psychopharmacol 25(11):1434–1452, 2011 20855349

Subramanian N, Doran M: Improvement of hallucinogen persisting perception disorder (HPPD) with oral risperidone: case report. Ir J Psychol Med 31(1):47–49, 2014 30189471

Talin P, Sanabria E: Ayahuasca's entwined efficacy: an ethnographic study of ritual healing from "addiction." Int J Drug Policy 44:23–30, 2017 28432902

Teixeira PJ, Johnson MW, Timmermann C, et al: Psychedelics and health behaviour change. J Psychopharmacol 36(1):12–19, 2022 34053342

Teksin ZS, Lee IJ, Nemieboka NN, et al: Evaluation of the transport, in vitro metabolism and pharmacokinetics of salvinorin A, a potent hallucinogen. Eur J Pharm Biopharm 72(2):471–477, 2009 19462483

Trulson ME, Crisp T, Henderson LJ: Mescaline elicits behavioral effects in cats by an action at both serotonin and dopamine receptors. Eur J Pharmacol 96(1–2):151–154, 1983 6581976

Tupper KW: The globalization of ayahuasca: harm reduction or benefit maximization? Int J Drug Policy 19(4):297–303, 2008 18638702

Upshall DG, Wailling DG: The determination of LSD in human plasma following oral administration. Clin Chim Acta 36(1):67–73, 1972 5007719

Uthaug MV, Davis AK, Haas TF, et al: The epidemiology of mescaline use: pattern of use, motivations for consumption, and perceived consequences, benefits, and acute and enduring subjective effects. J Psychopharmacol 36(3):309–320, 2022 33949246

van Amsterdam J, Nutt D, Phillips L, et al: European rating of drug harms. J Psychopharmacol 29(6):655–660, 2015 25922421

Vargas MV, Meyer R, Avanes AA, et al: Psychedelics and other psychoplastogens for treating mental illness. Front Psychiatry 12:727117, 2021 34671279

Vignon J, Chaudieu I, Allaoua H, et al: Comparison of [3H] phencyclidine ([3H] PCP) and [3H] N-[1-(2-thienyl) cyclohexyl] piperidine ([3H] TCP) binding properties to rat and human brain membranes. Life Sci 45(26):2547–2555, 1989 2615554

Vis PJ, Goudriaan AE, Ter Meulen BC, et al: On perception and consciousness in HPPD: a systematic review. Front Neurosci 15:675768, 2021 34456666

Vollenweider FX, Kometer M: The neurobiology of psychedelic drugs: implications for the treatment of mood disorders. Nat Rev Neurosci 11(9):642–651, 2010 20717121

Vollenweider FX, Preller KH: Psychedelic drugs: neurobiology and potential for treatment of psychiatric disorders. Nat Rev Neurosci 21(11):611–624, 2020 32929261

Vollenweider FX, Leenders KL, Scharfetter C, et al: Positron emission tomography and fluorodeoxyglucose studies of metabolic hyperfrontality and psychopathology in the psilocybin model of psychosis. Neuropsychopharmacology 16(5):357–372, 1997 9109107

Vollenweider FX, Vollenweider-Scherpenhuyzen MF, Bäbler A, et al: Psilocybin induces schizophrenia-like psychosis in humans via a serotonin-2 agonist action. Neuroreport 9(17):3897–3902, 1998 9875725

Wallach J, Brandt SD: Phencyclidine-based new psychoactive substances. Handb Exp Pharmacol 252:261–303, 2018 30105474

Wasko MJ, Witt-Enderby PA, Surratt CK: DARK classics in chemical neuroscience: ibogaine. ACS Chem Neurosci 9(10):2475–2483, 2018 30216039

Wasson R, Heim A: Les Champignon Hallucinogènes du Mexique: Etudes Ethnologiques, Taxinomiques, Biologiques, Physiologiques et Chimiques. Paris, Éditions du Muséum National D'Histoire Naturelle, 1958

Williams K, Romero OSG, Braunstein M, et al: Indigenous philosophies and the "psychedelic renaissance." Anthropology of Consciousness 33:506–527, 2022

Wu D, Otton SV, Inaba T, et al: Interactions of amphetamine analogs with human liver CYP2D6. Biochem Pharmacol 53(11):1605–1612, 1997 9264312

Wu JC, Buchsbaum MS, Bunney WE: Positron emission tomography study of phencyclidine users as a possible drug model of schizophrenia. Yakubutsu Seishin Kodo 11(1):47–48, 1991 1882590

Wu LT, Woody GE, Yang C, et al: Recent national trends in Salvia divinorum use and substance-use disorders among recent and former Salvia divinorum users compared with nonusers. Subst Abuse Rehabil 2011(2):53–68, 2011 21709724

Yaden DB, Berghella AP, Regier PS, et al: Classic psychedelics in the treatment of substance use disorder: potential synergies with twelve-step programs. Int J Drug Policy 98:103380, 2021 34329952

9

Club Drugs and Inhalants

Richard N. Rosenthal, M.D.
Marina Tsoy-Podosenin, M.D., Ph.D.

The use of club drugs, which include γ-hydroxybutyrate (GHB), 3,4-methylenedioxymethamphetamine (MDMA; ecstasy), and ketamine, particularly among adolescents and young adults, has raised concern (Chatlos 1996; Hill and Thomas 2011). Although more recent studies of adolescents (Johnston et al. 2022; National Institute on Drug Abuse 2021) and adults have shown a recent decrease in drug use overall, adolescent substance use remains a public health concern, particularly as it relates to the use of designer drugs (Armentano 1995; Johnston et al. 2010). Moreover, given their popularity among a subgroup of the LGBTQ+ community, club drugs also may represent a unique challenge in medical and psychotherapeutic work with patients in this group.

Club drugs originally received their name from their use in nightclubs and raves, the all-night dance parties that tend to attract adolescents and young adults ages 15–25 years (Koesters et al. 2002) and feature "techno" music intended to enhance drug effects. Ravers are often looking for "euphoric transcendence," which is reached through the combination of frenetic dancing and club drug use (Weir 2000). However, clinicians must also be concerned with nonclub uses of club drugs, particularly among high school and college students (Pedersen and Skrondal 1999). Although technically any drug used in a club could be considered a club drug, general interest has focused on three agents: GHB, MDMA, and ketamine. An additional concern is contamination of various club drugs with fentanyl and other high-potency synthetic opioids, which poses grave risk of overdose, poisoning, and death. Although a sampling of club drugs at Canadian music festivals suggested fentanyl and fentanyl analog contamination of only 2% (McCrae et al. 2019), other studies demonstrated a concerning increase in the presence of fentanyl or fentanyl analogs found in illicit drug seizures, including club drugs such as MDMA (Mema et al. 2018; Park et al. 2021).

Inhalants are typically volatile compounds, such as readily available organic solvents, anesthetics, nitrous oxide, and nitrites (Balster 2019), that are inhaled via various methods. Inhalants have various psychoactive or mind-altering effects, including reinforcing euphoric effects; however, inhalants also present a host of noteworthy negative medical consequences. Because they have low barriers to access and are frequently found in home settings, inhalants remain a low-prevalence but chronic public health problem, especially among children and early adolescents (Storck et al. 2016).

Club drug intoxication syndromes have various substance-specific psychopharmacological interventions to consider, whereas inhalant intoxication treatment is more typically focused on mitigation of acute medical sequela to prevent significant end-organ damage. Withdrawal syndromes have been documented for chronic use of club drugs (e.g., GHB, ketamine, and MDMA) and certain inhalants. There are no FDA-approved treatments for club drug or inhalant use disorders.

γ-Hydroxybutyrate and Related Compounds

GHB has been used both for legitimate clinical and clinical research purposes and for a range of illicit purposes. It was marketed legally in the United States until 1990, when the FDA banned its sale to consumers. Except for one FDA-approved indication (the treatment of cataplexy in patients

Club Drugs and Inhalants

with narcolepsy) described later in this section, GHB is a Schedule I controlled substance without other medical indications. The FDA also declared γ-butyrolactone (GBL) as a List I chemical and 1,4-butanediol (1,4-BD) as a Class I health hazard, practically designating these GHB precursors, which are also industrial solvents, as illicit and unapproved new drugs (Substance Abuse and Mental Health Services Administration 2013).

Pharmacology and Neurobiology: Biosynthetic and Metabolic Pathways

GHB is an endogenous, water-soluble, four-carbon fatty acid that is found in peripheral organs, including the heart, liver, kidney, and cardiac and skeletal muscle, as well as in the brain of mammals, where it is thought to play a role as a neurotransmitter (Maitre 1997; Nelson et al. 1981). This metabolite of GABA appears to be synthesized in the CNS, and it has been shown in rodents to bind to high-affinity receptors in neurons of the hippocampus, cortex, striatum, olfactory bulb and tubercle, and dopaminergic nuclei (Maitre 1997). In the mitochondria, GABA is transaminated by GABA transaminase into succinic semialdehyde (SSA) (Figure 9.1). Most of the SSA is oxidized into succinate in the mitochondria for use in the Krebs cycle, but a small amount (1%–2%) appears to be transported back into the cytosol, where it is reduced into GHB by SSA reductase, an enzyme found only in neurons (Maitre et al. 2000). In the brain, 1,4-BD is also converted into GHB (Snead et al. 1989), whereas peripheral lactonases appear to convert naturally occurring GBL into GHB, which then freely diffuses across the blood–brain barrier (Maitre 1997; Roth and Giarman 1968). In the liver, 1,4-BD is oxidized by alcohol dehydrogenase to γ-hydroxybutyraldehyde, which is oxidized to GHB by aldehyde dehydrogenase (Dyer et al. 2001).

Inhibiting the enzyme GABA transaminase will block the formation of GHB from GABA; however, neither this effect nor the blocking of alcohol dehydrogenase affects the formation of GHB from 1,4-BD in the brain, demonstrating at least two different pathways for GHB synthesis in the CNS (Snead et al. 1989). GHB is ultimately metabolized to carbon dioxide, which is eliminated through the lungs, although a small percentage is excreted in the urine (Galloway et al. 2000; Nicholson and Balster 2001).

GHB is rapidly absorbed from the gastrointestinal tract and is present in free form in the serum without protein binding (Li et al. 1998b), with peak plasma concentrations usually appearing 40–60 minutes after ingestion,

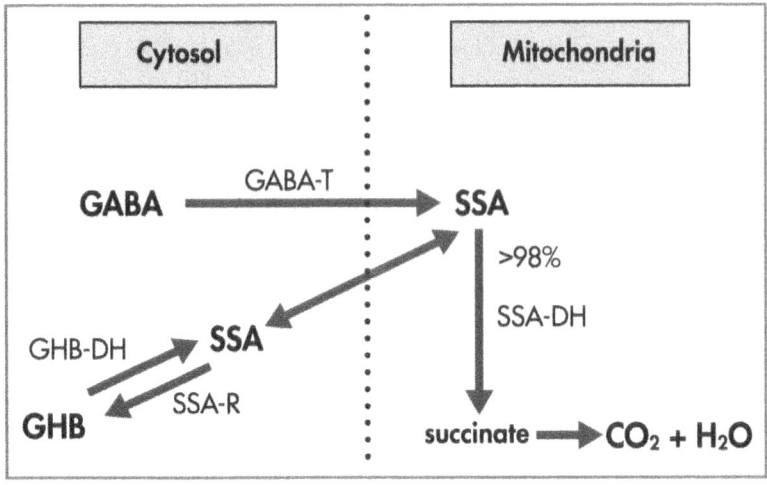

Figure 9.1 γ-Hydroxybutyrate synthesis in the neuron. Succinic semialdehyde (SSA) is synthesized in the mitochondria through transamination of GABA by GABA transaminase (GABA-T). Most of the SSA is oxidized by SSA-dehydrogenase (SSA-DH) to form succinate, which is used for energy metabolism and results in the end products CO_2 + H_2O, which are expired. A small portion of SSA (<2%) is converted by SSA reductase (SSA-R) in the cytosol to γ-hydroxybutyrate (GHB). GHB may also be oxidized back to SSA by GHB dehydrogenase (GHB-DH).

often more quickly (Borgen et al. 2003). However, absorption is capacity limited, and larger doses will increase the time to peak plasma concentration (Palatini et al. 1993). Food, especially that with high fat content, significantly reduces the bioavailability of GHB, reducing peak plasma concentration and increasing median time to peak concentration (Borgen et al. 2003).

Because the main enzyme for degradation of GHB is saturable and the elimination pharmacokinetics of GHB are nonlinear, plasma clearance of GHB decreases as the dose of GHB increases (Borgen et al. 2000). At low doses such as 12.5 mg/kg, the elimination half-life is as brief as 20 minutes, with clearance of 14 mL/min/kg, whereas at moderate doses such as 32 mg/kg, the mean clearance is reduced to 6.6 mL/min/kg and is further reduced by almost 40% with doses of approximately 60 mg/kg (Borgen et al. 2000; Roth and Giarman 1966; Scharf et al. 1998). Plasma levels of GHB are negligible 6 hours after a single 64-mg/kg (4.5 g) dose in healthy adults (Borgen et al. 2003). Because of the rapid elimination of GHB, the alteration in clearance with increased dose is not usually clinically relevant, except in the case of overdose, when high doses may result in coma, or when there is a pattern of high-dose administration at frequent intervals. The effect of the latter is discussed later in the section "Withdrawal Presentation."

GHB has sedative, anxiolytic, and euphoric effects similar to those of ethanol, likely because of potentiation of cerebral GABAergic and dopaminergic activities. In general, GHB is thought to exert tonic inhibitory control over dopamine and GABA release through high-affinity GHB receptors (Howard and Feigenbaum 1997; Kemmel et al. 2003). Increases in neuronal pools of dopamine are mediated by induction of tyrosine hydroxylase (Gessa et al. 1966), the rate-limiting enzyme in the catecholaminergic synthetic pathway. GHB may have a serotonergic effect that is mediated by increased transport of tryptophan into serotonergic cells (Gobaille et al. 2002). Although GHB does not interact directly with known sites of action of other drugs, including the $GABA_A$ receptor, in pharmacological doses it may be an agonist at $GABA_B$ sites (Nicholson and Balster 2001). It is likely that the rewarding properties of GHB occur mainly via disinhibition of ventral tegmental dopamine neurons rather than direct effects on the nucleus accumbens (Watson et al. 2010).

In addition, high-dose GHB causes epileptiform electroencephalogram (EEG) effects that are distinctly different from those of ethanol, and in preclinical studies it produced EEG changes that were more suggestive of petit mal absence seizures than of true sedation (Godschalk et al. 1977). However, the sedation caused by GHB is usually not thought to reflect absence seizures. Compared with benzodiazepine- and barbiturate-induced sedation, GHB-induced sedation at higher doses possesses distinct excitatory properties similar to those seen with dissociative anesthetics such as ketamine (Nicholson and Balster 2001; Winters and Kott 1979). This effect may contribute to its role as a club drug. GHB also differs from other sedative-hypnotics such as ethanol or benzodiazepines in that it consolidates rapid eye movement (REM) sleep.

Intoxication and Acute Presentation

Acute Effects

When GHB is taken for use as an intoxicant, typical acute effects described by users are euphoria, relaxation, and increased sexuality (Galloway et al. 1997; Kapitány-Fövény et al. 2015; Miotto et al. 2001). GHB is taken recreationally in capfuls or teaspoons of a salty/sour liquid, which, because of variations in concentration, may range in dose from 0.5 to 5.0 g. Common side effects are nausea, headache, itching, and vomiting (Borgen et al. 2003). GHB 10–20 mg/kg typically produces anxiolysis with hypotonia and amnesia, 20–30 mg/kg induces sleep, and 50–60 mg/kg induces anesthesia (Craig et al. 2000). In the context of rave-type parties, GHB or its precursors are often taken together with other, more stimulating club drugs (e.g., ketamine, MDMA) to offset the sedating properties of GHB and, conversely, modulate the stimulants' adverse effects such as teeth grinding and jaw clenching, while increasing the subjective euphoria and disinhibition. Reflecting street awareness of the side effects of loss of consciousness and decreased coordination, users usually avoid driving motor vehicles (Miotto et al. 2001).

Aside from the use of GHB and its analogs by bodybuilders for purported anabolic effects, the main nonmedical use of this class of compounds is recreational use, which produces sedation, euphoria, and sexual disinhibition (Miotto et al. 2001). The sedative effects of GHB may be related to inhibition of dopamine release and a subsequent increase in the intraneuronal dopamine level (Itzhak and Ali 2002). Although emergency department (ED) visits related to GHB are uncommon (<0.2% of drug/alcohol-related ED visits), the complaints that precipitate them may reflect the pattern of GHB sequelae in users in the community. A survey of 42 recreational users of GHB found that 66% reported episodes of unpredictable loss of consciousness, and 26% had experienced overdose (Miotto at al. 2001). Of daily users, 45% had experienced frequent amnesia during or after use of GHB, suggestive of blackouts typically attributed to high-volume alcohol use (Miotto at al. 2001). The rate of adverse events was greater among those who used higher GHB doses and among those who used GHB together with nonmedical use of other drugs. Because GHB potentially causes coma and anterograde amnesia (especially in conjunction with alcohol, with which its effects are synergistic), it has reportedly been used as a drug to facilitate sexual assault (Brennan and Van Hout 2014). In addition to disinhibition, GHB may cause impairment of judgment when used to facilitate sexuality—in one study among recreational users, almost a quarter of respondents experienced blackouts that can increase risk for sexual or acquisitory crimes (Kapitány-Fövény et al. 2015). GHB has also gained notoriety as a commonly used drug at gay circuit parties. In Liverpool, England, 61% of gay men identified in one study as having syphilis had used GHB as an aphrodisiac in the context of unprotected sex (Cook et al. 2001).

In an attempt to sidestep the FDA ban on human use of GHB and its precursors GBL and 1,4-BD, these drugs are frequently represented and sold on the internet as cleaning fluids (e.g., as wheel cleaner [GBL] and printer head cleaner) (Centers for Disease Control and Prevention 1999; Maxwell 2006; Zvosec et al. 2001).

Chronic Effects

In a conditioned place preference paradigm, mice treated repeatedly for a week with GHB 250 mg/kg showed place preference, suggesting that GHB cues are rewarding (Itzhak and Ali 2002). However, highly reinforcing drugs (e.g., cocaine, opioids) typically produce conditioned place preference after only two to three drug exposures; thus, GHB, which appears to require a greater number of exposures, may have a less reinforcing effect (Nicholson and Balster 2001). Nonetheless, it appears that a small percentage of human users of GHB or its precursors develop a substance use disorder or addiction syndrome. In addition to evidence of physiological dependence, including tolerance and withdrawal, patients may quickly experience a relapse to GHB or GBL use after complicated withdrawal (McDaniel and Miotto 2001), also meeting DSM-5 behavioral criteria (American Psychiatric Association 2022) for a substance use disorder. Part of the high relapse risk may be attributable to what McDaniel and Miotto (2001) described as a protracted abstinence syndrome, characterized by dysphoria, anxiety, memory problems, and insomnia, which may last for 3–6 months after the acute withdrawal has stabilized.

Because GHB induces slow-wave sleep, a peak period of sleep for release of growth hormone (Gerra et al. 1994; Takahara et al. 1977), it has been marketed as a nonregulated anabolic health-food supplement to bodybuilders since the 1980s. However, Addolorato and colleagues (1999b) found no evidence of purported anabolic effects during long-term administration of

GHB, and no other evidence from case reports or clinical trials exists for the efficacy of GHB in increasing muscle mass.

γ-Hydroxybutyrate as Medicine

GHB has been investigated as a potential treatment for several disorders, including those related to sleep, such as narcolepsy (Scrima et al. 1990) and sleep apnea (Sériès et al. 1992), and those postulated to involve dopamine and GABA systems, such as schizophrenia (Levy et al. 1983), alcohol withdrawal (Addolorato et al. 2000), and fibromyalgia (Staud 2011). GHB was developed under FDA orphan drug status as sodium oxybate (Xyrem), which was approved by the FDA in July 2002 as a Schedule III drug for the treatment of cataplexy in patients with narcolepsy. GHB reduces cataplexy and induces and consolidates the type of brain EEG changes seen in normal sleep, such as slow-wave sleep, without affecting REM sleep (Sériès et al. 1992). As such, GHB has shown efficacy in controlled clinical trials in patients with narcolepsy (Lammers et al. 1993; Scrima et al. 1990).

Another potential clinical use of GHB is in the treatment of alcohol withdrawal and alcohol dependence. In preclinical studies, GHB inhibited voluntary ethanol consumption in ethanol-preferring rats and suppressed the ethanol withdrawal syndrome in alcohol-dependent animals (Gessa et al. 2000). These results set the foundation for investigating the potential use of GHB in the clinical treatment of alcohol dependence. Although an alcohol treatment indication is not currently approved in the United States, in Europe several open studies and randomized clinical trials have suggested that GHB is efficacious in preventing or controlling symptoms of alcohol withdrawal (Addolorato et al. 1999a; Moncini et al. 2000; Nimmerrichter et al. 2002; van den Brink et al. 2018) and that GHB may have a role in reducing alcohol craving, increasing treatment retention (Moncini et al. 2000), and preventing relapse to drinking (Gallimberti et al. 1992, 2000) in detoxified alcoholic patients. In view of the addiction liability of GHB, it is not surprising that in some trials of GHB for alcohol dependence, more than 10% of the sample lost control over or became dependent on the study drug (Addolorato et al. 1996; Gallimberti et al. 2000). The potential role of GHB as a substitution pharmacotherapy for alcoholism is confounded by its short plasma half-life; the role of longer-acting GHB analogs remains to be explored (Galloway et al. 2000).

Toxicology

Overdose Effects

The most frequent presentation of GHB-related syndromes in EDs is that of overdose characterized by coma or stupor and respiratory depression and usually complicated by ingestion of other recreational drugs, but fatalities have been reported in the context of GHB and 1,4-BD use alone (Centers for Disease Control and Prevention 1997; Zvosec et al. 2001). Other common findings are bradycardia, respiratory acidosis, and vomiting (Chin et al. 1998). GHB is frequently taken together with other psychoactive substances, and alcohol acts synergistically with GHB to produce respiratory and CNS depression (Mamelak 1989). GHB overdose also presents certain unusual clinical characteristics: patients may rapidly shift from an unconscious, apneic state requiring respiratory support to a markedly agitated, combative state, and back again (Li et al. 1998b), as well as become combative on recovery of consciousness (Chin et al. 1998). These combative states are frequently triggered by the stimulus of intubation attempts, which indicate an exaggerated gag reflex (Li et al. 1998a; Ross 1995). Fortunately, since GHB became a Schedule I controlled substance in 2000, the prevalence of illicit GHB use, intoxication, and overdose declined (Carter et al. 2009), but evidence suggests a recrudescence.

Withdrawal Presentation

The development of tolerance for GHB has been repeatedly described in clinical vignettes and confirmed in animal models. For example, with repeated GHB treatment in mice, tolerance develops to both the hypolocomotion and the cataleptic effects of the drug (Itzhak and Ali 2002). There is also preclinical evidence of cross-tolerance and cross-dependence of GHB with alcohol (Colombo et al. 1995; Fadda et al. 1989). As described in the earlier subsection on clinical pharmacology, GHB and its analogs have been used in humans in the treatment of alcohol withdrawal. Nicholson and Balster (2001) reviewed the evidence for cross-tolerance and cross-dependence of GHB with alcohol.

In clinical trials with GHB, discontinuation syndromes were rarely mentioned (Addolorato et al. 1999c). However, numerous reports now exist of withdrawal syndromes clearly related to GHB or its precursors GBL and 1,4-BD (Alattas et al. 2022; Brunt et al. 2014; Craig et al. 2000; Dyer et al.

2001; McDaniel and Miotto 2001; Mycyk et al. 2001; Sivilotti et al. 2001). Craig and colleagues (2000) identified several probable antecedent factors that contribute to GHB withdrawal, including a history of prolonged nonmedical GHB use with gradual dose escalation, the experience of dysphoria, anxiety, and tremor on stopping, and numerous attempts to cut down or stop GHB use. Brunt et al. (2014) suggested that the threshold for GHB withdrawal is use of more than 18 g/day with a dosing frequency of at least four times daily over a 2- to 4-week period.

It is important for the clinician to obtain a clear history of the pattern of use of GHB or its precursors once the patient recovers from acute overdose. In the case of frequent dosing, the patient may be at high risk for severe withdrawal. A case series of 38 published reports stated that among heavily dependent users of GHB or its precursors, characterized by the use of 30 g/day or more of GHB or by a dosing frequency of at least every 8 hours, more than half deteriorated rapidly into delirium after initiating abstinence (McDonough et al. 2004). This high risk for severe withdrawal exists because a dose causing intoxication severe enough to require clinical treatment for overdose would have to be large enough to overcome the tolerance associated with repeated dosing. Most reports suggest that the distinguishing characteristic of patients presenting with the most clinically severe GHB withdrawal is a pattern of dosing at 2–4-hour intervals around the clock (Dyer et al. 2001; Hernandez et al. 1998; McDaniel and Miotto 2001; Miotto et al. 2001). This pattern of use is necessary in GHB-dependent patients because of the drug's short half-life. Severe withdrawal syndromes, which frequently include delirium in users of more than 25 g/day, have been described in numerous case studies and surveys (Alattas et al. 2022; Chin 2001; Craig et al. 2000; Hernandez et al. 1998; Hodges and Everett 1998; Sivilotti et al. 2001; Zvosec et al. 2001). Such withdrawal syndromes share similarities in symptom patterns to withdrawal from both alcohol and benzodiazepines.

The onset of GHB withdrawal symptoms typically begins 1–5 hours after the last dose; initial symptoms include anxiety, tremor, tachycardia, nausea, and insomnia (Table 9.1). Untreated, the symptoms may progress within 24 hours to a more severe pattern that is similar to delirium tremens, with dysfunction of cognition and sensorium, bouts of severe agitation, and autonomic dysregulation lasting up to 2 weeks (Dyer et al. 2001). Concurrent use of other sedative-hypnotics, in particular alcohol, may

Table 9.1 γ-Hydroxybutyrate withdrawal syndrome

Severity	Symptoms
Mild	Tremor, anxiety, insomnia, mood lability, abdominal cramping, nausea, vomiting, palpitations, diaphoresis, tachycardia, meiosis
Severe	Delirium with auditory or visual hallucinations and confusion, delusional thinking, autonomic instability with hypertension, increased temperature, severe agitation, horizontal nystagmus

Source. Dyer et al. (2001); Mycyk et al. (2001).

exacerbate the GHB withdrawal syndrome. The more severe forms of withdrawal typically occur within 48 hours of the last use and are characterized by delirium with auditory or visual hallucinations and confusion, horizontal nystagmus, autonomic instability with hypertension and increased temperature, and episodic agitation. Autonomic dysregulation characterized by tachycardia, fever, hypertension, and diaphoresis is generally milder than that seen in delirium tremens, and although generalized seizures are not reported, myoclonus resembling tonic-clonic movements has been described (see Dyer et al. 2001; Miotto and Roth 2001).

Pharmacological Management of Intoxication and Withdrawal

Overdose Management

The general treatment of GHB overdose is supportive medical care with a focus on the respiratory system. Patients typically regain consciousness in 2–5 hours. Commonly used coma reversal agents such as intravenous naloxone, glucose (50% dextrose in water), and flumazenil have had little benefit in GHB overdose (Li et al. 1998b). In addition, physostigmine has been suggested as a treatment for GHB overdose, but the risks of bradycardia and asystole in the context of GHB's short duration of action outweigh any purported benefits (Boyer et al. 2001).

Withdrawal Management

Milder forms of withdrawal, typically seen with a lower frequency of dosing or lower cumulative daily doses, may be successfully treated with benzodiazepines on an outpatient basis (Addolorato et al. 1999c; Galloway et al. 1997). Severe withdrawal states typically require medical support, high doses of intravenous benzodiazepines, and capacity for physical restraint to prevent the patient from harming themself or others during bouts of psychotic agitation (Dyer et al. 2001; Miotto and Roth 2001; Mycyk et al. 2001). Reports of the failure of benzodiazepines to adequately control symptoms of GHB withdrawal (Friedman et al. 1996; Mullins and Fitzmaurice 2001) have raised the question of how best to treat the disorder. The probable explanation for the observed lack of response is underdosing of the benzodiazepines. Many case reports have found that patients experiencing severe GHB withdrawal may require very high doses of intravenous benzodiazepines such as lorazepam, diazepam, or even midazolam to control agitation and autonomic dysregulation. The average intravenous dosage of lorazepam given over a 24-hour period in these cases has ranged from 8 to 10 mg/hour (Chin 2001; Craig et al. 2000). Craig and colleagues (2000) reported the case of a patient who needed 2,655 mg of diazepam equivalents (lorazepam 507 mg plus diazepam 120 mg) over 90 hours to control agitation. For patients taking high doses of benzodiazepines, Miotto and Roth (2001) suggested the use of pulse oximetry to monitor for oxygen desaturation. After a diagnosis of GHB withdrawal is established, it is likely that early aggressive dosing with benzodiazepines under careful medical supervision will reduce the severity and chronicity of acute GHB withdrawal, but this approach remains to be validated.

Other sedative-hypnotic medications, such as barbiturates, may play a useful role in severe withdrawal from this group of drugs. For example, in a case series of GBL withdrawal, use of intravenous pentobarbital in the range of 1–2 mg/kg/hour lowered the total requirement for intravenous lorazepam (Sivilotti et al. 2001). A recent case series ($N = 13$) reported the effectiveness of phenobarbital (wide range between 30 mg and 1,600 mg peak daily dosing before taper) administered to treat GHB-related withdrawal delirium following failure of benzodiazepine-based management (Freeman et al. 2023). In addition, several case reports describe the effectiveness of the $GABA_B$ receptor agonist baclofen in treatment of the GHB withdrawal syndrome (typical dosing of 10 mg tid) (Habibian et al. 2019; Lai et al. 2022).

Antipsychotic medications are often used to reduce psychotic agitation. However, because antipsychotic medications lower the seizure threshold and may contribute to loss of central control of temperature, leading to hyperthermia or neuroleptic malignant syndrome (NMS), they are not indicated as first-line medications for GHB withdrawal delirium (Dyer and Roth 2001; McDaniel and Miotto 2001; Sharma et al. 2001). Nonetheless, antipsychotic agents have been used most commonly as an adjunct to benzodiazepines in the management of GHB withdrawal (McDonough et al. 2004). In addition, Eiden and colleagues (2011) described a case of a patient tolerant to GBL who presented symptoms consistent with NMS, apparently precipitated by neuroleptics that were administered to control her symptoms of agitation and auditory and visual hallucinations. If antipsychotics are needed, second-generation agents are preferred because of their lower risk for dystonia, dyskinesia, and NMS (McDaniel and Miotto 2001; Olivera et al. 1990).

Freese et al. (2002) proposed that anticonvulsants such as gabapentin, which inhibit glutamate production, may reduce glutamate-induced excitotoxicity, thus reducing the severity of GHB withdrawal. However logical this may be, little evidence supports this intervention at present, except that the use of gabapentin, sodium valproate, or carbamazepine administered adjunctively with benzodiazepines has been described in a few published case reports (McDaniel and Miotto 2001).

Finally, evidence indicates that GHB itself can be used with a tapering dosage to detoxify individuals from GHB. In a prospective case series, de Jong and colleagues (2012) successfully stabilized 23 GHB-dependent inpatients by titrating to 70% of the estimated self-administration dose with pharmaceutical GHB (150 mg/mL). The drug was first administered within 1.5–2 hours after the last patient self-administration dose and then every 3 hours over 1–2 days, followed by tapering the dosage by 0.3–0.45 g/dose each day. Objective and subjective withdrawal symptoms were used to monitor withdrawal; although most patients experienced uncomfortable withdrawal symptoms during the GHB troughs in the first few days, none developed delirium or psychosis (de Jong et al. 2012). Wolf et al. (2021) examined data from two multisite trials of mostly successful inpatient GHB detoxification (mean length of stay = 11 days) in 285 patients with GHB use disorder who received a dose every 2–3 hours; the dose was then tapered off with pharmaceutical GHB at 70% of the patient's estimated street dose based on 650 mg/mL, dose adjusted to stabilize subjective and objective symptoms over the first 24–48 hours, then reduced by GHB 300 mg per dose daily. They reported that the most frequent withdrawal-related subjective symptoms were craving, fatigue, insomnia, sweating, and dysphoria, with objective symptoms of craving, fatigue, tremors, sweating, and bouts of rapid-onset cold or warm sensations.

Substance Use Disorder Presentation

GHB use disorder is frequently identified in the context of ED admissions for acute withdrawal, which de facto signals a use disorder (tolerance as a result of the need for frequent dosing and subsequent withdrawal). Although the evidence base for this relatively rare disorder compared with other substance use disorders is not well developed, patients who are dependent on GHB appear to benefit from cognitive and motivational psychosocial therapies and from support of recovery in a manner similar to that for alcohol-dependent patients. Given that subjective and objective measures of craving are marked by high frequency and high severity in conjunction with the extended features of the GHB withdrawal syndrome (Wolf et al. 2021), it is reasonable that post-detoxification psychosocial interventions include methods such as cognitive-behavioral therapy relapse prevention to support coping skills for navigating episodes of craving. However, because of the high likelihood of amnesia and cognitive dysfunction during the acute and subacute phases of GHB withdrawal, psychosocial interventions should, when possible, include significant others who can review and reinforce with the patient the negative consequences of physiological dependence on GHB and the typical impact of a use disorder.

3,4-Methylenedioxymethamphetamine

MDMA is commonly known as *ecstasy*, or in its pure form, *molly*. Other slang names for MDMA include XTC, X, E, adam, clarity, and lover's speed. MDMA is chemically similar to the stimulant amphetamine and the hallucinogen mescaline. It was developed in the early 1900s as a chemical precursor in the synthesis of pharmaceutical agents and was patented by Merck in 1914. MDMA was initially thought to have appetite-suppressant properties, but it was never marketed for that indication. The first reported "underground" synthesis of MDMA occurred in 1967 (Nichols 1986). MDMA is the *N*-methyl derivative of the entactogen precursor 3,4-methylenedioxyamphetamine (MDA), which has properties of both hallucinogens and amphetamines (Nozaki et al. 1977). Compared with the classic hallucinogens (lysergic acid diethylamine [LSD], mescaline, and psilocybin; see Chapter 8), MDA produces only minimal sensory effects (e.g., pseudo-hallucinations) but consistently increases feelings of elation, and modification by N-methylation to MDMA virtually eliminates hallucinogenic activity (Nichols 1986). The United Kingdom placed MDMA on Schedule I in 1977, and the United States did so in 1985.

During the 1970s and early 1980s, MDMA was used by some psychotherapists to enhance the therapy process in the treatment of depression, trauma, and other psychiatric disorders (Moonzwe et al. 2011). Although this use was based on the drug's purported entactogenic/empathogenic (relationship-enhancing) properties, it remains an illegal substance with no approved medical uses (Moonzwe et al. 2011). Until very recently, it had not been shown in high-quality studies to be effective in this role. A 2021 meta-analysis of 27 studies with 592 participants demonstrated a moderate to large effect (d = 0.86) of MDMA on sociability factors such as feeling loving, talkative, or friendly (Regan et al. 2021).

MDMA as Medicine

Small, randomized trials (Mithoefer et al. 2011, 2013; Oehen et al. 2013) demonstrated that at least two sessions of MDMA-assisted manualized psychotherapy appear safe and may be of both short- and longer-term benefit in patients with treatment-resistant PTSD. One study (N = 20) demonstrated significant reductions in clinician-rated PTSD symptoms at 2 months (Mithoefer et al. 2011) and long-term follow-up (mean = 3.5 years) (Mithoefer et al. 2013). The other study, using an active control over three sessions, demonstrated significant reductions in self-rated but not clinician-rated PTSD symptoms at 1-year follow-up (Oehen et al. 2013). More recent studies have further supported the pilot efficacy and safety of MDMA as a treatment adjunct to psychotherapeutic interventions for a few targeted mental disorders. A systematic review and meta-analysis of 10 studies including 190 participants receiving MDMA-assisted manualized psychotherapy for PTSD (Mithoefer et al. 2016) demonstrated a significant reduction of PTSD symptoms, and remission of PTSD diagnoses was observed in the randomized controlled trials (RCTs) (Tedesco et al. 2021). For example, Mitchell et al. (2021) conducted an RCT of MDMA-assisted (80–120 mg) versus placebo-assisted manualized psychotherapy among individuals with severe PTSD (N = 90) and demonstrated strong and significant reductions due to three MDMA sessions in measures of PTSD and depression severity as well as disability ratings, in addition to good safety and tolerability.

Regarding autism spectrum disorder, Danforth et al. (2018) demonstrated in a pilot RCT among adults with autism that MDMA-assisted (75–125 mg) psychotherapy in two 8-hour sessions produced quick and stable improvement in marked to very severe social anxiety symptoms. It is yet unclear whether the mechanism of benefit is attributable to the direct psychopharmacological effects of MDMA, such as decreased fear responding as demonstrated in animal models (Hake et al. 2019), or to general facilitation of targeted psychotherapeutic interventions delivered over extended (8-hour) sessions.

Brief Pharmacology and Neurobiology

MDMA is a weak agonist at serotonin (5-hydroxytryptamine [5-HT]) 5-HT_1 and 5-HT_2 receptors, targeting 5-HT_{2A}, 5-HT_{2B}, and 5-HT_{2C} receptors (Tedesco et al. 2021). Acutely, MDMA acts to increase serotonin through activity on the presynaptic serotonin transporter (SERT) (Rudnick and Wall 1992), but with chronic use, decreases in serotonin are noted, suggesting loss of serotonergic neurons (Montoya et al. 2002; Sprague et al. 1998). Decreases in SERT levels also have been reported (McCann et al. 1998; Schouw et al. 2012). MDMA use is also correlated with secondary increases in dopamine in the basal ganglia (Sprague et al. 1998). MDMA acts primarily in the frontal cortex, leading to effects on cognition and memory. It also works on the limbic system, leading to MDMA's effects on mood, anxiety, and emotions. Metabolism occurs through the cytochrome P450 (CYP) 2D6 enzyme system, although 20% is excreted unchanged in the urine (Karlsen et al. 2008; Tucker et al. 1994).

Given these proposed interactions with serotonergic systems, a complex relationship with serotonin reuptake–inhibiting medications (i.e., selective serotonin reuptake inhibitors [SSRIs]) has been observed; some reports support the ability of SSRI medications to block or mitigate the effects of MDMA (Liechti and Vollenweider 2000; Stein and Rink 1999), whereas others do not (McCann and Ricaurte 1993).

Intoxication and Acute Presentations

Toxicology

In the emergency setting, MDMA intoxication is usually seen in conjunction with dehydration, hyperthermia, tachycardia, hypertension, liver failure, rhabdomyolysis, or renal failure, often mimicking NMS (Jonas and Graeme-Cook 2001; Karlsen et al. 2008; Lester et al. 2000; Montoya et al. 2002;

Schwartz and Miller 1997). The physical symptoms may be accompanied by symptoms of anxiety, agitation, and even confusion (Montoya et al. 2002). Because these presentations are nonspecific, they lead to a wide differential diagnosis. Nevertheless, the clinician must have a high index of suspicion of a substance-induced basis for behavioral emergency presentations in most adolescents and young adults (Williams et al. 1998). The diagnosis is complicated by the fact that routine urine toxicology screens do not typically detect the presence of MDMA, although occasionally cross-reactivity with amphetamines may occur (Koesters et al. 2002; Shannon 2000). Although rare, death from MDMA overdose has been reported and is most commonly related to hyperthermia and hyponatremia (Jamt et al. 2022; Rogers et al. 2009).

MDMA's toxicity may be related to its effects on serotonergic neurons and to oxidative stress and free radical formation (Bolla et al. 1998; Gouzoulis-Mayfrank and Daumann 2006; McCann et al. 2000; Montoya et al. 2002). In animal studies, these processes are associated with exaggerated pruning in those regions of the brain with high serotonergic activity, particularly the hippocampus and amygdala (Green et al. 2012; Ricaurte et al. 1988, 2000). These changes may be long-lasting, persisting for as long as 7 years after MDMA exposure, although at least partial recovery may be possible with abstinence (Gouzoulis-Mayfrank and Daumann 2006; Hatzidimitriou et al. 1999).

The neurochemical changes caused by MDMA result in significant, observable functional impairment as well. These impairments occur in areas of the brain that have high concentrations of serotonergic neurons. Most notably affected are cognition and memory (Gouzoulis-Mayfrank and Daumann 2006; Montoya et al. 2002). Studies have shown decreases in word recall, as well as poorer functioning in general measures of memory (Montoya et al. 2002; Morgan 1999; Rodgers 2000; Verkes et al. 2001). It remains unclear whether this effect is dose related or independent of dose (Bolla et al. 1998). These effects may be compounded when MDMA and cannabis are combined (Gouzoulis-Mayfrank et al. 2000; Taffe 2012).

Clinical Presentation

Before its designation as a Schedule I drug in the United States in 1985, MDMA had a low level of use (Green et al. 2012). Use of MDMA tapered off in the period immediately following its designation as a Schedule I drug (Koesters et al. 2002). However, the 1990s saw a resurgence in the use of

MDMA, and its use continued to increase among adolescents in the early 2000s, with it becoming more commonly used than cocaine or crack. These numbers reached their peak in 2000–2002 and have generally declined since then. According to the Monitoring the Future survey, 3.0% of twelfth-grade students in 2022 reported they had used MDMA at least once in their lifetime (compared with 6.5% in 2009), and nearly 1% of twelfth-grade students had used MDMA in the month before they were surveyed (compared with nearly 2% in 2009) (Johnston et al. 2010; Miech et al. 2023). High school students generally view MDMA as easily accessible and as having a low harm potential (Johnston et al. 2010).

MDMA is a white, tasteless powder in its pure form that may be ingested orally, smoked, injected, or inhaled (Karlsen et al. 2008). It is commonly taken orally, usually in a tablet or capsule. The onset of effect is typically sudden, within 30–60 minutes. These effects generally last 3–6 hours, but they may persist as long as 8 hours (Baylen and Rosenberg 2006; Gouzoulis-Mayfrank and Daumann 2006; Jerrard 1990). Intoxication with MDMA is usually described as occurring in three stages (Koesters et al. 2002; Parrott and Lasky 1998). The initial stage consists of disorientation. This leads to the second stage of "yielding to tingling and spasmodic jerking" (Koesters et al. 2002). The final (target) stage of MDMA intoxication consists of the typical response of increased sociability, increased mental clarity, a feeling of emotional warmth and closeness to others, and a general sense of well-being (Cami et al. 2000; Koesters et al. 2002; Parrott and Lasky 1998). At higher doses, frank euphoria is experienced. A hangover is common the next day and can last for up to 48 hours. Side effects (including confusion, depression, insomnia, anxiety, and paranoia) have been reported to occur for weeks after ingestion (Curran and Travill 1997; Parrott and Lasky 1998).

The threshold dose of MDMA is 30 mg, but the average dose is 80–150 mg, with some users taking more than 200 mg. The lethal dose is estimated (from animal data) to be approximately 6,000 mg. On the street, concentrations of MDMA can vary greatly, and tablets may also contain other related substances such as MDA and methylenedioxyethylamphetamine (MDE) (Sherlock et al. 1999). The presence of these other substances is often associated with emergency presentations because of their narrower so-called therapeutic windows. As noted at the beginning of this chapter, the possible presence of fentanyl and other high-potency synthetic opioids in illicit MDMA preparations presents ever-increasing concerns.

Club Drugs and Inhalants 449

Pharmacological Management of Intoxication and Withdrawal
General principles of the treatment of MDMA intoxication are the same as those for intoxication with other stimulants, such as cocaine and methamphetamine. Overdoses of MDMA are generally treated with supportive care, because no specific pharmacological treatments have been identified (Shannon 2000; Solhkhah and Wilens 1998). This approach includes the use of routine laboratory tests to detect electrolyte abnormalities and to assess renal and hepatic functioning (Koesters et al. 2002). Adequate rehydration is crucial. Occasionally, the use of sedatives such as benzodiazepines is indicated, particularly when extreme agitation is present. If pronounced hyperthermia, hypertension, or rhabdomyolysis is present, observation in an ICU may be indicated. Observation may be combined with the use of dantrolene sodium (a skeletal muscle relaxant) at dosages of 2–3 mg/kg IV tid.

MDMA has been associated with significant increases in heart rate and blood pressure, similar to the increases associated with amphetamine use (Lester et al. 2000). This effect may require acute treatment with antihypertensive agents such as calcium channel blockers or nitroprusside (Koesters et al. 2002). The use of MDMA during raves may lead to dehydration, hypertension, intracerebral hemorrhage, heart failure, liver failure, kidney damage, and malignant hyperthermia (Barrett and Taylor 1993; Baylen and Rosenberg 2006; Harries and De Silva 1992; Jonas and Graeme-Cook 2001). Its use is often associated with jaw clenching (trismus) and bruxism (Jerrard 1990; Karlsen et al. 2008; Shannon 2000). This effect explains the use of pacifiers or lollipops by teenagers and other rave participants on the dance floor.

As was earlier described in the clinical presentation of MDMA, a hangover-like syndrome is common the next day after use of MDMA. MDMA withdrawal, which is thought to be caused by serotonin depletion, can last for weeks and includes symptoms of depression, anxiety, restlessness, and insomnia (Allen et al. 1993; McGuire et al. 1994). No specific treatments are currently indicated for this withdrawal syndrome, although the antidepressant bupropion may be helpful (Solhkhah and Wilens 1998; Solhkhah et al. 2001). Teenage lore has it that use of SSRIs may alleviate those symptoms acutely, but data to support this are lacking. In addition, MDMA use may be associated with sexual dysfunction (Baylen and Rosenberg 2006; Buffum and Moser 1986). This effect has led to use of a combination of MDMA and sildenafil (referred to colloquially as "sextasy").

Ketamine

Ketamine (2[2-chlorophenyl]-2-[methylamino]-cyclohexanone) is a Schedule III cyclohexane injectable anesthetic approved for human and veterinary use. It is known by slang names such as K, special K, vitamin K, and cat valium (Bobo and Miller 2002; Canet and Castillo 2012; Covvey et al. 2012). Despite its hallucinogenic effects and chemical similarity with phencyclidine (PCP), ketamine is included in this chapter rather than Chapter 8 ("Hallucinogens and Phencyclidine"), where PCP is discussed in detail, because ketamine has a history of being associated with use in club settings, similar to the use of MDMA and GHB. Ketamine is produced in a liquid form or as a white powder and is usually ingested orally or intranasally but is occasionally administered intramuscularly. It is a PCP analog that was first developed in 1962. Availability and nonmedical use of ketamine have increased over the past few decades; despite increasing media coverage and awareness of new medical indications, nonmedical use is still relatively uncommon but has been increasing globally (Barrios et al. 2025; Palamar et al. 2021).

Ketamine as Medicine

Ketamine has amnestic, analgesic, and anesthetic properties (Canet and Castillo 2012; Covvey et al. 2012) and has gained interest as an antidepressant (at a dose of 0.5 mg/kg), particularly for patients with treatment-resistant major depressive disorder or bipolar disorder (Bahji et al. 2021; Covvey et al. 2012; Diazgranados et al. 2010). The antidepressant effects of ketamine seem to be rapid and consistent and can be evident after a single dose (Covvey et al. 2012; Murrough 2012). Systematic reviews and meta-analyses of RCTs of ketamine, an N-methyl-D-aspartate (NMDA) glutaminergic receptor antagonist, demonstrate rapid but transient (days to weeks) effects in severe depression (FDA-approved indication) and suicidal ideation, as well as some evidence for its effects in social and general anxiety disorders, attributable to glutamate neuromodulation, increased prefrontal synaptic remodeling, neural plasticity, and altered functional connectivity (Iqbal et al. 2019; Walsh et al. 2021). Less robust but positive and short-lived effects of the use of ketamine for substance use disorders have been demonstrated, including reduced cravings, decreased self-administration of illicit drugs, and higher abstinence rates in 14 studies in alcohol use disorder, opioid use disorder, and cocaine use disorder (Walsh et al. 2021). For clinical treatment of depression, ketamine 0.4–0.5 mg/kg infused intravenously over 40–60 minutes is most common, with superior dose control and bioavailability, but oral, intramuscular, sublingual, and intranasal (e.g., esketamine or racemic ketamine) administration routes have advantages for repeated dosing and patient comfort. Higher dose ranges (0.71–2 mg/kg) have been used in substance use disorder studies with intravenous infusions.

Brief Pharmacology and Neurobiology

Ketamine is a noncompetitive NMDA receptor antagonist and is generally considered a psychotomimetic or schizophrenomimetic agent. Ketamine also appears to have cholinergic, opioidergic, and glutamatergic effects (Covvey et al. 2012; Koesters et al. 2002; Stone et al. 2012). This agent has been shown to increase plasma cortisol and prolactin levels, although the physiological significance of these effects is unclear (Krystal et al. 1994). Large doses of ketamine produce reactions similar to those produced by PCP, which include dream-like states, dissociation, and hallucinations (Koesters et al. 2002; Krystal et al. 1994; Murrough 2012). Important differences between ketamine and PCP include ketamine's lower potency, shorter duration of action, and tendency to cause less agitation. In general, the psychotic symptoms associated with ketamine include both positive and negative symptoms and may include catatonia (informally described as a "K-hole") (Koesters et al. 2002; Krystal et al. 1994). Functionally, ketamine leads to increased glutamatergic neurotransmission, predominantly in the anterior cingulate cortex (Stone et al. 2012). Ketamine is metabolized via the CYP system and has two major metabolites: dehydronorketamine and norketamine (Kalsi et al. 2011). Excretion is entirely via the urine.

Intoxication and Acute Presentations

As with the other club drugs, the use of ketamine has increased over the past decade. Although ketamine use remains much less common than use of MDMA, it is still an important cause of emergency presentations (Koesters et al. 2002). Estimates of lifetime use vary between 0.1% and 4% of the population (Kalsi et al. 2011), and studies have reported increases in past-year nonmedical use of ketamine, peaking at 0.9% of the general population in 2019 (Palamar et al. 2021). The use of ketamine leads to dose-dependent dissociative episodes (Bowdle et al. 1998). Emergence from ketamine-induced anesthetic effects leads to a variety of symptoms that are generally described as psychedelic or hallucinogenic by users, including "intense alterations in mood, perception, thinking, body awareness, and self-control" (Bowdle et al. 1998).

For nonmedical use, ketamine is often snorted, it is sometimes smoked with marijuana or tobacco products, and it also may be injected intramuscularly (Weiner et al. 2000). The typical street dose of ketamine ranges from 30 to 300 mg. These amounts are in contrast with the clinical doses used for anesthesia, which range from 2 to 10 mg/kg. Ketamine has a half-life of less than 2 hours (Koesters et al. 2002; Reich and Silvay 1989).

At low doses, ketamine may result in impairment of attention, learning ability, and memory; at high doses, it has been associated with delirium, amnesia, impaired motor function, hypertension, depression, and respiratory depression (Krystal et al. 1994). Another mechanism of action appears to be a blocking of the reuptake of catecholamines. This effect leads to an increase in heart rate and blood pressure (Reich and Silvay 1989).

Toxicology

In overdose, ketamine may lead to hyperthermia, seizures, hypertensive crisis, coma, and even death. Ketamine also may produce nonspecific abdominal pain (informally referred to as "K-cramps") (Kalsi et al. 2011). These symptoms are generally thought to result from ketamine's catecholaminergic effects (Reich and Silvay 1989). Ketamine is physically addicting, with a short-term (~48-hour) withdrawal syndrome (Critchlow 2006; Jansen and Darracot-Cankovic 2001; Winstock and Mitcheson 2012). Animal studies indicate that chronic ketamine use may lead to cognitive impairments (Kalsi et al. 2011; Venâncio et al. 2011). In the ED setting, the diagnosis of ketamine intoxication is a clinical one.

Ketamine is not routinely detected by urine toxicology tests, although it can be detected with high-performance liquid chromatography (Koesters et al. 2002). As with MDMA, the initial assessment for ketamine intoxication includes the use of routine laboratory tests to detect electrolyte abnormalities and to evaluate renal and hepatic functioning (Koesters et al. 2002). It is worth noting that although ketamine's median lethal dose in animals is 100 times the typical intravenous therapeutic dose, deaths due to ketamine overdose have been reported as mostly attributable to nonmedical use (Chaves et al. 2023; Kalsi et al. 2011).

Pharmacological Management of Intoxication/Withdrawal

No specific treatments for ketamine intoxication are currently indicated (Solhkhah and Wilens 1998). General supportive care, including providing the patient with a quiet, low-stimulus environment, can be helpful (Koesters et al. 2002; White et al. 1982). Benzodiazepines may be useful, particularly if agitation is present, although clinicians must be mindful of a possible interaction leading to a prolonged half-life for ketamine (Lahti et al. 1995; Lo and Cumming 1975). In general, because of the short half-life of ketamine, patients usually require observation only for several hours and then can be released home (Koesters et al. 2002).

As with many other hallucinogens, ketamine use may be associated with flashbacks. These flashbacks are generally milder and less frequent than those associated with PCP use (Fine and Finestone 1973). Generally, treatment with an antipsychotic is not required and can occasionally make symptoms worse (Solhkhah et al. 2000).

Inhalants

Inhalant use is the deliberate inhalation of volatile substances to induce a psychoactive or mind-altering effect (National Institute on Drug Abuse 2000). Inhalation is most commonly achieved by either breathing in a substance directly from its container (sniffing), placing a rag soaked in the substance over the nose and mouth and inhaling (huffing), or pouring the substance into a plastic bag and breathing the fumes (bagging). Rebreathing of exhaled air from a closed bag leads to hypercapnia and hypoxia, which potentiates the intoxicating effects of the solvent and increases the risk of suffocation. Inhalants encompass a broad range of volatile compounds, such as organic solvents (toluene, trichloroethylene, benzene, acetone, butane, propane, fluorocarbons, etc.), anesthetics (nitrous oxide, ether, chloroform, halothane), and nitrites (alkyl nitrites, informally referred to as "poppers") (Balster 2019).

Inhalants are legal products widely used in both household and industrial products and readily accessible to adolescents. According to the Substance Abuse and Mental Health Services Administration (Lipari 2017), the most commonly abused products containing inhalants include felt-tip pens or markers, glue, shoe polish, toluene, spray paints, gasoline or lighter fluid, computer cleaners or compressed-air dusters, correction fluid, paint solvents, amyl nitrite, poppers, locker room deodorizers, nitrous oxide (informally known as "laughing gas" or "whippets"), lighter fuels (butane or propane), halothane, ether, or other anesthetics.

All inhalants are highly lipophilic. They quickly cross the blood–brain barrier and cause CNS depression. For most abused solvents, 15–20 inhalations produce euphoria and subsequent drowsiness within seconds to minutes. Inhalants have a wide range of effects on neurotransmitter release, receptor activity, and membrane ion channels (Balster 2019). Like other drugs of abuse, inhalants seem to demonstrate reinforcing properties owing to their ability to modulate mesolimbic dopaminergic activity within both the ventral tegmental area and the nucleus accumbens (Bowen et al. 2006).

Most inhalants appear to have effects similar to those of alcohol and other CNS depressant drugs, stimulating GABA and glycine α_1 receptors and inhibiting NMDA receptors (Lubman et al. 2008). Toluene has the ability to produce visual and auditory hallucinations via activation of 5-HT$_{2A}$ receptors (Rivera-García et al. 2015). Nitrous oxide may also exhibit analgesic effects via direct stimulation of opioid receptors and NMDA antagonism. Nitrites primarily cause vasodilation and smooth muscle relaxation, which produce a sensation of floating, increased skin tactility, and warmth. Use of nitrites (poppers) has been popular among men who have sex with men to enhance sexual feelings, penile engorgement, and anal sphincter relaxation to intensify sexual experience (Brouette and Anton 2001).

Acute and chronic effects of different classes of inhalants are presented in Table 9.2. These effects are discussed in order in the following sections.

Intoxication and Acute Presentations

Acute intoxication includes initial euphoria and disinhibition, followed by sedation, slurred speech, dizziness, ataxia, diplopia, visual hallucinations, disorientation, and drowsiness or sleep within seconds to minutes (Howard et al. 2017). Volatile solvent use acutely causes respiratory mucosa irritation, sneezing, coughing, wheezing, excess salivation, and conjunctival erythema. Other acute complications include cardiac arrhythmias, respiratory depression, chemical and thermal burns, hypothermic injuries from propellants, and acute allergic reactions. Nitrous oxide intoxication can produce dissociation-like experiences, claustrophobia, and nausea and may lead to transient hypoxia. Acute intoxication with nitrites, especially combined with sildenafil, may result in tachycardia, blurred vision, headache, lightheadedness, and

Table 9.2 Acute and chronic effects of various classes of inhalants

Characteristic	Organic solvents	Anesthetics	Nitrites
Example sources	Toluene (airplane glue, paint thinner, nail polish remover), *n*-hexane (glue), trichloroethylene (correction fluid, stain remover, dry-cleaning chemicals, polyvinyl chloride cement), benzene (gasoline), acetone (nail polish remover, rubber cement), butane (lighter fuel), propane (lighter fuel), fluorocarbons (spray paint, hair spray, deodorant)	Nitrous oxide ("laughing gas," "whippets"), ether, chloroform, halothane	Alkyl nitrites (deodorizers, "poppers")
Acute effects	Euphoria, drowsiness, ataxia, slurred speech, diplopia, sneezing, coughing, salivation, conjunctival erythema	Euphoria, dissociation, nausea	Vasodilation and relaxation of smooth muscles, acute hypotension, headache, dizziness, nausea, vomiting, heightened sensation, sexual arousal, prolonged orgasm

Table 9.2 Acute and chronic effects of various classes of inhalants *(continued)*

Characteristic	Organic solvents	Anesthetics	Nitrites
Chronic effects	Hepatotoxicity, cardiac arrhythmia, myocarditis, teratogenic effect, white matter degeneration, peripheral neuropathy; toluene can cause cerebellar atrophy, sensorineural hearing loss, optic neuropathy, glomerulonephritis, renal tubular acidosis, hepatorenal failure, and emphysema; benzene may cause leukemia and aplastic anemia	Peripheral neuropathy (likely secondary to vitamin B_{12} deficiency), short-term memory impairment, depression, psychosis, bone marrow suppression	Hemolytic anemia, immunosuppression

severe hypotension, leading to syncope and cerebral or myocardial ischemia (Romanelli et al. 2004). Death may occur secondary to aspiration, accidental trauma, asphyxia, or so-called sudden sniffing death syndrome resulting from sensitization of the myocardium to endogenous catecholamines (Brouette and Anton 2001). Both tolerance and withdrawal may develop to volatile solvents. Withdrawal symptoms including fatigue, difficulty concentrating, palpitations, tremors, headache, nausea and vomiting, rhinorrhea, lacrimation, craving, irritability, sleep disturbance, anxiety, and depressed mood were reported among continuous users of volatile solvents (Perron et al. 2011).

Diagnosis of acute inhalant intoxication is based on clinical presentation, physical examination, and a detailed history. Signs of recent inhalant abuse include paint or oil stains on clothing or skin, spots or sores around the mouth, injected sclera, rhinorrhea, chemical odor on the breath, nystagmus, dazed appearance, slurred speech, difficulty concentrating, irritability, and excitability (Anderson and Loomis 2003). Decontamination of skin and clothing can reduce the risk of burns and extended harm. Because many inhalants may have nephrotoxic, hepatotoxic, and cardiotoxic effects, initial tests should include a laboratory panel (to determine complete blood count, serum electrolytes, methemoglobin, creatinine, blood urea nitrogen, and liver function), pulse oximetry, urinalysis, and electrocardiogram. Although inhalants are not detected in regular urine toxicology testing, one should screen for concomitant illicit drug use. Most volatiles can be detected within 10 hours of use by gas chromatography; however, this test is not routinely available (Broussard 2000). Treatment during acute intoxication includes medical monitoring and supportive care. Medical stabilization may involve cardiorespiratory monitoring, hydration, correction of metabolic and acid-base abnormalities, and control of agitation. Because of the sensitization of the myocardium to catecholamines, vasopressors and bronchodilators are relatively contraindicated. β-Blockers should be administered early to prevent arrhythmias (Anderson and Loomis 2003). Currently, no specific agents can reverse acute solvent intoxication.

Chronic Effects

Chronic solvent abuse has been associated with significant toxic effects, including neurological, renal, hepatic, cardiovascular, and pulmonary damage as well as immunosuppression. Regular long-term exposure to inhalants has been linked to significant cognitive deficits, cerebellar dysfunction, cortical atrophy, encephalopathy, focal neurological deficits, and dementia. There is consistent evidence that chronic abuse of inhalants during early adolescence is likely to result in cognitive impairment, including decreased IQ, personality changes, decreased concentration, memory and information-processing deficits, decreased problem-solving ability, speech and gait abnormalities, paranoid psychosis, temporal lobe epilepsy, tremors, and seizures (Cruz and Bowen 2021). Neuroimaging studies demonstrated structural abnormalities in specific brain areas (e.g., frontal cortex, hippocampus, and brain stem), enlargement of the ventricles, demyelination, and reduced brain perfusion and blood flow (Lubman et al. 2008). n-Hexane and n-butyl ketone (components of glues and paints) may cause peripheral neuropathy (Tenenbein et al. 1984). Chronic nitrous oxide abuse was related to short-term memory loss and peripheral neuropathy; the latter results from nitrous oxide inactivating vitamin B_{12}. The clinical picture resembles one of pernicious anemia, characterized by anemia, leukopenia, ataxia, broad-based gait, sensorimotor neuropathy, and posterior/lateral column spinal cord disease (Brouette and Anton 2001).

Nitrites have profound effects on hematological and immune systems. Inhalation of amyl nitrite increases methemoglobin and may result in hemolytic anemia. Nitrite use can produce carcinogenic nitrosamines and suppress T cell–mediated immune response. Chronic toluene abuse has been associated with renal tubular acidosis, urinary calculi, Fanconi's syndrome, glomerulonephritis, and renal failure (Anderson and Loomis 2003). The catecholamine-sensitizing effect of volatile solvents may increase the risk of arrhythmias, and direct toxic effects can cause cardiomyopathy (Vural and Ogel 2006). Long-term use of benzene has been associated with bone marrow suppression, leading to leukopenia, aplastic anemia, thrombocytopenia, and hemolysis (Anderson and Loomis 2003). Inhalant misuse during pregnancy increases risk of spontaneous abortion and premature labor, as well as withdrawal symptoms in the neonate. Teratogenic effects of toluene can result in fetal solvent syndrome, which encompasses developmental disorders and fetal malformations similar to those seen with fetal alcohol syndrome (Jones and Balster 1998).

Special Population Considerations

Higher levels of inhalant use in the United States are being observed for adolescents who are exposed to parental drug use, lack parental control, or live in a lower-resource household or in an isolated or rural area (Nonnemaker et al. 2011). Adolescent inhalant use has been associated with harmful use of alcohol, other substances, injectable drug use, co-occurring antisocial personality disorder, criminal behaviors, depression, and increased risk of suicide ideation and attempts (Nguyen et al. 2016). Studies of adolescents also have suggested some gender differences in the choice of inhalants used, with female adolescents preferring to use glue, shoe polish, spray paints, and correction fluid, whereas male adolescents were more likely to use gasoline, lighter fluid, and nitrous oxide (Wu et al. 2004). Use of nitrite among men who had sex with men has consistently been associated with risky sexual behaviors, use of other drugs, and transmission of sexually transmitted diseases, including HIV (Howard et al. 2017).

Despite highly prevalent inhalant use among adolescents, little research has been done on specific modalities of the diagnosis and treatment of inhalant use disorder. No evidence-based treatment options for inhalant abuse were identified (Konghom et al. 2010). The heterogeneity of inhalants and different mechanisms of action make the search for pharmacological treatment extremely challenging. Most clinicians apply treatment approaches used for other substance use disorders. Psychosocial approaches include individual counseling, family therapy, and activity and engagement programs (McWhirter 2008).

Key Points

- γ-Hydroxybutyrate (GHB) is an endogenous fatty acid that is believed to function as a neurotransmitter in the brain, with sedative, anxiolytic, and euphoric effects similar to alcohol; at high doses, GHB can have dissociative effects similar to ketamine.
- Because of its purported anabolic effects, GHB is often used by bodybuilders despite scant supporting scientific evidence. In addition, because of its ability to increase sexuality, GHB is often used as part of club or rave culture as well as gay circuit parties. GHB has also reportedly been used to facilitate sexual assault, because of its ability to produce anterograde amnesia.
- Pharmaceutical GHB is a Schedule III medication with an FDA-approved indication for the treatment of cataplexy in patients with

narcolepsy, because of its ability to consolidate slow-wave sleep. GHB is simultaneously a Schedule I drug, owing to its high misuse potential.
- GHB can be fatal in overdose, owing to its respiratory suppressive effects, and tolerance and withdrawal are possible in those who use GHB chronically. Overdose management is typically supportive of respiratory function, because no known reversal agents exist. Pharmacotherapy for withdrawal is typically with sedative-hypnotic medications, often in the form of high-dose intravenous benzodiazepine administration.
- 3,4-Methylenedioxymethamphetamine (MDMA) has structural similarities to both hallucinogens and amphetamine, although clinically it has very little (if any) hallucinogenic activity. MDMA increases serotonin neurotransmission through several mechanisms and has preferential effects on the frontal cortex and limbic systems. In overdose, MDMA can lead to dehydration, hyperthermia, tachycardia, hypertension, rhabdomyolysis, and death.
- Management of MDMA intoxication is typically supportive, including aggressive rehydration, end-organ monitoring, and sedative-hypnotic medications for agitation. Dantrolene and ICU-level care reportedly have been required in severe cases.
- Ketamine is often used as part of club or rave culture; this dissociative anesthetic exerts its effects mainly through N-methyl-D-aspartate glutaminergic receptor antagonism. It has also been used as a treatment for treatment-refractory depression.
- Ketamine intoxication can result in hyperthermia, seizures, hypertensive crisis, coma, and death, and treatment is generally supportive. Given its short half-life (unless combined with sedative-hypnotic medications), recovery from intoxication is often rapid.
- Inhalants are a diverse category of volatile chemicals that are inhaled and have psychoactive properties (most typically, CNS-depressive effects). Acutely, respiratory system irritation, cardiac arrhythmias, hypotension, and death have been reported. Chronic use can result in damage to many end-organ systems, most notably the CNS.
- There are no FDA-approved pharmacotherapies for club drug or inhalant use disorders.

References

Addolorato G, Castelli E, Stefanini GF, et al: An open multicentric study evaluating 4-hydroxybutyric acid sodium salt in the medium-term treatment of 179 alcohol dependent subjects. Alcohol Alcohol 31(4):341–345, 1996 8879280

Addolorato G, Balducci G, Capristo E, et al: Gamma-hydroxybutyric acid (GHB) in the treatment of alcohol withdrawal syndrome: a randomized comparative study versus benzodiazepine. Alcohol Clin Exp Res 23(10):1596–1604, 1999a 10549990

Addolorato G, Capristo E, Gessa GL, et al: Long-term administration of GHB does not affect muscular mass in alcoholics. Life Sci 65(14):PL191–PL196, 1999b 10530806

Addolorato G, Caputo F, Capristo E, et al: A case of gamma-hydroxybutyric acid withdrawal syndrome during alcohol addiction treatment: utility of diazepam administration. Clin Neuropharmacol 22(1):60–62, 1999c 10047936

Addolorato G, Caputo F, Capristo E, et al: Gamma-hydroxybutyric acid efficacy, potential abuse, and dependence in the treatment of alcohol addiction. Alcohol 20(3):217–222, 2000 10869862

Alattas IM, Alwajeeh SA, Alamoudi OO, et al: Withdrawal of gamma-Hydroxybutyrate in a Saudi male patient: a case report. Cureus 14(12):e32298, 2022

Allen RP, McCann UD, Ricaurte GA: Persistent effects of (+/-)3,4-methylenedioxymethamphetamine (MDMA, "ecstasy") on human sleep. Sleep 16(6):560–564, 1993 7901886

American Psychiatric Association: Diagnostic and Statistical Manual of Mental Disorders, 5th Edition, Text Revision. Washington, DC, American Psychiatric Association, 2022

Anderson CE, Loomis GA: Recognition and prevention of inhalant abuse. Am Fam Physician 68(5):869–874, 2003 13678134

Armentano ME: Assessment, diagnosis, and treatment of the dually diagnosed adolescent. Pediatr Clin North Am 42(2):479–490, 1995 7724271

Bahji A, Vazquez GH, Zarate CA Jr: Comparative efficacy of racemic ketamine and esketamine for depression: a systematic review and meta-analysis. J Affect Disord 278:542–555, 2021 33022440

Balster R: The pharmacology of inhalants, in The ASAM Principles of Addiction Medicine, 6th Edition. Edited by Miller S, Fiellin D, Rosenthal R, et al. New York, Wolters Kluwer, 2019, pp 681–702

Barrett PJ, Taylor GT: "Ecstasy" ingestion: a case report of severe complications. J R Soc Med 86(4):233–234, 1993 8099372

Barrios KP, Connolly DJ, Ferris JA, et al: Ketamine use in a large global sample: characteristics, patterns of use and emergency medical treatment. J Psychopharmacol 39(1):8–22, 2025 39420535

Baylen CA, Rosenberg H: A review of the acute subjective effects of MDMA/ecstasy. Addiction 101(7):933–947, 2006 16771886

Bobo WV, Miller SC: Ketamine as a preferred substance of abuse. Am J Addict 11(4):332–334, 2002 12584875

Bolla KI, McCann UD, Ricaurte GA: Memory impairment in abstinent MDMA ("Ecstasy") users. Neurology 51(6):1532–1537, 1998 9855498

Borgen L, Lane E, Lai A: Xyrem (sodium oxybate): a study of dose proportionality in healthy human subjects. J Clin Pharmacol 40:1053, 2000

Borgen LA, Okerholm R, Morrison D, et al: The influence of gender and food on the pharmacokinetics of sodium oxybate oral solution in healthy subjects. J Clin Pharmacol 43(1):59–65, 2003 12520629

Bowdle TA, Radant AD, Cowley DS, et al: Psychedelic effects of ketamine in healthy volunteers: relationship to steady-state plasma concentrations. Anesthesiology 88(1):82–88, 1998 9447860

Bowen SE, Batis JC, Paez-Martinez N, et al: The last decade of solvent research in animal models of abuse: mechanistic and behavioral studies. Neurotoxicol Teratol 28(6):636–647, 2006 17064879

Boyer EW, Quang L, Woolf A, et al: Use of physostigmine in the management of gamma-hydroxybutyrate overdose (letter). Ann Emerg Med 38(3):346, author reply 347–348, 2001 11524662

Brennan R, Van Hout MC: Gamma-hydroxybutyrate (GHB): a scoping review of pharmacology, toxicology, motives for use, and user groups. J Psychoactive Drugs 46(3):243–251, 2014 25052883

Brouette T, Anton R: Clinical review of inhalants. Am J Addict 10(1):79–94, 2001 11268830

Broussard LA: The role of the laboratory in detecting inhalant abuse. Clin Lab Sci 13(4):205–209, 2000 11586505

Brunt TM, van Amsterdam JG, van den Brink W: GHB, GBL and 1,4-BD addiction. Curr Pharm Des 20(25):4076–4085, 2014 24001290

Buffum J, Moser C: MDMA and human sexual function. J Psychoactive Drugs 18(4):355–359, 1986 2880951

Cami J, Farré M, Mas M, et al: Human pharmacology of 3,4-methylenedioxymethamphetamine ("ecstasy"): psychomotor performance and subjective effects. J Clin Psychopharmacol 20(4):455–466, 2000 10917407

Canet J, Castillo J: Ketamine: a familiar drug we trust. Anesthesiology 116(1):6–8, 2012 22080003

Carter LP, Pardi D, Gorsline J, et al: Illicit gamma-hydroxybutyrate (GHB) and pharmaceutical sodium oxybate (Xyrem): differences in characteristics and misuse. Drug Alcohol Depend 104(1–2):1–10, 2009 19493637

Centers for Disease Control and Prevention: Gamma hydroxy butyrate use—New York and Texas, 1995–96. MMWR Morb Mortal Wkly Rep 46(13):281–283, 1997 9121419

Centers for Disease Control and Prevention: Adverse events associated with ingestion of gamma-butyrolactone—Minnesota, New Mexico, and Texas, 1998–1999. MMWR Morb Mortal Wkly Rep 48(7):137–140, 1999 10077458

Chatlos JC: Recent trends and a developmental approach to substance abuse in adolescents. Child Adolesc Psychiatr Clin N Am 5:1–27, 1996

Chaves TV, Wilffert B, Sanchez ZM: Overdoses and deaths related to the use of ketamine and its analogues: a systematic review. Am J Drug Alcohol Abuse 49(2):141–150, 2023 36410032

Chin RL: A case of severe withdrawal from gamma-hydroxybutyrate. Ann Emerg Med 37(5):551–552, 2001 11326198

Chin RL, Sporer KA, Cullison B, et al: Clinical course of gamma-hydroxybutyrate overdose. Ann Emerg Med 31:716–722, 1998

Colombo G, Agabio R, Lobina C, et al: Cross-tolerance to ethanol and gamma-hydroxybutyric acid. Eur J Pharmacol 273(3):235–238, 1995 7737330

Cook PA, Clark P, Bellis MA, et al: Re-emerging syphilis in the UK: a behavioural analysis of infected individuals. Commun Dis Public Health 4(4):253–258, 2001 12109391

Covvey JR, Crawford AN, Lowe DK: Intravenous ketamine for treatment-resistant major depressive disorder. Ann Pharmacother 46(1):117–123, 2012 22190250

Craig K, Gomez HF, McManus JL, et al: Severe gamma-hydroxybutyrate withdrawal: a case report and literature review. J Emerg Med 18(1):65–70, 2000 10645841

Critchlow DG: A case of ketamine dependence with discontinuation symptoms. Addiction 101(8):1212–1213, 2006 16869851

Cruz SL, Bowen SE: The last two decades on preclinical and clinical research on inhalant effects. Neurotoxicol Teratol 87:106999, 2021 34087382

Curran HV, Travill RA: Mood and cognitive effects of +/-3,4-methylenedioxymethamphetamine (MDMA, "ecstasy"): week-end "high" followed by mid-week low. Addiction 92(7):821–831, 1997 9293041

Danforth AL, Grob CS, Struble C, et al: Reduction in social anxiety after MDMA-assisted psychotherapy with autistic adults: a randomized, double-blind, placebo-controlled pilot study. Psychopharmacology (Berl) 235(11):3137–3148, 2018 30196397 de Jong CA, Kamal R, Dijkstra BA, et al: Gamma-hydroxybutyrate detoxification by titration and tapering. Eur Addict Res 18(1):40–45, 2012 22142784

Diazgranados N, Ibrahim L, Brutsche NE, et al: A randomized add-on trial of an N-methyl-D-aspartate antagonist in treatment-resistant bipolar depression. Arch Gen Psychiatry 67(8):793–802, 2010 20679587

Dyer JE, Roth B: In reply (letter). Ann Emerg Med 38:606, 2001

Dyer JE, Roth B, Hyma BA: Gamma-hydroxybutyrate withdrawal syndrome. Ann Emerg Med 37(2):147–153, 2001 11174231

Eiden C, Capdevielle D, Deddouche C, et al: Neuroleptic malignant syndrome-like reaction precipitated by antipsychotics in a patient with gamma-butyrolactone withdrawal. J Addict Med 5(4):302–303, 2011 21817917

Fadda F, Colombo G, Mosca E, et al: Suppression by gamma-hydroxybutyric acid of ethanol withdrawal syndrome in rats. Alcohol Alcohol 24(5):447–451, 1989 2818752

Fine J, Finestone SC: Sensory disturbances following ketamine anesthesia: recurrent hallucinations. Anesth Analg 52(3):428–430, 1973 4735997

Freeman G, Siefried KJ, Roberts DM, et al: Phenobarbital to manage severe gamma-hydroxybutyrate withdrawal: a case series. Drug Alcohol Rev 42(1):27–32, 2023 36269081

Freese TE, Miotto K, Reback CJ: The effects and consequences of selected club drugs. J Subst Abuse Treat 23(2):151–156, 2002 12220613

Friedman J, Westlake R, Furman M: "Grievous bodily harm": gamma hydroxybutyrate abuse leading to a Wernicke-Korsakoff syndrome. Neurology 46(2):469–471, 1996 8614515

Gallimberti L, Ferri M, Ferrara SD, et al: Gamma-hydroxybutyric acid in the treatment of alcohol dependence: a double-blind study. Alcohol Clin Exp Res 16(4):673–676, 1992 1326902

Gallimberti L, Spella MR, Soncini CA, et al: Gamma-hydroxybutyric acid in the treatment of alcohol and heroin dependence. Alcohol 20(3):257–262, 2000 10869867

Galloway GP, Frederick SL, Staggers FE Jr, et al: Gamma-hydroxybutyrate: an emerging drug of abuse that causes physical dependence. Addiction 92(1):89–96, 1997 9060200

Galloway GP, Frederick-Osborne SL, Seymour R, et al: Abuse and therapeutic potential of gamma-hydroxybutyric acid. Alcohol 20(3):263–269, 2000 10869868

Gerra G, Caccavari R, Fontanesi B, et al: Flumazenil effects on growth hormone response to gamma-hydroxybutyric acid. Int Clin Psychopharmacol 9(3):211–215, 1994 7814832

Gessa G, Vargiu L, Crabai F, et al: Selective increase of brain dopamine induced by gamma-hydroxybutyrate. Life Sci 5:1921–1930, 1966

Gessa GL, Agabio R, Carai MA, et al: Mechanism of the antialcohol effect of gamma-hydroxybutyric acid. Alcohol 20(3):271–276, 2000 10869869

Gobaille S, Schleef C, Hechler V, et al: Gamma-hydroxybutyrate increases tryptophan availability and potentiates serotonin turnover in rat brain. Life Sci 70(18):2101–2112, 2002 12002803

Godschalk M, Dzoljic MR, Bonta IL: Slow wave sleep and a state resembling absence epilepsy induced in the rat by gamma-hydroxybutyrate. Eur J Pharmacol 44(2):105–111, 1977 407087

Gouzoulis-Mayfrank E, Daumann J: Neurotoxicity of methylenedioxyamphetamines (MDMA; ecstasy) in humans: how strong is the evidence for persistent brain damage? Addiction 101(3):348–361, 2006 16499508

Gouzoulis-Mayfrank E, Daumann J, Tuchtenhagen F, et al: Impaired cognitive performance in drug free users of recreational ecstasy (MDMA). J Neurol Neurosurg Psychiatry 68(6):719–725, 2000 10811694

Green AR, King MV, Shortall SE, et al: Lost in translation: preclinical studies on MDMA provide mechanisms of action, but do not allow accurate prediction of adverse events in humans. Br J Pharmacol 166:1521–1522, 2012

Habibian S, Ahamad K, McLean M, et al: Successful management of gamma-hydroxybutyrate (GHB) withdrawal using baclofen as a standalone therapy: a case report. J Addict Med 13(5):415–417, 2019 30907765

Hake HS, Davis JKP, Wood RR, et al: 3,4-Methylenedioxymethamphetamine (MDMA) impairs the extinction and reconsolidation of fear memory in rats. Physiol Behav 199:343–350, 2019 30529341

Harries DP, De Silva R: "Ecstasy" and intracerebral haemorrhage. Scott Med J 37(5):150–152, 1992 1492208

Hatzidimitriou G, McCann UD, Ricaurte GA: Altered serotonin innervation patterns in the forebrain of monkeys treated with (+/-)3,4-methylenedioxymethamphetamine seven years previously: factors influencing abnormal recovery. J Neurosci 19(12):5096–5107, 1999 10366642

Hernandez M, McDaniel CH, Costanza CD, et al: GHB-induced delirium: a case report and review of the literature of gamma hydroxybutyric acid. Am J Drug Alcohol Abuse 24(1):179–183, 1998 9513637

Hill SL, Thomas SH: Clinical toxicology of newer recreational drugs. Clin Toxicol (Phila) 49(8):705–719, 2011 21970769

Hodges B, Everett J: Acute toxicity from home-brewed gamma hydroxybutyrate. J Am Board Fam Pract 11(2):154–157, 1998 9542708

Howard M, Bowen S, Garland E: Inhalant-related disorders, in Kaplan and Sadock's Comprehensive Textbook of Psychiatry, 10th Edition. Edited by Sadock B, Sadock V, Ruiz P. Baltimore, MD, Lippincott Williams & Wilkins, 2017, pp 1328–1342

Howard SG, Feigenbaum JJ: Effect of gamma-hydroxybutyrate on central dopamine release in vivo: a microdialysis study in awake and anesthetized animals. Biochem Pharmacol 53(1):103–110, 1997 8960069

Iqbal MN, Levin CJ, Levin FR: Treatment for substance use disorder with co-occurring mental illness. Focus Am Psychiatr Publ 17(2):88–97, 2019 31975963

Itzhak Y, Ali SF: Repeated administration of gamma-hydroxybutyric acid (GHB) to mice: assessment of the sedative and rewarding effects of GHB. Ann NY Acad Sci 965:451–460, 2002 12105120

Jamt R, Edvardsen H, Middelkoop G, et al: Deaths associated with MDMA in the period 2000–2019 [in Norwegian]. Tidsskr Nor Laegeforen 19:142(8), 2022

Jansen KL, Darracot-Cankovic R: The nonmedical use of ketamine, part two: a review of problem use and dependence. J Psychoactive Drugs 33(2):151–158, 2001 11476262

Jerrard DA: "Designer drugs": a current perspective. J Emerg Med 8(6):733–741, 1990 2096172

Johnston LD, O'Malley PM, Bachman JG, et al: Monitoring the Future: National Results on Adolescent Drug Use: Overview of Key Findings, 2009 (NIH Publ No 10-7583). Bethesda, MD, National Institute on Drug Abuse, 2010. Available at: https://monitoringthefuture.org/wp-content/uploads/2022/08/mtf-overview2011.pdf. Accessed February 10, 2025.

Johnston LD, Miech RA, O'Malley PM, et al: Monitoring the Future: National Survey Results on Drug Use, 1975–2021: Overview, Key Findings on Adolescent Drug Use. Ann Arbor, Institute for Social Research, University of Michigan, 2022. Available at: https://monitoringthefuture.org/wp-content/uploads/2022/08/mtf-overview2021.pdf. Accessed February 10, 2025.

Jonas MM, Graeme-Cook FM: Case records of the Massachusetts General Hospital: weekly clinicopathological exercises: case 6-2001—a 17-year-old girl with marked jaundice and weight loss. N Engl J Med 344(8):591–599, 2001 11207356

Jones HE, Balster RL: Inhalant abuse in pregnancy. Obstet Gynecol Clin North Am 25(1):153–167, 1998 9547765

Kalsi SS, Wood DM, Dargan PI: The epidemiology and patterns of acute and chronic toxicity associated with recreational ketamine use. Emerg Health Threats J 4:7107, 2011 24149025

Kapitány-Fövény M, Mervó B, Corazza O, et al: Enhancing sexual desire and experience: an investigation of the sexual correlates of gamma-hydroxybutyrate (GHB) use. Hum Psychopharmacol 30(4):276–284, 2015 26216563
Karlsen SN, Spigset O, Slørdal L: The dark side of ecstasy: neuropsychiatric symptoms after exposure to 3,4-methylenedioxymethamphetamine. Basic Clin Pharmacol Toxicol 102(1):15–24, 2008 18047478
Kemmel V, Taleb O, Andriamampandry C, et al: Gamma-hydroxybutyrate receptor function determined by stimulation of rubidium and calcium movements from NCB-20 neurons. Neuroscience 116(4):1021–1031, 2003 12617943
Koesters SC, Rogers PD, Rajasingham CR: MDMA ("ecstasy") and other "club drugs." The new epidemic. Pediatr Clin North Am 49(2):415–433, 2002 11993291
Konghom S, Verachai V, Srisurapanont M, et al: Treatment for inhalant dependence and abuse. Cochrane Database Syst Rev 12(12):CD007537, 2010 21154379
Krystal JH, Karper LP, Seibyl JP, et al: Subanesthetic effects of the noncompetitive NMDA antagonist, ketamine, in humans: psychotomimetic, perceptual, cognitive, and neuroendocrine responses. Arch Gen Psychiatry 51(3):199–214, 1994 8122957
Lahti AC, Koffel B, LaPorte D, et al: Subanesthetic doses of ketamine stimulate psychosis in schizophrenia. Neuropsychopharmacology 13(1):9–19, 1995 8526975
Lai W, Raposa JT, Parlapalli R: Treatment of poorly responsive gamma-hydroxybutyrate withdrawal with baclofen: a case report. Cureus 14(6):e25728, 2022 35812608
Lammers GJ, Arends J, Declerck AC, et al: Gammahydroxybutyrate and narcolepsy: a double-blind placebo-controlled study. Sleep 16(3):216–220, 1993 8506453
Lester SJ, Baggott M, Welm S, et al: Cardiovascular effects of 3,4-methylenedioxymethamphetamine: a double-blind, placebo-controlled trial. Ann Intern Med 133(12):969–973, 2000 11119398
Levy MI, Davis BM, Mohs RC, et al: Gamma-hydroxybutyrate in the treatment of schizophrenia. Psychiatry Res 9(1):1–8, 1983 6193548
Li J, Stokes SA, Woeckener A: A tale of novel intoxication: a review of the effects of gamma-hydroxybutyric acid with recommendations for management. Ann Emerg Med 31:729–736, 1998a
Li J, Stokes SA, Woeckener A: A tale of novel intoxication: seven cases of gamma-hydroxybutyric acid overdose. Ann Emerg Med 31(6):723–728, 1998b 9624312

Liechti ME, Vollenweider FX: The serotonin uptake inhibitor citalopram reduces acute cardiovascular and vegetative effects of 3,4-methylenedioxymethamphetamine ("Ecstasy") in healthy volunteers. J Psychopharmacol 14(3):269–274, 2000 11106307

Lipari RN: Understanding adolescent inhalant use, in The CBHSQ Report. Center for Behavioral Health Statistics and Quality, Substance Abuse and Mental Health Services Administration, Rockville, MD, June 13, 2017. Available at: https://www.ncbi.nlm.nih.gov/books/NBK441821/pdf/Bookshelf_NBK441821.pdf. Accessed February 10, 2025.

Lo JN, Cumming JF: Interaction between sedative premedicants and ketamine in man in isolated perfused rat livers. Anesthesiology 43(3):307–312, 1975 1163830

Lubman DI, Yücel M, Lawrence AJ: Inhalant abuse among adolescents: neurobiological considerations. Br J Pharmacol 154(2):316–326, 2008 18332858

Maitre M: The gamma-hydroxybutyrate signalling system in brain: organization and functional implications. Prog Neurobiol 51(3):337–361, 1997 9089792

Maitre M, Andriamampandry C, Kemmel V, et al: Gamma-hydroxybutyric acid as a signaling molecule in brain. Alcohol 20(3):277–283, 2000 10869870

Mamelak M: Gammahydroxybutyrate: an endogenous regulator of energy metabolism. Neurosci Biobehav Rev 13(4):187–198, 1989 2691926

Maxwell JC. Substance Abuse Trends in Texas, January 2006. The Gulf Coast Addiction Technology Transfer Center (GCATTC), Center for Social Work Research at The University of Texas at Austin, 2006. Available at: https://socialwork.utexas.edu/wp-content/uploads/2021/06/trends106.pdf Accessed June 3, 2025.

McCann UD, Ricaurte GA: Reinforcing subjective effects of (+/-) 3,4-methylenedioxymethamphetamine ("ecstasy") may be separable from its neurotoxic actions: clinical evidence. J Clin Psychopharmacol 13(3):214–217, 1993 8102623

McCann UD, Szabo Z, Scheffel U, et al: Positron emission tomographic evidence of toxic effect of MDMA ("Ecstasy") on brain serotonin neurons in human beings. Lancet 352(9138):1433–1437, 1998 9807990

McCann UD, Eligulashvili V, Ricaurte GA: (+/-)3,4-Methylenedioxymethamphetamine ("Ecstasy")-induced serotonin neurotoxicity: clinical studies. Neuropsychobiology 42(1):11–16, 2000 10867551

McCrae K, Tobias S, Tupper K, et al: Drug checking services at music festivals and events in a Canadian setting. Drug Alcohol Depend 205:107589, 2019 31605958

McDaniel CH, Miotto KA: Gamma hydroxybutyrate (GHB) and gamma butyrolactone (GBL) withdrawal: five case studies. J Psychoactive Drugs 33:143–149, 2001

McDonough M, Kennedy N, Glasper A, et al: Clinical features and management of gamma-hydroxybutyrate (GHB) withdrawal: a review. Drug Alcohol Depend 75:3–9, 2004 15225884

McGuire PK, Cope H, Fahy TA: Diversity of psychopathology associated with use of 3,4-methylenedioxymethamphetamine ("Ecstasy"). Br J Psychiatry 165(3):391–395, 1994 7994514

McWhirter PT: Enhancing adolescent substance abuse treatment engagement. J Psychoactive Drugs 40(2):173–182, 2008 18720667

Mema SC, Sage C, Xu Y, et al: Drug checking at an electronic dance music festival during the public health overdose emergency in British Columbia. Can J Public Health 109(5–6):740–744, 2018 30251119

Miech R, Johnston L, Patrick M, et al: Monitoring the Future National Survey Results on Drug Use, 1975–2022: Secondary School Students. Ann Arbor, MI, Institute for Social Research, The University of Michigan, 2023. Available at: https://monitoringthefuture.org/wp-content/uploads/2022/12/mtf2022.pdf. Accessed February 10, 2025.

Miotto K, Roth B: GHB Withdrawal Syndrome. Austin, Texas Commission on Alcohol and Drug Abuse, 2001. Available at: https://drugs-forum.com/data/attachment-files/2012/02/145126_ghb_addiction2.pdf. Accessed June 3, 2025.

Miotto K, Darakjian J, Basch J, et al: Gamma-hydroxybutyric acid: patterns of use, effects and withdrawal. Am J Addict 10(3):232–241, 2001 11579621

Mitchell JM, Bogenschutz M, Lilienstein A, et al: MDMA-assisted therapy for severe PTSD: a randomized, double-blind, placebo-controlled phase 3 study. Nat Med 27(6):1025–1033, 2021 33972795

Mithoefer MC, Wagner MT, Mithoefer AT, et al: The safety and efficacy of +/-3,4-methylenedioxymethamphetamine-assisted psychotherapy in subjects with chronic, treatment-resistant posttraumatic stress disorder: the first randomized controlled pilot study. J Psychopharmacol 25(4):439–452, 2011 20643699

Mithoefer MC, Wagner MT, Mithoefer AT, et al: Durability of improvement in post-traumatic stress disorder symptoms and absence of harmful effects or drug dependency after 3,4-methylenedioxymethamphetamine-assisted psychotherapy: a prospective long-term follow-up study. J Psychopharmacol 27(1):28–39, 2013 23172889

Mithoefer M, Mithoefer A, Jerome L, et al: A Manual for MDMA-Assisted Psychotherapy in the Treatment of Posttraumatic Stress Disorder. Santa Cruz,

CA, Multidisciplinary Association for Psychedelic Studies, 2016. Available at: https://maps.org/2014/01/27/a-manual-for-mdma-assisted-therapy-in-the-treatment-of-ptsd/. Accessed February 10, 2025.

Moncini M, Masini E, Gambassi F, et al: Gamma-hydroxybutyric acid and alcohol-related syndromes. Alcohol 20(3):285–291, 2000 10869871

Montoya AG, Sorrentino R, Lukas SE, et al: Long-term neuropsychiatric consequences of "ecstasy" (MDMA): a review. Harv Rev Psychiatry 10(4):212–220, 2002 12119307

Moonzwe LS, Schensul JJ, Kostick KM: The role of MDMA (Ecstasy) in coping with negative life situations among urban young adults. J Psychoactive Drugs 43(3):199–210, 2011 22111403

Morgan MJ: Memory deficits associated with recreational use of "ecstasy" (MDMA). Psychopharmacology (Berl) 141(1):30–36, 1999 9952062

Mullins ME, Fitzmaurice SC: Lack of efficacy of benzodiazepines in treating gamma-hydroxybutyrate withdrawal. J Emerg Med 20(4):418–420, 2001 11396429

Murrough JW: Ketamine as a novel antidepressant: from synapse to behavior. Clin Pharmacol Ther 91(2):303–309, 2012 22205190

Mycyk MB, Wilemon C, Aks SE: Two cases of withdrawal from 1,4-butanediol use. Ann Emerg Med 38(3):345–346, 2001 11524661

National Institute on Drug Abuse: Inhalant Abuse (DHHS Publ No 000-3818). Rockville, MD, National Institute of Health, 2000

National Institute on Drug Abuse: Percentage of adolescents reporting drug use decreased significantly in 2021 as the COVID-19 pandemic endured. Bethesda, MD, National Institutes of Health, 2021. Available at: https://www.NIH.gov/news-events/news-releases/percentage-of-adolescents-reporting-drug-use-decreased-significantly-in-2021-as-the-covid-19-pandemic-endured. Accessed June 6, 2025.

Nelson T, Kaufman E, Kline J, et al: The extraneural distribution of gamma-hydroxybutyrate. J Neurochem 37(5):1345–1348, 1981 7299403

Nguyen J, O'Brien C, Schapp S: Adolescent inhalant use prevention, assessment, and treatment: a literature synthesis. Int J Drug Policy 31:15–24, 2016 26969125

Nichols DE: Differences between the mechanism of action of MDMA, MBDB, and the classic hallucinogens. Identification of a new therapeutic class: entactogens. J Psychoactive Drugs 18(4):305–313, 1986 2880944

Nicholson KL, Balster RL: GHB: a new and novel drug of abuse. Drug Alcohol Depend 63(1):1–22, 2001 11297827

Nimmerrichter AA, Walter H, Gutierrez-Lobos KE, et al: Double-blind controlled trial of gamma-hydroxybutyrate and clomethiazole in the treatment of alcohol withdrawal. Alcohol Alcohol 37(1):67–73, 2002 11825860

Nonnemaker JM, Crankshaw EC, Shive DR, et al: Inhalant use initiation among U.S. adolescents: evidence from the National Survey of Parents and Youth using discrete-time survival analysis. Addict Behav 36(8):878–881, 2011 21481544

Nozaki M, Vaupel DB, Martin WR: A pharmacologic comparison of 3,4-methylenedioxyamphetamine and LSD in the chronic spinal dog. Eur J Pharmacol 46(4):339–349, 1977 590343

Oehen P, Traber R, Widmer V, et al: A randomized, controlled pilot study of MDMA (±3,4-methylenedioxymethamphetamine)-assisted psychotherapy for treatment of resistant, chronic post-traumatic stress disorder (PTSD). J Psychopharmacol 27(1):40–52, 2013 23118021

Olivera AA, Kiefer MW, Manley NK: Tardive dyskinesia in psychiatric patients with substance use disorders. Am J Drug Alcohol Abuse 16(1–2):57–66, 1990 1970451

Palamar JJ, Rutherford C, Keyes KM: Trends in ketamine use, exposures, and seizures in the United States up to 2019. Am J Public Health 111(11):2046–2049, 2021 34618543

Palatini P, Tedeschi L, Frison G, et al: Dose-dependent absorption and elimination of gamma-hydroxybutyric acid in healthy volunteers. Eur J Clin Pharmacol 45(4):353–356, 1993 8299669

Park JN, Rashidi E, Foti K, et al: Fentanyl and fentanyl analogs in the illicit stimulant supply: results from U.S. drug seizure data, 2011–2016. Drug Alcohol Depend 218:108416, 2021 33278761

Parrott AC, Lasky J: Ecstasy (MDMA) effects upon mood and cognition: before, during and after a Saturday night dance. Psychopharmacology (Berl) 139(3):261–268, 1998 9784083

Pedersen W, Skrondal A: Ecstasy and new patterns of drug use: a normal population study. Addiction 94(11):1695–1706, 1999 10892008

Perron BE, Glass JE, Ahmedani BK, et al: The prevalence and clinical significance of inhalant withdrawal symptoms among a national sample. Subst Abuse Rehabil 2011(2):69–76, 2011 21709745

Regan A, Margolis S, de Wit H, et al: Does ±3,4-methylenedioxymethamphetamine (ecstasy) induce subjective feelings of social connection in humans? A multilevel meta-analysis. PLoS One 16(10):e0258849, 2021 34695117

Reich DL, Silvay G: Ketamine: an update on the first twenty-five years of clinical experience. Can J Anaesth 36(2):186–197, 1989 2650898

Ricaurte GA, Forno LS, Wilson MA, et al: (+/-)3,4-Methylenedioxymethamphetamine selectively damages central serotonergic neurons in nonhuman primates. JAMA 260(1):51–55, 1988 2454332

Ricaurte GA, Yuan J, McCann UD: (+/-)3,4-Methylenedioxymethamphetamine ("Ecstasy")-induced serotonin neurotoxicity: studies in animals. Neuropsychobiology 42(1):5–10, 2000 10867550

Rivera-García MT, López-Rubalcava C, Cruz SL: Preclinical characterization of toluene as a non-classical hallucinogen drug in rats: participation of 5-HT, dopamine and glutamate systems. Psychopharmacology (Berl) 232(20):3797–3808, 2015 26255180

Rodgers J: Cognitive performance amongst recreational users of "ecstasy." Psychopharmacology (Berl) 151(1):19–24, 2000 10958112

Rogers G, Elston J, Garside R, et al: The harmful health effects of recreational ecstasy: a systematic review of observational evidence. Health Technol Assess 13(6):iii–iv, ix–xii, 2009

Romanelli F, Smith KM, Thornton AC, et al: Poppers: epidemiology and clinical management of inhaled nitrite abuse. Pharmacotherapy 24(1):69–78, 2004 14740789

Ross TM: Gamma hydroxybutyrate overdose: two cases illustrate the unique aspects of this dangerous recreational drug. J Emerg Nurs 21(5):374–376, 1995 7500561

Roth RH, Giarman NJ: Gamma-butyrolactone and gamma-hydroxybutyric acid, I: distribution and metabolism. Biochem Pharmacol 15:1333–1348, 1966

Roth RH, Giarman NJ: Evidence that central nervous system depression by 1,4-butanediol is mediated through a metabolite, gamma-hydroxybutyrate. Biochem Pharmacol 17(5):735–739, 1968 5649891

Rudnick G, Wall SC: The molecular mechanism of "ecstasy" [3,4-methylenedioxymethamphetamine (MDMA)]: serotonin transporters are targets for MDMA-induced serotonin release. Proc Natl Acad Sci U S A 89(5):1817–1821, 1992 1347426

Scharf MB, Lai AA, Branigan B, et al: Pharmacokinetics of gammahydroxybutyrate (GHB) in narcoleptic patients. Sleep 21(5):507–514, 1998 9703591

Schouw ML, Gevers S, Caan MW, et al: Mapping serotonergic dysfunction in MDMA (ecstasy) users using pharmacological MRI. Eur Neuropsychopharmacol 22(8):537–545, 2012 22209360

Schwartz RH, Miller NS: MDMA (Ecstasy) and the rave: a review. Pediatrics 100(4):705–708, 1997 9310529

Scrima L, Hartman PG, Johnson FH Jr, et al: The effects of gamma-hydroxybutyrate on the sleep of narcolepsy patients: a double-blind study. Sleep 13(6):479–490, 1990 2281247

Sériès F, Sériès I, Cormier Y: Effects of enhancing slow-wave sleep by gamma-hydroxybutyrate on obstructive sleep apnea. Am Rev Respir Dis 145(6):1378–1383, 1992 1596007

Shannon M: Methylenedioxymethamphetamine (MDMA, "Ecstasy"). Pediatr Emerg Care 16(5):377–380, 2000 11063374

Sharma AN, Lombardi MH, Illuzzi FA, et al: Management of gamma-hydroxybutyrate withdrawal. Ann Emerg Med 38(5):605–607, 2001 11679881

Sherlock K, Wolff K, Hay AW, et al: Analysis of illicit ecstasy tablets: implications for clinical management in the accident and emergency department. J Accid Emerg Med 16(3):194–197, 1999 10353046

Sivilotti ML, Burns MJ, Aaron CK, et al: Pentobarbital for severe gamma-butyrolactone withdrawal. Ann Emerg Med 38(6):660–665, 2001 11719746

Snead OC III, Furner R, Liu CC: In vivo conversion of gamma-aminobutyric acid and 1,4-butanediol to gamma-hydroxybutyric acid in rat brain: studies using stable isotopes. Biochem Pharmacol 38(24):4375–4380, 1989 2604740

Solhkhah R, Wilens TE: Pharmacotherapy of adolescent alcohol and other drug use disorders. Alcohol Health Res World 22(2):122–125, 1998 15706786

Solhkhah R, Finkel J, Hird S: Possible risperidone-induced visual hallucinations. J Am Acad Child Adolesc Psychiatry 39(9):1074–1075, 2000 10986801

Solhkhah R, Wilens TE, Prince JB, et al: Bupropion sustained release for substance abuse, ADHD, and mood disorders in adolescents (NR31), in New Research Abstracts of the 154th Annual Meeting of the American Psychiatric Association, New Orleans, LA, May 7, 2001. Washington, DC, American Psychiatric Association, 2001

Sprague JE, Everman SL, Nichols DE: An integrated hypothesis for the serotonergic axonal loss induced by 3,4-methylenedioxymethamphetamine. Neurotoxicology 19(3):427–441, 1998 9621349

Staud R: Sodium oxybate for the treatment of fibromyalgia. Expert Opin Pharmacother 12(11):1789–1798, 2011 21679091

Stein DJ, Rink J: Effects of "Ecstasy" blocked by serotonin reuptake inhibitors. J Clin Psychiatry 60(7):485, 1999 10453804

Stone JM, Dietrich C, Edden R, et al: Ketamine effects on brain GABA and glutamate levels with 1H-MRS: relationship to ketamine-induced psychopathology. Mol Psychiatry 17(7):664–665, 2012 22212598

Storck M, Black L, Liddell M: Inhalant abuse and dextromethorphan. Child Adolesc Psychiatr Clin N Am 25(3):497–508, 2016 27338970

Substance Abuse and Mental Health Services Administration: Drug Abuse Warning Network, 2011: National Estimates of Drug-Related Emergency Department Visits (HHS Publ No SMA-13-4760, DAWN Series D-39). Rockville, MD, Substance Abuse and Mental Health Services Administration, 2013. Available at: https://www.samhsa.gov/data/sites/default/files/DAWN2k11ED/DAWN2k11ED/DAWN2k11ED.pdf. Accessed February 10, 2025.

Taffe MA: Δ9-Tetrahydrocannabinol attenuates MDMA-induced hyperthermia in rhesus monkeys. Neuroscience 201:125–133, 2012 22138434

Takahara J, Yunoki S, Yakushiji W, et al: Stimulatory effects of gamma-hydroxybutyric acid on growth hormone and prolactin release in humans. J Clin Endocrinol Metab 44(5):1014–1017, 1977 858775

Tedesco S, Gajaram G, Chida S, et al: The efficacy of MDMA (3,4-methylenedioxymethamphetamine) for post-traumatic stress disorder in humans: a systematic review and meta-analysis. Cureus 13(5):e15070, 2021

Tenenbein M, deGroot W, Rajani KR: Peripheral neuropathy following intentional inhalation of naphtha fumes. Can Med Assoc J 131(9):1077–1079, 1984 6093978

Tucker GT, Lennard MS, Ellis SW, et al: The demethylenation of methylenedioxymethamphetamine ("ecstasy") by debrisoquine hydroxylase (CYP2D6). Biochem Pharmacol 47(7):1151–1156, 1994 7909223

van den Brink W, Addolorato G, Aubin HJ, et al: Efficacy and safety of sodium oxybate in alcohol-dependent patients with a very high drinking risk level. Addict Biol 23(4):969–986, 2018 30043457

Venâncio C, Magalhães A, Antunes L, et al: Impaired spatial memory after ketamine administration in chronic low doses. Curr Neuropharmacol 9(1):251–255, 2011 21886600

Verkes RJ, Gijsman HJ, Pieters MS, et al: Cognitive performance and serotonergic function in users of ecstasy. Psychopharmacology (Berl) 153(2):196–202, 2001 11205419

Vural M, Ogel K: Dilated cardiomyopathy associated with toluene abuse. Cardiology 105(3):158–161, 2006 16479101

Walsh Z, Mollaahmetoglu OM, Rootman J, et al: Ketamine for the treatment of mental health and substance use disorders: comprehensive systematic review. BJPsych Open 8(1):e19, 2021 35048815

Watson J, Guzzetti S, Franchi C, et al: Gamma-hydroxybutyrate does not maintain self-administration but induces conditioned place preference when injected in the ventral tegmental area. Int J Neuropsychopharmacol 13(2):143–153, 2010 19573264

Weiner AL, Vieira L, McKay CA, et al: Ketamine abusers presenting to the emergency department: a case series. J Emerg Med 18(4):447–451, 2000 10802423

Weir E: Raves: a review of the culture, the drugs and the prevention of harm. CMAJ 162(13):1843–1848, 2000 10906922

White PF, Way WL, Trevor AJ: Ketamine: its pharmacology and therapeutic uses. Anesthesiology 56(2):119–136, 1982 6892475

Williams H, Dratcu L, Taylor R, et al: "Saturday night fever": ecstasy related problems in a London accident and emergency department. J Accid Emerg Med 15(5):322–326, 1998 9785160

Winstock AR, Mitcheson L: New recreational drugs and the primary care approach to patients who use them. BMJ 344:e288, 2012 22337751

Winters WD, Kott KS: Continuum of sedation, activation and hypnosis or hallucinosis: a comparison of low dose effects of pentobarbital, diazepam or gamma-hydroxybutyrate in the cat. Neuropharmacology 18(11):877–884, 1979 575917

Wolf CJH, Beurmanjer H, Dijkstra BAG, et al: Characterization of the GHB withdrawal syndrome. J Clin Med 10(11):2333, 2021 34073640

Wu LT, Pilowsky DJ, Schlenger WE: Inhalant abuse and dependence among adolescents in the United States. J Am Acad Child Adolesc Psychiatry 43(10):1206–1214, 2004 15381887

Zvosec DL, Smith SW, McCutcheon JR, et al: Adverse events, including death, associated with the use of 1,4-butanediol. N Engl J Med 344(2):87–94, 2001 11150358

10

Behavioral Addictions

Luis C. Farhat, M.D., Ph.D.
Marc N. Potenza, M.D., Ph.D.

Gambling disorder (GD) and internet gaming disorder (IGD) are behavioral addictions formally recognized by such entities as DSM-5 (American Psychiatric Association 2022) and ICD-11 (World Health Organization 2019). Both conditions have been associated with negative functional, general health, and psychiatric outcomes. Therefore, proper treatment of these conditions is an important topic for mental health practitioners and researchers, especially those specializing in addictions.

In this chapter, we provide an overview of the pharmacological agents that have been evaluated against placebo for the treatment of GD and IGD in randomized controlled trials (RCTs). Tables 10.1 and 10.2 summarize findings of RCTs for GD and IGD, respectively, and describe important study-level characteristics, such as sources of sponsorship, numbers of

Table 10.1 Randomized controlled trials of pharmacological agents against placebo for the treatment of gambling disorder

Agent, reference	N	Country	Sponsorship	Study design	Sex (% male)	Mean age (SD)(y)	Dosage (mg/d)[a]	Duration (wk)	Outcome assessment tool
Antidepressants									
Hollander et al. 2000	15	U.S.	Industry	Crossover	100	38.9 (10.3)	Fluvoxamine 250	8	PG-CGI-I; PG-YBOCS
Blanco et al. 2002	32	Spain	Industry	Parallel	65.63	42.1 (11.7)	Fluvoxamine 200	24	Expenditure; frequency
Kim et al. 2002	45	U.S.	Industry	Parallel	33.33	49.3 (10.3)	Paroxetine 60	8	G-SAS; PG-CGI
Grant et al. 2003	76	U.S. and Spain	Industry	Parallel	60.52	45.4 (10.6)	Paroxetine 60	16	PG-CGI-I; PG-YBOCS; G-SAS; PGI-CGI-S

Table 10.1 Randomized controlled trials of pharmacological agents against placebo for the treatment of gambling disorder *(continued)*

Agent, reference	N	Country	Sponsorship	Study design	Sex (% male)	Mean age (SD)(y)	Dosage (mg/d)[a]	Duration (wk)	Outcome assessment tool
Grant et al. 2006	13	U.S.	Industry	Parallel	53.8	55.8 (8.1)	Escitalopram 30	8	PG-YBOCS; PG-CGI-I; G-SAS
Saiz-Ruiz et al. 2005	66	Spain	Industry	Parallel	90	38.9 (11.6)	Sertraline 150	24	CCPGQ; PG-CGI-I
Hollander et al. 1992	1	U.S.	NR	Crossover	0	31	Clomipramine 150	10	CGI-I; self-reported improvement
Black et al. 2007	39	U.S.	NIMH	Parallel	71.72	43.2 (18.8)	Bupropion 375	12	PG-YBOCS; G-SAS; PG-CGI-I; PG-CGI-S

Table 10.1 Randomized controlled trials of pharmacological agents against placebo for the treatment of gambling disorder *(continued)*

Agent, reference	N	Country	Sponsorship	Study design	Sex (% male)	Mean age (SD)(y)	Dosage (mg/d)[a]	Duration (wk)	Outcome assessment tool
Opioid receptor antagonists									
Kim et al. 2001	45	U.S.	National Center for Responsible Gambling	Parallel	35.55	48.6 (9.6)	Naltrexone 250	11	PG-CGI-I; G-SAS
Grant et al. 2008	77	U.S.	NIMH	Parallel	38.96	47.0 (9.7)	Naltrexone 50, 100, or 250	18	PG-YBOCS; G-SAS; PG-CGI-S
Toneatto et al. 2009	52	Canada	Ontario Problem Gambling Research Centre	Parallel	93	40 (NR)	Naltrexone 250	10	Gambling episodes; expenditure

Table 10.1 Randomized controlled trials of pharmacological agents against placebo for the treatment of gambling disorder *(continued)*

Agent, reference	N	Country	Sponsorship	Study design	Sex (% male)	Mean age (SD)(y)	Dosage (mg/d)[a]	Duration (wk)	Outcome assessment tool
Kovanen et al. 2016	101	Finland	National Institute for Health and Welfare	Parallel	68.3	45.9 (15.2)	Naltrexone 50	20	PG-YBOCS; expenditure; episodes
Grant et al. 2006	207	U.S.	Industry	Parallel	56.5	45.9 (11.4)	Nalmefene 25, 50, or 100	16	PG-YBOCS; G-SAS; PG-CGI
Grant et al. 2010a	233	U.S.	Industry	Parallel	58.4	46.5 (12.0)	Nalmefene 20 or 40	10	PG-YBOCS; PG-CGI
Glutamate modulators									
Grant et al. 2007	27	U.S.	NIMH	Parallel	55.6	50.8 (12.1)	NAC 1,800	6	PG-YBOCS; G-SAS
Grant et al. 2014	28	U.S.	NIMH	Parallel	82.1	47.6 (10.9)	NAC 3,000	24	PG-YBOCS

Table 10.1 Randomized controlled trials of pharmacological agents against placebo for the treatment of gambling disorder *(continued)*

Agent, reference	N	Country	Sponsorship	Study design	Sex (% male)	Mean age (SD)(y)	Dosage (mg/d)[a]	Duration (wk)	Outcome assessment tool
Mood stabilizers and anticonvulsants									
Hollander et al. 2005	40	U.S.	NIMH	Parallel	58	44.5 (8.9)	Lithium 0.6–1.2 mEq/L	10	PG-YBOCS; PG-CGI-I
Berlin et al. 2013	42	U.S.	Industry	Parallel	45.2	47.5 (9.6)	Topiramate 300	14	PG-YBOCS; G-SAS/ PG-CGI-I
de Brito et al. 2017	38	Brazil	NR	Parallel	53.3	48.2 (11)	Topiramate 300	12	G-SAS; PG-YBOCS

Table 10.1 Randomized controlled trials of pharmacological agents against placebo for the treatment of gambling disorder *(continued)*

Agent, reference	N	Country	Sponsorship	Study design	Sex (% male)	Mean age (SD)(y)	Dosage (mg/d)[a]	Duration (wk)	Outcome assessment tool
Atypical antipsychotics									
McElroy et al. 2008	42	U.S.	Industry	Parallel	57.1	49.2 (10)	Olanzapine 15	12	PG-YBOCS; PG-CGI-S
Fong et al. 2008	23	U.S.	NIMH	Parallel	52	44.9 (10.5)	Olanzapine 10	7	Expenditure; frequency

Note. CCPGQ = Criteria for Control of Pathological Gambling Questionnaire; G-SAS = Gambling Symptom Assessment Scale; NAC = *N*-acetylcysteine; NIMH = National Institute of Mental Health; NR = not reported; PG-CGI = Pathological Gambling Clinical Global Impressions; PG-CGI-I = Pathological Gambling Clinical Global Impressions—Improvement; PG-CGI-S = Pathological Gambling Clinical Global Impressions—Severity; PG-YBOCS = Yale Brown Obsessive Compulsive Scale adapted for Pathological Gambling.
[a]Typically maximal. Also see the section "Psychopharmacology" for more details regarding dosing.

Table 10.2 Randomized controlled trials of pharmacological agents against placebo for the treatment of internet gaming disorder

Characteristic	Han and Renshaw 2012	Song et al. 2016
Country	South Korea	South Korea
Sponsorship	Korea Research Foundation	Korean Mental Health Technology
Study design	Parallel	Parallel
N	57	122
Sex (% male)	100	100
Age (y), mean (SD)	20.16 (7.2)	19.81 (3.9)
Medication dosage (typically maximal)[a]	Bupropion 300 mg/d	Bupropion 300 mg/d or escitalopram 20 mg/d
Duration (wk)	8	6
Outcome assessment tool	Young Internet Addiction Scale	Young Internet Addiction Scale

[a]See the section "Psychopharmacology" for more details regarding dosing.

participants randomized, participant mean (SD) ages, percentages of male subjects, maximum dosages allowed (in milligrams per day), durations of intervention (in weeks), and main outcomes evaluated. For both GD and IGD, we provide a critical summary of the available literature, highlighting limitations and providing guidance that may be particularly useful for routine practice.

We argue here that the treatment literature for both conditions is scant and has considerable limitations that hamper our ability to draw definitive conclusions from the data. Nonetheless, we note that some medications, such as naltrexone and bupropion, may be efficacious for GD and IGD, respectively, and additional studies should be performed to clarify their roles in the treatment of these conditions. We also highlight that targeting comorbid symptomatology, such as depression, anxiety, ADHD, and substance-related addictions, may be informative in the pharmacological management of GD and IGD and should be further evaluated by studies in the field.

The umbrella term *behavioral addictions* has been used to describe patterns of engagement with short-term rewarding behaviors other than psychoactive substance intake; examples include gambling, gaming, internet use, sex, shopping, and eating, although in the last case, debate exists as to whether the term *food addiction* or *eating addiction* is more appropriate (Lacroix et al. 2018; Schulte et al. 2018). These behaviors or conditions are characterized by core elements of addiction, including poor control, sustained engagement despite adverse consequences, and cravings or urges before engagement (Grant et al. 2010b; Petry et al. 2018). Although clinicians have recognized the negative personal, social, academic, occupational, physical, and mental health consequences of excessive engagement with these behaviors over decades (Potenza 2017), classificatory manuals such as DSM-5 (American Psychiatric Association 2022) and ICD-11 have only recently recognized the existence of novel or previously described disorders as *behavioral addictions* in their official classification of diagnoses. More specifically, GD (previously known as *pathological gambling*) and IGD (also termed *gaming disorder* in ICD-11) were the two conditions formally recognized by DSM-5 as non-substance-related or behavioral addictions and by ICD-11 as disorders due to addictive behaviors.

GD and IGD define persistent, recurrent patterns of gambling and gaming, respectively, that are associated with substantial distress, impairment, or both (Potenza et al. 2019; Saunders et al. 2017). We encourage readers to refer to DSM-5 or DSM-5-TR for a detailed description of the diagnostic criteria for GD and research criteria for IGD. Both GD and IGD have been associated with multiple negative functional, general health, and psychiatric outcomes, such as interpersonal/familial problems (Dowling et al. 2009; Hodgins et al. 2007; Kalischuk et al. 2006; Teng et al. 2020), financial concerns (Carey et al. 2022; Grant and Kim 2001), physical/somatic health problems (e.g., hypertension, obesity, sedentarism) (Black et al. 2013; Männikkö et al. 2015; Morasco et al. 2006), and other psychiatric conditions, including depressive/anxiety disorders, ADHD, and substance use disorders (Cowlishaw and Hakes 2015; Cowlishaw et al. 2016; Desai et al. 2010; Gentile et al. 2011; Pilver et al. 2013; Van Rooij et al. 2011, 2014).

Gambling Disorder

Neurobiology

The neurobiology of GD is complex and a subject of ongoing studies. Several neurotransmitters and hormones have been studied as candidates in the pathophysiology of GD, with some having implications for treatment development for GD. In this section, we review several neurotransmitters, including serotonin, dopamine, endorphins/opioids, and glutamate.

Serotonin (5-hydroxytryptamine), a neurotransmitter derived from the amino acid tryptophan, has been implicated in the pathophysiology of GD. Low levels of metabolites of serotonin and peripheral markers of serotonin have been found in the cerebrospinal fluid and serum samples, respectively, of individuals with GD (Nordin and Eklundh 1999). Additionally, individuals with GD reported feeling euphoric when administered *meta*-chlorophenyl piperazine, a partial agonist of serotonin receptors, whereas individuals without GD reported experiencing unpleasant sensations (Pallanti et al. 2006). The potential role of serotonin in the pathophysiology of GD was a basis for multiple RCTs evaluating the effects of serotonin reuptake inhibitors in the treatment of GD.

Dopamine is a catecholamine neurotransmitter derived from the amino acid tyrosine. Dopaminergic brain pathways, such as the mesolimbic pathway, have been implicated in rewarding and reinforcing behaviors (Everitt and Robbins 2005). However, currently available findings are relatively mixed regarding the involvement of dopamine in the pathophysiology of GD (Potenza 2018), and more research is required to clarify its role in GD (Potenza 2013). Clinical researchers have evaluated the effects of bupropion, a dopamine and norepinephrine reuptake inhibitor, against placebo in one RCT involving people with GD.

Opioid systems have also been implicated in the pathophysiology of GD: challenge studies with oral amphetamine showed a blunted opioid response in individuals with GD (Mick et al. 2016), a transdiagnostic finding that was also observed among individuals with other addictive behaviors, such as substance use disorders (Gorelick et al. 2005). The potential role of the opioid system in the pathophysiology of GD, in conjunction with the observation that other psychiatric conditions whose phenomenology was also marked by the presence of urges were successfully managed with opioid receptor antagonists, served as a basis for RCTs evaluating the effects of opioid receptor antagonists in the treatment of GD. Thus far, naltrexone has been the most widely studied medication in double-blind RCTs versus placebo for the treatment of GD, with some RCTs also evaluating other opioid receptor antagonists (e.g., nalmefene).

Glutamate is an amino acid and the principal excitatory neurotransmitter in the adult brain (Pittenger et al. 2011). Disruption of glutamatergic synapses (e.g., through certain knockout mice experiments) has implicated glutamate in learning and memory. Glutamate may also have a key role in repetitive behaviors including, but not limited to, addictive behaviors (Chambers et al. 2003; Kalivas and Volkow 2005). Among individuals with GD, cerebrospinal fluid levels of glutamic acid and aspartic acid have been found to be higher than those in nonaffected control subjects (Nordin et al. 2007). The glutamatergic agent N-acetylcysteine (NAC), a modulator of extrasynaptic glutamate, has also been studied for the treatment of GD in RCTs.

Psychopharmacology

Antidepressants

Two small RCTs have investigated fluvoxamine in the treatment of GD. In a crossover RCT, Hollander et al. (2000) evaluated the effects of fluvoxamine (mean [SD] dosage = 195 [50] mg/day) and showed that individuals taking the medication were more likely to experience global improvement compared with those taking placebo. However, in a second study by Blanco et al. (2002), there were no statistically significant differences between fluvoxamine (100 mg bid) and placebo in the gambling outcomes of the study at the end of treatment. There were also larger dropout rates in the fluvoxamine arm (seven subjects [47%]) compared with the placebo arm (four subjects [23%]), including dropout attributable to adverse events (three subjects [20%] vs. one subject [5%]).

One small RCT and one medium-sized RCT have been conducted to investigate the role of paroxetine in the treatment of GD. Kim et al. (2002) initially evaluated the effects of paroxetine (mean [SD] dosage = 51.7 [13.1] mg/day). Individuals taking paroxetine experienced greater reductions in problem-gambling symptoms and greater global improvement during treatment. However, in a larger, multicenter RCT by Grant et al. (2003), paroxetine (mean [SD] dosage = 50 [8.3] mg/day) did not differ significantly from placebo on any problem-gambling outcomes. Individuals in the paroxetine treatment arm were less likely to tolerate the medication and demonstrated higher dropout attributable to adverse events (16.7% vs. 2.5%).

Although there are no RCTs evaluating the acute effects of starting escitalopram against placebo for the treatment of GD, Grant and Potenza (2006) conducted a double-blind discontinuation study in which individuals with GD and clinically significant anxiety were started on escitalopram after a 1-week placebo lead-in phase. Individuals received a mean (SD) dosage of 25.4 (6.6) mg/day and experienced considerable reductions in problem-gambling severity and large global improvement. Of note, the improvement in problem-gambling symptoms occurred concurrently with improvement in anxiety. After a 3-month period, individuals who were considered responders were then randomly assigned to either continue the medication or switch to placebo. However, only six participants were deemed responders, and only four agreed to enter the discontinuation phase, limiting the data available from the double-blinded period.

Saiz-Ruiz et al. (2005) conducted an RCT evaluating the effects of sertraline (mean dosage = 95 mg/day) and showed that individuals taking either sertraline or placebo experienced considerable improvements at the end of treatment, with 74% and 72% response rates, respectively. There were no significant differences between sertraline and placebo.

Other Antidepressants

Hollander et al. (1992) conducted a trial in a 31-year-old woman with a 12-year history of GD. After a 10-week trial of clomipramine (125 mg/day), the woman reported larger and considerable self-reported improvement in problem-gambling behaviors versus when she was taking placebo for the same treatment duration. Clinical ratings of global improvement supported the greater self-reported improvement during treatment with clomipramine.

Black et al. (2007) evaluated the effects of bupropion (mean dosage = 324 mg/day) against placebo. At the end of treatment, subjects receiving either bupropion or placebo had experienced significant improvements, and active treatment did not separate from placebo in any problem-gambling outcomes. There was frequent discontinuation in both arms (56% in bupropion and 33% in placebo), including that due to adverse events.

Opioid Receptor Antagonists

In an initial report, Kim et al. (2001) conducted a parallel RCT to evaluate the effects of naltrexone (mean [SD] dosage = 187.50 [96.45] mg/day). The findings indicated that naltrexone was more effective than placebo in all problem-gambling outcome measures. In a second study, Grant et al. (2008) corroborated the initial findings from Kim et al. (2001) by conducting a fixed-dose study of naltrexone against placebo, in which participants were randomly assigned to receive naltrexone at three different dosages or placebo. The study failed to demonstrate a clear beneficial dose, because outcomes did not differ significantly between the three doses (50, 100, and 250 mg/day). However, subjects assigned to naltrexone had significantly greater reductions in problem-gambling symptoms and had greater global improvement and an increase in psychosocial functioning compared with individuals taking placebo.

However, two other RCTs did not support the efficacy of naltrexone treatment for GD. Toneatto et al. (2009) evaluated the effects of naltrexone in a sample of individuals whose symptoms met diagnostic criteria for both alcohol use disorder and GD. The investigators randomized participants to naltrexone (mean [SD] dosage = 100 [59.4] mg/day) or placebo as adjuvant treatment to cognitive-behavioral therapy for both gambling and alcohol use problems. At the end of the trial, participants had reduced alcohol use (frequency and quantity consumed) and gambling (frequency and expenditure) behaviors, but there were no significant differences between the groups who received active drug compared with placebo. Kovanen et al. (2016) conducted an RCT in which as-needed naltrexone (50 mg) was compared with placebo. Participants were instructed to take the medication when they intended to gamble, when they experienced a strong urge to gamble, or both. No dose adjustments were made throughout the study. At the end of the 20-week follow-up period, the naltrexone group did not differ from the placebo group on any of the problem-gambling outcomes.

Two large RCTs have evaluated the effects of nalmefene against placebo for the treatment of GD. Grant et al. (2006) conducted a multicenter RCT in the United States, in which participants were randomly assigned to placebo or fixed doses of nalmefene. The study demonstrated that nalmefene was efficacious in reducing gambling symptoms and promoting global improvement. There were no differences between the 25-mg/day dosage and the 50- or 100-mg/day dosages in the primary outcome of efficacy, and the 25-mg/day dosage was the only one that differentiated from placebo on global improvement. The lower dose also appeared to be more well tolerated, because the dropout rates attributable to side effects were smaller than those for the higher doses (36.4% for 25 mg/day, 45.9% for 50, and 56.8% for

100). However, in a second, confirmatory large study by Grant et al. (2010a) with similar fixed doses, active drug did not differ from placebo on any of the problem-gambling outcome measures unless analyses were restricted to individuals who had full titration of nalmefene for at least 1 week (73% of participants).

Glutamatergic Agents

To date, two small RCTs have evaluated the effects of NAC in the management of GD. Grant et al. (2007) initially performed a maintenance study with responders from an uncontrolled administration of NAC for 8 weeks (mean [SD] dosage = 1,476.9 [311.3] mg/day). There were 27 and 23 participants who started and completed the uncontrolled trial, respectively. Of these, 16 participants (59.3%) had symptom ratings that met the criteria of treatment response, and 13 of them were randomly assigned to either maintain NAC treatment or switch to placebo for the next 6 weeks. At the end of the 6-week maintenance trial, individuals who were randomly assigned to receive NAC had better problem-gambling outcomes than their counterparts who had been allocated to placebo.

Grant et al. (2014) conducted a parallel RCT in which participants with co-occurring tobacco use disorder and GD were randomly assigned to NAC or placebo in a 12-week augmentation trial of behavioral therapies targeting tobacco use and gambling. Imaginal desensitization, a relaxation-based technique in which individuals are oriented to visualize being exposed to gambling triggers and then leaving the situation in a state of continued relaxation, targeted GD symptoms. The Ask-Advise-Refer therapeutic approach targeted tobacco use. At the end of the 4-month follow-up, participants in the NAC group had better problem-gambling outcomes compared with individuals in the placebo group, and more rapid within-treatment response was noted for smoking cessation.

Mood Stabilizers

Given the success of lithium and valproate in impulse-control disorders in uncontrolled trials, Hollander et al. (2005) conducted a small RCT to investigate the efficacy of lithium for GD in participants with bipolar spectrum disorders (largely bipolar II disorder). The mean (SD) dosage and lithium levels at end point were 1,150 (215) mg/day and 0.87 (0.1) mEq/L, respectively. At the end of treatment, lithium was more efficacious than placebo in some problem-gambling outcomes (those assessed through rating scales but not functional outcomes, such as expenditure or frequency).

Other Mood-Stabilizing Agents

Following successful treatment studies of topiramate for other psychiatric conditions characterized by impulsivity, two RCTs have evaluated the effects of topiramate against placebo for the management of GD. Berlin et al. (2013) conducted a multicenter study in the United States, in which participants were randomly assigned to either topiramate (mean [SD] dosage = 222.5 [108.49] mg/day) or placebo. At the end of the 14-week follow-up period, individuals receiving topiramate had similar problem-gambling outcomes as those taking placebo. However, de Brito et al. (2017) administered topiramate (mean [SD] dosage = 180.7 [95.5] mg/day) combined with brief cognitive restructuring for GD, and they reported that individuals who received topiramate experienced greater reductions in gambling-related expenditures and gambling frequency.

Antipsychotic Agents

Two small RCTs have investigated the effects of olanzapine in the treatment of GD. McElroy et al. (2008) evaluated the effects of olanzapine (mean [SD] dosage = 8.9 [5.2] mg/day) and reported no differences between active and placebo groups on primary outcomes for efficacy. Individuals in the olanzapine (versus placebo) arm demonstrated greater discontinuation rates for any reason (52% vs. 29%) and because of adverse events (14.3% vs. 9.5%). In an independent study, Fong et al. (2008) also did not observe significant differences between olanzapine and placebo in problem-gambling outcomes.

Critical Summary and Clinical Perspectives

The literature regarding pharmacological treatments of GD is scant, findings are mixed, and there are limitations that create difficulties when attempting to draw definitive conclusions about the efficacy of any medication that has been evaluated in RCTs against placebo for GD. First, most RCTs have included a relatively small number of individuals, limiting the statistical power to detect significant differences, particularly for dichotomous outcomes (e.g., response rates). Second, few medications have been investigated in more than one RCT or in two similarly designed studies. For instance, although naltrexone was evaluated by four RCTs, two (Kovanen et al. 2016; Toneatto et al. 2009) involved considerably different interventions compared with the two previous studies (Grant et al. 2008; Kim et al. 2001), and the extent to which these differences are responsible for mixed findings regarding the efficacy of naltrexone is unclear. Third, some trials (Black et al. 2013; Grant et al. 2006; Hollander et al. 2000) had large discontinuation rates, which were often imbalanced between active and control conditions and related to adverse events. Because statistical methods that do not account for nonrandom patterns of missing data (e.g., completer, last-observation-carried-forward analyses) are common and have been used in some trials, some findings may show bias in favor of active treatments (Sterne et al. 2019). Fourth, most trials were sponsored by industry. Industry-sponsored trials are more likely to show statistically significant findings, such as with the addition of post hoc analyses and outcomes (Barber and Cipriani 2017). Therefore, findings of stated significance involving such analyses (e.g., Grant et al. 2010a; Kim et al. 2001) should be interpreted with caution, although several negative trials have been industry sponsored (Berlin et al. 2013; Grant et al. 2003, 2010a). Fifth, uncontrolled phases of RCTs (e.g., Grant and Potenza 2006; Grant et al. 2007) are important for dosing and safety considerations but provide limited evidence for efficacy when subjective outcomes such as gambling behaviors are evaluated, because one cannot account for regression to the mean of problem-gambling behaviors or placebo responses over the course of treatment, and caution is required regarding these findings. Indeed, a sizable number of trials have demonstrated considerable response rates in the placebo group (Black et al. 2007; Saiz-Ruiz et al. 2005). The issue of placebo response in GD RCTs has been raised previously (e.g., by Grant and Chamberlain 2017) and deserves more attention, because it may be one factor underlying negative findings of pharmacological treatments in double-blind RCTs for GD. Finally, N-of-1 studies (e.g., Hollander et al. 1992), in which the medication is tested in just one individual, are particularly limited, and caution is required when extrapolating these findings to other individuals.

The limitations of existing studies highlight the need for more, and better, RCTs for GD in the future. Regardless, practitioners are currently faced with patients who require assistance and may still desire some practical guidance regarding the pharmacological treatment of GD. Bullock and Potenza (2012) provided an empirically informed algorithm that may be helpful for these practitioners, and we encourage readers to refer to their work for additional details. Briefly, because some pharmacotherapy trials have selected patients based on patterns of co-occurring disorders (e.g., anxiety, substance use disorders), pharmacotherapy recommendations stemming from the presence or absence of specific disorders may be generated. Importantly, in some of the RCTs discussed in this chapter, improvements in problem-gambling symptoms occurred concurrently with the improvement in comorbid symptomatology (e.g., anxiety, mood, or substance use improvement), suggesting that targeting co-occurring symptomatology could be a valid therapeutic strategy for the management of GD. This approach of employing pharmacological interventions based on co-occurring disorders is likely to resonate with prescribing physicians trained to evaluate patients systematically for the presence or absence of specific disorders, and hence it may be particularly useful. Analysis of data across trials has provided additional clinical insights. For example, the pharmacotherapy treatment algorithm from Bullock and Potenza (2012) incorporated information from an analysis of two studies suggesting that better response to opioid receptor antagonists was associated with a family history of alcoholism and strong gambling urges at treatment onset (Grant et al. 2008). Additionally, the algorithm considered the willingness of individuals with GD to take a medication and offered over-the-counter dietary supplements (e.g., NAC) for people less willing to take medications. Furthermore, the algorithm has been updated to include behavioral therapies (Potenza et al. 2019), because behavioral therapies are often the mainstay of treatment for GD.

Internet Gaming Disorder

Neurobiology

Research on IGD (or gaming disorder in ICD-11) is still in early stages, and multiple aspects need to be examined. Most studies of the neurobiology of IGD have focused on brain structures or circuits, in line with the National Institute of Mental Health Research Domain Criteria initiative. For an in-depth review, see Kuss et al. (2018). Briefly, studies seem to support that individuals with IGD have prefrontal cortical differences that may be associated with impairments in response inhibition, emotion regulation, working memory, and decision-making. Individuals with IGD may also differ in subcortical structure and function—for example, with respect to reward processing. Therefore, currently available studies support the role of dual-process models (i.e., reward and control systems) in IGD, which is similar to what has been found in individuals with GD and substance-related addictions. It is hoped that these neurobiological findings will contribute to treatment development in IGD, particularly with respect to neuromodulation.

Psychopharmacology

To date, bupropion and escitalopram have been the only medications evaluated in placebo-controlled RCTs for IGD. Han and Renshaw (2012) evaluated the effects of bupropion in a sample of individuals with major depressive disorder (MDD) and co-occurring problematic internet gaming, defined as 1) more than 4 hours/day or 30 hours/week of internet game play; 2) a score greater than 50 on the Young Internet Addiction Scale (Young 1998); and 3) impaired behaviors or distress attributable to gaming behavior. Participants in both treatment arms were administered weekly sessions of psychoeducation about internet use. At the end of treatment, bupropion versus placebo was associated with significantly greater reductions in problem-gaming severity, and these changes in gaming behavior occurred in parallel with reductions in depressive symptoms. Song et al. (2016) evaluated effects of bupropion (mean [SD] dosage = 159.3 [48.5] mg/day) and escitalopram (mean [SD] dosage = 15.6 [6.1] mg/day) in individuals with symptoms meeting DSM-5 diagnostic criteria for IGD. Both escitalopram and bupropion were able to separate from placebo at the treatment end point. However, the study's findings are of limited value because the participants were not blinded to treatment, and internet gaming symptoms represent a subjective outcome that could be influenced by lack of blinding.

Other medications have been evaluated for the treatment of problematic internet gaming behavior in head-to-head trials. For instance, Park et al. (2016) compared methylphenidate and atomoxetine for individuals with ADHD and problematic internet gaming behavior, whereas Nam et al. (2017) compared bupropion and escitalopram for individuals with MDD and problematic internet gaming behaviors. In each trial, the two medications were associated with improvements in IGD symptoms. Nevertheless, the utility of head-to-head comparisons without a placebo at this stage of IGD research (i.e., without clear effective mediations) is unclear.

Clinical Perspective

Research in IGD is in its early stages, and additional clinical trials are needed. To date, available evidence in favor of a specific medication is almost nonexistent. For instance, considering bupropion, only one double-blind RCT has been conducted to date. Besides, some studies suggest that targeting co-occurring disorders (e.g., ADHD, MDD) may be an effective therapeutic strategy, but this specific question has yet to be fully answered by empirical research. Therefore, additional RCTs are needed to properly help guide practitioners treating individuals with IGD.

Key Points

- The term *behavioral addiction* refers to an emerging clinical concept that encompasses a group of pathological behaviors, such as gambling disorder (GD) and internet gaming disorder (IGD), that do not necessarily involve the consumption of a substance. Although GD and IGD are currently the most researched, behavioral addictions may also include such activities as internet use, sex, and shopping.
- The neurobiological etiology of GD is not certain, but endogenous serotonin, glutamate, and opioid neurotransmission have all been implicated.
- Research on pharmacotherapies for GD are scant and methodologically limited. Trials that have been conducted using antidepressant, opioid antagonist, and glutamatergic medications for GD have yielded largely mixed outcomes, which, when combined with the wide methodological variability, limit the generalizability of these results.
- IGD research is still in the early stages, with studies suggesting that reward and control system pathologies may contribute to the development of IGD.
- To date, randomized controlled trials of only bupropion and escitalopram have been undertaken in the treatment of IGD, with outcomes suggesting potential benefit, but methodological considerations limit the generalizability of these studies.
- Studies on both GD and IGD suggest that targeting of co-occurring psychiatric disorders may provide collateral benefit for GD and IGD

behaviors, thus providing a possible clinical decision pathway for clinicians in the absence of a robust treatment evidence base.

References

American Psychiatric Association: Diagnostic and Statistical Manual of Mental Disorders, 5th Edition. Arlington, VA, American Psychiatric Association, 2013

American Psychiatric Association: Diagnostic and Statistical Manual of Mental Disorders, 5th Edition, Text Revision. Washington, DC, American Psychiatric Association, 2022

Barber S, Cipriani A: Lessons learned from Restoring Study 329: transparent reporting, open databases and network meta-analyses as the way forward. Aust N Z J Psychiatry 51(4):407–409, 2017 27864343

Berlin HA, Braun A, Simeon D, et al: A double-blind, placebo-controlled trial of topiramate for pathological gambling. World J Biol Psychiatry 14(2):121–128, 2013 21486110

Black DW, Arndt S, Coryell WH, et al: Bupropion in the treatment of pathological gambling: a randomized, double-blind, placebo-controlled, flexible-dose study. J Clin Psychopharmacol 27(2):143–150, 2007 17414236

Black DW, Shaw M, McCormick B, et al: Pathological gambling: relationship to obesity, self-reported chronic medical conditions, poor lifestyle choices, and impaired quality of life. Compr Psychiatry 54(2):97–104, 2013 22938650

Blanco C, Petkova E, Ibáñez A, et al: A pilot placebo-controlled study of fluvoxamine for pathological gambling. Ann Clin Psychiatry 14(1):9–15, 2002 12046642

Bullock SA, Potenza MN: Pathological gambling: neuropsychopharmacology and treatment. Curr Psychopharmacol 1(1):67–85, 2012 24349964

Carey PAK, Delfabbro P, King D: An evaluation of gaming-related harms in relation to gaming disorder and loot box involvement. Int J Ment Health Addict 20(5):2906–2921, 2022 34121958

Chambers RA, Taylor JR, Potenza MN: Developmental neurocircuitry of motivation in adolescence: a critical period of addiction vulnerability. Am J Psychiatry 160(6):1041–1052, 2003 12777258

Cowlishaw S, Hakes JK: Pathological and problem gambling in substance use treatment: results from the National Epidemiologic Survey on Alcohol and Related Conditions (NESARC). Am J Addict 24(5):467–474, 2015 25950376

Cowlishaw S, Hakes JK, Dowling NA: Gambling problems in treatment for affective disorders: results from the National Epidemiologic Survey on Alcohol and Related Conditions (NESARC). J Affect Disord 202:110–114, 2016 27261840 de Brito AMC, de Almeida Pinto MG, Bronstein G, et al: Topiramate combined with cognitive restructuring for the treatment of gambling disorder: a two-center, randomized, double-blind clinical trial. J Gambl Stud 33(1):249–263, 2017 27256372

Desai RA, Krishnan-Sarin S, Cavallo D, et al: Video-gaming among high school students: health correlates, gender differences, and problematic gaming. Pediatrics 126(6):e1414–e1424, 2010 21078729

Dowling N, Smith D, Thomas T: The family functioning of female pathological gamblers. Int J Ment Health Addict 7:29–44, 2009

Everitt BJ, Robbins TW: Neural systems of reinforcement for drug addiction: from actions to habits to compulsion. Nat Neurosci 8(11):1481–1489, 2005 16251991

Fong T, Kalechstein A, Bernhard B, et al: A double-blind, placebo-controlled trial of olanzapine for the treatment of video poker pathological gamblers. Pharmacol Biochem Behav 89(3):298–303, 2008 18261787

Gentile DA, Choo H, Liau A, et al: Pathological video game use among youths: a two-year longitudinal study. Pediatrics 127(2):e319–e329, 2011 21242221

Gorelick DA, Kim YK, Bencherif B, et al: Imaging brain mu-opioid receptors in abstinent cocaine users: time course and relation to cocaine craving. Biol Psychiatry 57(12):1573–1582, 2005 15953495

Grant JE, Chamberlain SR: The placebo effect and its clinical associations in gambling disorder. Ann Clin Psychiatry 29(3):167–172, 2017 28738096

Grant JE, Kim SW: Demographic and clinical features of 131 adult pathological gamblers. J Clin Psychiatry 62(12):957–962, 2001 11780876

Grant JE, Potenza MN: Escitalopram treatment of pathological gambling with co-occurring anxiety: an open-label pilot study with double-blind discontinuation. Int Clin Psychopharmacol 21(4):203–209, 2006 16687991

Grant JE, Kim SW, Potenza MN, et al: Paroxetine treatment of pathological gambling: a multi-centre randomized controlled trial. Int Clin Psychopharmacol 18(4):243–249, 2003 12817159

Grant JE, Potenza MN, Hollander E, et al: Multicenter investigation of the opioid antagonist nalmefene in the treatment of pathological gambling. Am J Psychiatry 163(2):303–312, 2006 16449486

Grant JE, Kim SW, Odlaug BL: N-acetyl cysteine, a glutamate-modulating agent, in the treatment of pathological gambling: a pilot study. Biol Psychiatry 62(6):652–657, 2007 17445781

Grant JE, Kim SW, Hartman BK: A double-blind, placebo-controlled study of the opiate antagonist naltrexone in the treatment of pathological gambling urges. J Clin Psychiatry 69(5):783–789, 2008 18384246

Grant JE, Odlaug BL, Potenza MN, et al: Nalmefene in the treatment of pathological gambling: multicentre, double-blind, placebo-controlled study. Br J Psychiatry 197(4):330–331, 2010a 20884959

Grant JE, Potenza MN, Weinstein A, et al: Introduction to behavioral addictions. Am J Drug Alcohol Abuse 36(5):233–241, 2010b 20560821

Grant JE, Odlaug BL, Chamberlain SR, et al: A randomized, placebo-controlled trial of N-acetylcysteine plus imaginal desensitization for nicotine-dependent pathological gamblers. J Clin Psychiatry 75(1):39–45, 2014

Han DH, Renshaw PF: Bupropion in the treatment of problematic online game play in patients with major depressive disorder. J Psychopharmacol 26(5):689–696, 2012 21447539

Hodgins DC, Shead NW, Makarchuk K: Relationship satisfaction and psychological distress among concerned significant others of pathological gamblers. J Nerv Ment Dis 195(1):65–71, 2007 17220742

Hollander E, Frenkel M, Decaria C, et al: Treatment of pathological gambling with clomipramine. Am J Psychiatry 149(5):710–711, 1992 1575267

Hollander E, DeCaria CM, Finkell JN, et al: A randomized double-blind fluvoxamine/placebo crossover trial in pathologic gambling. Biol Psychiatry 47(9):813–817, 2000 10812040

Hollander E, Pallanti S, Allen A, et al: Does sustained-release lithium reduce impulsive gambling and affective instability versus placebo in pathological gamblers with bipolar spectrum disorders? Am J Psychiatry 162(1):137–145, 2005 15625212

Kalischuk RG, Nowatzki N, Cardwell K, et al: Problem gambling and its impact on families: a literature review. Int Gambl Stud 6:31–60, 2006

Kalivas PW, Volkow ND: The neural basis of addiction: a pathology of motivation and choice. Am J Psychiatry 162(8):1403–1413, 2005 16055761

Kim SW, Grant JE, Adson DE, et al: Double-blind naltrexone and placebo comparison study in the treatment of pathological gambling. Biol Psychiatry 49(11):914–921, 2001 11377409

Kim SW, Grant JE, Adson DE, et al: A double-blind placebo-controlled study of the efficacy and safety of paroxetine in the treatment of pathological gambling. J Clin Psychiatry 63(6):501–507, 2002 12088161

Kovanen L, Basnet S, Castrén S, et al: A randomised, double-blind, placebo-controlled trial of as-needed naltrexone in the treatment of pathological gambling. Eur Addict Res 22(2):70–79, 2016 26339899

Kuss DJ, Pontes HM, Griffiths MD: Neurobiological correlates in internet gaming disorder: a systematic literature review. Front Psychiatry 9:166, 2018 29867599

Lacroix E, Tavares H, von Ranson KM: Moving beyond the "eating addiction" versus "food addiction" debate: comment on Schulte et al. (2017). Appetite 130:286–292, 2018 29936021

Männikkö N, Billieux J, Kääriäinen M: Problematic digital gaming behavior and its relation to the psychological, social and physical health of Finnish adolescents and young adults. J Behav Addict 4(4):281–288, 2015 26690623

McElroy SL, Nelson EB, Welge JA, et al: Olanzapine in the treatment of pathological gambling: a negative randomized placebo-controlled trial. J Clin Psychiatry 69(3):433–440, 2008 18251624

Mick I, Myers J, Ramos AC, et al: Blunted endogenous opioid release following an oral amphetamine challenge in pathological gamblers. Neuropsychopharmacology 41(7):1742–1750, 2016 26552847

Morasco BJ, Pietrzak RH, Blanco C, et al: Health problems and medical utilization associated with gambling disorders: results from the National Epidemiologic Survey on Alcohol and Related Conditions. Psychosom Med 68(6):976–984, 2006 17132843

Nam B, Bae S, Kim SM, et al: Comparing the effects of bupropion and escitalopram on excessive internet game play in patients with major depressive disorder. Clin Psychopharmacol Neurosci 15(4):361–368, 2017 29073748

Nordin C, Eklundh T: Altered CSF 5-HIAA disposition in pathologic male gamblers. CNS Spectr 4(12):25–33, 1999 18311105

Nordin C, Gupta RC, Sjödin I: Cerebrospinal fluid amino acids in pathological gamblers and healthy controls. Neuropsychobiology 56(2–3):152–158, 2007 18259089

Pallanti S, Bernardi S, Quercioli L, et al: Serotonin dysfunction in pathological gamblers: increased prolactin response to oral m-CPP versus placebo. CNS Spectr 11(12):956–964, 2006 17146409

Park JH, Lee YS, Sohn JH, et al: Effectiveness of atomoxetine and methylphenidate for problematic online gaming in adolescents with attention deficit hyperactivity disorder. Hum Psychopharmacol 31(6):427–432, 2016 27859666

Petry NM, Zajac K, Ginley MK: Behavioral addictions as mental disorders: to be or not to be? Annu Rev Clin Psychol 14:399–423, 2018 29734827

Pilver CE, Libby DJ, Hoff RA, et al: Problem gambling severity and the incidence of Axis I psychopathology among older adults in the general population. J Psychiatr Res 47(4):534–541, 2013 23333039

Pittenger C, Bloch MH, Williams K: Glutamate abnormalities in obsessive compulsive disorder: neurobiology, pathophysiology, and treatment. Pharmacol Ther 132(3):314–332, 2011 21963369

Potenza MN: How central is dopamine to pathological gambling or gambling disorder? Front Behav Neurosci 7:206, 2013 24391562

Potenza MN: Clinical neuropsychiatric considerations regarding nonsubstance or behavioral addictions. Dialogues Clin Neurosci 19(3):281–291, 2017 29302225

Potenza MN: Searching for replicable dopamine-related findings in gambling disorder. Biol Psychiatry 83(12):984–986, 2018 29804589

Potenza MN, Balodis IM, Derevensky J, et al: Gambling disorder. Nat Rev Dis Primers 5(1):51, 2019 31346179

Saiz-Ruiz J, Blanco C, Ibáñez A, et al: Sertraline treatment of pathological gambling: a pilot study. J Clin Psychiatry 66(1):28–33, 2005 15669885

Saunders JB, Hao W, Long J, et al: Gaming disorder: its delineation as an important condition for diagnosis, management, and prevention. J Behav Addict 6(3):271–279, 2017 28816494

Schulte EM, Potenza MN, Gearhardt AN: Specific theoretical considerations and future research directions for evaluating addictive-like eating as a substance-based, food addiction: comment on Lacroix et al. (2018). Appetite 130:293–295, 2018 29935292

Song J, Park JH, Han DH, et al: Comparative study of the effects of bupropion and escitalopram on Internet gaming disorder. Psychiatry Clin Neurosci 70(11):527–535, 2016 27487975

Sterne JAC, Savović J, Page MJ, et al: RoB 2: a revised tool for assessing risk of bias in randomised trials. BMJ 366:l4898, 2019 31462531

Teng Z, Griffiths MD, Nie Q, et al: Parent-adolescent attachment and peer attachment associated with internet gaming disorder: a longitudinal study of first-year undergraduate students. J Behav Addict 9(1):116–128, 2020 32359235

Toneatto T, Brands B, Selby P: A randomized, double-blind, placebo-controlled trial of naltrexone in the treatment of concurrent alcohol use disorder and pathological gambling. Am J Addict 18(3):219–225, 2009 19340640

Van Rooij AJ, Schoenmakers TM, Vermulst AA, et al: Online video game addiction: identification of addicted adolescent gamers. Addiction 106(1):205–212, 2011 20840209

Van Rooij AJ, Kuss DJ, Griffiths MD, et al: The (co-)occurrence of problematic video gaming, substance use, and psychosocial problems in adolescents. J Behav Addict 3(3):157–165, 2014 25317339

World Health Organization: International Statistical Classification of Diseases and Related Health Problems, 11th Edition. Geneva, World Health Organization, 2019

Young KS: Internet addiction: the emergence of a new clinical disorder. Cyberpsychol Behav 1:237–244, 1998

11

Integrative Medicine Approaches to Addiction Treatment

Sita Yerramsetti, M.D., M.P.H.
Carla Marienfeld, M.D.
Jeffrey DeVido, M.D., M.T.S.

Complementary, alternative, and *integrative* are terms often used to describe a range of ever-evolving health care approaches that are not typically part of conventional medical care. Survey data revealed that the use of these approaches to medical care is common, with 38.3% of adults reporting use of some form of unconventional approach to their health care (Clarke et al. 2015). Unsurprisingly, complementary, alternative, and integrative approaches to health care are big business, with Americans spending between $27 and $34 billion annually on these services (Eisenberg et al.

1993; Nahin et al. 2009). Given the high prevalence of these nonmainstream approaches to health care, coupled with the significant largely unregulated consumer marketplace, the National Institutes of Health established the National Center for Complementary and Integrative Health (NCCIH) in 2014 to advance research and provide information for consumers and practitioners (Substance Abuse and Mental Health Services Administration 2015). Research on (and consumer and provider information about) the role of complementary, alternative, and integrative approaches to a range of behavioral health conditions, including addictive disorders, is supported by the NCCIH and is available on the NCCIH website (www.nccih.nih.gov). The NCCIH is but one of many institutions and organizations aiming to advance our understanding of these unconventional approaches to health care.

The terms *complementary*, *alternative*, and *integrative* require some clarification because they are often used (incorrectly) interchangeably. The term *complementary* refers to a nonmainstream approach that is used together with conventional medicine, whereas the term *alternative* refers to a nonmainstream approach that is used in place of conventional medicine. The term *integrative health* brings together conventional and complementary approaches in a coordinated way and aims for well-coordinated care among various providers from multiple backgrounds and approaches. Broadly, therapies can be physical (e.g., massage and acupuncture), psychological (e.g., meditation and relaxation therapies), nutritional (e.g., dietary and herbal supplements), or a combination (e.g., yoga) (National Center for Complementary and Integrative Health 2021).

Overall, the research on complementary, alternative, and integrative approaches to the treatment of addictive disorders is severely lacking relative to the evidence base amassed for conventional medical and behavioral health treatment approaches. Nonetheless, inclusion of a summary outline of some of the more widely researched and prevalent nonconventional approaches to the treatment of addictive disorders is warranted in this book for two important reasons. First, many patients may be considering (or already) partaking in these approaches; therefore, providers can benefit from knowing about these treatments and their potential benefits and harms or cautions. Second, being able to communicate more openly and honestly with patients about the full range of treatment approaches they may encounter or consider can help develop a positive, destigmatizing rapport and support recovery.

Nutritional Approaches: Supplements

The use of dietary supplements is rising in the general population. An analysis using 2017–2018 National Health and Nutrition Examination Survey data revealed that among adults age 20 or older, 57.8% had used a dietary supplement within the past 30 days, with use increasing with age and higher in women than men (Mishra et al. 2021).

Supplements are increasingly being utilized in the treatment of mental health conditions as well, based on the proposed association of some psychiatric conditions with elevated oxidative stress and inflammatory markers or with nutritional deficiencies. The perception of relative safety of dietary supplements also encourages their use. In a review of meta-analyses of randomized controlled trials (RCTs) evaluating the safety and efficacy of supplements in mental health disorders, the authors found that all nutritional supplements within the studies analyzed had good safety profiles (Firth et al. 2019).

Even if the compounds themselves are relatively safe, there is little monitoring of the over-the-counter, commercially available preparations that tend to be purchased by individuals, and these products are not regulated by the FDA. As a result, supplements can vary widely in quality, potency, and composition. Therefore, those taking over-the-counter supplements and botanicals run the risk of inadvertent exposure to products that are adulterated or contaminated with other substances or ingestion of active ingredients in excess of labeled amounts (Bailey 2020). Multiple factors can affect the potency of botanical supplements, including the part of the plant used, the age of the harvested plant, and the method of preparation (Shipkowski et al. 2018).

The U.S. Dietary Supplement Health and Education Act (DSHEA) of 1994 attempted to regulate dietary supplements through the creation of guidelines regarding marketing and health claims that supplement manufacturers are allowed to make. However, supplements are treated more like food than prescription medications under the DSHEA and are not held to the same standards of quality, safety, and efficacy as pharmaceuticals. The DSHEA also allowed the FDA to establish the Good Manufacturing Guidelines in an attempt to regulate supplements such that the actual composition of the supplement is consistent with the labeled product. However, there is no premarket approval process for supplements, and manufacturers can ultimately set their own quality standards.

The Food Safety Modernization Act of 2011 provided the FDA with recall authority to remove products determined to be unsafe from the market. This postmarket approach leaves consumers at risk of exposure to potentially dangerous supplements (Bailey 2020). Nonetheless, as described earlier in this section, use of dietary supplements overall is on the rise, and despite the limitations in regulatory oversight, resources of varying rigor and quality do exist to help guide patients in selecting supplements. There are several industry-driven, independent third-party certification companies such as ConsumerLab, the United States Pharmacopoeia Convention, and NSF (formerly the National Sanitation Foundation) to help health care professionals and consumers determine what products have been tested for contaminants and had their compositions verified. Federal resources are available as well, including the Dietary Supplement Ingredient Database and the Dietary Supplement Label Database from the National Institutes of Health Office of Dietary Supplements. Nonetheless, these products remain less tightly regulated than other pharmaceutical products.

There is increasing interest in the role of nutrition and dietary supplement use in the treatment of substance use disorders. In the following sections, we highlight several of note.

N-Acetylcysteine

N-acetylcysteine (NAC) is a prodrug to the amino acid cysteine and, therefore, a precursor to glutathione. NAC has clinical efficacy for a variety of medical conditions, including acetaminophen toxicity and bronchopulmonary disorders.

NAC is thought to have several mechanisms of action via regulation of several neurotransmitters, oxidative homeostasis, and inflammatory mediators (Smaga et al. 2021). Because these processes have been proposed to contribute to several neuropsychiatric processes, there has been increasing interest in the utilization of NAC to treat mental health disorders. In the context of substance use disorders, one potential neurobiological mechanism of action of interest is NAC's role in modulating glutamate dysregulation, a dysregulation that has been implicated in the genesis and maintenance of several addictive disorders (Schmaal et al. 2012). The clinical mechanism of NAC's effectiveness remains unclear; however, a review of the efficacy of NAC in substance use treatment suggests that NAC may be associated with decreased cravings to use or seek out substances such as stimulants (Tomko et al. 2018).

In a 2021 meta-analysis of RCTs, Chang et al. evaluated the impact of NAC use on clinical symptoms related to substance use (specifically, craving, depressive symptoms, and withdrawal syndrome) measured in studies of multiple different types of substances, including alcohol, tobacco, methamphetamine, cannabis, and cocaine. The meta-analysis of trials evaluating craving symptoms demonstrated a statistically significant decrease in symptoms of craving in the NAC intervention groups versus the control groups (Chang et al. 2021).

A double-blind, placebo-controlled study evaluated the impact of NAC in cocaine dependence (per DSM-IV criteria [American Psychiatric Association 1994]). The findings indicated that those who were able to achieve abstinence from cocaine at the beginning of treatment with NAC reported lower craving and achieved longer abstinence (LaRowe et al. 2013).

There is some evidence for the utility of NAC in cannabis and alcohol use disorders as well, with the results from a randomized double-blind trial indicating that adolescents with cannabis dependence (per DSM-IV criteria) who received NAC had more than twice the odds of subsequent negative urine screens during treatment relative to those taking placebo (Gray et al. 2012). A randomized double-blind study on the impact of NAC on alcohol use in cannabis-dependent individuals revealed that those in the NAC group had decreased numbers of drinks and drinking days per week, along with increased between-visit abstinence from alcohol (Squeglia et al. 2018).

Despite the popularity of NAC, its availability as a supplement is in question. In July 2020, the FDA sent warning letters to several manufacturers of supplements or products containing NAC asserting that NAC could not be lawfully marketed as a supplement because acetylcysteine had previously been approved as a medication in 1963.

Kudzu

Kudzu extract, also known as *Pueraria,* has long been utilized as a treatment for alcohol use and intoxication within traditional Chinese medicine (TCM), with evidence of its use dating back to AD 600 (Liang and Olsen 2014). Kudzu's proposed efficacy is due to its bioactive isoflavones, specifically, puerarin, daidzein, and diadzin. The kudzu herbal preparation has two components with differing proposed mechanisms of action: *Pueraria flos,* the flower, is proposed to enhance the removal of acetaldehyde and is a traditional hangover cure, typically in combination with several other herbs. *Pueraria lobata*, the root, has been proposed to inhibit mitochondrial aldehyde dehydrogenase and therefore lead to increased acetaldehyde levels, causing an aversive response to alcohol similar to that from disulfiram (McGregor 2007; Wang et al. 2016).

Human research into kudzu has been limited, but some small studies have postulated that kudzu may alter the bioavailability of alcohol and lead to early satiety while drinking. One study found that despite not increasing the subjective intoxicating effects of alcohol, pretreatment with a standardized kudzu extract before ingestion of alcohol resulted in a more rapid rise in plasma ethanol levels and increased heart rate and skin temperature compared with placebo (Penetar et al. 2011). Other studies have found that use of kudzu for several weeks may lead to reductions in alcohol consumption (Lukas et al. 2013), and a single dose before consumption may lead to a reduction in the amount of alcohol ingested during a binge drinking episode (Penetar et al. 2015). Also encouraging is some evidence that kudzu does not appear to affect sleep quality or quantity (Bracken et al. 2011).

Although research into the use of kudzu has been promising, existing studies are small, and some study sites and authors had potential conflicts of interest attributable to patents for and involvement in the production of kudzu extract. Furthermore, the potential increase in acetaldehyde with this herbal supplement raises concerns for a potential increase in acetaldehyde-related neoplasms or other negative health effects (McGregor 2007). Although kudzu remains a supplement of interest in the potential treatment of alcohol use disorder, it and its potential side effects warrant further study.

Kava

Kava, a psychoactive drink prepared from the rhizome of the *Piper methysticum* plant, has been used throughout the South Pacific and Pacific Island region in multiple contexts ranging from the social to the ceremonial. Several methods of preparation exist that alter the potency of kava; in general, it is primarily used in small doses for its anxiolytic and muscle relaxant properties, and it is used in large doses for its narcotic-like properties, including euphoria and alterations in sensorium (Cairney et al. 2002).

The pharmacological effects of kava are due to the action of lipid-soluble compounds called *kavalactones*, or *kavapyrones*, which are concentrated mostly within the roots and rhizomes of the plant, with decreased concentration in the aerial parts of the plant. Studies suggest multiple mechanisms of action of kavalactones, including enhancement of GABA and acetylcholine transmission, inhibition of sodium and calcium channels, reversible inhibition of monoamine oxidase B, and decreased reuptake of dopamine and norepinephrine (Sarris et al. 2011; White 2018).

Given these pharmacological effects and its traditional use, kava has been studied as an intervention for anxiety, with some promising evidence. A 6-week double-blind, placebo-controlled study in participants with generalized anxiety disorder (GAD) revealed significant reductions in anxiety for the kava group versus the placebo group, with a more pronounced effect in those characterized to have moderate to severe GAD (Sarris et al. 2013).

Kava's anxiolytic properties do not appear to be attributable to direct GABA receptor binding, from evidence that the GABA-enhancing effect of one of the most abundant kavalactones, kavain, was unaffected by flumazenil (Chua et al. 2016). Given this, as well as kava's antinociceptive effects but apparent lack of direct opioid receptor agonism (Jamieson and Duffield 1990), kava has been proposed as a potential adjunctive treatment for opioid withdrawal (Toce et al. 2018).

In a study following up on experimental data that kava could potentially reduce lung cancer risk, Wang et al. (2020) found that a weeklong course of kava among smokers was associated with a statistically significant reduction in ratings of smoking satisfaction and enjoyment of respiratory tract sensation on the Modified Cigarette Evaluation Questionnaire, as well as decreased urinary total nicotine equivalents. These findings suggest that kava consumption could support tobacco smoking cessation (Wang et al. 2020). Moreover, the study demonstrated significant reductions in plasma cortisol and urinary total cortisol levels. Because elevated cortisol levels can be indicative of increased stressed states, which can reinforce smoking behaviors, Wang et al. (2020) hypothesized that kava-mediated anxiolysis and stress reduction may have contributed to the decrease in smoking behaviors observed in the study.

Despite encouraging evidence of kava's clinical effectiveness, concerns about safety have led to its restriction in multiple countries. The most concerning adverse effect associated with kava is hepatotoxicity, likely secondary to excessive or prolonged kava use, adulteration of products, or use of substandard kava cultivars. There is also evidence that the medium used for kava extraction, such as acetone or ethanol, may increase this risk, but kava itself is also increasingly recognized as a risk factor for hepatotoxicity

(Teschke and Schulze 2010; White 2018). Dermatopathy is another well-documented side effect of kava in regular and heavy users that is generally reversible with discontinuation of use (White 2018).

Kratom

Kratom (*Mitragyna speciosa*) is a tropical tree native to Southeast Asia, whose leaves have been traditionally consumed for its stimulant and pain-relieving properties. Kratom use is on the rise in the United States, with 2020 data from the National Survey on Drug Use and Health (NSDUH) revealing that an estimated 0.8% of those age 12 years or older in this nationally representative sample reported kratom use within the past year (U.S. Department of Health and Human Services 2020). The NSDUH asks questions regarding misuse of various substances, and it then poses additional lines of questioning to determine whether those participants who reported misuse also met criteria for a proxy diagnosis of a substance use disorder. Of relevance here, individuals identified through the NSDUH as carrying a proxy diagnosis of prescription opioid use disorder were found to have higher odds of kratom use (~10.4% of this population) (Palamar 2021). This finding is consistent with clinical practice, in which patients who report kratom use also report opioid use and, in some cases, turn to kratom as a means of detoxifying from use of other opioids.

Kratom has several bioactive alkaloids, with mitragynine being the most abundant. This compound, and the less-abundant 7-hydroxymitragynine alkaloid, are thought to be the most potent psychoactive components of kratom, with both compounds having affinity for opioid receptors. Kratom alkaloids have also been shown to have action at serotonergic 5-hydroxytryptamine receptor 2A and postsynaptic α_2-adrenergic receptors, with the latter, in particular, potentially accounting for kratom's reported stimulant activity (Warner et al. 2016).

As introduced at the beginning of this section, kratom has been theorized to be helpful for opioid withdrawal, given its μ opioid receptor activity along with its potential clonidine-like effects owing to its α_2 agonist activity (Boyer et al. 2008). In Southeast Asia, there has been evidence of kratom's use in the treatment of opium withdrawal dating back to the nineteenth century, with more recent evidence for its use in the treatment of morphine addiction (Hassan et al. 2013). Kratom continues to be used for both opioid withdrawal symptoms and mood-elevating effects in those who are opioid abstinent (Singh et al. 2020).

Research into the motivation for kratom use has shown that among kratom users, it is less preferred than other substances of misuse, suggesting that kratom may not be an attractive primary substance of misuse (Smith and Lawson 2017). Although it may be less preferred than other substances, there is still growing evidence that kratom can lead to physiological dependence. Regular kratom users surveyed in Malaysia endorsed cravings, and those who discontinued use after chronic use endorsed withdrawal symptoms consistent with opioid withdrawal, with the severity of withdrawal symptoms correlating with the amount, duration, and frequency of use (Singh et al. 2014). A case series of individuals with kratom withdrawal documented that using symptom management–based opioid withdrawal management protocols led to improvement in and, in some instances, resolution of kratom withdrawal symptoms (Stanciu et al. 2019). A review of the literature on the management of kratom use disorder, along with clinical expert consensus, indicates that it is reasonable to use medications for addiction treatment (buprenorphine or methadone) such as one might use for the long-term management of opioid use disorder (Stanciu et al. 2021).

Despite some potential utility for the treatment of opioid use disorder, kratom clearly carries its own risks of physiological dependence and the potential for its own use disorder. Safety concerns persist regarding potential toxicity of kratom in overdose—although evidence suggests that kratom carries a lower risk of significant respiratory depression than other opioids (Kruegel and Grundmann 2018). Nonetheless, there have been several case reports of overdose deaths implicating kratom as the cause of death (Olsen et al. 2019).

Furthermore, given the lack of regulation of kratom because of its status as a dietary supplement, there are significant concerns of contamination in kratom products. The FDA has issued multiple warnings regarding kratom, including a mandatory recall for kratom products in 2018 after finding evidence of salmonella contamination (U.S. Food and Drug Administration 2018), as well as a warning about the risk of heavy metal poisoning after laboratory testing revealed significant lead and nickel concentrations in various kratom products (U.S. Food and Drug Administration 2019). An analysis of eight kratom products legally purchased in Chicago was consistent with the FDA's warnings, and although the evaluation did not demonstrate evidence of salmonella, the investigators found that six of eight samples were positive for bacteria and fungi, and seven of eight products showed significant levels of heavy metals (Prozialeck et al. 2020).

Ibogaine and Hallucinogens

Both ibogaine and hallucinogens are reviewed in more detail in Chapter 8 ("Hallucinogens and Phencyclidine"). Therefore, only a brief mention of these nonconventional treatment approaches to addictive disorders will be provided here.

Ibogaine is an indole alkaloid found predominantly in the root of the *Tabernanthe iboga* shrub that is widely used in traditional African medicine. Low doses are used to prevent fatigue, whereas high doses have hallucinogenic properties that are used in religious and initiatory celebrations. Ibogaine was brought to France in the 1800s, and the isolated psychoactive compound ibogaine was marketed there as an antidepressant with stimulant properties under the trade name Lambarene until the 1960s (Wasko et al. 2018). Ibogaine started to gain popularity in the West during that time, when heroin users claimed that it allowed for a smooth detoxification from, and near resolution of cravings for, opioids.

There have been few clinical trials to date evaluating the clinical impact of ibogaine, although clinical trials outside of the United States are underway. Most data regarding the effectiveness of ibogaine have been observational, with findings that require further study. In an observational study of 30 individuals seeking opioid use disorder treatment in Mexico, individuals reported a significant reduction in symptoms of withdrawal after ibogaine administration, and half of the study population reported abstinence from opioids at 1-month follow-up (Brown and Alper 2018). These findings are consistent with other observational studies, including a larger (N = 191) open-label case series that evaluated the effects of ibogaine on individuals who self-referred for inpatient treatment of substance use and whose symptoms met DSM-IV criteria for either opioid or cocaine dependence (Mash et al. 2018). Both groups reported significantly decreased drug craving and had improved depressive symptoms immediately post ibogaine treatment and at 1-month follow-up (Mash et al. 2018).

Another small observational study conducted in New Zealand showed longer-term effects after ibogaine treatment, with participants completing treatment showing a significant reduction in drug use and depression at 12-month follow-up (Noller et al. 2018). In an online survey of patients who had received ibogaine treatment in Mexico, 80% reported that ibogaine had significantly reduced or eliminated withdrawal symptoms, and 30% reported no relapses since treatment (Davis et al. 2017).

The duration of action for ibogaine's effects is quite long and said to be characterized by three distinct stages: 1) an acute stage, characterized by a dream-like quality with visions or hallucinations when patients have their eyes closed (as opposed to traditional hallucinogens); 2) an evaluative stage, in which visual imagery abates and a period of self-reflection and personal insight is prominent; and 3) a residual stimulation phase, in which individuals report decreased need for sleep and a feeling of mental clarity that can last more than 24 hours. The totality of these stages typically completes within 3–4 days.

One proposed mechanism for ibogaine's efficacy for substance use is the strong psychological transformation that many individuals report undergoing. Specifically, users have reported powerful subjective experiences while under the effects of ibogaine, in which they confront feelings of regret and experience a sense of clarity and insight into their substance use, which can be a motivator for abstinence (Brown 2013).

Despite encouraging data, research into ibogaine has been limited because of concerns over serious adverse effects, the most well known of which is cardiotoxicity. Ibogaine is known to induce bradycardia and, at higher doses, can prolong the QT interval via blockade of voltage-gated cardiac potassium channels, leading to cardiac arrest. There have been several reports of sudden death in the setting of ibogaine use. Given the length of noribogaine's duration of action, cardiac complications can occur days to weeks after a single dose (Corkery 2018). Other common side effects included ataxia and nausea during the active phase after administration and headache after dose administration (Mash et al. 2018).

Research into the use of other hallucinogens as treatments for various behavioral health conditions has had a resurgence recently. Studies of psilocybin, for example, have signaled promising positive effects on the severity of a variety of psychiatric symptoms ranging from cancer-related existential distress and depression/anxiety (Griffiths et al. 2016; Ross et al. 2016) to symptoms of OCD (Moreno et al. 2006) and substance use disorders. The evidence for psilocybin has been so encouraging that the FDA granted it breakthrough therapy status in 2018, facilitating further research into this substance.

Interest in psilocybin's potential as a treatment for substance use disorders has also increased. Small studies on the impact of psilocybin on tobacco smoking and alcohol use disorder have been promising (Bogenschutz et al. 2015, 2022; Johnson et al. 2014, 2017).

Although current research has focused on psilocybin, extensive research was undertaken in the 1950s through 1970s on the impact of lysergic acid diethylamide (LSD) use in alcohol use disorder. In a systematic review of these historical studies evaluating the effectiveness of LSD, the authors concluded that despite the heterogeneity of therapeutic approaches and methodologies, there was evidence to support the utility of LSD in improving abstinence and reducing alcohol use (Fuentes et al. 2020). A prior meta-analysis of six of these older studies found that a single dose of LSD was associated with a decrease in alcohol consumption, with a statistically significant treatment effect up to 6 months after administration (Krebs and Johansen 2012).

Increased cognitive flexibility, beneficial effects on negative emotional states, and hallucinogen-induced mystical experiences are thought to be important mediators for the decreases in substance use found in trials of hallucinogen-assisted treatments (de Veen et al. 2017; Garcia-Romeu et al. 2014). Hallucinogens also appear to offer patients more insight into their problematic use of substances (Krebs and Johansen 2012). It is important to note that many study protocols involve hallucinogen-assisted psychotherapy, in which therapists are present in a supportive capacity during the treatment and in postsession integration, with the focus being on the internal experiences of the patient.

In terms of safety, hallucinogens seem to have a low rate of overdose toxicity and a relatively limited side-effect profile, and most psychedelic side effects appear to be transient. A systematic review of systematic reviews reported that the most common adverse reactions in controlled research settings were transient and moderate increases in blood pressure and heart rate, gastrointestinal discomfort, and less commonly, transient anxiety and psychotic-like reactions (Dos Santos et al. 2018).

Physical Approaches

Acupuncture

Acupuncture is an increasingly popular integrative medicine intervention within the United States. The 2012 National Health Interview Survey, the largest and most recent survey addressing complementary health approaches, revealed that 1.5% of those surveyed reported use of acupuncture (Clarke et al. 2015). With the increasing acceptance and adoption of integrative health and wellness strategies, this number has likely risen in the decade since the survey was conducted.

In TCM, health and wellness are thought to arise from the balance between *yin* and *yang* and the free flow of vital energy (also known as *chi* or *qi*) through energetic pathways called *meridians* throughout the body. Within this conception, disease is thought to be due to deficiency, excess, or blockage of qi that leads to disharmony between yin and yang (Kaptchuk 2002). Acupuncture entails the manipulation of certain points in the body to facilitate the unblocking or balancing of qi. Although this can be done through the application of manual pressure, heat, or even electrical stimulation, acupuncture is typically performed through the insertion of very fine needles into the skin (Van Hal et al. 2022). Of note, the clinical effectiveness of acupuncture is thought to be related to a sensation of heaviness or soreness at the acupuncture point, called *de qi* (Lu et al. 2008). Overall, acupuncture has a relatively good safety profile, with a systematic review revealing that the most common adverse events were needle pain, some feelings of tiredness, and mild bleeding (Ernst and White 2001). Many practitioners now utilize sterile, solid, single-use needles, which has reduced the risk of infection from acupuncture.

Acupuncture has found growing acceptance within the Western medical community, owing to evidence of its effectiveness in multiple conditions, including cancer care for chemotherapy-related side effects (Lu et al. 2008) and pain complaints. Acupuncture was among the American College of Physicians' 2017 practice guidelines for nonpharmacological treatment of low back pain (Hauk 2017). It is thought to be useful in psychiatric complaints as well because within TCM, physical and mental health are interdependent such that mental health symptoms and dysregulation are similarly thought to result from blockage, excess, or deficiency of qi (Aung et al. 2013). Several studies have attempted to assess the impact of acupuncture on mental health, particularly depression. In a Cochrane review of available studies, Smith et al. (2018) found that evidence suggested that acupuncture was associated with a reduction in severity of depression, although they noted that studies indicating this effect were of low quality.

Study design and methodology can be variable in acupuncture research, because it can be difficult to conduct RCTs with this intervention. Clinical acupuncture treatments are individualized to the patient, and it is therefore difficult to standardize a given acupuncture protocol for study purposes (Van Hal et al. 2022). Furthermore, control conditions may consist of sham acupuncture, wherein an acupuncture point is stimulated with nonpenetrating needles or stimulation of nonindicated or nonactive points is carried out; sham control subjects may therefore not be true inactive control subjects. A meta-analysis assessing the nonspecific effects of sham intervention found that sham had moderately large nonspecific effects, which could limit the ability to detect potentially small specific effects from true acupuncture (Linde et al. 2010).

The difficulty ascertaining the specific effect of acupuncture is reflected in the difficulty determining a clear mechanism of action for this intervention. Many mechanisms have been proposed, with an early hypothesis implicating the involvement of the endogenous opioid system (How does acupuncture work? 1981; Kaptchuk 2002). A 2021 review of the available literature, including animal model studies, postulated that acupuncture may be efficacious in substance use disorder treatment by inhibiting neuronal and behavioral sensitization of the mesolimbic pathway via mechanical activation of somatosensory afferents (this may explain the belief that the de qi sensation, which suggests stimulation of the somatosensory afferent, is important for clinical benefit) (Lee et al. 2021). The review also postulated that acupuncture attenuates the negative emotional state related to hypoactivity of this pathway during withdrawal (Lee et al. 2021). The psychological effects of acupuncture treatment as they relate to symptoms of interest have also been hypothesized to contribute to its efficacy, particularly the relaxing and calming effect associated with acupuncture. These effects may lead to reductions in impulsivity that can hallmark addictive disorders (Carter and Olshan-Perlmutter 2015).

One of the most popular acupuncture protocols for substance use treatment is a 5-point auricular acupuncture protocol known as *NADA*, named after the organization that promoted its use (National Acupuncture Detoxification Association). The NADA protocol has been taught to more than 25,000 health professionals worldwide and is utilized in "more than 1,000 publicly licensed addiction treatment programs" in the United States (National Acupuncture Detoxification Association 2025). This protocol was developed in response to early research in the 1970s by Hong Kong neurosurgeon H.L. Wen and his colleague S.Y.C. Cheung, which indicated that acupuncture (both manual and electrically stimulated) helped relieve withdrawal symptoms in individuals with heroin and opium addiction. This finding led to the addition of auricular acupuncture to the methadone-assisted detoxification program at the Lincoln Hospital in the South Bronx, New York, which ultimately evolved into a 5-point auricular acupuncture protocol that is now known as the NADA protocol (Smith and Khan 1988).

Studies evaluating the NADA protocol have been mixed but have found some support for its use as an adjunctive treatment for substance use. A randomized prospective trial performed in an intensive outpatient setting compared a control group of patients receiving traditional substance use treatment with those receiving traditional treatment along with biweekly NADA sessions (Carter et al. 2017). The authors found a statistically significant reduction in self-reported alcohol use in the NADA group at 3- and 6-month follow-up and decreased tobacco use at 6-month follow-up, although these results were self-reported (Carter et al. 2017). A 2002 randomized sham-controlled trial used a 5-point NADA protocol along with one wrist acupuncture point to evaluate acupuncture's efficacy in tobacco cessation. Researchers compared this intervention alone versus the intervention plus education and sham plus education. They found that the NADA intervention plus education was associated with statistically significant reductions in self-reported smoking after treatment compared with the other two groups (Bier et al. 2002).

Other studies using different acupuncture protocols have also revealed encouraging data for the use of acupuncture in conjunction with stan-dard substance use disorder treatments. A 4-week randomized trial evaluated the impact of acupuncture in individuals receiving outpatient methadone maintenance treatment by comparing biweekly sessions of acupuncture (a combination of electroacupuncture plus auricular acupuncture) versus sham acupuncture. The authors found a significant decrease in daily methadone dosage in the acupuncture group starting after week 2 of the study period, as well as statistically significant pre/post improvements in sleep quality, sleep latency, and daytime dysfunction scores, as measured by the Pittsburgh Sleep Quality Index (Chan et al. 2014).

Despite promising data, the overall body of evidence regarding acupuncture's effectiveness in substance use disorder treatment can be characterized as inconsistent. A review of RCTs evaluating the effectiveness of acupuncture for heroin and other opiate use determined that although acupuncture showed potential for improving withdrawal symptoms, 8 of the 10 studies meeting inclusion criteria were of low quality (Lin et al. 2012). A large 2002 RCT evaluating the impact of a 4-point version of NADA auricular acupuncture in patients with cocaine dependence (per DSM-IV criteria) found no evidence of benefit over both a control condition (with auricular needles inserted in points not associated with addiction treatment) and a relaxation control condition when assessing for a reduction in cocaine use (Margolin et al. 2002). White (2013) conducted a review of that study, as well as other studies of acupuncture and substance use disorders available at the time, to evaluate the discrepancy between research findings and clinical observation of acupuncture's effectiveness in treatment settings. White (2013) concluded that the inconsistency in the results of these studies was likely due to a "large number of variables in treatment and outcomes," (p. 301) and that there was evidence in RCTs that acupuncture could in fact be helpful for cravings and withdrawal.

Studies of acupuncture's utility in substance use treatment appear to be plagued by significant methodological issues and publication bias (Grant et al. 2016), resulting in an inconsistent and variable body of evidence for its effectiveness in substance use disorder. Despite this, there are anecdotal reports from patients regarding its effectiveness for protracted withdrawal symptoms ranging from craving to anxiety (Bergdahl et al. 2014). Although acupuncture's mechanism of action and clinical impact require further elucidation, it is a relatively safe, accessible, and low-cost intervention (particularly in community acupuncture settings) that may provide clinical utility in conjunction with other substance use treatments.

Other Considerations

The genesis and the maintenance of addictive disorders are typically multifactorial, with individuals often citing various physical and mental health maladies as factors that contribute to their current conditions. For instance, individuals may point to their anxiety, insomnia, or pain issues as the primary driving force in the development of their addictive disorder, the resolution of which is seen as central to their recovery. It is beyond the scope of this chapter to discuss the full range of complementary, alternative, and integrative approaches that have been studied in relation to improving those conditions indirectly tied to an individual's addictive disorder. However, it bears mentioning here that although there may not be a strong evidence base for various complementary, alternative, or integrative approaches in the direct treatment of a particular addictive disorder, there may nonetheless be a role for various nonconventional approaches in treating the array of other conditions that affect individuals with addictive disorders. For instance, the literature supporting the use of yoga or chiropractic adjustment sessions in the treatment of addictive disorders is scant; however, the literature is more robust supporting the benefits of yoga or chiropractic in the treatment of various pain disorders that may be complicating a person's recovery from an addictive disorder.

It is therefore incumbent on providers to think holistically about the array of conditions that their patients present with and to seek to understand and support (where appropriate) how complementary, alternative, or integrative approaches may be beneficial to their overall recovery.

Key Points

- Although these terms are sometimes used interchangeably, *complementary* refers to a nonmainstream approach that is used together with conventional medicine, whereas *alternative* refers to a nonmainstream approach that is used in place of conventional medicine. *Integrative health* brings together conventional and complementary approaches in a coordinated way and aims for well-coordinated care among various providers from multiple backgrounds and approaches. Research indicates that complementary, alternative, and integrative health approaches are commonly used in the United States.
- Broadly, complementary, alternative, and integrative health approaches can be physical in nature (e.g., massage and acupuncture), psychological (e.g., meditation, relaxation therapies), nutritional (e.g., dietary and herbal supplements), or a combination (e.g., yoga).
- Overall, robust research on complementary, alternative, and integrative health approaches to the treatment of addictive disorders is scant and prone to methodological limitations.
- Supplements studied in the treatment of addictive disorders include *N*-acetylcysteine, kudzu, kava, and kratom, with mixed results. Despite their perceived safety, supplements may carry their own risks

through either interactions with other substances or their own misuse potential (e.g., kratom).
- Hallucinogens have demonstrated some promise in studies looking at their utility in the treatment of substance use disorders, with psilocybin and LSD being the most studied. Ibogaine, another hallucinogen, has a smaller research base supporting its effect on opioid use disorder treatment, in particular; however, ibogaine also carries serious toxicity concerns.
- Physical interventions for substance use disorders, such as acupuncture, chiropractic, and yoga, also have mixed results in a literature that consists mainly of small, unblinded, methodologically inconsistent studies.
- Dietary supplements are not regulated by the FDA; there may be significant variability between these commercially available products and the quality controls in their production processes. Therefore, caution is advised.
- Despite the lack of direct evidence to support the utility of complementary, alternative, or integrative therapeutic approaches to the treatment of substance use disorders, a growing literature looking at the role of these interventions in the treatment of co-occurring conditions (whether psychiatric or medical) may provide indirect benefits to those seeking to achieve recovery from substance use.

References

American Psychiatric Association: Diagnostic and Statistical Manual of Mental Disorders, 4th Edition. Washington, DC, American Psychiatric Association, 1994

Aung SK, Fay H, Hobbs RF III: Traditional Chinese medicine as a basis for treating psychiatric disorders: a review of theory with illustrative cases. Med Acupunct 25(6):398–406, 2013 24761185

Bailey RL: Current regulatory guidelines and resources to support research of dietary supplements in the United States. Crit Rev Food Sci Nutr 60(2):298–309, 2020 30421981

Bergdahl L, Berman AH, Haglund K: Patients' experience of auricular acupuncture during protracted withdrawal. J Psychiatr Ment Health Nurs 21(2):163–169, 2014 23230968

Bier ID, Wilson J, Studt P, et al: Auricular acupuncture, education, and smoking cessation: a randomized, sham-controlled trial. Am J Public Health 92(10):1642–1647, 2002 12356614

Bogenschutz MP, Forcehimes AA, Pommy JA, et al: Psilocybin-assisted treatment for alcohol dependence: a proof-of-concept study. J Psychopharmacol 29(3):289–299, 2015 25586396

Bogenschutz MP, Ross S, Bhatt S, et al: Percentage of heavy drinking days following psilocybin-assisted psychotherapy vs placebo in the treatment of adult patients with alcohol use disorder: a randomized clinical trial. JAMA Psychiatry 79(10):953–962, 2022 36001306

Boyer EW, Babu KM, Adkins JE, et al: Self-treatment of opioid withdrawal using kratom (Mitragynia speciosa korth). Addiction 103(6):1048–1050, 2008 18482427

Bracken BK, Penetar DM, Maclean RR, et al: Kudzu root extract does not perturb the sleep/wake cycle of moderate drinkers. J Altern Complement Med 17(10):961–966, 2011 22010780

Brown TK: Ibogaine in the treatment of substance dependence. Curr Drug Abuse Rev 6(1):3–16, 2013 23627782

Brown TK, Alper K: Treatment of opioid use disorder with ibogaine: detoxification and drug use outcomes. Am J Drug Alcohol Abuse 44(1):24–36, 2018 28541119

Cairney S, Maruff P, Clough AR: The neurobehavioural effects of kava. Aust N Z J Psychiatry 36(5):657–662, 2002 12225450

Carter K, Olshan-Perlmutter M: Impulsivity and stillness: NADA, pharmaceuticals, and psychotherapy in substance use and other DSM-5 disorders. Behav Sci (Basel) 5(4):537–546, 2015 26703743

Carter K, Olshan-Perlmutter M, Marx J, et al: NADA ear acupuncture: an adjunctive therapy to improve and maintain positive outcomes in substance abuse treatment. Behav Sci (Basel) 7(2):37, 2017 28621706

Chan YY, Lo WY, Li TC, et al: Clinical efficacy of acupuncture as an adjunct to methadone treatment services for heroin addicts: a randomized controlled trial. Am J Chin Med 42(3):569–586, 2014 24871652

Chang CT, Hsieh PJ, Lee HC, et al: Effectiveness of N-acetylcysteine in treating clinical symptoms of substance abuse and dependence: a meta-analysis of randomized controlled trials. Clin Psychopharmacol Neurosci 19(2):282–293, 2021 33888657

Chua HC, Christensen ET, Hoestgaard-Jensen K, et al: Kavain, the major constituent of the anxiolytic kava extract, potentiates $GABA_A$ receptors: functional characteristics and molecular mechanism. PLoS One 11(6):e0157700, 2016 27332705

Clarke TC, Black LI, Stussman BJ, et al: Trends in the use of complementary health approaches among adults: United States, 2002–2012. Natl Health Stat Rep (79):1–16, 2015 25671660

Corkery JM: Ibogaine as a treatment for substance misuse: potential benefits and practical dangers. Prog Brain Res 242:217–257, 2018 30471681

Davis AK, Barsuglia JP, Windham-Herman AM, et al: Subjective effectiveness of ibogaine treatment for problematic opioid consumption: short- and long-term outcomes and current psychological functioning. J Psychedelic Stud 1(2):65–73, 2017 30272050

de Veen BT, Schellekens AF, Verheij MM, et al: Psilocybin for treating substance use disorders? Expert Rev Neurother 17(2):203–212, 2017 27684102

Dos Santos RG, Bouso JC, Alcázar-Córcoles MÁ, et al: Efficacy, tolerability, and safety of serotonergic psychedelics for the management of mood, anxiety, and substance-use disorders: a systematic review of systematic reviews. Expert Rev Clin Pharmacol 11(9):889–902, 2018 30102078

Eisenberg DM, Kessler RC, Foster C, et al: Unconventional medicine in the United States: prevalence, costs, and patterns of use. N Engl J Med 328(4):246–252, 1993 8418405

Ernst E, White AR: Prospective studies of the safety of acupuncture: a systematic review. Am J Med 110(6):481–485, 2001 11331060

Firth J, Teasdale SB, Allott K, et al: The efficacy and safety of nutrient supplements in the treatment of mental disorders: a meta-review of meta-analyses of randomized controlled trials. World Psychiatry 18(3):308–324, 2019 31496103

Fuentes JJ, Fonseca F, Elices M, et al: Therapeutic use of LSD in psychiatry: a systematic review of randomized-controlled clinical trials. Front Psychiatry 10:943, 2020 32038315

Garcia-Romeu A, Griffiths RR, Johnson MW: Psilocybin-occasioned mystical experiences in the treatment of tobacco addiction. Curr Drug Abuse Rev 7(3):157–164, 2014 25563443

Grant S, Kandrack R, Motala A, et al: Acupuncture for substance use disorders: a systematic review and meta-analysis. Drug Alcohol Depend 163:1–15, 2016 26968093

Gray KM, Carpenter MJ, Baker NL, et al: A double-blind randomized controlled trial of N-acetylcysteine in cannabis-dependent adolescents. Am J Psychiatry 169(8):805–812, 2012 22706327

Griffiths RR, Johnson MW, Carducci MA, et al: Psilocybin produces substantial and sustained decreases in depression and anxiety in patients with life-threatening cancer: a randomized double-blind trial. J Psychopharmacol 30(12):1181–1197, 2016 27909165

Hassan Z, Muzaimi M, Navaratnam V, et al: From Kratom to mitragynine and its derivatives: physiological and behavioural effects related to use, abuse, and addiction. Neurosci Biobehav Rev 37(2):138–151, 2013 23206666

Hauk L: Low back pain: American College of Physicians practice guideline on noninvasive treatments. Am Fam Physician 96(6):407–408, 2017 28925633

How does acupuncture work? Br Med J (Clin Res Ed) 283(6294):746–748, 1981 6268241

Jamieson DD, Duffield PH: The antinociceptive actions of kava components in mice. Clin Exp Pharmacol Physiol 17(7):495–507, 1990 2401103

Johnson MW, Garcia-Romeu A, Cosimano MP, et al: Pilot study of the 5-HT2AR agonist psilocybin in the treatment of tobacco addiction. J Psychopharmacol 28(11):983–992, 2014 25213996

Johnson MW, Garcia-Romeu A, Griffiths RR: Long-term follow-up of psilocybin-facilitated smoking cessation. Am J Drug Alcohol Abuse 43(1):55–60, 2017 27441452

Kaptchuk TJ: Acupuncture: theory, efficacy, and practice. Ann Intern Med 136(5):374–383, 2002 11874310

Krebs TS, Johansen PØ: Lysergic acid diethylamide (LSD) for alcoholism: meta-analysis of randomized controlled trials. J Psychopharmacol 26(7):994–1002, 2012 22406913

Kruegel AC, Grundmann O: The medicinal chemistry and neuropharmacology of kratom: a preliminary discussion of a promising medicinal plant and analysis of its potential for abuse. Neuropharmacology 134(Pt A):108–120, 2018 28830758

LaRowe SD, Kalivas PW, Nicholas JS, et al: A double-blind placebo-controlled trial of N-acetylcysteine in the treatment of cocaine dependence. Am J Addict 22(5):443–452, 2013 23952889

Lee MY, Lee BH, Kim HY, et al: Bidirectional role of acupuncture in the treatment of drug addiction. Neurosci Biobehav Rev 126:382–397, 2021 33839169

Liang J, Olsen RW: Alcohol use disorders and current pharmacological therapies: the role of GABA(A) receptors. Acta Pharmacol Sin 35(8):981–993, 2014 25066321

Lin JG, Chan YY, Chen YH: Acupuncture for the treatment of opiate addiction. Evid Based Complement Alternat Med 2012:739045, 2012 22474521

Linde K, Niemann K, Schneider A, et al: How large are the nonspecific effects of acupuncture? A meta-analysis of randomized controlled trials. BMC Med 8:75, 2010 21092261

Lu W, Dean-Clower E, Doherty-Gilman A, et al: The value of acupuncture in cancer care. Hematol Oncol Clin North Am 22(4):631–648, 2008 18638692

Lukas SE, Penetar D, Su Z, et al: A standardized kudzu extract (NPI-031) reduces alcohol consumption in nontreatment-seeking male heavy drinkers. Psychopharmacology (Berl) 226(1):65–73, 2013 23070022

Margolin A, Kleber HD, Avants SK, et al: Acupuncture for the treatment of cocaine addiction: a randomized controlled trial. JAMA 287(1):55–63, 2002 11754709

Mash DC, Duque L, Page B, et al: Ibogaine detoxification transitions opioid and cocaine abusers between dependence and abstinence: clinical observations and treatment outcomes. Front Pharmacol 9:529, 2018 29922156

McGregor NR: Pueraria lobata (Kudzu root) hangover remedies and acetaldehyde-associated neoplasm risk. Alcohol 41(7):469–478, 2007 17980785

Mishra S, Stierman B, Gahche JJ, et al: Dietary supplement use among adults: United States, 2017–2018. NCHS Data Brief (399):1–8, 2021 33663653

Moreno FA, Wiegand CB, Taitano EK, et al: Safety, tolerability, and efficacy of psilocybin in 9 patients with obsessive-compulsive disorder. J Clin Psychiatry 67(11):1735–1740, 2006 17196053

Nahin RL, Barnes PM, Stussman BJ, et al: Costs of complementary and alternative medicine (CAM) and frequency of visits to CAM practitioners: United States, 2007. Natl Health Stat Rep (18):1–14, 2009 19771719

National Acupuncture Detoxification Association: NADA Protocol. Available at: https://acudetox.com/about-nada/. Accessed April 3, 2025.

National Center for Complementary and Integrative Health: Complementary, Alternative, or Integrative Health: What's in a Name? Bethesda, MD, National Center for Complementary and Integrative Health, April 2021. Available at: https://www.nccih.nih.gov/health/complementary-alternative-or-integrative-health-whats-in-a-name. Accessed August 13, 2021.

Noller GE, Frampton CM, Yazar-Klosinski B: Ibogaine treatment outcomes for opioid dependence from a twelve-month follow-up observational study. Am J Drug Alcohol Abuse 44(1):37–46, 2018 28402682

Olsen EO, O'Donnell J, Mattson CL, et al: Notes from the field: unintentional drug overdose deaths with kratom detected—27 states, July 2016–December 2017. MMWR Morb Mortal Wkly Rep 68(14):326–327, 2019 30973850

Palamar JJ: Past-year kratom use in the U.S.: estimates from a nationally representative sample. Am J Prev Med 61(2):240–245, 2021 34027890

Penetar DM, Maclean RR, McNeil JF, et al: Kudzu extract treatment does not increase the intoxicating effects of acute alcohol in human volunteers. Alcohol Clin Exp Res 35(4):726–734, 2011 21244439

Penetar DM, Toto LH, Lee DY, et al: A single dose of kudzu extract reduces alcohol consumption in a binge drinking paradigm. Drug Alcohol Depend 153:194–200, 2015 26048637

Prozialeck WC, Edwards JR, Lamar PC, et al: Evaluation of the mitragynine content, levels of toxic metals and the presence of microbes in kratom products purchased in the western suburbs of Chicago. Int J Environ Res Public Health 17(15):5512, 2020 32751712

Ross S, Bossis A, Guss J, et al: Rapid and sustained symptom reduction following psilocybin treatment for anxiety and depression in patients with life-threatening cancer: a randomized controlled trial. J Psychopharmacol 30(12):1165–1180, 2016 27909164

Sarris J, LaPorte E, Schweitzer I: Kava: a comprehensive review of efficacy, safety, and psychopharmacology. Aust N Z J Psychiatry 45(1):27–35, 2011 21073405

Sarris J, Stough C, Bousman CA, et al: Kava in the treatment of generalized anxiety disorder: a double-blind, randomized, placebo-controlled study. J Clin Psychopharmacol 33(5):643–648, 2013 23635869

Schmaal L, Veltman DJ, Nederveen A, et al: N-acetylcysteine normalizes glutamate levels in cocaine-dependent patients: a randomized crossover magnetic resonance spectroscopy study. Neuropsychopharmacology 37(9):2143–2152, 2012 22549117

Shipkowski KA, Betz JM, Birnbaum LS, et al: Naturally complex: perspectives and challenges associated with botanical dietary supplement safety assessment. Food Chem Toxicol 118:963–971, 2018 29626579

Singh D, Müller CP, Vicknasingam BK: Kratom (Mitragyna speciosa) dependence, withdrawal symptoms and craving in regular users. Drug Alcohol Depend 139:132–137, 2014 24698080

Singh D, Yeou Chear NJ, Narayanan S, et al: Patterns and reasons for kratom (Mitragyna speciosa) use among current and former opioid poly-drug users. J Ethnopharmacol 249:112462, 2020 31816368

Smaga I, Frankowska M, Filip M: N-acetylcysteine as a new prominent approach for treating psychiatric disorders. Br J Pharmacol 178(13):2569–2594, 2021 33760228

Smith CA, Armour M, Lee MS, et al: Acupuncture for depression. Cochrane Database Syst Rev 3(3):CD004046, 2018 29502347

Smith KE, Lawson T: Prevalence and motivations for kratom use in a sample of substance users enrolled in a residential treatment program. Drug Alcohol Depend 180:340–348, 2017 28950240

Smith MO, Khan I: An acupuncture programme for the treatment of drug-addicted persons. Bull Narc 40(1):35–41, 1988 3219455

Squeglia LM, Tomko RL, Baker NL, et al: The effect of N-acetylcysteine on alcohol use during a cannabis cessation trial. Drug Alcohol Depend 185:17–22, 2018 29413434

Stanciu CN, Gnanasegaram SA, Ahmed S, et al: Kratom withdrawal: a systematic review with case series. J Psychoactive Drugs 51(1):12–18, 2019 30614408

Stanciu C, Ahmed S, Hybki B, et al: Pharmacotherapy for management of "kratom use disorder": a systematic literature review with survey of experts. WMJ 120(1):54–61, 2021 33974767

Substance Abuse and Mental Health Services Administration: Complementary Health Approaches: Advising Clients About Evidence and Risks (HHS Publ No SMA-15-4921). Rockville, MD, Substance Abuse and Mental Health Services Administration, 2015. Available at: https://library.samhsa.gov/sites/default/files/sma15-4921.pdf. Accessed February 10, 2025.

Teschke R, Schulze J: Risk of kava hepatotoxicity and the FDA consumer advisory. JAMA 304(19):2174–2175, 2010 21081732

Toce MS, Chai PR, Burns MM, et al: Pharmacologic treatment of opioid use disorder: a review of pharmacotherapy, adjuncts, and toxicity. J Med Toxicol 14(4):306–322, 2018 30377951

Tomko RL, Jones JL, Gilmore AK, et al: N-acetylcysteine: a potential treatment for substance use disorders. Curr Psychiatr 17(6):30–55, 2018 30016376

U.S. Department of Health and Human Services, Substance Abuse and Mental Health Services Administration, Center for Behavioral Health Statistics and Quality: National Survey on Drug Use and Health 2020. Rockville, MD, Substance Abuse and Mental Health Services Administration, 2020. Available at: https://www.samhsa.gov/data/sites/default/files/reports/rpt35323/NSDUHDetailedTabs2020/NSDUHDetailedTabs2020/NSDUHDetTabsAppB2020.htm. Accessed February 10, 2025.

U.S. Food and Drug Administration: FDA orders mandatory recall for kratom products due to risk of salmonella. Silver Spring, MD, U.S. Food and Drug Administration, April 3, 2018. Available at: https://www.fda.gov/news-events/press-announcements/fda-orders-mandatory-recall-kratom-products-due-risk-salmonella. Accessed January 17, 2025.

U.S. Food and Drug Administration: Laboratory Analysis of Kratom Products for Heavy Metals. Silver Spring, MD, U.S. Food and Drug Administration, 2019. Available at: https://www.fda.gov/news-events/public-health-focus/laboratory-analysis-kratom-products-heavy-metals. Accessed January 17, 2025.

Van Hal M, Dydyk AM, Green MS: Acupuncture. Treasure Island, FL, StatPearls, 2022. Available at: https://www.ncbi.nlm.nih.gov/books/NBK532287/. Accessed February 10, 2025.

Wang F, Li Y, Zhang YJ, et al: Natural products for the prevention and treatment of hangover and alcohol use disorder. Molecules 21(1):64, 2016

Wang Y, Narayanapillai SC, Tessier KM, et al: The impact of one-week dietary supplementation with kava on biomarkers of tobacco use and nitrosamine-based carcinogenesis risk among active smokers. Cancer Prev Res (Phila) 13(5):483–492, 2020 32102948

Warner ML, Kaufman NC, Grundmann O: The pharmacology and toxicology of kratom: from traditional herb to drug of abuse. Int J Legal Med 130(1):127–138, 2016 26511390

Wasko MJ, Witt-Enderby PA, Surratt CK: DARK classics in chemical neuroscience: ibogaine. ACS Chem Neurosci 9(10):2475–2483, 2018 30216039

White A: Trials of acupuncture for drug dependence: a recommendation for hypotheses based on the literature. Acupunct Med 31(3):297–304, 2013 23665887

White CM: The pharmacology, pharmacokinetics, efficacy, and adverse events associated with kava. J Clin Pharmacol 58(11):1396–1405, 2018 29791008

12

Circuit-Based Interventions for Substance Use Disorders

Zafiris Daskalakis, M.D., Ph.D.
Hewa Artin, M.D.

First-line treatment options for substance use disorders (SUDs), such as pharmacotherapy or psychosocial interventions, are not always effective or may be difficult to tolerate for some patients, which has led to a search for novel treatment options for SUDs. Interventional neuromodulatory approaches (also called *circuit-based interventions*) have been investigated as one such set of options. There are many such approaches; for the purposes of this book, we limit the scope to neuromodulation techniques with the most evidence in SUDs, including transcranial magnetic stimulation (TMS), transcranial direct-current stimulation (tDCS), and deep brain stimulation (DBS). We also focus on the most common SUDs that have been investigated with these modalities, including alcohol, nicotine, cocaine, and opioid use disorders. We conclude by reviewing future interventional techniques under investigation for SUDs.

Transcranial Magnetic Stimulation

TMS is a noninvasive method of brain stimulation that involves placement of an electromagnetic coil against the scalp and projection of fluctuating magnetic fields (pulses) into the brain. Employing Faraday's principle of electromagnetic induction, these pulses generate an electrical current that, in turn, is capable of modulating neuronal firing (Klomjai et al. 2015; Rossini and Rossi 2007). Magnetic pulses may be delivered with varying frequency, either as a single pulse or pair of pulses or as a repetitive train. With single or paired pulse stimulation, the effects do not last beyond the stimulation period, and this modality is used in research and diagnostic settings to explore brain functioning (Rossi et al. 2009; Tremblay et al. 2019). In contrast, delivery of repetitive trains of pulses, known as *repetitive transcranial magnetic stimulation* (rTMS), can have longer-lasting effects on underlying brain circuitry that extend beyond the period of acute stimulation. In general, high-frequency rTMS, defined as greater than 1 pulse per second (1 Hz), is associated with increased cortical excitability; in contrast, low-frequency TMS, defined as less than 1 pulse per second (<1 Hz), is associated with a decrease in cortical excitability (Speer et al. 2000). Standard rTMS involves the use of a figure-8 coil, although different coil types have been developed, including an H-coil commonly employed in deep transcranial magnetic stimulation (dTMS), which is thought to stimulate deeper and larger brain volumes (Levkovitz et al. 2015). Different patterns of stimulation have also been developed, such as 1) continuous theta-burst stimulation (cTBS), which is associated with inducing long-term depression (LTD), a persistent reduction of efficacy in synaptic transmission; and 2) intermittent theta-burst stimulation (iTBS), which is associated with inducing long-term potentiation (LTP), an enhancement in efficacy of synaptic transmission.

TMS has been investigated in a range of psychiatric disorders, including depression, bipolar disorder, OCD, PTSD, schizophrenia, and autism spectrum disorder. In these studies, TMS was well tolerated, with common side effects including headache. The most serious complications associated with TMS are seizures, although these are extremely rare in modern treatments (Rossi et al. 2009). Despite the rarity of seizures associated with

TMS treatment, careful consideration of medications that can theoretically lower seizure thresholds, such as bupropion, amitriptyline, and clozapine, is warranted. Rather than necessitating discontinuation, these medications typically require diligent monitoring, especially when adjustments to medication regimens are made (Dobek et al. 2015). Such monitoring may include periodic reassessment of the resting motor threshold. Additionally, providers must remain cautious with the use of substances known to decrease the seizure threshold, such as amphetamines and alcohol; they must also consider other factors that increase seizure risk, such as sleep deprivation and a history of seizure disorders (Stultz et al. 2020). A thorough risk-benefit analysis is recommended, focusing on vigilant monitoring to maintain both safety and the ongoing efficacy of TMS treatment.

Supportive findings led the FDA to approve rTMS in 2008 for treatment-resistant depression. Since then, various rTMS devices have been approved for treatment-resistant depression and OCD (Homan et al. 2021). dTMS was also approved by the FDA for the indication of short-term smoking cessation (Young et al. 2021).

The use of TMS for SUD treatment is being investigated. Initial findings in this area are promising, although more research is needed to discover the optimal treatment parameters of TMS for SUDs, including frequency of administration, site of stimulation, and pattern of stimulation. The mechanism of action of TMS in the treatment of SUDs also needs to be further elucidated. A 2021 review of the efficacy of TMS in the treatment of alcohol, tobacco, and cocaine use disorders highlighted that rTMS in particular showed promise in reducing craving and consumption of these substances. The authors proposed that neurotransmitter changes brought about by rTMS in the mesolimbic and mesostriatal systems may facilitate increased release of dopamine, which may account for the positive effects documented (Antonelli et al. 2021). Furthermore, a 2024 systematic review and meta-analysis of neuromodulation techniques (rTMS, DBS, and tDCS) reported that rTMS had a positive impact on alcohol and tobacco craving, consumption, and relapse, especially if multiple stimulation sessions were applied and the left dorsolateral prefrontal cortex (DLPFC) was targeted (Mehta et al. 2024). These findings are discussed in further detail in "Deep Brain Stimulation."

A final practical consideration of TMS is price. TMS availability is becoming more widespread, but there is wide variability in insurance coverage for it. For example, although Medicare covers TMS treatment for major depressive disorder (MDD) (as of 2022), Medicaid coverage may vary from state to state (Centers for Medicare and Medicaid Services 2022). Private-pay treatment options are also available, with costs varying significantly, sometimes into the thousands of dollars. As stated earlier in this section, TMS is not approved by the FDA for the treatment of SUDs outside of short-term smoking cessation.

Tobacco Craving and Use

TMS has been investigated in targeting tobacco use and cravings, and dTMS has been approved for short-term smoking cessation. One of the first studies investigating the effect of TMS on cigarette smoking was conducted in patients randomly assigned with crossover using a single day of high-frequency (20-Hz) rTMS over the left DLPFC versus sham (Eichhammer et al. 2003). Active rTMS significantly reduced the number of cigarettes consumed over sham TMS, although cravings were not affected (Eichhammer et al. 2003). Similar effects occurred in a study of smokers randomly assigned to 10 days of active high-frequency (10-Hz) rTMS or sham. In this study, active treatment reduced cigarette consumption and picture-induced cravings, although these effects dissipated with time (Amiaz et al. 2009). Another study looked at smoking outcomes in smokers who were abstinent for 6 hours and randomly assigned with crossover to high-frequency (10-Hz) rTMS to the left DLPFC with electroencephalography (Pripfl et al. 2014). The study reported that both nicotine craving and electroencephalography delta power, which has been linked to dopaminergic activity and may provide a mechanistic understanding of rTMS in SUDs, were significantly reduced after active stimulation versus sham. However, these changes did not directly correlate with each other (Pripfl et al. 2014).

Other stimulation parameters and treatment locations have been investigated for smoking cessation. dTMS was investigated in a large placebo-controlled study with 115 participants randomly assigned to 13 sessions of dTMS at high frequency, low frequency, or sham. High-frequency dTMS, but not low-frequency or sham dTMS, reduced the number of cigarettes smoked and increased abstinence rates up to 6 months after treatment. Interestingly, half of participants were shown a smoking cue just before stimulation; the study found that exposure to this cue increased abstinence rates, suggesting a possible augmenting tool that may be employed with TMS (Dinur-Klein et al. 2014).

rTMS has also been investigated as a tool for tobacco use and cravings in specific patient populations. In a randomized controlled trial on schizophrenia that was conducted over 10 weeks, six participants received active bilateral 20-Hz stimulation to the DLPFC and nine received sham. The patients receiving active stimulation had reduced cravings after the first week, although abstinence rates did not increase (Wing et al. 2012). A subsequent study of the effects of rTMS in patients with schizophrenia found that after 21 sessions of high-frequency rTMS (10-Hz) over the left DLPFC, cigarette smoking was significantly lower in patients who received active stimulation versus sham (Prikryl et al. 2014). However, negative results have also been demonstrated in this patient population (Kozak et al. 2018). rTMS can improve smoking outcomes in populations with comorbid depression and anxiety. In a 2021 randomized controlled trial investigating the effects of 10 days of high-frequency (20-Hz) rTMS over the left DLPFC on smoking, anxiety, and depression, Abdelrahman et al. (2021) found that cigarette consumption per day decreased in both the active and sham groups, but improvement persisted for 3 months longer in the active group versus the sham group. Furthermore, there was a significant decrease in Hamilton Rating Scale for Depression and Hamilton Anxiety Scale scores (measures of depressive and anxiety symptoms, respectively) in the active group (Abdelrahman et al. 2021).

TMS has shown promise as an adjunct to nicotine replacement therapy and psychotherapy. In a study using high-frequency (20-Hz) rTMS to the left DLPFC for 10 treatment sessions along with an evidence-based self-help intervention, active rTMS was found to reduce the relative risk of relapse, increase abstinence rates, increase the use of the self-help intervention, and decrease delay discounting, which is associated with cigarette smoking (Sheffer et al. 2018). A pilot study showed that four sessions of add-on iTBS to cognitive-behavioral therapy did not affect craving but increased the abstinence rate in the active treatment group versus the sham group at 3 months, although not at 6 and 12 months. The authors suggested that four treatment sessions may not be sufficient to achieve durable effects (Dieler et al. 2014). A study investigating the combination of 2 weeks of low-frequency (1-Hz) rTMS of the right DLPFC with nicotine replacement therapy found an increase in the rate of abstinence with active rTMS versus sham 2 weeks after quitting. Nicotine patches were then continued, although no further increase in the rate of abstinence was seen at 6 or 12 weeks, suggesting that with these stimulation parameters, the effects of rTMS were not long lasting (Trojak et al. 2015). Finally, in a multicenter, double-blind, randomized controlled trial, 262 chronic smokers were randomly assigned to 3 weeks of daily bilateral rTMS or sham to the lateral prefrontal cortex (PFC) and insular cortex, then weekly rTMS for 3 weeks (Zangen et al. 2021). The investigators found a significantly greater reduction in craving and cigarette consumption with active stimulation than with sham (Zangen et al. 2021). This study ultimately was important in the FDA approving dTMS for smoking cessation.

Further investigation is warranted on whether other parameters will be approved for this indication, how long the effects of treatment last, and how to maximize efficacy of treatment by pairing it with other evidence-based modalities.

Alcohol Craving and Use

TMS has also been investigated in various studies as a treatment for alcohol craving and use. One of the first studies investigating the use of TMS in patients with alcohol dependence was conducted in 2010, in which 30 patients and 15 control subjects were randomly assigned (2:1) to either active high-frequency (10-Hz) rTMS or sham targeted to the right DLPFC for 10 treatment sessions (Mishra et al. 2010). The investigators found a reduction of alcohol craving (measured with the Alcohol Craving Questionnaire) with active TMS after the last session and at 1-month follow-up (Mishra et al. 2010). This finding was further supported in a 2015 open-label study of high-frequency (20-Hz) rTMS to the right DLPFC in patients with alcohol use disorder (AUD) who had undergone recent detoxification from alcohol (Herremans et al. 2015). They found a decrease in general cravings after 15 sessions of rTMS, although cue-induced cravings were not affected (Herremans et al. 2015). In another study of patients with alcohol dependence who received 10 sessions of high-frequency (10-Hz) stimulation to the right versus left DLPFC, subjects showed a significant reduction in craving scores with either right-sided or left-sided rTMS. The study noted that there was no difference in craving between groups (Mishra et al. 2015).

Bilateral stimulation with dTMS has also been investigated for AUD. In a 2013 study of dTMS in patients with comorbid dysthymic disorder and AUD, three patients underwent high-frequency stimulation (20 Hz) of the DLPFC with dTMS for 28 days. They showed improvement in both anxiety and depressive symptoms as well as alcohol craving at the end of treatment and at 6-month follow-up (Rapinesi et al. 2013). This work was further supported by a follow-up study of 23 patients (12 with MDD and 11 with comorbid MDD and AUD) employing 20-Hz dTMS (Rapinesi et al. 2015). The authors found improvements in clinical status in both groups as well as reductions in Obsessive-Compulsive Drinking Scale scores in patients with comorbid AUD and MDD, which were maintained at 6 months (Rapinesi et al. 2015). Building on these studies and pointing to a possible mechanism of action, a sham-controlled study with 11 patients utilizing dTMS and SPECT imaging demonstrated that at baseline, patients with AUD had higher dopamine transporter availability than healthy control subjects and that patients treated with 12 days of 10-Hz real dTMS targeted to the DLPFC showed a reduction of dopamine transporter availability as well as a decrease in alcohol intake versus the sham control (Addolorato et al. 2017). Beyond targeting the DLPFC, the medial prefrontal cortex (mPFC) has also been investigated as a potential therapeutic target. One sham-controlled study conducted targeting the mPFC found that 10 sessions of 20-Hz treatments using real dTMS led to decreases in craving visual analog scale scores and mean number of drinks per day, as well as reduced blood cortisol and prolactin (Ceccanti et al. 2015). In a 2022 study of 51 patients with AUD randomly assigned to sham or active dTMS over the mPFC and anterior cingulate cortex (ACC), craving and percentage of heavy drinking days were significantly lower in the active group versus the sham control group (Harel et al. 2022).

Additionally, different stimulation patterns have been tested in studies on alcohol craving and use. In a sham-controlled study using cTBS targeting the mPFC of 49 substance-dependent individuals (24 of these specifically with AUD), a decreased blood-oxygen-level–dependent (BOLD) signal in the orbitofrontal cortex, as well as in other cortical nodes associated with reactivity to drug cues, was found with real cTBS (Hanlon et al. 2017). Although these studies are supportive of a potential role of TMS in treatment of alcohol craving and use, not all studies have demonstrated positive findings. A 2012 sham-controlled study failed to show a reduction in alcohol craving with one single high-frequency (20-Hz) stimulation of the right DLPFC in hospitalized patients who had recently undergone alcohol detoxification (Herremans et al. 2012). Another sham-controlled study of 10 days of high-frequency (20-Hz) stimulation of the left DLPFC in 19 female subjects who had been detoxified from alcohol failed to find a significant difference in alcohol craving between active and sham treatments (Höppner et al. 2011). A sham-controlled study by Del Felice et al. (2016) in subjects with alcohol dependence showed that after four sessions of high-frequency (10-Hz) rTMS over the left DLPFC, subjects were able to improve performance on an inhibitory control task, had reduced symptoms of depression, and had a decrease of fast electroencephalography frequencies compared with the sham group. However, real TMS was not more effective than sham at reducing alcohol intake and craving (Del Felice et al. 2016). Finally, a 2018 study showed that cTBS of the right DLPFC compared with sham actually led to an impairment of inhibitory control and increased alcohol consumption (McNeill et al. 2018).

Overall, the efficacy of TMS in alcohol craving and use remains to be determined. There is methodological heterogeneity within positive and negative studies, and this warrants further exploration. Interestingly, some of the positive trials point to a potential role for modulation of dopaminergic neurotransmission. Furthermore, even some of the negative findings of craving and alcohol intake point toward effects of TMS on neurocognitive function, which may have relevance in the treatment of AUD.

Cocaine Craving and Use

TMS has also been explored in the setting of cocaine craving and use. The first study investigating the use of rTMS on cocaine craving consisted of a randomized crossover design, with six male subjects meeting criteria for cocaine dependence (Camprodon et al. 2007). Participants received two sessions of high-frequency (10-Hz) rTMS over the left or right DLPFC, with a week between sessions. Cravings were measured with visual scales 10 minutes before, directly after, and 4 hours after rTMS. Right-sided but not left-sided rTMS led to significant decreases in craving by 19% after treatment, but these effects returned to pre-TMS baseline after 4 hours (Camprodon et al. 2007). A 2008 study with 36 subjects (31 male and 5 female) with symptoms meeting DSM-IV criteria (American Psychiatric Association 1994) for cocaine dependence underwent high-frequency (15-Hz) rTMS directed at the left DLPFC for 10 treatment sessions (Politi et al. 2008). rTMS gradually reduced cocaine cravings, with a notable decrease by the seventh session. Of note, this study was not sham controlled (Politi et al. 2008). Another study was conducted with 32 patients whose symptoms met DSM-5 criteria

(American Psychiatric Association 2013) for cocaine use disorder. They were randomly assigned to either high-frequency (15-Hz) rTMS directed to the left DLPFC or to a control of pharmacological agents including pramipexole 0.35 mg tid, bupropion 150 mg/day, oxazepam 15 mg tid, triazolam 0.25 mg/day, and γ-hydroxybutyrate 1.75 g/day for 29 days. Patients who received rTMS had a higher number of cocaine-free urine samples as well as significantly decreased cravings. In the second stage of the study, patients were offered the choice to continue their current treatment or to switch to the other treatment. There was no significant difference in results between patients who switched to rTMS from the control and those in the original rTMS group (Terraneo et al. 2016). Similarly, another study reported benefit from 10 sessions of high-frequency (15-Hz) stimulation of the left DLPFC in patients with cocaine use disorder (Pettorruso et al. 2018). Promisingly, a 2020 retrospective study of 284 outpatients demonstrated that 3 months of high-frequency (15-Hz) stimulation of the left DLPFC led to a reduction of cocaine use. Long-term follow-up of these subjects showed that the median time to first relapse was 91 days (Madeo et al. 2020).

dTMS has also been investigated in cocaine use disorder. In a 2016 study by Bolloni et al., 18 subjects (16 male and 2 female) whose symptoms met DSM-IV criteria for cocaine use disorder were recruited and randomly assigned to receive either active high-frequency (10-Hz) rTMS or sham delivered to the bilateral PFC. Four subjects were excluded because of an extremely high amount of cocaine measured by hair analysis before treatment, and three subjects from the sham group and one from the active group dropped out before completing the study. Hair was analyzed at the end of treatment and 3 and 6 months later. The study found no difference at individual time points in the amount of cocaine detected but found a significant decrease in cocaine use from baseline to 3 and 6 months later in the active group versus the sham group (Bolloni et al. 2016).

Other sites of the brain have also been investigated as potential targets of stimulation. In a study using dTMS targeting the mPFC and the dorsal ACC, subjects with cocaine use disorder were admitted to an inpatient unit and randomly assigned to high-frequency (10-Hz) stimulation, low-frequency (1-Hz) stimulation, or sham stimulation for 3 weeks. The study findings suggested that high-frequency stimulation could reduce the amount of smoked cocaine over low-frequency stimulation or sham (Martinez et al. 2018).

TBS has also been explored as a novel modality to target cocaine cravings and use. In a single-blind, sham-controlled crossover trial, Hanlon et al. (2017) investigated cTBS targeting the mPFC in subjects with cocaine use disorder. Subjects underwent TMS-BOLD scanning before and after treatment. Craving was monitored with self-report before and after treatment. The study found that active cTBS to the mPFC led to a decrease in activity in the striatum and anterior insula, and active stimulation was more likely to reduce craving than sham TMS (Hanlon et al. 2017). The safety and tolerability of iTBS was also tested in a study of individuals with cocaine use disorder given three sessions of iTBS targeting the left DLPFC per day for 10 days. Accelerated iTBS to the left DLPFC reduced both the frequency and the amount of cocaine use (Steele et al. 2019). Finally, a study attempting to shed light on optimal treatment parameters for TMS in cocaine use disorder compared bilateral iTBS versus high-frequency rTMS (15 Hz) in subjects seeking treatment for cocaine use. This study found nearly equivalent effects on cocaine intake, evaluated with urine tests at the end of treatment; these findings suggested potential equivalence in efficacy between the two treatment modalities in the setting of cocaine use disorder (Sanna et al. 2019).

Opioid Craving and Use

There is limited published literature on the use of rTMS for opioid use disorder. The first published study investigating the effect of rTMS on opioid use was conducted in 2016 in subjects with a history of heroin abuse. This study found that 5 days of high-frequency (10-Hz) stimulation over the left DLPFC reduced cue-induced heroin cravings (Shen et al. 2016). In a case report, a 25-year-old man with opioid use disorder and cocaine use disorder was administered seven treatments of high-frequency (10-Hz) rTMS targeting the left DLPFC over the course of 3 weeks. The authors found a large reduction of approximately 60%–82% in cue-induced cravings for heroin and cocaine (Mahoney et al. 2020).

A larger recent randomized controlled trial of rTMS in the setting of opioid use was conducted to further characterize the effects and optimal parameters. A total of 118 male patients with a history of recurrent heroin use disorder were recruited, and 112 patients were randomly assigned to high-frequency (10-Hz) rTMS, low-frequency (1-Hz) rTMS, or a waitlist control group (Liu et al. 2020). Patients receiving rTMS received 20 sessions over a month, directed at the left DLPFC. The study found that in the 10- and 1-Hz-treated groups, cue-induced cravings were significantly decreased compared with the control group, and this effect lasted up to 60 days after cessation of rTMS treatment. The study suggested that given the right parameters, TMS may prove to be a beneficial treatment option in opioid use disorder, with potentially durable effects. It is interesting to note that both high-frequency and low-frequency rTMS had a beneficial effect. The authors proposed that the mechanism of rTMS efficacy in opioid use may be related to changes in metabolism, plasticity, or modulation of monoamine concentration, and that the benefit derived from both 10- and 1-Hz frequency stimulation may be attributable to the varying effect that these frequencies have on the brain. Further work is warranted to better characterize the treatment effects and mechanism of action of rTMS in opioid use and cravings.

Transcranial Direct-Current Stimulation

tDCS is another interventional approach that is being investigated for SUDs. tDCS is a noninvasive method of brain stimulation that involves placement of electrodes on the scalp with delivery of a low-amplitude electrical current (Thair et al. 2017). One proposed mechanism of action of tDCS is a shift in resting membrane potential of neurons. tDCS can be delivered as positive stimulation (anodal), which is associated with shifting membrane potentials toward depolarization, or as negative stimulation (cathodal), which is associated with shifting membrane potentials toward hyperpolarization. Additionally, tDCS has been suggested to promote LTP-like effects at the anode and LTD-like effects at the cathode (Woods et al. 2016). These effects and their durability appear to be dependent on factors including the duration and intensity of the current. tDCS has been investigated in the settings of Parkinson's disease, chronic pain, depression, and anxiety; early studies suggested potential benefit in these settings, although there are no FDA-approved indications for tDCS at this time (Lefaucheur et al. 2017). There are no serious adverse effects reported in the tDCS literature, although the treatment has been associated with headache and irritation at the site of stimulation (Bikson et al. 2016). tDCS has begun to be studied in the setting of SUDs. Although evidence is somewhat limited, preliminary results show a potential benefit of tDCS in targeting substance cravings and use. Research thus far has mostly focused on targeting the

DLPFC, with the hypothesis that stimulation of this area with tDCS may serve to enhance executive control that may be impaired in the setting of substance use. Further research is needed to define the optimal treatment parameters, including laterality and number of sessions associated with therapeutic benefit. Additionally, research is needed to elucidate the mechanism of action of the therapeutic effect of tDCS in SUDs.

Tobacco Craving and Use

tDCS has been investigated in the setting of tobacco craving and use. One study used a crossover design in 24 subjects, in which they received three different types of brain stimulation: active anodal tDCS over the left DLPFC, active anodal tDCS over the right DLPFC, and sham. Active tDCS of the left or right DLPFC significantly reduced smoking cravings in the presence of smoking-related cues compared with sham (Fregni et al. 2008). Based on these preliminary data, the same group designed a follow-up study investigating the effects of repeated tDCS sessions, in which subjects were randomly assigned to receive either sham or active anodal tDCS over 5 consecutive days of stimulation (Boggio et al. 2009). The authors showed a cumulative effect of tDCS on modifying cue-induced cravings and found that active stimulation led to a decrease in cravings after exposure to smoking cues compared with sham. Additionally, they noted that the active tDCS group had a small but significant reduction in number of cigarettes smoked (Boggio et al. 2009). In a third study by this group, participants were randomly assigned with crossover to two 5-day courses of active anodal tDCS over the right DLPFC or sham. Active stimulation led to a decrease in the number of cigarettes smoked (as tracked by a cigarette diary), and this effect lasted 4 days after the end of active stimulation (Fecteau et al. 2014).

Another placebo-controlled randomized study was conducted using anodal tDCS to the left DLPFC versus sham, along with monitoring of functional neuroimaging changes, heart rate variability, and subjective measurements of craving. The authors observed that during cue exposures, participants had increased connectivity between the orbitofrontal cortex and the DLPFC after active tDCS versus sham, although active tDCS did not significantly alter cravings or heart rate variability (Kroczek et al. 2016). In a study of 40 daily and social smokers using 10 sessions of sham versus active tDCS over the left DLPFC, the authors found a significant decrease in number of cigarettes smoked by daily smokers as well as by social smokers in the active group versus the sham group (Hajloo et al. 2019). One promising study of 210 male subjects randomly assigned to five groups (bupropion 300 mg/day for 8 weeks, active tDCS for 4 or 12 weeks, and sham tDCS for 4 or 12 weeks) found that 12 weeks of active tDCS had a clinical effect similar to that of bupropion (Ghorbani Behnam et al. 2019).

However, not all results for tDCS are supportive. A study in smokers randomly assigned to sham versus anodal tDCS to the left DLPFC found a reduction in scores for mood disturbance and other measures of mood and anxiety with active tDCS; there was no difference in cigarette craving (Xu et al. 2013). In a study in subjects randomly assigned to either active anodal tDCS to the right DLPFC or sham, the authors found that active stimulation reduced cravings, but this did not translate to a difference in number of cigarettes smoked or exhaled carbon monoxide after 1 month (Mondino et al. 2018). Finally, a study was conducted in 106 smokers randomly assigned to three sessions of sham or anodal 1- or 2-mA tDCS to the left DLPFC. The investigators found no effect of active tDCS on the ability to maintain abstinence during a 7-day quitting period, nor was there any change in the number of cigarettes smoked per day (Falcone et al. 2019). Overall, although there may be a role for tDCS in reducing tobacco craving, further research is needed, and optimal treatment parameters remain to be determined.

Alcohol Craving and Use

tDCS has also been investigated in the setting of alcohol craving and use. One study investigating the effect of tDCS on cravings was conducted in 13 subjects with alcohol dependence. Subjects were randomly assigned with crossover to receive active anodal tDCS to the left DLPFC/cathodal tDCS to the right DLPFC, anodal tDCS to the right DLPFC/cathodal tDCS to the left DLPFC, or sham tDCS after observing a video with alcohol cues. The study found that active stimulation to either the left or right DLPFC significantly decreased cravings for alcohol compared with sham stimulation (Boggio et al. 2008). Another sham-controlled study of subjects with alcohol dependence randomly assigned to either anodal tDCS to the left DLPFC or sham tDCS, repeated once a week for 5 weeks, found a larger reduction in cravings and depressive symptoms in subjects receiving active tDCS than sham after treatment (da Silva et al. 2013). The authors also obtained event-related potentials (ERPs) before and after treatment and found that active tDCS led to less neural activation in the PFC than sham after exposure to alcohol-related and neutral cues. Of note, however, da Silva et al. (2013) highlighted an increased trend toward relapse in the active tDCS group. The same group conducted a study using repetitive tDCS over 5 consecutive days in alcohol-dependent subjects randomly assigned to either active bilateral left cathodal/right anodal or sham tDCS. Significantly less relapse was found in the active tDCS group at 6-month follow-up. Interestingly, no differences in cravings, depressive or anxious symptoms, or global mental status were observed between the two groups; however, the active tDCS group reported improved perception of overall quality of life and subjective assessment of their environment (Klauss et al. 2014). The same group carried out a similar study but extended it to 10 sessions every other day. Here, 49 patients with AUD were randomly assigned to either active cathodal left/anodal right tDCS or sham tDCS. Craving scores were found to decrease in both groups, but this reached significance only in the active tDCS group. Additionally, at 3-month follow-up, 72.7% of patients in the real tDCS group were abstinent, whereas 72.2% of patients in the sham tDCS group had experienced alcohol relapse (Klauss et al. 2018). In another study in 30 patients with alcohol dependence randomly assigned to either active left cathodal/right anodal or sham tDCS, subjects receiving active stimulation had decreased cravings and increased startle amplitudes after being presented with alcohol-related cues compared with sham (Wietschorke et al. 2016).

Although these studies suggest a possible role of tDCS in the setting of alcohol dependence, other studies have had negative findings. Two studies combining tDCS with cognitive bias modification (CBM), an intervention that aims to retrain cognitive biases that are linked to alcohol use and has shown an improvement in clinical outcomes, found that in a design that included random assignment to control/active tDCS over the left DLPFC, control/sham tDCS, CBM/active tDCS, or CBM/sham tDCS, there was a limited positive effect of active tDCS on cue-induced cravings but not on overall cravings, and no enhancement of the effects of CBM was observed with tDCS (den Uyl et al. 2016). A follow-up study by the same group showed similar results, although den Uyl et al. (2017) noted that relapse rates showed a trend toward decreasing with active tDCS versus sham after a year.

Cocaine Craving and Use

tDCS has been investigated in the setting of cocaine craving and use. A few early studies in this area measured brain changes induced by tDCS in the setting of crack-cocaine addiction. In the first study, 13 crack-cocaine users were randomly assigned to receive a single session of either cathodal left/anodal right tDCS to DLPFC or sham (Conti and Nakamura-Palacios 2014). Subjects were monitored with electroencephalography. The authors found that the N2 component of the ERP of the ACC was decreased during exposure to crack-related cues in the active tDCS group, whereas the opposite effect was observed in the sham-treated group. No difference was seen on exposure to neutral cues (Conti and Nakamura-Palacios 2014). In another study, 13 crack-cocaine users were randomly assigned to five sessions of left cathodal/right anodal tDCS or sham tDCS once every other day. A single stimulation of active tDCS was found to lead to a decrease in the intensity of the P3 segment of the ERP after crack-related cues, as well as to an increase in intensity with neutral cues, which was the opposite of what was observed with sham. On the other hand, repeated active tDCS stimulation led to increased current density in a wide variety of prefrontal areas when visualizing crack-related cues but to decreased current density in prefrontal areas other than the DLPFC when visualizing neutral cues (Conti et al. 2014). These studies suggested the possibility of modulation of brain processes in cocaine use with tDCS, which may have important clinical applications.

Another study observing changes in risk-taking behavior was conducted with recently abstinent cocaine users versus control subjects (Gorini et al. 2014). Subjects were randomly assigned with crossover to active anodal tDCS to the right DLPFC/cathodal tDCS to the left DLPFC, anodal left/cathodal right tDCS, and sham, spaced 48 hours apart, and were tasked with a balloon analog risk task (BART) and game of dice task (GDT). Gorini et al. found that right and left active tDCS reduced risky behaviors in those who completed the BART task. In the GDT task, cocaine-dependent subjects and control subjects both decreased risk-taking behavior after stimulation of the right DLPFC; interestingly, risk-taking behavior increased in cocaine-dependent subjects after stimulation of the left DLPFC (Gorini et al. 2014).

Beyond effects on brain function, the effects of tDCS on craving and quality of life in cocaine users has also been assessed. In a study conducted in crack-cocaine users randomly assigned to five sessions of active left cathodal/right anodal tDCS versus sham, investigators found a decrease in craving and positive trends in anxiety and quality of life in the group treated with active tDCS (Batista et al. 2015). In a previous study, however, patients with symptoms meeting

DSM-5 diagnostic criteria for cocaine use disorder were randomly assigned to active cathodal left/anodal right tDCS to the DLPFC versus sham, applied once every other day for 10 days. Researchers found no difference between active versus sham tDCS in terms of effect on cravings (Klauss et al. 2018).

Verveer et al. (2020) further explored the use of tDCS in the setting of cocaine use disorder. In this study, 59 patients were randomly assigned to 10 sessions over 5 days of either active left cathodal/right anodal or sham tDCS. Researchers found no significant effect on days of cocaine use or cravings, and they found no differences on measures of inhibitory control and decision-making as measured by a go/no-go task and a two-choice gambling task between active tDCS and sham (Verveer et al. 2020). Although there is limited evidence for the benefit of tDCS in the setting of cocaine use and cravings, objective changes after active tDCS have been observed with changes in components of ERPs in cocaine users. The clinical utility of this measurement remains to be determined, and further studies are needed to determine the role of tDCS in the setting of cocaine use.

Opioid Craving and Use

There are limited studies investigating the use of tDCS in the setting of opioid craving and use. One of the first studies to investigate this was conducted in heroin-using participants randomly assigned to either active tDCS or sham, with the cathode electrode placed bilaterally over the frontal-parietal-temporal area and the anode over the occipital lobe. Real tDCS was found to reduce craving scores significantly over sham after exposure to heroin cues (Wang et al. 2016). Another study investigating the effect of tDCS on cravings in heroin users was conducted in male heroin users randomly assigned to receive two administrations of either active anodal tDCS over the right DLPFC/cathodal left tDCS or sham. Investigators found that cravings significantly decreased in the group treated with active tDCS (Sharifi-Fardshad et al. 2018).

A 2019 study was conducted to investigate the effect of tDCS on the primary outcome of opium craving and the secondary outcome of depression and anxiety when combined with standard methadone maintenance. Sixty participants were randomly assigned to receive either active anodal right/cathodal left tDCS with methadone, sham tDCS with methadone, or standard methadone maintenance alone. The group treated with active tDCS with methadone had decreases in opium cravings and depression and anxiety symptoms compared with the other two treatment groups (Taremian et al. 2019). These studies suggest a potential benefit of tDCS in the setting of opioid craving and, intriguingly, a potential role for tDCS in augmenting the effect of standard methadone therapy.

Deep Brain Stimulation

DBS is an invasive method of brain stimulation that involves implanting electrodes directly within the brain to stimulate specific areas of the brain and affect brain function. DBS was approved for Parkinson's disease in 1997, and has since been approved for dystonia, epilepsy, Tourette syndrome, and OCD under a humanitarian device exemption. Given the invasive nature of the procedure, DBS is typically reserved for the setting of severe treatment-refractory conditions, and safety considerations include those that are typically considered in the setting of an invasive neurosurgery.

Some reports have found that DBS also provides a benefit in comorbid SUDs, and limited trials have been conducted exploring potential benefits of DBS in the setting of addiction. In these studies, the nucleus accumbens (NAc) is often targeted as a site of stimulation because it is a key node in reward circuitry and is thought to play an important role in addictive behavior (Salgado and Kaplitt 2015). These studies suggest that DBS may have a potential role in the setting of severe treatment-resistant SUDs. A 2024 systematic review and meta-analysis also cited support for DBS's potential positive impact on substance use, summarizing that four studies examining the effects of DBS on AUD all showed significant decreases in alcohol consumption and/or craving after treatment, and that similar results were seen in individuals with tobacco and opioid use disorder who underwent DBS (albeit there were fewer total studies) (Mehta et al. 2024).

Tobacco Craving and Use

One retrospective study of patients who had been treated in Germany with DBS of the NAc for severe anxiety, OCD, and Tourette syndrome found that of the patients with comorbid nicotine dependence, those who were highly motivated to quit and less nicotine dependent were more likely to quit after DBS of the NAc (Kuhn et al. 2009). Another case report from the Netherlands described a 47-year-old woman treated with DBS to the NAc for refractory OCD. After treatment, the patient experienced improvements in OCD symptoms; interestingly, 10 months after treatment with DBS, she found she was no longer interested in smoking and was able to stop without cravings or withdrawal. She also began dieting 2 weeks later and reached her goal weight (Mantione et al. 2010).

Alcohol Craving and Use

DBS has also been studied in the setting of alcohol use. One of the first case reports suggesting a possible benefit of DBS in addiction was in a 54-year-old patient with severe anxiety, depression, and comorbid alcohol dependence who underwent DBS of the NAc to target anxiety and depression (Kuhn et al. 2007). Interestingly, the patient demonstrated minimal change in anxiety and depressive symptoms but a profound change in alcohol use after treatment—from a more than 10-year history of drinking and consuming more than 10 drinks per day to only occasional consumption of alcohol (1–2 drinks on average). Positive effects were observed even 12 months after treatment (Kuhn et al. 2007). One small study investigating DBS in alcohol dependence showed positive effects with stimulation of the NAc. In the initial study of three patients, two maintained abstinence and one had a reduction in drinking days at 1-year follow-up (Müller et al. 2009). In a follow-up study of up to 8 years in these three patients, along with follow-up of two additionally treated patients, all patients were reported to have a reduction in cravings, and two patients were able to remain abstinent for years after follow-up. Two patients died after 4 and 8 years; these deaths were not considered to be attributable to DBS and were suspected to be due to use of alcohol (Müller et al. 2016). One case report pointed to the possible mechanism of DBS in the treatment of addiction (Heldmann et al. 2012). A 38-year-old man with severe alcohol dependence was treated with DBS with electrodes stimulating the NAc, the bed nucleus of the stria terminalis, and the ventral pallidum. Treatment with DBS led to abstinence, and the subject made less risky, more careful choices in decision-making tasks than when his DBS was switched off. PET imaging also showed activation in areas implicated in behavioral control, including the paracingulate cortex, precuneus, hippocampus, and temporal poles, with active DBS (Heldmann et al. 2012).

Cocaine Craving and Use

DBS has also been investigated in the setting of cocaine dependence in a double-blind trial composed of three phases (Gonçalves-Ferreira et al. 2016). The subject in this study was a 36-year-old man with a history of polysubstance abuse and symptoms meeting DSM-IV criteria for cocaine dependence. In the first phase, lasting 9 months, DBS was implanted; during this phase, stimulation parameters were optimized and refractoriness from cocaine was confirmed. In the next phase, lasting 9 months, stimulation was randomly assigned to either on/off with crossover, and there were 3 months of single-blind off-stimulation. Finally, in the last phase, lasting 12 months, continuous stimulation was delivered. The study investigators found that after 2.5 years, DBS resulted in significant improvement in terms of cocaine dependence (measured by subjective impression, rating scales, and number of negative urinalysis results). The study particularly noted that useful anatomical targets of stimulation appeared to be the posterior NAc and the bed nucleus of the stria terminalis (Gonçalves-Ferreira et al. 2016).

Opioid Craving and Use

Building on studies conducted in China demonstrating that ablating the NAc with stereotactic surgery had beneficial effects in the setting of opioid addiction, one case study was conducted with DBS to target the NAc in a patient who had been using heroin 1–1.5 g/day for 5 years and for whom numerous attempts at detoxification had failed. DBS leads were implanted bilaterally into the NAc, and pulses were delivered consistently over 2.5 years. After 3 years, the patient and family requested that the pulse generator be removed. Interestingly, there was no relapse at 6-year follow-up with the pulse generator removed, and the patient was able to resume working and experienced improvements in depression and anxiety self-rating scale scores. Additionally, the patient was noted to have reduced cigarette smoking from approximately 40 to 10 cigarettes per day (Zhou et al. 2011).

Another study with DBS targeting the NAc was conducted in China in eight patients with a long-term history of heroin use and multiple relapses (Chen et al. 2019). Stimulation continued for 24 months, and five patients were able to remain abstinent for 3 years, even after the stimulation had ended. Two of the eight patients experienced relapse at 10 months and 7 months following surgery, and one patient was lost to follow-up. The authors noted that the patients who were able to maintain abstinence also experienced decreased cravings and improved subjective quality of life, as well as changes in metabolism in the inferior frontal gyrus, the middle temporal gyrus, and the angular, precuneus, and supramarginal gyri (Chen et al. 2019). These early results are promising, although further research is warranted.

Future Directions

Directions for future research to consider include identifying therapeutic mechanisms of interventional techniques, further investigating the use of interventional techniques in SUDs and in SUDs with psychiatric comorbidities, and developing novel treatment modalities. One modality that may allow for a clearer understanding of the mechanism of action of interventional techniques includes the concurrent use of TMS and functional MRI imaging. This promising modality may allow for a more direct mapping of the effect of rTMS stimulation and the behavioral effects of rTMS to changes in brain activity (Bergmann et al. 2021). Another area of future research could involve investigating the use of interventional techniques in SUDs with comorbid psychiatric disorders. Given the high prevalence of comorbidities with SUDs and the established efficacy of rTMS in the setting of psychiatric conditions such as depression, clinical trials to assess the use of rTMS in SUDs with comorbid conditions are needed.

Beyond the techniques reviewed in this chapter, novel interventional techniques are also currently under investigation with limited studies in the setting of SUDs. One noninvasive interventional technique under investigation is focused ultrasound, which uses converging beams of ultrasound that, depending on frequency, can either ablate or alter the functioning of normal neuronal structures. This treatment has been approved by the FDA for Parkinson's disease and essential tremor, and it is now under investigation in certain psychiatric conditions. Another invasive interventional technique being investigated is vagus nerve stimulation (VNS). VNS involves the use of an implantable device that stimulates the vagus nerve to modulate brain function. Additionally, noninvasive methods of VNS are being studied. Currently, invasive VNS is approved by the FDA for epilepsy and depression, and the FDA has approved a noninvasive device for the treatment of cluster headaches. Investigations are now underway for the use of VNS in SUDs.

Key Points

- For individuals who have not benefited (or only partially so) from pharmacotherapies or psychosocial interventions for substance use disorders (SUDs), circuit-based interventions such as transcranial

magnetic stimulation (TMS), transcranial direct-current stimulation (tDCS), and deep brain stimulation (DBS) are alternative approaches for which there is an emerging evidence base.
- TMS is a noninvasive method of brain stimulation that involves electromagnetic induction of electrical currents that are capable of strategically modulating neuronal firing. Of the circuit-based interventions considered in this chapter, TMS has the most evidence to date, with recent FDA approval of deep transcranial magnetic stimulation (dTMS) as an aid in the setting of short-term smoking cessation.
- Repetitive transcranial magnetic stimulation (rTMS) and dTMS have both been studied in the treatment of tobacco, cocaine, opioid, and alcohol use disorders, with results in some studies suggesting some relief from cravings in particular. However, the results are inconsistent, and mechanisms of action and methodologies need to be further elucidated and standardized.
- tDCS involves application of low-amplitude electrical current across the scalp to modulate neuronal resting membrane potentials. Studies of tDCS in SUD treatment have focused on modulating neuronal potentials in the dorsolateral prefrontal cortex; similar to TMS, some studies have demonstrated positive effects of tDCS on cravings and use patterns in individuals using tobacco, alcohol, cocaine, and opioids. The results are inconsistent, and mechanisms of action and methodologies need to be further elucidated and standardized.
- Aside from dTMS for smoking cessation, no other TMS or tDCS intervention has received FDA approval for SUD treatment.
- DBS is an invasive intervention that involves implanting electrodes directly within the brain to stimulate specific areas of the brain and affect brain function. Although it was initially piloted in the treatment of other neurological and psychiatric conditions, DBS was found to have benefits in relieving SUD symptoms in some of these individuals, especially if the stimulation was provided to the nucleus accumbens.
- DBS has been studied in the treatment of tobacco, alcohol, cocaine, and opioid use disorders, with some positive results warranting further study. Given the highly invasive nature of DBS, its consideration should be reserved for only the most severely affected individuals.

- Although the mechanisms of action of these interventional modalities in SUDs are unclear, the studies described herein point to the potential role of modulating dopaminergic neurotransmission, enhancing executive control, and altering crucial nodes in the brain's reward circuitry.

References

Abdelrahman AA, Noaman M, Fawzy M, et al: A double-blind randomized clinical trial of high frequency rTMS over the DLPFC on nicotine dependence, anxiety and depression. Sci Rep 11(1):1640, 2021 33452340

Addolorato G, Antonelli M, Cocciolillo F, et al: Deep transcranial magnetic stimulation of the dorsolateral prefrontal cortex in alcohol use disorder patients: effects on dopamine transporter availability and alcohol intake. Eur Neuropsychopharmacol 27(5):450–461, 2017 28390775

American Psychiatric Association: Diagnostic and Statistical Manual of Mental Disorders, 4th Edition. Washington, DC, American Psychiatric Association, 1994

American Psychiatric Association: Diagnostic and Statistical Manual of Mental Disorders, 5th Edition. Arlington, VA, American Psychiatric Association, 2013

Amiaz R, Levy D, Vainiger D, et al: Repeated high-frequency transcranial magnetic stimulation over the dorsolateral prefrontal cortex reduces cigarette craving and consumption. Addiction 104(4):653–660, 2009 19183128

Antonelli M, Fattore L, Sestito L, et al: Transcranial magnetic stimulation: a review about its efficacy in the treatment of alcohol, tobacco and cocaine addiction. Addict Behav 114:106760, 2021 33316590

Batista EK, Klauss J, Fregni F, et al: A randomized placebo-controlled trial of targeted prefrontal cortex modulation with bilateral tDCS in patients with crack-cocaine dependence. Int J Neuropsychopharmacol 18(12):pyv066, 2015 26065432

Bergmann TO, Varatheeswaran R, Hanlon CA, et al: Concurrent TMS-fMRI for causal network perturbation and proof of target engagement. Neuroimage 237:118093, 2021 33940146

Bikson M, Grossman P, Thomas C, et al: Safety of transcranial direct current stimulation: evidence based update 2016. Brain Stimul 9(5):641–661, 2016 27372845

Boggio PS, Sultani N, Fecteau S, et al: Prefrontal cortex modulation using transcranial DC stimulation reduces alcohol craving: a double-blind, sham-controlled study. Drug Alcohol Depend 92(1–3):55–60, 2008 17640830

Boggio PS, Liguori P, Sultani N, et al: Cumulative priming effects of cortical stimulation on smoking cue-induced craving. Neurosci Lett 463(1):82–86, 2009 19619607

Bolloni C, Panella R, Pedetti M, et al: Bilateral transcranial magnetic stimulation of the prefrontal cortex reduces cocaine intake: a pilot study. Front Psychiatry 7:133, 2016 27551268

Camprodon JA, Martínez-Raga J, Alonso-Alonso M, et al: One session of high frequency repetitive transcranial magnetic stimulation (rTMS) to the right prefrontal cortex transiently reduces cocaine craving. Drug Alcohol Depend 86(1):91–94, 2007 16971058

Ceccanti M, Inghilleri M, Attilia ML, et al: Deep TMS on alcoholics: effects on cortisolemia and dopamine pathway modulation: a pilot study. Can J Physiol Pharmacol 93(4):283–290, 2015 25730614

Centers for Medicare and Medicaid Services: Local Coverage Determination: Transcranial Magnetic Stimulation (TMS) in the Treatment of Adults with Major Depressive Disorder. Baltimore, MD, Centers for Medicare and Medicaid Services, December 11, 2022. Available at: https://www.cms.gov/medicare-coverage-database/view/lcd.aspx?LCDId=34998. Accessed May 5, 2024.

Chen L, Li N, Ge S, et al: Long-term results after deep brain stimulation of nucleus accumbens and the anterior limb of the internal capsule for preventing heroin relapse: an open-label pilot study. Brain Stimul 12(1):175–183, 2019 30245163

Conti CL, Nakamura-Palacios EM: Bilateral transcranial direct current stimulation over dorsolateral prefrontal cortex changes the drug-cued reactivity in the anterior cingulate cortex of crack-cocaine addicts. Brain Stimul 7(1):130–132, 2014 24139147

Conti CL, Moscon JA, Fregni F, et al: Cognitive related electrophysiological changes induced by non-invasive cortical electrical stimulation in crack-cocaine addiction. Int J Neuropsychopharmacol 17(9):1465–1475, 2014 24776374

da Silva MC, Conti CL, Klauss J, et al: Behavioral effects of transcranial direct current stimulation (tDCS) induced dorsolateral prefrontal cortex plasticity in alcohol dependence. J Physiol Paris 107(6):493–502, 2013 23891741

Del Felice A, Bellamoli E, Formaggio E, et al: Neurophysiological, psychological and behavioural correlates of rTMS treatment in alcohol dependence. Drug Alcohol Depend 158:147–153, 2016 26679060 den Uyl TE, Gladwin TE, Wiers RW: Electrophysiological and behavioral effects of combined transcranial direct current stimulation and alcohol approach bias retraining in hazardous drinkers. Alcohol Clin Exp Res 40(10):2124–2133, 2016 27558788

den Uyl TE, Gladwin TE, Rinck M, et al: A clinical trial with combined transcranial direct current stimulation and alcohol approach bias retraining. Addict Biol 22(6):1632–1640, 2017 27790791

Dieler AC, Dresler T, Joachim K, et al: Can intermittent theta burst stimulation as add-on to psychotherapy improve nicotine abstinence? Results from a pilot study. Eur Addict Res 20(5):248–253, 2014 24924851

Dinur-Klein L, Dannon P, Hadar A, et al: Smoking cessation induced by deep repetitive transcranial magnetic stimulation of the prefrontal and insular cortices: a prospective, randomized controlled trial. Biol Psychiatry 76(9):742–749, 2014 25038985

Dobek CE, Blumberger DM, Downar J, et al: Risk of seizures in transcranial magnetic stimulation: a clinical review to inform consent process focused on bupropion. Neuropsychiatr Dis Treat 11:2975–2987, 2015 26664122

Eichhammer P, Johann M, Kharraz A, et al: High-frequency repetitive transcranial magnetic stimulation decreases cigarette smoking. J Clin Psychiatry 64(8):951–953, 2003 12927012

Falcone M, Bernardo L, Wileyto EP, et al: Lack of effect of transcranial direct current stimulation (tDCS) on short-term smoking cessation: results of a randomized, sham-controlled clinical trial. Drug Alcohol Depend 194:244–251, 2019 30497056

Fecteau S, Agosta S, Hone-Blanchet A, et al: Modulation of smoking and decision-making behaviors with transcranial direct current stimulation in tobacco smokers: a preliminary study. Drug Alcohol Depend 140:78–84, 2014 24814566

Fregni F, Liguori P, Fecteau S, et al: Cortical stimulation of the prefrontal cortex with transcranial direct current stimulation reduces cue-provoked smoking craving: a randomized, sham-controlled study. J Clin Psychiatry 69(1):32–40, 2008 18312035

Ghorbani Behnam S, Mousavi SA, Emamian MH: The effects of transcranial direct current stimulation compared to standard bupropion for the treatment of tobacco dependence: a randomized sham-controlled trial. Eur Psychiatry 60:41–48, 2019 31100611

Gonçalves-Ferreira A, do Couto FS, Rainha Campos A, et al: Deep brain stimulation for refractory cocaine dependence. Biol Psychiatry 79(11):e87–e89, 2016 26235303

Gorini A, Lucchiari C, Russell-Edu W, et al: Modulation of risky choices in recently abstinent dependent cocaine users: a transcranial direct-current stimulation study. Front Hum Neurosci 8:661, 2014 25221496

Hajloo N, Pouresmali A, Alizadeh Goradel J, et al: The effects of transcranial direct current stimulation of dorsolateral prefrontal cortex on reduction of craving in daily and social smokers. Iran J Psychiatry 14(4):291–296, 2019 32071602

Hanlon CA, Dowdle LT, Correia B, et al: Left frontal pole theta burst stimulation decreases orbitofrontal and insula activity in cocaine users and alcohol users. Drug Alcohol Depend 178:310–317, 2017 28686990

Harel M, Perini I, Kämpe R, et al: Repetitive transcranial magnetic stimulation in alcohol dependence: a randomized, double-blind, sham-controlled proof-of-concept trial targeting medial prefrontal and anterior cingulate cortex. Biol Psychiatry 91(12):1061–1069, 2022 35067356

Heldmann M, Berding G, Voges J, et al: Deep brain stimulation of nucleus accumbens region in alcoholism affects reward processing. PLoS One 7(5):e36572, 2012 22629317

Herremans SC, Baeken C, Vanderbruggen N, et al: No influence of one right-sided prefrontal HF-rTMS session on alcohol craving in recently detoxified alcohol-dependent patients: results of a naturalistic study. Drug Alcohol Depend 120(1–3):209–213, 2012 21855234

Herremans SC, Van Schuerbeek P, De Raedt R, et al: The impact of accelerated right prefrontal high-frequency repetitive transcranial magnetic stimulation (rTMS) on cue-reactivity: an fMRI study on craving in recently detoxified alcohol-dependent patients. PLoS One 10(8):e0136182, 2015 26295336

Homan S, Muscat W, Joanlanne A, et al: Treatment effect variability in brain stimulation across psychiatric disorders: a meta-analysis of variance. Neurosci Biobehav Rev 124:54–62, 2021 33482243

Höppner J, Broese T, Wendler L, et al: Repetitive transcranial magnetic stimulation (rTMS) for treatment of alcohol dependence. World J Biol Psychiatry 12(Suppl 1):57–62, 2011 21905997

Klauss J, Penido Pinheiro LC, Silva Merlo BL, et al: A randomized controlled trial of targeted prefrontal cortex modulation with tDCS in patients with alcohol dependence. Int J Neuropsychopharmacol 17(11):1793–1803, 2014 25008145

Klauss J, Anders QS, Felippe LV, et al: Multiple sessions of transcranial direct current stimulation (tDCS) reduced craving and relapses for alcohol use: a randomized placebo-controlled trial in alcohol use disorder. Front Pharmacol 9:716, 2018 30018558

Klomjai W, Katz R, Lackmy-Vallée A: Basic principles of transcranial magnetic stimulation (TMS) and repetitive TMS (rTMS). Ann Phys Rehabil Med 58(4):208–213, 2015 26319963

Kozak K, Sharif-Razi M, Morozova M, et al: Effects of short-term, high-frequency repetitive transcranial magnetic stimulation to bilateral dorsolateral prefrontal cortex on smoking behavior and cognition in patients with schizophrenia and non-psychiatric controls. Schizophr Res 197:441–443, 2018 29486960

Kroczek AM, Häußinger FB, Rohe T, et al: Effects of transcranial direct current stimulation on craving, heart-rate variability and prefrontal hemodynamics during smoking cue exposure. Drug Alcohol Depend 168:123–127, 2016 27639130

Kuhn J, Lenartz D, Huff W, et al: Remission of alcohol dependency following deep brain stimulation of the nucleus accumbens: valuable therapeutic implications? J Neurol Neurosurg Psychiatry 78(10):1152–1153, 2007 17878197

Kuhn J, Bauer R, Pohl S, et al: Observations on unaided smoking cessation after deep brain stimulation of the nucleus accumbens. Eur Addict Res 15(4):196–201, 2009 19622886

Lefaucheur J-P, Antal A, Ayache SS, et al: Evidence-based guidelines on the therapeutic use of transcranial direct current stimulation (tDCS). Clin Neurophysiol 128(1):56–92, 2017 27866120

Levkovitz Y, Isserles M, Padberg F, et al: Efficacy and safety of deep transcranial magnetic stimulation for major depression: a prospective multicenter randomized controlled trial. World Psychiatry 14(1):64–73, 2015 25655160

Liu X, Zhao X, Liu T, et al: The effects of repetitive transcranial magnetic stimulation on cue-induced craving in male patients with heroin use disorder. EBioMedicine 56:102809, 2020 32512513

Madeo G, Terraneo A, Cardullo S, et al: Long-term outcome of repetitive transcranial magnetic stimulation in a large cohort of patients with cocaine-use disorder: an observational study. Front Psychiatry 11:158, 2020 32180745

Mahoney JJ, Marshalek PJ, Rezai AR, et al: A case report illustrating the effects of repetitive transcranial magnetic stimulation on cue-induced craving in an individual with opioid and cocaine use disorder. Exp Clin Psychopharmacol 28(1):1–5, 2020 31647279

Mantione M, van de Brink W, Schuurman PR, et al: Smoking cessation and weight loss after chronic deep brain stimulation of the nucleus accumbens: therapeutic and research implications: case report. Neurosurgery 66(1):E218, 2010 20023526

Martinez D, Urban N, Grassetti A, et al: Transcranial magnetic stimulation of medial prefrontal and cingulate cortices reduces cocaine self-administration: a pilot study. Front Psychiatry 9:80, 2018 29615935

McNeill A, Monk RL, Qureshi AW, et al: Continuous theta burst transcranial magnetic stimulation of the right dorsolateral prefrontal cortex impairs inhibitory control and increases alcohol consumption. Cogn Affect Behav Neurosci 18(6):1198–1206, 2018 30132267

Mehta DD, Praecht A, Ward HB, et al: A systematic review and meta-analysis of neuromodulation therapies for substance use disorders. Neuropsychopharmacology 49(4):649–680, 2024 38086901

Mishra BR, Nizamie SH, Das B, et al: Efficacy of repetitive transcranial magnetic stimulation in alcohol dependence: a sham-controlled study. Addiction 105(1):49–55, 2010 20078462

Mishra BR, Praharaj SK, Katshu MZUH, et al: Comparison of anticraving efficacy of right and left repetitive transcranial magnetic stimulation in alcohol dependence: a randomized double-blind study. J Neuropsychiatry Clin Neurosci 27(1):e54–e59, 2015 25255169

Mondino M, Luck D, Grot S, et al: Effects of repeated transcranial direct current stimulation on smoking, craving and brain reactivity to smoking cues. Sci Rep 8(1):8724, 2018 29880873

Müller UJ, Sturm V, Voges J, et al: Successful treatment of chronic resistant alcoholism by deep brain stimulation of nucleus accumbens: first experience with three cases. Pharmacopsychiatry 42(6):288–291, 2009 19924591

Müller UJ, Sturm V, Voges J, et al: Nucleus accumbens deep brain stimulation for alcohol addiction: safety and clinical long-term results of a pilot trial. Pharmacopsychiatry 49(4):170–173, 2016 27145161

Pettorruso M, Spagnolo PA, Leggio L, et al: Repetitive transcranial magnetic stimulation of the left dorsolateral prefrontal cortex may improve symptoms of anhedonia in individuals with cocaine use disorder: a pilot study. Brain Stimul 11(5):1195–1197, 2018 29885861

Politi E, Fauci E, Santoro A, et al: Daily sessions of transcranial magnetic stimulation to the left prefrontal cortex gradually reduce cocaine craving. Am J Addict 17(4):345–346, 2008 18612892

Prikryl R, Ustohal L, Kucerova HP, et al: Repetitive transcranial magnetic stimulation reduces cigarette consumption in schizophrenia patients. Prog Neuropsychopharmacol Biol Psychiatry 49:30–35, 2014 24211840

Pripfl J, Tomova L, Riecansky I, et al: Transcranial magnetic stimulation of the left dorsolateral prefrontal cortex decreases cue-induced nicotine craving and EEG delta power. Brain Stimul 7(2):226–233, 2014 24468092

Rapinesi C, Kotzalidis GD, Serata D, et al: Efficacy of add-on deep transcranial magnetic stimulation in comorbid alcohol dependence and dysthymic disorder: three case reports. Prim Care Companion CNS Disord 15(1):PCC.12m01438, 2013 23724355

Rapinesi C, Curto M, Kotzalidis GD, et al: Antidepressant effectiveness of deep transcranial magnetic stimulation (dTMS) in patients with major depressive disorder (MDD) with or without alcohol use disorders (AUDs): a 6-month, open label, follow-up study. J Affect Disord 174:57–63, 2015 25484178

Rossi S, Hallett M, Rossini PM, et al: Safety, ethical considerations, and application guidelines for the use of transcranial magnetic stimulation in clinical practice and research. Clin Neurophysiol 120(12):2008–2039, 2009 19833552

Rossini PM, Rossi S: Transcranial magnetic stimulation: diagnostic, therapeutic, and research potential. Neurology 68(7):484–488, 2007 17296913

Salgado S, Kaplitt MG: The nucleus accumbens: a comprehensive review. Stereotact Funct Neurosurg 93(2):75–93, 2015 25720819

Sanna A, Fattore L, Badas P, et al: Intermittent theta burst stimulation of the prefrontal cortex in cocaine use disorder: a pilot study. Front Neurosci 13:765, 2019 31402851

Sharifi-Fardshad M, Mehraban-Eshtehardi M, Shams-Esfandabad H, et al: Modulation of drug craving in crystalline-heroin users by transcranial direct current stimulation of dorsolateral prefrontal cortex. Addict Health 10(3):173–179, 2018 31105915

Sheffer CE, Bickel WK, Brandon TH, et al: Preventing relapse to smoking with transcranial magnetic stimulation: feasibility and potential efficacy. Drug Alcohol Depend 182:8–18, 2018 29120861

Shen Y, Cao X, Tan T, et al: 10-Hz repetitive transcranial magnetic stimulation of the left dorsolateral prefrontal cortex reduces heroin cue craving in long-term addicts. Biol Psychiatry 80(3):e13–e14, 2016 26995024

Speer AM, Kimbrell TA, Wassermann EMD, et al: Opposite effects of high and low frequency rTMS on regional brain activity in depressed patients. Biol Psychiatry 48(12):1133–1141, 2000 11137053

Steele VR, Maxwell AM, Ross TJ, et al: Accelerated intermittent theta-burst stimulation as a treatment for cocaine use disorder: a proof-of-concept study. Front Neurosci 13:1147, 2019 31736689

Stultz DJ, Osburn S, Burns T, et al: Transcranial magnetic stimulation (TMS) safety with respect to seizures: a literature review. Neuropsychiatr Dis Treat 16:2989–3000, 2020 33324060

Taremian F, Nazari S, Moradveisi L, et al: Transcranial direct current stimulation on opium craving, depression, and anxiety: a preliminary study. J ECT 35(3):201–206, 2019 30664050

Terraneo A, Leggio L, Saladini M, et al: Transcranial magnetic stimulation of dorsolateral prefrontal cortex reduces cocaine use: a pilot study. Eur Neuropsychopharmacol 26(1):37–44, 2016 26655188

Thair H, Holloway AL, Newport R, et al: Transcranial direct current stimulation (tDCS): a beginner's guide for design and implementation. Front Neurosci 11:641, 2017 29213226

Tremblay S, Rogasch NC, Premoli I, et al: Clinical utility and prospective of TMS-EEG. Clin Neurophysiol 130(5):802–844, 2019 30772238

Trojak B, Meille V, Achab S, et al: Transcranial magnetic stimulation combined with nicotine replacement therapy for smoking cessation: a randomized controlled trial. Brain Stimul 8(6):1168–1174, 2015 26590478

Verveer I, van der Veen FM, Shahbabaie A, et al: Multi-session electrical neuromodulation effects on craving, relapse and cognitive functions in cocaine use disorder: a randomized, sham-controlled tDCS study. Drug Alcohol Depend 217:108429, 2020 33250383

Wang Y, Shen Y, Cao X, et al: Transcranial direct current stimulation of the frontal-parietal-temporal area attenuates cue-induced craving for heroin. J Psychiatr Res 79:1–3, 2016 27115508

Wietschorke K, Lippold J, Jacob C, et al: Transcranial direct current stimulation of the prefrontal cortex reduces cue-reactivity in alcohol-dependent patients. J Neural Transm (Vienna) 123(10):1173–1178, 2016 27038632

Wing VC, Bacher I, Wu BS, et al: High frequency repetitive transcranial magnetic stimulation reduces tobacco craving in schizophrenia. Schizophr Res 139(1–3):264–266, 2012 22464727

Woods AJ, Antal A, Bikson M, et al: A technical guide to tDCS, and related non-invasive brain stimulation tools. Clin Neurophysiol 127(2):1031–1048, 2016 26652115

Xu J, Fregni F, Brody AL, et al: Transcranial direct current stimulation reduces negative affect but not cigarette craving in overnight abstinent smokers. Front Psychiatry 4:112, 2013 24065930

Young JR, Galla JT, Appelbaum LG: Transcranial magnetic stimulation treatment for smoking cessation: an introduction for primary care clinicians. Am J Med 134(11):1339–1343, 2021 34407423

Zangen A, Moshe H, Martinez D, et al: Repetitive transcranial magnetic stimulation for smoking cessation: a pivotal multicenter double-blind randomized controlled trial. World Psychiatry 20(3):397–404, 2021 34505368

Zhou H, Xu J, Jiang J: Deep brain stimulation of nucleus accumbens on heroin-seeking behaviors: a case report. Biol Psychiatry 69(11):e41–e42, 2011 21489407

Index

Page numbers printed in **boldface type** *refer to tables and figures.*

3,4-MDMA (ecstasy), 431, 444–445
5-hydroxytryptamine 5-HT$_1$, 446
  as medicine, 445–446
  for PTSD treatment, 445
  for treatment of autism spectrum disorder, 446
  for treatment of mental disorders, 445
  pharmacology and neurobiology of, 446
  selective serotonin reuptake inhibitors (SSRIs), interaction with, 446
3,4-MDMA (ecstasy) intoxication, 446
  clinical presentation of, 447–448
  illicit MDMA preparations, 448
  three stages of, 448
  pharmacological management of, 449, 453
  physical symptoms of, 447
  side effects of, 448
  toxicology of, 446–447
    neurochemical changes, 447
    treatment with antihypertensive agents, 449
3,4-MDMA (ecstasy) withdrawal, 449
  bupropion for, 449
  use of SSRIs for, 449
12-step facilitation programs, 16
  alcohol use disorder, 17

Abstinence-based treatment, 9

and agonist-based MOUD, 10
  opioid use disorder, 10
Acetaldehyde dehydrogenases (ALDHs), 74
Addiction Severity Index, 19
Addiction treatment, 501
  acupuncture, 512–516
    clinical effectiveness of, 513
    cocaine dependence, 516
    endogenous opioid system, 514
    National Acupuncture Detoxification Association (NADA) protocol, 514
    physical and mental health, 513
    psychological effects of, 514
    substance use disorder treatments, 515–516
    for substance use treatment, 514
    tobacco cessation, 515
  complementary, alternative, integrative differences, 502
  hallucinogens for, 511–512
    hallucinogen-assisted psychotherapy, 512
    psilocybin, 511
    psychedelic side effects, 512
    psychiatric symptoms, 511
  ibogaine, 510–511
    ataxia and nausea, 511
    cardiotoxicity, 511
    clinical impact of, 510
    drug use and depression, 510

Addiction treatment *(continued)*
  duration of action, 511
  opioid treatment, 510
  nutritional and dietary supplements approach to, 503–512
    kava, 506–507
    kratom (mitragyna speciosa), 508–509
    kudzu (pueraria) extract, 505–506
    N-acetylcysteine (NAC), 504–505
    potency of, 503
    regulatory oversight, 503–504
    third-party certification companies, 504
    types of, 502
Alcohol, 72
  alcohol pharmacokinetics, 74
    ALDH*2, 74
    sex and population group differences in, 74
  behavioral effects of, 72
  effects of, 75
  ingestion of, 72
  pharmacodynamics, 74–75
  primary route of ethanol metabolism, 73
Alcohol Craving Questionnaire, 532
Alcohol dehydrogenases (ADHs), 72, 74
  metabolism of alcohol, 72
Alcohol dependence, 78
  administration of mGluRs, 78
Alcohol detoxification, 93
Alcoholics Anonymous (AA), 15
Alcohol relapse, 82
Alcohol-sensitizing medications, 96–99
Alcohol use disorder (AUD), 16, 74
  antipsychotic medications, 116
    aripiprazole, 116
    quetiapine, 116
  citalopram, 114
  drug dependence and psychiatric disorders, 119
  effects of prazosin, 85
  fluoxetine, 114
  medication selection and treatment goals, 119
  neurobiology of, 75–81
    adenosinergic receptor systems, 78
    dopaminergic receptor systems, 79
    GABA type A ($GABA_A$) receptors, 75–76
    GABA type B ($GABA_B$) receptor, 112
    glutamatergic receptor systems, 76–78
    kainate receptors, 77
    opioidergic receptor systems, 79–81
  neuropeptide and hormone systems in, 81–84
    corticotropin-releasing factor (CRF), 81–83
    hypothalamic-pituitary-adrenal (HPA) axis dysfunction, 81
    neuropeptide Y, 83
    orexin receptors, 82
    vasopressin and oxytocin, 83–84
  psychotropic medications, 119
  serotonergic medications, 113–115
    ondansetron, 115
    pharmacogenetics of, 115
    selective serotonin reuptake inhibitors (SSRIs), 113–114
Alcohol use disorder treatment, 87, 100–117
  acamprosate, 87, 106–108, 117–118
  alcohol abstinence, 108
  alcohol dependence treatment, 107
  alcohol withdrawal, 107
  efficacy in AUD treatment, 107
  reduction of drinking, 107
  reduction of relapse risk, 108
  use in combination with disulfiram, 108
  anticonvulsants, 109–113
    baclofen, 112–113
    carbamazepine, 109
    gabapentin, 110–111, 118
    topiramate, 109, 117

Index 559

valproate, 109
zonisamade, 110
baclofen, 112–113, 118
  adverse effects, 112
  alcohol dependence, 112
  efficacy in, 113
  reward signaling, 112
  and co-occurring psychiatric symptoms, 120–123
  antidepressants, 120–121
  anxiety symptoms, 121
  depression, 120
  naltrexone, 120
  sertraline, 120
  SSRI fluvoxamine, 121
  SSRI paroxetine, 121
  SSRIs and depression, 121
  SSRIs vs. antidepressants, 121
disulfiram, 87, 98–99, 117, 119
long-acting injectable naltrexone, 87
medications approved by the FDA for treating alcohol use disorder, 88
medications for AUD treatment, 117
lysergic acid diethylamide (LSD), 512
NAC, 505
nalmefene, 87, 100, 105–106
  efficacy in treating AUD, 106
  relapse to heavy drinking, 105
naltrexone, 87, 100–105, 117
  alcohol craving, 100
  alcohol drinking relapse, 100
  combination with other medications, 104
  effectiveness for treating AUD, 101, 106
  individuals experiencing homelessness and AUD, 101
  intramuscular XR-NTX formulation, 103
  reduction of heavy drinking, 102
  relapse to heavy drinking, 105
  vs. XR-NTX, 103

non-FDA-approved medications for treating alcohol use disorder, 90
use of kudzu for, 506
Alcohol withdrawal, 75, 82, 120
  administration of CRF_1, 82
  gabapentin, 111
  medications to manage, 93
  noradrenergic systems, 85
  subacute withdrawal, 120
  symptom reduction with vasopressin and oxytocin, 84
  symptoms of, 93
Alcohol withdrawal syndrome (AWS), 93–96
  agent selection considerations, 96
  anticonvulsants for treating, 94–95
  benzodiazepines for treating, 95
  detoxification, 94
  epidemiology of, 93
  $GABA_A$ receptor complex for, 94–95
  medical problems of, 94
  medications to treat, 95–96
  objectives of treating, 93
Alprazolam, 333
American Academy of Addiction Psychiatry (AAAP), 293, 310
American College of Obstetricians and Gynecologists, 178
American Geriatrics Society, 352
American Psychiatric Association, 117
American Psychiatric Association Benzodiazepine Dependence, Toxicity, and Abuse Task Force, 332
American Society of Addiction Medicine (ASAM), 8, 293, 310
  patient placement criteria, 14
Amphetamine intoxication, 280
  acute agitation, 280
  pharmacological management of, 280
  pharmacological interventions for, 280
  psychopharmacological approach to, 280

Amphetamines, 275, 287
  for cocaine use disorder, 287
  effects of, 279
  monoaminergic neurotransmission, 277
Amphetamine use disorder, 276
Amphetamine withdrawal, 285
Anticonvulsants, 166
  for cannabis use disorder treatment, 166–167
Antidepressants, 157
  for cannabis use disorder, 157–162
Antipsychotics, 152
  for amphetamine intoxication, 285
  for cannabinoid hyperemesis syndrome, 173
  for cannabis-induced psychosis treatment, 171
  for cannabis use disorder treatment, 166
  for cannabis use treatment, 152
  for CUD in individuals with psychiatric comorbidities, 176
  for PCP intoxication, 405
Aripiprazole, 171
  for cannabis-induced psychosis treatment, 171

Barbiturates, 329
  for GHB withdrawal treatment, 442
Behavioral addictions, 485
  characteristics of, 485
  negative outcomes of, 485
Behavioral therapy, 17
  treatment response, 17
Behavioral treatment, 14
Benzodiazepine, 10
Benzodiazepine intoxication, 333
  features of, 341
  flumazenil-induced seizures, 335
  pathognomonic signs of, 333
  presentation of, 333–335
Benzodiazepine receptor agonists (BzRAs), 327
  for anxiety and insomnia, 328
  chronic BzRA exposure, 331
  GABA type A receptor ($GABA_A$), 329

Benzodiazepines, 15, 328
  for acute agitation in amphetamine intoxication, 280
  for acute alcohol withdrawal treatment, 121
  for acute mania, agitation, and seizures, 327
  for alcohol withdrawal syndrome, 94
  for anxiety and depression treatment, 121
  for AUD treatment, 122
  benzodiazepine-specific $GABA_A$ receptor, 330
  for cannabinoid hyperemesis syndrome, 172
  for cannabinoid hyperemesis syndrome (CHS) treatment, 152
  for cannabis-induced psychosis treatment, 171
  depressive symptoms, 122
  for GBH withdrawal treatment, 442
  initial marketing of, 329
  long-acting, 338
  lorazepam, 96
  for MDMA treatment, 449
  other substance use disorders (SUDs), 329
  oxazepam, 96
  for PCP intoxication, 405
  short-acting, 339
  vs. barbiturates, 330
Benzodiazepine use disorder, 330–335
  Approximate oral benzodiazepine receptor agonist dose equivalency, **333**
  long-term management of, 347–352
  medical or physiological considerations for, 352–355
  in individuals with co-occurring OUD, 353–354
  in older adults, 352–353
  in pregnancy, 353
  in women, 354
  in young adults, 354–355
  Model $GABA_A$ receptor showing drug binding sites, **331**

Index 561

oxidative metabolism, 333
physiological dependence, 332
physiological dependence vs SUD, 331
Benzodiazepine withdrawal, 335–337
  acute withdrawal presentation, 335–336
  inpatient management of, 339–341
  kindling effect, 337, 340
  onset symptoms, 336
  pharmacological management of, 338–346
    benzodiazepine tapers, 338
    carbamazepine, 342
    clonidine for, 345–346
    fixed-dose diazepam tapering, 340
    gabapentin and pregabalin for, 343–344
    oxcarbazepine for, 344
    propranolol for, 345
    summary of inpatient and outpatient pharmacotherapies for benzodiazepine withdrawal, 346
    valproate, 343
  postacute withdrawal syndrome, 337
  symptoms of, 338
  pseudowithdrawal presentation, 337
    etiology for pseudowithdrawal, 337
  symptoms of, 336
Blood alcohol concentrations (BACs), 72, 74–75, 77
Brief Addiction Monitor, 19
Buprenorphine, 15, 192, 199, 293
  initiation of, 230
  for MOUD, 17
  for opioid withdrawal treatment, 209
  for OUD, 206
  OUD treatment in pregnancy, 245
  for pain treatment, 224
  for respiratory depression, 199
  sublingual tablets for OUD, 225

  treatment response, 17
  for withdrawal syndrome, 202
Bupropion, 275, 293
  abstinence in cocaine-dependent, 293
  for cocaine dependence treatment, 299
  for cocaine use disorder treatment, 293, 535
  for gambling disorder, 484, 486, 488
  for internet gaming disorder, 484
  for methamphetamine/amphetamine use disorder, 299
Buspirone, 121, 170
  anxiety, 122
  for anxiety and depression treatment, 121
  anxiolytic effects, 122
  AUD and co-occurring generalized anxiety disorder, 122

Cannabinoid hyperemesis syndrome (CHS), 152, 171–173
  cannabis abstinence, 172
  cyclic vomiting syndrome (CVS), 173
  diagnostic criteria for, 171
  phases of, 171
  presentation of, 171
  supportive measures for, 172
Cannabinoids, 151
  endocannabinoids, 153, 174
  endogenous cannabinoids, 151, 178
  exogenous, 174
  phytocannabinoids, 151, 153
    cannabidiol (CBD), 151
    tetrahydrocannabinol (THC), 151
  synthetic cannabinoids, 151, 153
    naphthoylindole JWH-018, 153
    vs. THC, 154
Cannabinoid system–based treatments, 152
Cannabis, 10
Cannabis cessation, 152

Cannabis-induced psychosis (CIP), 151, 170
  antipsychotics, 151
  anxiolytics, 151
  chronic cannabis use and schizophrenia, 170
Cannabis intoxication, 155, 170
  signs and symptoms of, 155
  symptoms of, 170
  toxicology of, 155
Cannabis medical complications, 170–173
Cannabis use disorder (CUD), 152
  in adolescents, 173–174
    CB_1 receptors, 174
    glutamate transmission, 174
    use of NAC, 174
  anxiety disorder, 175
  for breastfeeding individuals, 177–178
    marijuana use, 178
    pharmacotherapies for, 178
  cannabidiol (CBD), 177
  in individuals with psychiatric comorbidities, 174–177
    ADHD, 175
    adjuvant gabapentin use, 175
    fluoxetine for, 175
    personality disorders, 175
    pharmacotherapy for, 175
    psychosis, 176
    PTSD, 175
  N-acetylcysteine (NAC) for treatment, 152
  neurobiology of, 152–153
    cannabinoid receptor types (CB_1 and CB_2), 153
    pharmacology of, 153–154
    pharmacotherapies, 152
    THC potency, 154
  in pregnancy, 152, 177–178
    adverse effects, 177
    CHS, 178
    marijuana, 177
    psychosocial interventions for treatment, 178
  presentation of, 156–157
  and psychiatric comorbidities, 152
  psychotic disorders, 176
  relaxation and anxiety seeking, 157
  signs and symptoms, 156
  and substance use disorder, 157
Cannabis use disorder treatment, 157
  antipsychotics, 166
  cannabidiol (CBD) for, 168
  cannabinoid-based treatments, 167–168
  cannabinoid degradative enzyme inhibitors (FAAH inhibitors) for, 168
  hormone therapy, 170
  nabiximols for, 168
  NAC, 505
  N-acetylcysteine for, 169
  THC-based, 167
  with antidepressants, 157–162
Cannabis withdrawal, 152, 155
  buspirone for, 170
  dronabinol for, 167
  DSM-5-TR signs and symptoms, 155
Carbamazepine, 342, 344
  for benzodiazepine withdrawal, 342
Characteristics of some common opioids, **195**
Chlordiazepoxide, 96
  for treating AWS, 95
Chlorpromazine, 156
Circuit-based interventions. *See* Interventional neuromodulatory approaches, treatment of SUDs
Clinical Institute Withdrawal Assessment for Alcohol—Revised (CIWA-Ar), 95, 340
Clinical Institute Withdrawal Assessment for Alcohol Scale, 13
Clinical Institute Withdrawal Assessment for Benzodiazepines (CIWA-B), 340
Clinical Opiate Withdrawal Scale, 13
Clinical Opiate Withdrawal Scale (COWS), 203
Clinician cultural competency, 11
  ideal vs. behavioral norms, 11
  subculture membership, 12
  SUD treatment, 11

Clonazepam, 156
Clonidine, 345
  efficacy for benzodiazepine
      withdrawal, 346
Club drug intoxication syndromes, 432
Club drugs, 431
  3,4-MDMA (ecstasy), 432
  concerns about, 432
  fentanyl (analog) contamination,
      432
  ketamine, 432
  pharmacology and neurobiology of,
      433–435
    GABA transaminase, 433
    γ-hydroxybutyrate synthesis in
        the neuron, 434
  populations and age groups using,
      431
  γ-Hydroxybutyrate (GHB),
      431–432, 435
    effects of, 435
    epileptiform
        electroencephalogram
        (EEG), 435
    $GABA_A$ and $GABA_B$ receptors,
        435
Club drug use disorder, 432
Cocaine, 10, 275
  duration of action, 278
  monoamine transmission, 276
  non-monoaminergic
      neurotransmitter effects of,
      277
Cocaine and amphetamine use
    disorder, 276
  medical and psychiatric
      considerations, 303–308
    cardiovascular diseases, 307
    cerebral vascular accidents, 307
    cocaine-induced psychosis, 308
    coronary artery diseases, 307
    depression and anxiety, 308
    development of psychotic
        symptoms, 308
    lung diseases, 307
  neuropharmacology of, 276–278
  special populations, 308–309
    MSM population risks, 308

Cocaine intoxication, 278
  acute agitation, 280
  presentation of, 278
Cocaine Selective Severity Assessment
    (CSSA), 285
Cocaine use disorder, 275
  and alcohol use disorder, 278
  hedonic dysregulation model, 286
  incentive sensitization, 286
  medications to treat, 287–298
    bupropion, 293
    disulfiram, 292–293
    dopamine antagonists, 297–298
    dopaminergic and GABA/
        glutamate medications,
        296–297
    GABAergic and glutamatergic
        medications, 294–296
    methylphenidate and
        amphetamines, 287–290
    modafinil, 290–291
    N-acetylcysteine (NAC), 298,
        505
  medications to treat cocaine
      use disorder (all non-FDA-
      approved indications), 287
  neurotransmitter systems, 276
  pharmacotherapies for, 275
  vaccine (TACD) for, 311
Cocaine withdrawal, 279, 285
  presentation of, 279–280
  symptoms, 280
Cognitive-behavioral therapy (CBT),
    15
  SUDs, 16
  SUD treatment, 15
Consolidated Appropriations Act of
    2023, 228
Contingency management, 15
Cyclic vomiting syndrome (CVS)
  amitriptyline for, 173
Cyclic vomiting syndrome (CVS), 173

Default-mode network (DMN), 373
  hallucinogen ingestion, 382
Designer drugs, 431
Dextroamphetamine, 290
  for cocaine use disorder, 287

Diazepam, 96, 328, 332
  for HPPD, 384
  lipophilic agents, 96
  for panic reactions, 393
  for PCP intoxication, 405
  for treating AWS, 96
Disulfiram, 97–99
  abstinence from alcohol, 99
  alcohol consumption, 99
  aldehyde dehydrogenase (ALDH), 97
  clinical use of, 98–99
  for cocaine use disorder treatment, 292
  disulfiram-ethanol reaction (DER), 97
  frequency of drinking, 98
  fulminant hepatic failure, 292
  pharmacology of, 97–98
  for treating alcohol use disorder, 97–98
Dorsolateral prefrontal cortex (DLPFC), 529
Dosing and use: treatments with some or limited benefit for the treatment of cannabis use and withdrawal, **157**
Drug counseling, 16
DSHEA. *See* U.S. Dietary Supplement Health and Education Act of 1994
DSM-5-TR
  behavioral addictions in, 485
  cocaine use symptoms, 534
  gambling and internet gaming disorders in, 477
  IGD in, 494
  substance use disorder, 286
DSM-5-TR criteria for substance use disorders, 347

E-cigarette or vaping use–associated lung injury (E-VALI), 52
E-cigarettes. *See* Electronic nicotine delivery systems
Ecstasy. *See* 3,4-MDMA (ecstasy)
Electronic cigarettes. *See* Electronic nicotine delivery systems
Electronic cigarettes (e-cigarettes), 33

Electronic nicotine delivery systems (ENDS), 51–53
  cannabis use with, 52
  during pregnancy, 56
  erectile dysfunction medication with, 52
  prevalence of, 51
  weight loss medications with, 52
Eszopiclone, 327
Extended-release naltrexone (XR-NTX), 101, 103
  adverse effects of, in AUD treatment, 103
  for opioid use disorder treatment, 103

FDA Drug Safety Communication of 2020, 329
Fentanyl, 198, 201
  consumer-based drug supply testing for, 198
  overdose prevention, 198
  rapid complete vocal cord closure (VCC), 206
  withdrawal from, 202
Flumazenil, 335
  optimal dosing of, 335

Gambling disorder (GD), 477
  neurobiology of, 486–487
  glutamate, 487
  involvement of dopamine in, 486
  opioid systems, 486
  serotonin, 486
  randomized controlled trials of pharmacological agents against placebo for the treatment of gambling disorder, 478
Gambling disorder (GD) treatment, 487–491
  antidepressants for, 487–488
  bupropion, 488
  clomipramine, 488
  escitalopram, 488
  fluvoxamine, 487
  paroxetine, 487
  sertraline, 488

antipsychotic agents for, 491
  olanzapine, 491
glutamatergic agents for, 490
  N-acetylcysteine (NAC), 490
mood stabilizers for, 490–491
  lithium and valproate, 490
  topiramate, 491
opioid receptor antagonists for, 488–489
  cognitive-behavioral therapy, 489
  nalmefene, 490
  naltrexone, 489
pharmacological limitations of, 491–492
practical recommendations for, 492
Gaming disorder. *See* Internet gaming disorder

Hallucinogenic substances, 385
dimethyltryptamine (DMT and related chemicals), 391
  5-methoxy-*N*,*N*-dimethyltryptamine (5-MeO-DMT), 391
  pharmacodynamics of, 392
  pharmacokinetics of, 392
  psychological effects of, 392
  somatic effects of, 393
  traditional use in Latin America, 391
ibogaine (12-methoxyibogamine), 398–401
  acute and chronic effects of, 400–401
  intoxication phases, 400
  pharmacodynamics of, 399
  pharmacokinetics of, 399
  psychostimulatory effects of, 399
  traditional use of, 398
lysergic acid diethylamide (LSD), 385–387
  complications of, 387
  intoxication and treatment, 387
  pharmacodynamics of, 385
  pharmacokinetics of, 385–386
  physiological effects of, 386
  psychological effects of, 386–387
  typical sensory and psychological effects under the influence of a medium dose of LSD, 388
mescaline, 393–395
  mescaline intoxication, 393–394
  mescaline poisoning, 395
  pharmacodynamics of, 394
  pharmacokinetics of, 394
  psychological effects of, 394
plant alkaloids, 397
  psychological and physiological effects of, 398
psilocybin, 387–388
  acute and chronic effects of, 389–390
  complications of, 390
  pharmacodynamics of, 389
  pharmacokinetics of, 389
salvia divinorum and salvinorin A, 395–397
  acute and chronic effects of, 396–397
  pharmacodynamics of, 395
  pharmacokinetics of, 396
Hallucinogen intoxication, 373
  management of, 382
  benzodiazepine sedative-hypnotic medications, 382
  neuroleptics, 383
Hallucinogens, 369–372
  addiction treatment, 372
  Alice in Wonderland Syndrome (AIWS), 384
  categories of, 370
  classic hallucinogens, 372
  consequences of, 371
  for depression/anxiety, 511
  flashback phenomena, 383–384
  hallucinogen persisting perception disorder (HPPD), 383–384
  management strategies for, 384
  historical use in human societies, 370
  nonclassic hallucinogens, 372
  psychedelic medicine, 370

Hallucinogens *(continued)*
 psychoactive and physiological
  effects of, 373
 alterations of consciousness,
  373
 hallucinogen physiological and
  psychological effects, 381
 sociopolitical settings, 371
 substances classified as, 372
 for substance use disorder (SUD)
  treatment, 406–408
 traditional cultural settings, 370
Hallucinogen withdrawal, 383
Haloperidol, 156
Hamilton Anxiety Scale, 531
Hamilton Rating Scale for Depression,
 531
Harm-reduction interventions, 6, 9
 housing-first initiatives, 6
 naloxone distribution, 6
 overdose deaths, 6
 overdose education, 6
 supervised consumption sites, 6
 syringe-needle access programs, 6
Himmelsbach scale, 203
Hydroxyzine, 156
Hypnotics, 327

Illicit opioid drug supply, 249
 adulterants and additives, 249
 benzimidazole-opioids (nitazenes),
  250–251
 fentanyl test strips, 251
 overdose and poisoning, 251
 fentanyl and xylazine combination,
  249
 overdose and poisoning, 249
Indoleamines, 372
Ineffective treatments for cannabis use,
 157–162
Inhalant intoxication, 454
 acute complications of, 454
 acute presentations of, 454–457
 signs of inhalant abuse, 457
 treatment of, 457
Inhalants, 432, 453–454
 acute and chronic effects of various
  classes of inhalants, 455
 among children and early
  adolescents, 432
 anesthetics, 432
 chronic effects of, 457–458
 chronic nitrous oxide abuse, 458
 chronic toluene abuse, 458
 effects of, 454
 nitrites, 432, 458
 nitrites (poppers), 454
 nitrous oxide, 432, 454
 organic solvents, 432
 special population considerations,
  458–459
 in adolescents, 459
 toluene, 454
Inhalant use disorder, 432
 abnormalities in brain, 458
Inhalant withdrawal, 457
 symptoms of, 457
Internet gaming disorder (IGD), 477
 neurobiology of, 493
 psychopharmacology of, 494
 bupropion, 494
 bupropion for, 494
 escitalopram, 494
 randomized controlled trials of
  pharmacological agents against
  placebo for the treatment of
  internet gaming disorder, 484
Interventional neuromodulatory
 approaches, treatment of SUDs,
 527
 deep brain stimulation (DBS), 527,
  543
 for alcohol use and cravings, 544
 for cocaine use and cravings,
  544
 for opioid use and cravings, 545
 for tobacco use and cravings,
  543
 future research areas in, 546
 transcranial direct-current
  stimulation (tDCS), 527, 537
 for alcohol use and cravings,
  539–540
 anodal tDCS stimulation, 538
 for cocaine use and cravings,
  540–542

Index 567

for opioid use and cravings,
   542–543
as positive or negative
   stimulation, 537
for tobacco use and cravings,
   538–539
transcranial magnetic stimulation
   (TMS), 527–529
for alcohol use and cravings,
   532–534
for cocaine use and cravings,
   534–536
deep transcranial magnetic
   stimulation (dTMS), 528
Faraday's principle of
   electromagnetic induction,
   528
for opioid use and cravings,
   536
for psychiatric disorders, 528
repetitive transcranial magnetic
   stimulation (rTMS),
   528–529
for tobacco use and cravings,
   530–532
Intoxication, 82

Ketamine, 372, 431, 450
effects on substance use disorders,
   450
flashbacks, 453
low-dose effects, 452
for major depressive disorder or
   bipolar disorder, 450
as medicine, 450
pharmacology and neurobiology
   of, 451
similarities/differences with PCP,
   451
for treatment of GHB, 450
for treatment of MDMA, 450
Ketamine intoxication, 451
acute presentations of, 451–452
anesthetic effects of, 452
assessment of, 452
symptoms of, 452
toxicology of, 452
Kratom use disorder, 509

Lithium, 123
for AUD and co-occuring bipolar
   disorder treatment, 123
for gambling disorder, 490
Lorazepam, 156
for acute agitation in amphetamine
   intoxication, 280
for benzodiazepine detoxification,
   340
for GHB withdrawal treatment,
   442
for HPPD, 384
for PCP intoxication, 405
Lysergic acid diethylamide (LSD),
   385–387

Medically supervised withdrawal
   (MSW), 191, 207
naltrexone, 239
vs. long-term medication for OUD,
   222
Medication for opioid use disorder
   (MOUD), 7
agonist-based, 10
buprenorphine, 15
first- and second-line agonist-based,
   7
treatment retention, 19
Methadone, 15, 192
for MOUD, 16
as opioid agonist, 201
for opioid withdrawal treatment,
   208
for OUD, 216
OUD treatment in pregnancy, 245
craving and withdrawal, 244
Methamphetamine/amphetamine use
   disorder, 287, 299
contingency management for, 287,
   302
selective serotonin reuptake
   inhibitor (SSRI)
   citalopram, 303
Voucher-based reinforcement
   therapy (VBRT), 302–303
medications to treat, 287, 299–301
buproprion, 299–300
dextroamphetamine, 301

Methamphetamine/amphetamine use
disorder *(continued)*
methamphetamine/
amphetamine use disorder
(all non-FDA-approved
indications), **304**
methylphenidate, 302
naltrexone, 300
psychostimulant replacement
therapy, 302
topiramate, 301
XRNT-bupropion combination
for, 301
vaccines for, 311
Methamphetamines, 248
effects of, 279
monoaminergic neurotransmission,
277
release of norepinephrine, 278
Methamphetamine use disorder, 275
Methamphetamine withdrawal, 285
Methylenedioxymethamphetamine. *See*
3,4-MDMA (ecstasy)
Methylphenidate, 287
for cocaine use disorder, 287
Mirtazapine, 276, 309
for methamphetamine craving and
withdrawal symptoms, 309
for methamphetamine use disorder,
276, 309
Modafinil, 290
Modified Cigarette Evaluation
Questionnaire, 507
Mood stabilizers, 166
for cannabis use disorder treatment,
166–167
Motivational interviewing, 11
SUDs, 16
MOUD. *See* Medication for opioid use
disorder

N-acetylcysteine (NAC), 169
for cannabis use disorder, 169
Naloxone, 6
agonist opioids from MORs, 205
bioavailability of, 226
for fentanyl-involved overdoses,
205

for high-potency synthetic opioids
(HPSOs), 204
methadone overdose, 205
for opioid intoxication, 203
for opioid overdose, 205
for OUD treatment, 226
OUD treatment in pregnancy, 244
Naltrexone, 152, 169, 300
for cannabis use disorder, 169
for CUD treatment, 152
for gambling disorder, 484, 489
for internet gaming disorder, 485
for methamphetamine/
amphetamine use disorder, 301
oral naltrexone and LAI naltrexone,
237
OUD treatment in pregnancy, 244
relapse treatment in OUD, 241
Narcotics Anonymous, 15
National Center for Complementary
and Integrative Health (NCCIH),
502
National Institute of Mental Health
Research Domain Criteria, 493
National Survey on Drug Use and
Health (NSDUH), 508
NCCIH. *See* National Center for
Complementary and Integrative
Health
Neonatal opioid withdrawal syndrome
(NOWS), 245
buprenorphine vs. methadone, 245
respiratory depression, 245
taper of opioid agonist, 245
Neuropeptide Y, 83
Nicotine cessation, 39
sustained-release bupropion, 44
transdermal nicotine patch, 41
Nicotine dependence, 43
nicotine cravings, 46
Nicotine replacement therapies (NRTs),
34, 39–42
combined nicotine replacement
therapy formulations, 43
during pregnancy, 56
nicotine gum, 39–40
treatment duration, 40
nicotine inhaler, 42

Index 569

nicotine lozenge, 40
nicotine nasal spray, 42
transdermal nicotine patch, 41
Nicotinic acetylcholine receptors, 86–87
  alcohol consumption regulation, 87
Nicotinic receptors, 34, 43
N-methyl-D-aspartate (NMDA), 372
Nonbenzodiazepine hypnotic medications, 329–330
Non-nicotine pharmacotherapies, 43–51
  clonidine, 48
  cytisine, 49–50
  during pregnancy, 55–57
    adverse pregnancy outcomes, 55
    nicotine metabolism, 56
  monoamine oxidase inhibitors (MAO-A and -B), 49
  naltrexone, 48
  neuromodulation, 50
  nicotine vaccines, 50
  nortriptyline, 47
  selective serotonin reuptake inhibitors (SSRIs), 49
  in smokers with cardiovascular disease, 53
  in smokers with psychiatric disorder, 54–55
  smoking relapse, 46
  sustained-release bupropion, 43–45
    adverse effects of, 45
    effects of, 46
    goals of bupropion therapy, 44
  Varenicline (tartrate), 45–46
    effects of, 47
Noradrenergic systems, 84–85
  stress-related alcohol-seeking, 85
  treatment with prazosin, 85
Norepinephrine, 277
  relapse to cocaine, 276
  stimulant sensitization, 277
NSDUH. *See* National Survey on Drug Use and Health

Olanzapine, 156
Opioid addiction, 5

Opioid dependence, 192, 201
Opioid intoxication, 200
  pharmacological management of, 203–206
  presentation of, 200–201
Opioid relapse, 191
  craving and, 192
Opioids, 193
  considerations for chronic pain treatment, 242–243
  complex opioid dependence, 243
  hyperalgesia and hyperkatifeia, 243
  opioid-induced chronic pain syndrome (OICP), 243
  effects of, 192–193
  hypogonadism, 193
  miosis, 193
  pain and opioid therapy, 242
  opioid-induced hyperalgesia (OIH), 242
  pharmacokinetics of, 194
  fentanyl, 198
  heroin, 194
  morphine, 194
  pharmacology of, 194
  release of norepinephrine, 200
  respiratory depression, 193, 203, 206
  naloxone for, 203
  serotonin syndrome, 201
  synthetic and semisynthetic, 198
Opioid use disorder, 14
  pharmacotherapy, 14
Opioid use disorder (OUD), 191
  abstinence, 214
  adverse outcomes of, 213
  craving and withdrawal, 215
  development stages of, 192
  in DSM-5, 210
  efficacy of medication for, 215
  maintenance pharmacological management of, 214–215
  opioid treatment program (OTP), 215
  presentation of, 210–213
  repeated reinforcements, 213

Opioid use disorder treatment, 237
  buprenorphine treatment for,
    224–230
    initiation protocols, 231–235
    traditional initiation on
      sublingual buprenorphine/
      naloxone tablets, 232
    in individuals with psychiatric
      comorbidities, 246–248
    ADHD, 248
    cocaine use disorders, 246
    co-occurring alcohol use
      disorder, 247
    depression and anxiety, 246
    psychotherapy, 248
    PTSD, 246
    use of benzodiazepine, 247
    use of methadone,
      buprenorphine, or
      naltrexone, 246
  methadone treatment for, 215–223
    methadone metabolism and
      interacting medications,
      219
    naltrexone vs. methadone/
      buprenorphine, 238
  opioid antagonists, 237–241
    naltrexone, 237–241
    naltrexone microinitiation, 241
    Vivitrol, 239
  in pregnancy, 244–245
Opioid withdrawal, 167, 192
  buprenorphine for, 209
  chronic changes, 200
  clonidine and lofexidine for,
    209–210
  codeine withdrawal, 202
  commonly used symptomatic
    nonopioid medications to treat
    opioid withdrawal, 211
  dronabinol for, 167
  galantamine for, 167
  lofexidine for, 167
  medications for symptoms of, 191
  meperidine withdrawal, 202
  pharmacological approaches to,
    207
    agonist opioid replacement, 207

    agonist opioid taper approach,
      208–209
    symptomatic management, 207,
      209–210
    pharmacological management of,
      206–210
    precipitated, 201
    presentation of, 201–203
    signs of, 203
    symptoms of, 202
Opioid withdrawal syndrome, 193
  methadone for, 208
  protracted abstinence, 202
Oxazepam, 156
  for cocaine use disorder treatment,
    535
Oxcarbazepine, 344

Pathological gambling. *See* Gambling
  disorder
Peer-based recovery communities, 5
Peer recovery support, 17
Pharmacological and neuromodulation
  treatments for tobacco use
  disorder, **35**
Pharmacological treatment of cannabis
  use: outcomes, direction of effect,
  and level of evidence, **157**
Pharmacotherapy, 14
  SUDs, 16
Phencyclidine intoxication, 405
  management of, 405–406
  urinary acidification, 406
Phencyclidine (PCP), 401
  acute and chronic effects of,
    403–405
  dextromethorphan, 402
  effects of phencyclidine, 407
  pharmacodynamics of, 403
  pharmacokinetics of, 402–403
Phenethylamines, 372
Phenobarbital, 340, 342
  for barbiturate dependence, 340
  for GHB withdrawal treatment,
    442
  for severe benzodiazepine
    withdrawal, 341
Polygenic risk scores (PRSs), 118

Prediction of Alcohol Withdrawal
    Severity Scale, 13
Pregabalin, 344
  for anxiety disorder, 344
  for benzodiazepine withdrawal and
    dependence, 344
Propranolol, 345
  for benzodiazepine withdrawal, 345
Psychodynamic therapy, 16
Psychostimulant therapy, 15

Quetiapine, 156

Recovery coaching, 17
Risperidone, 156

Sedative-hypnotics, 327
  barbiturates, 327
  chloral hydrate, 327
Sedatives, 327
Selective serotonin reuptake inhibitors
    (SSRIs), 43
Serotonergic systems, 85–86
  alcohol craving, 86
  ondansetron treatment, 86
Signs and symptoms of opioid
    withdrawal, **204**
Smoking cessation, 39
  abstinence, 58
  behavioral counseling, 59
  cytisine, 49–50
  ENDS for, 53
  monoamine oxidases A and B
    (MAO-A and -B), 49
  naltrexone, 48
  nicotine gum, 40
  nortriptyline, 47
  selective serotonin reuptake
    inhibitors (SSRIs), 49
  sustained-release bupropion, 44, 54
  in patients with schizophrenia,
    55
  varenicline tartrate, 45
  in smokers with schizoaffective
    disorder, 55
Stigma and bias, 4
  opioid use, 4
  substance use disorders, 1

  in substance use disorders, 4–5
Stimulant intoxication, 280
  examples of psychopharmacological
    interventions for stimulant
    intoxication (adults), 280
Stimulants, 248
  use of NAC for treating, 504
Stimulant use disorder, 248
Stimulant use disorder treatment,
    248
  ASAM and AAAP clinical
    guidelines for, 310
  contingency management therapy,
    249
Substance Abuse and Mental Health
    Services Administration
    (SAMHSA), 229, 453
Substance Use Disorders (SUDs)
  access to LOCs, 9
  assessment of patients presenting
    for, 12–14
  clinical interview, 13
  withdrawal states, 13
  carceral systems, 7
  co-occurring, 10
  drug craving and liking, 286
  epidemiology of, 2
  hallucinogens and dissolution of
    ego, 411
  involuntary treatment, 8
  legislation of, 5
  length of stay (LOS), 8
  levels of care (LOC), 8, 15
  medical management approaches
    to, 14
  overdose deaths, 3
  pharmacotherapy, 8
  presentation of, 285–286
  psychological treatment modalities,
    15
  sedative, hypnotic, or anxiolytic use
    disorder presentation, 346
  shifting perceptions, 5
  trauma exposure, 12
  treatment approaches, 16–17
  treatment goals, 9–10
  meaningful outcomes, 10
  prevalence of co-use, 11

Substance use disorders (SUDs)
  (continued)
  treatment in the legal and carceral systems, 7
  treatment of, 3–4
    abstinence-based psychosocial approaches, 7
    polysubstance use, 3
    treatment retention, 19
  treatment with ayahuasca, 409
    alcohol use disorder, 410
  treatment with ibogaine, 410
  treatment with lysergic acid diethylamide (LSD), 408
  treatment with mescaline, 410
  treatment with psilocybin, 408–409
    alcohol use disorder, 409
    tobacco use disorder, 409
Substance use disorder (SUD)
  use of NAC for treating, 505
Sustained-release (SR) bupropion, 34, 53
  in patients with schizophrenia, 54
  in smokers with schizophrenia, 54

Tobacco use disorder, 16
Tobacco use disorder (TUD), 33
  in people experiencing homelessness, 57–58
  as a coping mechanism, 57
  quit attempts, 58
  RCT interventions, 58
  smoking abstinence, 58
  treatment-resistant, 34
  withdrawal symptoms, 39
Topiramate, 275
  for cocaine dependence, 294
  for cocaine use disorder, 275, 294
  for comorbid cocaine and alcohol use disorders, 285
  for gambling disorder, 491
  for methamphetamine/amphetamine use disorder, 301
Tranquilizers. *See* Hypnotics
Transcranial magnetic stimulation (TMS), 34
Treatment response, 18
  assessment in SUDs, 18–19

toxicology and drug testing, 18
TUD. *See* Tobacco use disorder
U.S. Department of Veterans Affairs, 117
U.S. Dietary Supplement Health and Education Act (DSHEA) of 1994, 503
U.S. Drug Enforcement Administration (DEA), 228, 329
U.S. Veterans Health Administration, 87

Valproate, 343
  for benzodiazepine withdrawal, 343
Vapes. *See* Electronic nicotine delivery systems
Varenicline, 34, 53, 169
  for AUD treatment, 117
  for cannabis use disorder, 169
  and CBT in relapse prevention, 55
  for CUD treatment, 152
  for nicotine dependence, 87
  in smokers with mental illness, 55
Ventral tegmental area (VTA), 75
Veterans Administration Cooperative Studies Group, 98

Xylazine, 249
  test strips, 250
  withdrawal syndrome, 250

Young Internet Addiction Scale, 494

Zaleplon, 327
Z drugs, 328. *See* Zaleplon
  $GABA_{A1}$ receptors, 331
  vs. benzodiazepines, 330
Zolpidem, 327, 330
  COVID-19 pandemic, 330
γ-Hydroxybutyrate (GHB), 432
  acute effects of, 436–437
  chronic effects of, 437
  for cocaine use disorder treatment, 535
  common side effects of, 436
  conditioned place preference, 437
  as medicine, 438

alcohol withdrawal/dependence, 438
for narcolepsy treatment, 438
sleep apnea treatment, 438
nonmedical use of, 436
as Schedule I controlled substance, 439
sexual or acquisitory crimes, 437
toxicology of, 439–440
cross-tolerance and cross-dependence with alcohol, 439
overdose effects, 439
γ-Hydroxybutyrate (GHB) intoxication, 441
overdose management, 441
γ-Hydroxybutyrate (GHB) substance use disorder, 444
presentation of, 444
psychosocial interventions, 444
γ-Hydroxybutyrate (GHB) withdrawal syndrome, 439
delirium, 440–441, 443
detoxification of, 443
gabapentin for treatment of, 443
medical management of, 441–443
presentation of, 439–440
dosing frequency, 440
use of sedative-hypnotics, 440
γ-hydroxybutyrate withdrawal syndrome, 441
δ opioid receptor (DOR), 199–200
κ opioid receptor (KOR), 199–200, 372
withdrawal from, 202
μ opioid receptor (MOR) agonists, 199
μ opioid receptors (MORs), 79, 191, 199
nalbuphine, 200